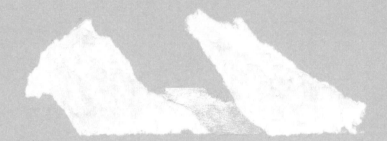

# Pediatric Dentistry

## Infancy Through Adolescence

# Pediatric Dentistry

## Infancy Through Adolescence

### *Fourth Edition*

**Jimmy R. Pinkham, DDS, MS**
Professor Emeritus
Department of Pediatric Dentistry
College of Dentistry
University of Iowa
Iowa City, Iowa

**Paul S. Casamassimo, DDS, MS**
Professor and Chair
Section of Pediatric Dentistry
College of Dentistry
The Ohio State University
Chief, Department of Dentistry
Columbus Children's Hospital
Columbus, Ohio

**Dennis J. McTigue, DDS, MS**
Professor
Section of Pediatric Dentistry
College of Dentistry
The Ohio State University
Attending, Department of Dentistry
Columbus Children's Hospital
Columbus, Ohio

**Henry W. Fields, Jr, DDS, MS, MSD**
Professor
Section of Orthodontics
College of Dentistry
The Ohio State University
Attending, Department of Dentistry
Columbus Children's Hospital
Columbus, Ohio

**Arthur J. Nowak, DMD**
Professor Emeritus
Departments of Pediatric Dentistry and Pediatrics
Colleges of Dentistry and Medicine
University of Iowa
Executive Director
American Board of Pediatric Dentistry
Iowa City, Iowa

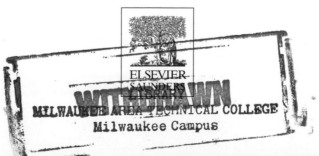

## ELSEVIER
## SAUNDERS

11830 Westline Industrial Drive
St. Louis, Missouri 63146

Pediatric Dentistry: Infancy Through Adolescence,                    ISBN 0-7216-0312-2
**Copyright © 2005, 1999, 1994, 1988 Elsevier Inc. All rights reserved.**

---

### NOTICE

Pediatric Dentistry is an ever-changing field. Standard safety precautions must be followed, but as new research and clinical experience broaden our knowledge, changes in treatment and drug therapy may become necessary or appropriate. Readers are advised to check the most current product information provided by the manufacturer of each drug to be administered to verify the recommended dose, the method and duration of administration, and contraindications. It is the responsibility of the licensed prescriber, relying on experience and knowledge of the patient, to determine dosages and the best treatment for each individual patient. Neither the publisher nor the author assumes any liability for any injury and/or damage to persons or property arising from this publication.

---

FOURTH EDITION

**International Standard Book Number 0-7216-0312-2**

*Executive Editor:* Penny Rudolph
*Senior Developmental Editor:* Jaime Pendill
*Publishing Services Manager:* Patricia Tannian
*Project Manager:* John Casey
*Book Design Manager:* Julia Dummitt

Printed in China

Last digit is the print number: 9  8  7  6  5  4  3  2  1

# Contributors

**STEVEN M. ADAIR, DDS, MS**
Professor and Chairman
Department of Pediatric Dentistry
School of Dentistry
Medical College of Georgia
Augusta, Georgia

**THOMAS H. BELHORN, MD, PHD**
Assistant Professor
Department of Pediatrics
Division of Infectious Diseases
School of Dentistry
University of North Carolina
Chapel Hill, North Carolina

**JOEL H. BERG, DDS, MS**
Professor and Lloyd Kay Chapman Chair for
   Oral Health
Department of Pediatric Dentistry
School of Dentistry
University of Washington
Seattle, Washington

**WILLIAM CHAMBERS, DDS, MS**
Private Practice
Ashville, North Carolina

**JOHN R. CHRISTENSEN, DDS, MS**
Adjunct Professor
Department of Pediatric Dentistry and
   Orthodontics
School of Dentistry
University of North Carolina
Chapel Hill, North Carolina

**JAMES J. CRALL, DDS, ScD**
Professor and Chair of Pediatric Dentistry
UCLA School of Dentistry
Los Angeles, California

**THEODORE P. CROLL, DDS**
Adjunct Professor
Department of Pediatric Dentistry
Dental School
University of Texas Health Science Center at San
   Antonio
San Antonio, Texas
Private Practice
Doylestown, Pennsylvania

**MARCIO A. DA FONSECA, DDS, MS**
Clinical Associate Professor
Department of Orthodontics and Pediatric
   Dentistry
School of Dentistry
University of Michigan
Ann Arbor, Michigan

**PETER C. DAMIANO, DDS, MPH**
Professor
Department of Preventive and Community
   Dentistry
Director, Health Policy Research Program
Public Policy Center
University of Iowa
Iowa City, Iowa

**DIANE C. DILLEY, DDS**
Associate Professor
Department of Pediatric Dentistry
School of Dentistry
University of North Carolina
Chapel Hill, North Carolina

**KEVIN JAMES DONLY, DDS, MS**
Professor and Postdoctoral Program Director
Department of Pediatric Dentistry
Dental School
University of Texas Health Science Center at San
   Antonio
San Antonio, Texas

**CLIFTON O. DUMMETT, JR, DDS, MSD, MED**
Professor and Head
Department of Pediatric Dentistry
School of Dentistry
Louisiana State University
Chief, Pediatric Dentistry Section
Charity Hospital of New Orleans
New Orleans, Louisiana

**CATHERINE M. FLAITZ, DDS, MS**
Dean and Professor, Oral and Maxillofacial
    Pathology and Pediatric Dentistry
Department of Diagnostic Sciences
University of Texas—Houston Health Science
    Center Dental Branch
Houston, Texas

**ANNA B. FUKS, CD**
Professor
Hadassah School of Dental Medicine
Hebrew University
Jerusalem, Israel

**CLEMENS A. FULL, DDS, MS**
Professor Emeritus
Department of Pediatric Dentistry
College of Dentistry
University of Iowa
Iowa City, Iowa

**GAYLE J. GILBAUGH, RDH, BS**
Program Assistant
Department of Pediatric Dentistry
College of Dentistry
University of Iowa
Iowa City, Iowa

**ANN L. GRIFFEN, DDS, MS**
Professor
Department of Pediatric Dentistry
College of Dentistry
The Ohio State University
Columbus, Ohio

**IIANA HELING, DMD, MSC**
Clinical Associate Professor
Endodontics
Hadassah School of Dental Medicine
The Hebrew University
Jerusalem, Israel

**JOHN HICKS, DDS, MS, PHD, MD**
Professor and Medical Director of Surgical and
    Ultrastructural Pathology
Department of Pathology
Texas Children's Hospital and Baylor College of
    Medicine
Adjunct Professor and Director of Caries
    Research
University of Texas—Houston Health Science
    Center Dental Branch
Houston, Texas

**GIDEON HOLAN, DMD**
Senior Lecturer, Director of Postgraduate
    Program
Pediatric Dentistry
Hadassah School of Dental Medicine
The Hebrew University
Jerusalem, Israel

**MICHAEL J. KANELLIS, DDS, MS**
Associate Professor and Head
Department of Pediatric Dentistry
College of Dentistry
University of Iowa
Iowa City, Iowa

**DIANNE M. MCBRIEN, MD**
Assistant Professor
Department of Pediatrics
University of Iowa Hospitals and Clinics
Iowa City, Iowa

**R. DENNY MONTGOMERY, DDS**
Clinical Assistant Professor
Department of Oral and Maxillofacial Surgery
College of Dentistry
The Ohio State University
Columbus, Ohio

**EILEEN OLDEROG-HERMISTON, RDH, BS**
Research Assistant
Department of Pediatric Dentistry
College of Dentistry
University of Iowa
Iowa City, Iowa

**DENNIS N. RANALLI, DDS, MDS**
Senior Associate Dean
Professor
Department of Pediatric Dentistry
School of Dental Medicine
University of Pittsburgh
Pittsburgh, Pennsylvania

**JOHN W. REINHARDT, DDS, MS**
Dean
College of Dentistry
University of Nebraska Medical Center
Lincoln, Nebraska

**MICHAEL W. ROBERTS, DDS, MSCD**
Henson Distinguished Professor
Department of Pediatric Dentistry
School of Dentistry
University of North Carolina
Chapel Hill, North Carolina

**SUE SEALE, DDS, MSD**
Professor and Chair
Department of Pediatric Dentistry
Baylor College of Dentistry
Texas A&M University System Health Science
   Center
Dallas, Texas

**ADRIANA SEGURA, DDS, MS**
Professor and Predoctoral Program Director
Department of Pediatric Dentistry
Dental School
University of Texas Health Science Center at San
   Antonio
San Antonio, Texas

**MARK D. SIEGAL, DDS, MPH**
Bureau Chief
Bureau of Oral Health Services
Ohio Department of Health
Columbus, Ohio

**M. CATHERINE SKOTOWSKI, RDH, MS**
Preventive Dentistry Program Director
Department of Pediatric Dentistry
College of Dentistry
University of Iowa
Iowa City, Iowa

**REBECCA L. SLAYTON, DDS, PHD**
Associate Professor
Department of Pediatric Dentistry
University of Washington
Seattle, Washington

**WILLIAM F. VANN, JR, DMD, MS, PHD**
Demeritt Distinguished Professor and Graduate
   Program Director
Department of Pediatric Dentistry
School of Dentistry
University of North Carolina
Dental Staff UNC Children's Hospital, Director
   MCH center for Leadership
Pediatric Dentistry
School of Dentistry
University of North Carolina
Chapel Hill, North Carolina

**KAAREN G. VARGAS, DDS, PHD**
Assistant Professor
Department of Pediatric Dentistry and Dows
   Institute for Dental Research
College of Dentistry
University of Iowa
Iowa City, Iowa

**MARCOS A. VARGAS, DDS, MS**
Associate Professor
Department of Operative Dentistry
College of Dentistry
University of Iowa
Iowa City, Iowa

**WILLIAM F. WAGGONER, DDS, MS**
Private Practice
Las Vegas, Nevada

**JERRY WALKER, DDS, MA**
Professor
Department of Pediatric Dentistry
College of Dentistry
University of Iowa
Staff Dentist
University of Iowa Hospital and Clinics
Iowa City, Iowa

**JOHN J. WARREN, DDS, MS**
Associate Professor
Department of Preventive and Community
   Dentistry
College of Dentistry
University of Iowa
Iowa City, Iowa

**KARIN WEBER-GASPARONI, DDS, MS, PHD**
Assistant Professor
Department of Pediatric Dentistry
College of Dentistry
University of Iowa
Iowa City, Iowa

**JAMES S. WEFEL, PHD**
Professor
Department of Pediatric Dentistry
Director
Department of Pediatric Dentistry and Dows
   Institute for Dental Research
College of Dentistry
University of Iowa
Iowa City, Iowa

**STEPHEN WILSON, DMD, MA, PHD**
Professor and Chairperson
Department of Pediatric Dentistry
School of Dentistry
University of Colorado
Professor and Chief of Dentistry
Department of Dentistry
   The Children's Hospital
   Denver, Colorado

# Orientation to the Textbook

Topics discussed in this textbook are divided by age group. Certain examination considerations and preventive issues are pertinent to all ages; in such situations the information is addressed again as necessary. As much as possible, issues are discussed only once at the point in a child's development at which they are first most appropriate, in the editors' judgment, to be addressed. For instance, fluoride supplementation, which is certainly pertinent for a very young child, is discussed in Part 2: Conception to Age Three. It is only referred to in following sections, even though supplementation is certainly a fundamental feature of preventive programs in older age groups. Using the same guideline, the stainless steel crown technique is discussed in the restorative chapter of Part 3: The Primary Dentition Years: Three to Six Years. This is because it is rare for dentists to treat children younger than 3 years restoratively but is commonplace after age 3.

The following represent the locations of the topics that occur in at least two parts of the textbook:

Dynamics of change: Chapters 12, 17, 29, 36
Examination: Chapters 13, 18, 30, 37
Treatment planning: Chapters 13, 18, 30, 37
Radiographic concerns: Chapters 18, 30, 37
Prevention: Chapters 14, 19, 31, 38
Trauma: Chapters 15, 34, 39, 40
Restorative dentistry: Chapters 20, 21, 32, 39
Pulp therapy: Chapters 22, 23
Orthodontic therapy: Chapters 27, 35
Orthodontic diagnosis: Chapters 18, 30, 37
Behavior management: Chapters 6, 23
Public health: Chapters 1, 11

If a student is using the text as a reference and wants to find a certain issue or technique, he or she is encouraged to first review the table of contents and then the index. A quick perusal of the text should also help in orienting a student to the location of certain information.

We have also included a brief introduction to each part of the textbook. It is recommended that the student who is trying to gain or enhance a perspective on a dentist's responsibilities for a child in any age group read these before trying to assimilate the information in any of the age-related chapters.

# Preface

Pediatric Dentistry: Infancy Through Adolescence has been favorably received around the world since its first edition in 1988. Now in its fourth edition, we are excited to offer nine chapters in full color. Color images in select chapters will help readers to better visualize topics such as oral pathology, dental anomalies, and aesthetics. We have continued with the popular format of dividing age groups to emphasize age appropriate themes. Just as we maintained in the 1980s, we submit that it is even more true today, "that pediatric dentistry now approaches children of varying ages with such specificity that a book portraying the realistic differences between dentistry for various age groups is needed."

The textbook is divided into a total of five parts. *Part 1: Fundamentals of Pediatric Dentistry* deals with the basic information and topics pertinent to children of all ages. The four remaining parts of the textbook divide childhood into four age groups and address each of these age groups according to the changes that children experience physically, cognitively, emotionally, and socially; the epidemiology of dental diseases; examination requirements; prevention needs; and possible treatment considerations.

*Part 2: Conception to Age Three* discusses an age group that was historically not involved in dental supervision. It is deeply believed by the editors and contributors that prevention programs must be started well before age three to ensure success and that much more can be done for this age group. This section focuses on the needs of an age group that was overlooked for so many years.

*Part 3: The Primary Dentition Years: Three to Six Years* deals with children with a complete primary dentition who generally are capable of going into the dental office as cooperative patients. Indeed, most of the literature on techniques useful for behavior management of children is directed at this age group. The clinician who works with this age group needs to understand the morphology and anatomy of the primary dentition, how to preserve dental arch integrity if teeth are lost, and how to intercept malocclusions in the primary dentition. The primary dentition presents its own challenges regarding restoration and pulpal therapy. The primary dentition also serves as a template for the permanent dentition and contains many clues to the final form of the permanent dentition. Because of the management concerns related to age and the importance of maintaining an intact primary dentition, the information in this section is critical to the family dentist.

*Part 4: The Transitional Years: Six to Twelve Years* focuses on the "transition" to permanent dentition. Orthodontic and aesthetic considerations become more and more important in this age group. Although the prevention needs of a preschool child remain pertinent in the transitional years, these years also see children taking on more responsibility for their own oral hygiene.

*Part 5: Adolescence* deals with another age group that many in dentistry believe has been largely overlooked by the profession. The needs of the adolescent in regard to prevention and treatment planning considerations, the seriousness of dental and facial aesthetics at this age, and the increasing concerns about periodontal disease certainly justify a major section in any pediatric dental textbook.

One of the conclusions of the first edition was that pediatric dentistry had matured as a clinical offering based on substantial gains in science and technologies. Now, in the early twenty-first century, hindsight shows that even more enormous strides were made since publication of the first edition in 1988. Those attainments, to varying degrees, have happened all over the world. There is every indication that the discipline called pediatric dentistry will continue to define and refine itself in a most positive manner as its participants—clinicians, scientists, and teachers—strive for the betterment of the dental and oral health of children. What good news this truly is!

**Jimmy R. Pinkham, DDS, MS**

# Contents

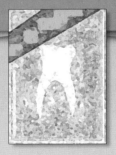

# PART 1

## FUNDAMENTALS OF PEDIATRIC DENTISTRY

This section deals with information and themes pertinent to dentistry for children at virtually all ages. Much of this information has been, or will be, covered in other aspects of dental education. However, because of the uniqueness of children, their physiologic differences from adults, and other age-related issues, no textbook on pediatric dentistry would be complete without a discussion of the topics covered in this section of the textbook.

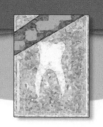

# CHAPTER 1
## The Practical Importance of Pediatric Dentistry
*Jimmy R. Pinkham and Joel H. Berg*

Pediatric dentistry is synonymous with dentistry for children. Pediatric dentistry exists because children have dental and orofacial problems. The genesis of dentistry for children unquestionably is allied to dental decay, pulpitis, and the inflammation and pain associated with infected pulpal tissue and suppuration in alveolar bone.

From its extraction-oriented beginnings, pediatric dentistry phased into an era of decay interception with an emphasis on diagnostic procedures and the maintenance of arch integrity in instances of tooth loss due to decay or trauma. Restorative techniques, pulpal therapy, space maintenance, and interceptive orthodontics were the main themes of this era. This era is not over. Tooth decay still exists, although its prevalence is significantly lower in certain areas of the United States than it was several decades ago. Therefore, these treatment techniques are covered in detail in this book. A new emphasis incorporating modern restorative materials and adhesive dentistry is detailed.

Today, however, pediatric dentistry also emphasizes prevention. Unquestionably, the prevention of dental diseases is a primary focus of this book, and it is addressed specifically for each of the four age groups that determine the organization of this book. A newer perspective, that of risk assessment, is also featured in this edition. The ability and need to categorize children into risk groups in terms of the likelihood of caries progression is presented to us because of improved technology and greater awareness among the total health care community.

## HISTORICAL PERSPECTIVE

Until the mid-1950s, in at least one state of the United States, a major dental supplier gave all new clients opening dental offices a very handsome sign that said: *No children under age 13 treated in this office.* Fortunately, such attitudes and such signs are now gone. Over the past several decades, specific educational guidelines for pediatric dentistry have been adopted and are imposed on all dental schools accredited by the American Dental Association's Commission on Accreditation. Graduates of all accredited dental schools have not only a didactic education in dentistry for children but also a clinical education. Furthermore, through the efforts of organized dentistry and other organizations and individuals interested in the oral health of children, the ignorant notion that the "baby teeth don't deserve care because you lose them anyway" has largely disappeared save for the most uninformed persons.

Indeed, at the writing of the first edition of this book in the 1980s, it was asserted that dentistry seemed to be on the brink of advocating routine "well baby" dental consultations and examinations for children younger than 3 years. In fact, both the American Academy of Pediatric Dentistry and the American Society of Dentistry for Children now advocate a routine dental appointment on or before the first birthday. In addition, in May 2003, after printing of the previous edition of this book, the American Academy of Pediatrics (AAP) issued a guidance asking its 50,000-plus pediatrician member base to invoke the practice of oral health assessment at 6 months of age. Unquestionably, the appropriateness of this recommendation for earlier dental care is due to the quality of prevention information, treatment, and techniques available to the profession today. This recommendation parallels the change in the voices within the dental profession that for years questioned the best age for a child to enter professional supervision. When dentistry was treatment oriented, age was a consideration because of behavioral reasons and the inability of the clinician and the child patient to communicate. For these reasons the customary age of the first dental appointment was on or after the third birthday. With the maturity of the dental profession in the area of preventive dentistry for the child patient, however, this age became far too old for the initiation of appropriate preventive services. Prevention of disease can never be started too early. The importance of dentistry's involvement with infants on or before their first birthday cannot be overstated. Despite the truth of this conclusion, addressing the needs of this age group remains a relevant challenge to the dental profession. It is clear even today that in subsequent editions of this textbook we will be discussing maternal intervention as a means of preventing disease in her offspring.

## MILESTONES IN DENTISTRY FOR CHILDREN IN THE UNITED STATES

1900   Few children are treated in dental offices. Little or no instruction in the care of "baby teeth" is given in the 50 dental schools in the United States.

1924   First comprehensive textbook on dentistry for children is published.

1926   The Gies Report on dental education notes that only 5 of the 43 dental schools in the United States have facilities especially designed for treating children.

1927   After almost a decade of frustration in getting a group organized to promote dentistry for children, the American Society for the Promotion of Dentistry for Children is established at the meeting of the American Dental Association (ADA) in Detroit.

1932   A report of the College Committee of the American Society for the Promotion of Dentistry for Children states that in 1928, 15 dental schools provided no clinical experience with children and 22 schools had no didactic information in this area.

1935   Six graduate programs and eight postgraduate programs exist in pedodontics.

1940   The American Society for the Promotion of Dentistry for Children changes its name to the American Society of Dentistry for Children.

1941   Children's Dental Health Day is observed in Cleveland, and Children's Dental Health Week is observed in Akron, Ohio.

1942   The effectiveness of topical fluoride applications at preventing caries is described. The Council on Dental Education recommends that all dental schools have pedodontics as part of their curriculum.

1945    First artificial water fluoridation plant is begun at Grand Rapids, Michigan.

1947    The American Academy of Pedodontics is formed. (To a large degree, the start of the Academy was prompted by the need for a more scientifically focused organization concerned with the dental health of children.)

1948    The American Board of Pedodontics, a group formulated to certify candidates in the practice of dentistry for children, is formally recognized by the Council on Dental Education of the ADA.

1949    The first full week of February is designated National Children's Dental Health Week.

1955    The acid-etch technique is described.

1960    Eighteen graduate programs and 17 postgraduate programs in pedodontics exist.

1964    Crest becomes the first ADA-approved fluoridated toothpaste.

1974    The International Workshop on Fluorides and Dental Caries Reductions recommends that appropriate fluoride supplementation begin as soon after birth as possible. (This recommendation was later modified by authorities to start at 6 months of age.)

1981    February is designated National Children's Dental Health Month.

1983    A Consensus Development Conference held at the National Institutes of Dental Health endorses the effectiveness and usefulness of sealants.

1984    The American Academy of Pedodontics changes its name to the American Academy of Pediatric Dentistry.

1995    A new definition is adopted for the specialty of pediatric dentistry by the ADA's House of Delegates.
Pediatric dentistry is an age-defined specialty that provides both primary and comprehensive preventive and therapeutic oral health care for infants and children through adolescence, including those with special health care needs.

2003    The AAP establishes "Policy Statement on Oral Health Risk Assessment Timing and Establishment of a Dental Home." The issuance of this policy statement will be manifested in several outcomes including the need to identify effective means for rapid screening in pediatricians' offices, and the mechanisms for swift referral and intervention for high-risk children.

## APPLICATION OF OTHER DISCIPLINES

Unquestionably, pediatric dentistry, as a body of knowledge and as a clinical discipline, has borrowed heavily from other aspects of dental schools' curricula and from breakthroughs in other specialty areas of dentistry. To be a complete clinician capable of handling the majority of needs of the children of any community, a dentist needs to know thoroughly preventive dentistry techniques, pulpal therapy, instrumentation and restoration of teeth, dental materials, oral surgery, preventive and interceptive orthodontics, and principles of prosthetics. In addition, to really be knowledgeable about the best needs of child patients, the dentist must know certain basics in pediatric medicine, general and oral pathology, and growth and development. Knowledge of nutrition and an understanding of both systemic and topical fluorides are essential in the development of appropriate prevention strategies for the child patient. Lastly, it is inconceivable that a person would be happy dedicating a significant amount of practice time to children without understanding their emotional and psychological needs as well as their processes of emotional change and social maturation.

The child has to be treated differently from the adult and, in fact, the modes of management are extremely age related. Immediately prior to publication of this edition, the American Academy of Pediatric Dentistry held a consensus conference on Behavior Management in Children. Although the proceedings of the conference are not yet published, it can be noted that the conference highlighted the need for (1) careful examination of evidence base in dental care for children (discussed later on) and (2) a clear understanding of the diagnostic aspects of behavior management before employing the most appropriately determined behavior management techniques. Advanced (specialty) training in pediatric dentistry calls for a clear understanding of the above-stated practices of behavior management, including both nonpharmacologic and pharmacologic approaches.

Pediatric dentistry does in fact borrow a lot from other disciplines, but beyond this borrowing it is a discipline unto itself. The student who wishes to master intellectually and clinically the challenges that this age group presents must understand and be able to discern when simple transfers from one discipline can be made to the child patient and when transfers must be modified because of the age requirements or limitations that the child patient presents. The student must also understand that these requirements and limitations may vary from one age group to another.

## CHALLENGES FOR PEDIATRIC DENTISTRY IN THE 21ST CENTURY

In the first two editions of this textbook this introductory chapter contained a section that addressed recent trends in dentistry for children. In the second edition, published in 1994, the following 15 trends were highlighted:

- Preventive dentistry, including understanding the caries process as it relates to such factors as nutrition, sealants, water fluoridation, topical fluorides, fluoridated toothpastes, and home care
- Infant oral health
- Acid-etch techniques, sealants, and composite resins
- Dentistry for the disabled patient and other children with special needs
- Early orthodontic diagnosis and treatment
- More sophisticated modalities of pain and anxiety control such as sedation techniques
- Sophistication of radiographic techniques and machinery
- Expanding problem with fluorosis
- Eating disorders and their dental implications
- Smokeless tobacco use, particularly by adolescent boys
- Informed consent and risk management
- Infection control, barrier techniques, sterilization methods, and concerns about the transmission of disease from patient to clinician and from clinician to patient
- Early predisposing factors to temporomandibular joint problems in adolescents and adults
- Possible diminishing numbers of children who are generally and dreadfully afraid of dentists
- Abused and neglected children

None of these issues has gone away, but most are so much a part of the landscape of contemporary pediatric dentistry today that addressing them in this fourth edition as recent trends seems unnecessary. All of these themes are addressed in this textbook.

Eight phenomena that will have to be addressed in the 21st century are deemed important enough to be reviewed in this introductory chapter. These are child abuse and neglect, the children of poverty, informed consent and risk management, evidence-based dental practice, technology, health care delivery strategies/ payment strategies, caries risk assessment, and emergence of pediatric dentistry as a worldwide community.

### Child Abuse and Neglect

Child abuse and child neglect are ugly and emotionally charged aspects of the more general problem of family dysfunction in our society. Since the 1960s these themes have received increased attention from the legal and health science professions. By 1966, each of the 50 states had drafted legislation describing the responsibilities of professionals to report suspected abuse of children. The same laws that mandate dentists to report suspected abuse often also protect them from legal litigation, often brought by angry and vengeful parents.

These laws also spell out the legal implications for the dentist who knowingly and willfully fails to report suspected child abuse. Although the laws vary from state to state, generally the dentist who fails to report such cases is considered guilty of a simple misdemeanor and is subject to a fine or jail sentence, usually 30 days in length. The law usually also makes the dentist civilly liable for any damages to the child caused by a failure to report abuse. In other words, litigation for damages can be conducted against the dentist for any further abuse sustained by the child.

If while performing an examination on a child something questionable like a bruise becomes apparent, the child should be interviewed for his or her analysis and explanation of the injury. Obviously, this approach is more effective for the older child. Next, after the examination is completed, the parents should be interviewed separately from the child to see whether the two stories correlate. If there is no correlation between the two accounts of the injury, the appropriate authorities should be informed.

Abuse can be documented in terms of the trauma caused by burning, slapping, hitting, choking, twisting, pulling, and pinching. Broken teeth, burns, lacerations, bruises, and broken bones alert the dentist that something may be wrong. Neglect, however, is more subtle. The dentist should look at the child's overall hygiene as well as dental hygiene and clothing worn. Suspicion of poor nutrition, apparent lack of medical care, and absence of previous dental care are situations that should alert the dentist to consider neglect. The dentist is responsible for taking the same approach to neglect as to abuse; reporting of such cases is mandatory. The American Academy of Pediatric Dentistry defines dental neglect as failure of the parent or guardian to seek treatment for caries, oral infections, or oral pain or failure of the parent or guardian to follow through with treatment once he or she is informed that the aforementioned conditions exist.

## Milestones in the American Recognition and Approach to Family Dysfunction and Other Cruelties to Children

19th century    House of refuge movement. This movement occurred in many major cities and enabled the state to place abandoned or neglected children somewhere safe.

1870s    Formation of the New York Society for the Prevention of Cruelty to Children. This was the first of many groups that worked in cooperation with the houses of refuge to rescue endangered children.

1899–1920    Establishment of juvenile courts. The first juvenile court was begun in Illinois in 1899. By 1920, all but three states had such courts.

1946    Medical discovery of child abuse. A paper by Caffey[2] concludes that the origin of many long bone fractures in children could not be specifically documented.

1957    Caffey asserts that injuries such as fractures in long bones of infants have often been deliberately inflicted.

1961    First conference is held on the battered child syndrome.

1962    Article on battered children[4] is published in the *Journal of the American Medical Association*. The concept of parental cruelty is made public. By this time, there is a movement to do something about this problem.

1966    All 50 states have passed laws describing the responsibilities of health science professionals in reporting suspected abuse.

1971    Fontana[3] proposes a more global definition of the mistreatment of children. Neglect is now considered a potential parental shortcoming.

1974    A National Center on Child Abuse and Neglect is established by Congress to provide further leadership in improving the potential protection of children. Sexual abuse is added as a category of child abuse.

1976–1979    The number of cases of child abuse reported nationally rises 71% from 1976 to 1979, when 711,142 cases are reported.[1]

1995    The number of reported cases of child abuse continues to increase to approximately 1 million. It is estimated that approximately 2000 children die from abuse each year.

1996    Nearly all states have child death review teams. Mental injury and passive exposure of children to illegal drugs are increasingly recognized as other forms of child abuse.

## Children of Poverty

Even though there is great news about the success of dentistry in addressing the dental diseases of children and the fact that preventive dentistry is today a successful phenomenon for literally millions of children, students reading this book are urged to understand that this is not true for all children. Those children who come from the circumstances of poverty are at substantial risk for the ravages of dental decay despite all the preventive dentistry accomplishments of the last 30 years.

The children of poverty have always presented unique problems to the dental profession.[5] First, certain forms of poverty make accessibility to dental care by poor patients difficult. Poverty also may predict a lack of knowledge about home care, prevention techniques, proper diet, and even when professional dental care should be started. The decay rates among the children of poverty are higher today than they are among more fortunate children. Unfortunately, the number of poor children continues to increase.

The recent publication[6] of the first-ever Surgeon General's Report on Oral Health elucidated a multitude of socioeconomic issues related to the general picture of oral health in America and highlighted the problem of disparities in access to care. Already, this disparities issue has led to a host of outcomes including research in the field of access, programs to engage in better access to care among the underserved population, and enhanced predoctoral education for all members of the dental community toward addressing this ever-important problem.

The editors and contributors to this text hope that the dental profession, government agencies, and other advocacy groups for children in general and particularly children in special circumstances, such as poverty, will act responsibly to solve the growing need for a more vigorous and determined policy of health care, dental as well as medical, for these children.

## Informed Consent and Risk Management

Informed consent is the legal mechanism that protects a patient's right not to be touched or in any way treated without the patient's authorization. The issue assumes that it is a right of a mentally competent adult human being to determine what, if anything, a practitioner of health sciences may do to his or her body.

There are two kinds of consent: expressed and implied. Implied consent is determined by the behavior of the patient. For instance, the patient got in the chair, opened his mouth, but said nothing. Expressed consent is written or oral. A signed written consent to treatment is the most substantial consent for protecting a dentist from litigation.

Informed consent also implies that the patient is aware of the nature of the treatment, alternatives to treatment, probable sequelae to treatment, and potential benefits and possible risks of any treatment. In other words, an "uninformed" patient is incapable of giving informed consent. A signature, if the patient is uninformed, is legally useless also.

The law assumes that minors cannot take the responsibility for giving informed consent. To avoid liability, the dentist must secure consent from the parent or the person acting *in loco parentis*. An exception to this would be the rendering of emergency care that preserves life or avoids severe compromise to the child's health when the parents cannot be located in the time available.

Obtaining informed consent can be a difficult problem for the dentist who treats children. It is not unusual for older children and adolescents to come to the dental office unaccompanied by a parent. In such cases, it is advised that only very safe, limited-risk procedures be performed.

Risk management is a broad term that describes the attitudes, processes, and techniques that a dentist and the staff can have and can do to minimize legal involvement in the circumstances that arise in the course of treating patients. Obviously, in pediatric dentistry this management involves not only how the dentist and child interact but also, importantly, how the dentist and child's parents or guardians interact.

The practice of informed consent is basic to risk management. However, risk management involves issues other than those that are technically legal. It involves a satisfaction in communication between the clinician and the public, community, or individuals with whom he or she works. In the area of dentistry for children, risk management encourages open dialogue between the dentist and the people who bring children to the clinic.

Although much of risk management centers on actual treatment, in the area of pediatric dentistry behavioral management of the child and the perception of how the dentist appropriately or inappropriately reacts to the developing psyche of the child are important issues. These issues are addressed in Chapter 23.

## Evidence-Based Dental Practice

Much of dental practice is founded either on evidence gathered from former times when treatment regimens differed and devices and delivery systems differed from today, or on collections of historically sound practices wherein practitioners and scientists have de facto warranted such treatments the "standards of care," based on their prevalence of use in the practice community. Today there is a stronger call for practice based on evidence collected in prospective clinical trials designed to scientifically scrutinize the techniques to be employed. In spite of this loud voice asking for evidence behind all four treatments, it is also known that not all clinically employed practices can be entirely based on the highest levels of evidence, such as those based on outcomes of prospective, randomized, controlled clinical trials. There are often ethical or time constraints that preclude such intense evaluation. Nevertheless, evidence-based dentistry is here to stay. Therefore, today's practitioners must have a good understanding of the levels of evidence behind the scientific research leading to our treatments and must be trained to ask questions about how evidence is collected in the determination of appropriate treatment protocols for children.

## Technology

The technologies currently available and those that are on the horizon will remain a constant challenge for dentists to better serve their patients. The 21st century promises new materials, changes in techniques, electronic records, further use of lasers, advanced x-ray machinery, and further use of computers. Even the Internet has affected dentistry.

Recent technologies include enhancements in adhesive dentistry and dental adhesive products along with improved, lower shrinkage resin composites and improved glass ionomer materials. Such combinations, discussed later in this book, will undoubtedly allow additional alternatives to the use of amalgam and stainless steel crowns.

## Health Care Delivery Strategies/Payment Strategies

Health care delivery and payment strategies was not a theme in the first or second edition of this book; however, health care reform initiatives in the United States in recent years and the promise of continuing dialogue at the federal, state, and corporate levels on the issues of delivery and payment demand that a responsible education in pediatric dentistry today include these themes. Some of these are covered in Chapter 11.

## Caries Risk Assessment

The Surgeon General's Report on Oral Health placed considerable emphasis on the fact that "80% of the caries disease resides in 20% of the population." Being cognizant of this scenario is essential to effectively manage the population as a whole and to reduce the dental disease in our communities. However, awareness of this fact alone will not mitigate the problem. The "call to action" originating from the Report asks that we employ modern, validated mechanisms of risk assessment in the entire population, and in particular in individuals at greatest risk of disease, to identify those in the highest risk categories and to get them to treatment. Practitioners today must therefore keep abreast of the latest technological and scientific discoveries in the field of risk

assessment, as new findings are emerging rapidly. These authors believe that the uniform implementation of appropriate risk assessment tools will change the way we practice dentistry for children more profoundly than anything in recent years.

Some of the many outcomes of risk assessment-based practice will be (1) introduction of early caries treatments that are medicinally based, (2) closer interaction and referral among the entire health care team, and (3) broader development of dental devices and materials used in restorative dentistry that will provide therapeutic as well as restorative approaches to management of caries.

## Emergence of Pediatric Dentistry as a Worldwide Community

Children are a resource of the world. They are a promise of what our future is going to be. A healthy child is a better promise of a better world than an unhealthy child. Therefore, the dental health of any child is a concern to the world's dental community regardless of the child's nationality, ethnicity, and geographic location. Dentistry for children is now an international community with international initiatives, concerns, strategies, and cooperation.

## REFERENCES

1. American Humane Association: National Analysis of Official Child Neglect and Abuse Reporting (1979). DHHS Publication No. (OHDS) 81-30232, revised 1981. Washington, DC, U.S. Government Printing Office, 1981.
2. Caffey J: Multiple fractures in the long bones of infants suffering from chronic subdural hematoma. *Am J Roentgenol* 56:163, 1946.
3. Fontana V: *The Maltreated Child: The Maltreatment Syndrome in Children.* Springfield, IL, Charles C Thomas, 1971.
4. Kempe CH, Silverman EN, Steele BF, et al: The battered child syndrome. *JAMA* 181:17, 1962.
5. Pinkham JR, Casamassimo P, Levy S: Dentistry and the children of poverty. *J Dent Child* 55(1):17-23, 1988.
6. U.S. Department of Health and Human Services. *Oral Health in America: A Report of the Surgeon General.* Rockville, MD: National Institute of Dental and Craniofacial Research, National Institutes of Health, 2000.

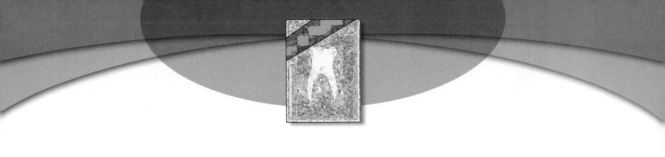

# CHAPTER 2

## Differential Diagnosis of Oral Lesions and Developmental Anomalies

### *Catherine M. Flaitz*

A wide variety of oral lesions and soft tissue anomalies occur in children. The purpose of this chapter is to highlight selected lesions that are most commonly found in children or pathologic entities that primary develop in this age group. In addition, oral lesions associated with several genetic disorders and specific malignancies, which may mimic benign or inflammatory conditions, are included to broaden the disease scope. The material is outlined in tables in order to make this comprehensive subject more succinct and easier to review. The brief description for each entity summarizes the most important clinical information that is relevant to the child patient. Representative examples of these conditions are included to illustrate the characteristic clinical or radiographic features.

Each oral lesion is described according to key points: (1) the most common pediatric age group affected and the gender predilection; (2) the characteristic clinical and radiographic findings of the lesion; (3) the typical location for the lesion; (4) the pediatric significance of the lesion; (5) the treatment and prognosis for the lesion; and (6) the differential diagnosis that is pertinent to this age group.

Except for the first table on selected developmental anomalies, the other tables are arranged to capture the primary clinical or radiographic characteristics for the purpose of comparison. The sequential headings for each of the tables include the following disease categories:

Developmental anomalies (Table 2-1, Fig. 2-1)
White soft tissue lesions (Table 2-2, Fig. 2-2)
    White surface thickening lesions
    White surface material lesions
    White subsurface lesions
Dark soft tissue lesions (Table 2-3, Fig. 2-3)
    Red or purple-blue lesions
    Brown-black lesions
Ulcerative lesions (Table 2-4, Fig. 2-4)
Soft tissue enlargements (Table 2-5, Fig. 2-5)
    Papillary lesions
    Acute inflammatory lesions
    Tumor and tumor-like lesions
Radiolucent lesions of bone (Table 2-6, Fig. 2-6)
Mixed radiolucent and radiopaque lesions of
    bone (Table 2-7, Fig. 2-7)
Radiopaque lesions of bone (Table 2-8, Fig. 2-8)

**TABLE 2-1**

**Developmental Anomalies (Fig. 2-1)**

| CONDITION | PEDIATRIC AGE AND GENDER | CLINICAL FINDINGS | LOCATION | PEDIATRIC SIGNIFICANCE | TREATMENT AND PROGNOSIS | DIFFERENTIAL DIAGNOSIS |
|---|---|---|---|---|---|---|
| Fissured tongue | First and second decades No gender predilection | Multiple furrows or grooves; tender, if irritated; may occur with *erythema migrans* | Dorsal tongue | Polygenic or autosomal dominant trait; occurs in *Down syndrome,* dry mouths; detected in 1% of children; source of halitosis | Brush tongue; becomes more prominent with age | Erythema migrans Crenated tongue |
| Partial ankyloglossia (tongue-tie) | Present at birth Male predilection | Short, thick lingual frenum or attachment to tip of tongue; may cause slight cleft at tip | Ventral tongue and floor of mouth | Occurs in 2% to 4% of children; rarely causes speech, swallowing or periodontal problems; multiple frenula associated with *oral-facial-digital* syndrome | Infrequently frenectomy is indicated; may self-correct | Complete ankyloglossia Bifid tongue |
| Lingual thyroid | Second decade Female predilection | Nodular mass with pink or red, smooth surface; may cause dysphagia, dysphonia, or dyspnea | Midline base of tongue; *thyroglossal duct cyst* is variant that occurs in midline neck | Symptoms develop during puberty or pregnancy; normal thyroid absent in 70%; important cause of infantile hypothyroidism | Thyroid hormone therapy, excision or radioactive iodine ablation; carcinomas arise in 1% of cases | Lymphoid hyperplasia Hemangioma Lymphangioma Velecula |
| Commissural lip pits | Second decade Male predilection | Unilateral or bilateral invaginations; fluid may be expressed | Corners of mouth | Occurs in <1% of children; associated with preauricular pits | None required | Paramedian lip pits Angular chelitis |

*Continued*

| Condition | Pediatric Age and Gender | Clinical Findings | Location | Pediatric Significance | Treatment and Prognosis | Differential Diagnosis |
|---|---|---|---|---|---|---|
| Paramedian lip pits (Congenital lip pits) | Present at birth<br>No gender predilection | Bilateral and symmetric depressions or swellings; fluid may be expressed | Adjacent to the midline of the lower lip vermilion | Autosomal dominant trait; associated with cleft lip and palate | None required; surgery if cosmetic problem | Mucocele<br>Soft tissue abscess<br>Median lip fissure |
| Retrocuspid papilla | First and second decades<br>Female predilection | Asymptomatic, pink, sessile papule or nodule; usually bilateral | Lingual attached gingiva, adjacent to mandibular canines | Very common in children and regresses with age | None required; normal anatomic structure | Irritation fibroma<br>Giant cell fibroma<br>Soft tissue abscess |
| Bifid uvula | Present at birth<br>No gender predilection | Midline groove or splitting of uvula | Midline, posterior soft palate | Minimal expression of cleft palate; may be associated with submucous palatal cleft | None required; genetic counseling may be indicated | Traumatic defect |
| Hyperplastic labial frenum | Present at birth<br>No gender predilection | Thick triangular band of pink soft tissue; may be associated with gingival recession or diastema | Midline labial mucosa and gingiva; both maxillary and mandibular lip | Bleeds freely when lacerated; multiple frenula associated with *oral-facial-digital syndrome* | None required; frenectomy reserved for correction of large diastema or gingival recession | Traumatic scar |

**TABLE 2-1**

**Developmental Anomalies (Fig. 2-1)–cont'd**

| Condition | Pediatric Age and Gender | Clinical Findings | Location | Pediatric Significance | Treatment and Prognosis | Differential Diagnosis |
|---|---|---|---|---|---|---|
| Torus palatinus (Palatal torus) | Second decade Female predilection | Bony hard mass that varies in size and shape; asymptomatic, unless traumatized; rarely seen as radiopacity on radiographs | Midline hard palate | Most tori in this age group are slightly elevated with a smooth surface; autosomal dominant inheritance or multifactorial influence | None required; will continue to grow during adulthood | Prominent median palatal raphe Palatal exostosis |
| Torus mandibularis (Mandibular torus) | Second decade Male predilection | Bony hard mass that varies in size and shape; asymptomatic, unless traumatized; radiopacity may be superimposed over roots of teeth | Bilateral, lingual mandible | Less common that torus palatinus; genetic and environmental influence | None required; will continue to grow during adulthood | Osteomyelitis with proliferative periostitis Osteoma Fibrous dysplasia Condensing osteitis |
| Exostoses | Second decade No gender predilection | Single or multiple bony hard nodules; asymptomatic, unless traumatized; radiopacity may be superimposed over roots of teeth | Maxillary and mandibular alveolar ridge on the facial aspect; usually bilateral; may occur on the palate | Exostoses that are traumatized mimic odontogenic infection because of the location | None required; will continue to grow during adulthood | Osteomyelitis with proliferative periostitis Osteoma Fibrous dysplasia Condensing osteitis |

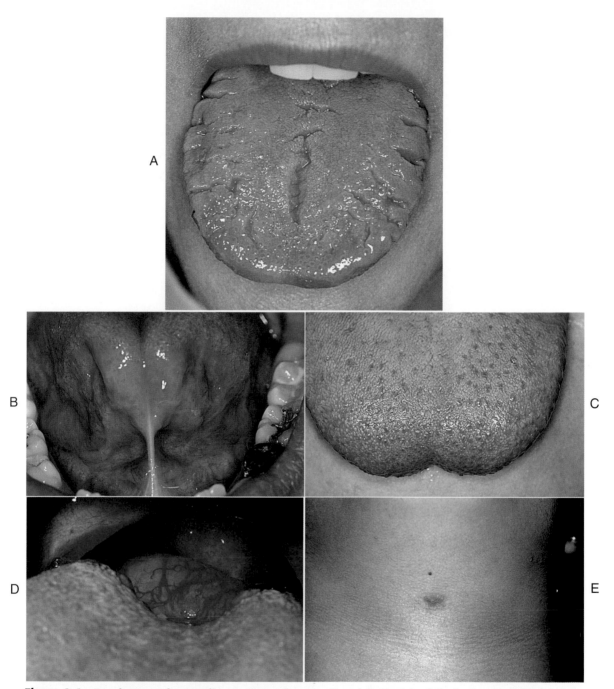

**Figure 2-1**  Developmental anomalies. **A,** Fissured tongue. **B** and **C,** Partial ankyloglossia with lingual frenum attachment at the tip of the tongue (**B**). Note the restricted mobility of the tongue with extension (**C**). **D,** Lingual thyroid of the midline base of the tongue. **E,** Thyroglossal duct cyst with sinus tract, midline neck. (**D** courtesy Dr. G. E. Lilly, University of Iowa College of Dentistry.)                                            *Continued*

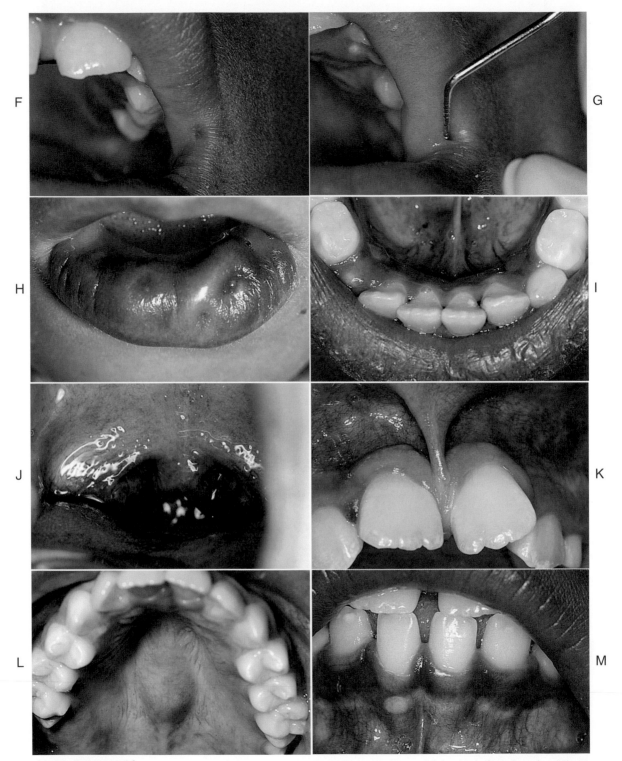

**Figure 2-1—cont'd**   F and G, Commissural lip pit (F) with depth illustrated by periodontal probe (G). H, Paramedian lip pits. I, Retrocuspid papilla of the lingual mandibular gingiva. J, Bifid uvula. K, Hyperplastic maxillary labial frenum. L, Torus palatinus of the midline hard palate. M, Small exostosis of the anterior mandibular alveolus, facial aspect.

## TABLE 2-2
### White Soft Tissue Lesions (Fig. 2-2)

| Lesion | Pediatric Age and Gender | Clinical Findings | Location | Pediatric Significance | Treatment and Prognosis | Differential Diagnosis |
|---|---|---|---|---|---|---|
| **White Surface Thickening Lesions** | | | | | | |
| Frictional keratosis | First and second decades<br>No gender predilection | Localized to diffuse, white, rough or shredded patches; adherent; asymptomatic | Mucosa adjacent to occlusal plane, including buccal, labial mucosa, lateral tongue; attached gingiva | Caused by chronic biting or sucking habits, irritation from orthodontic appliances, fractured teeth and improper tooth brushing | Elimination of cause; lesion regresses | Leukoedema<br>Linea alba<br>Smokeless tobacco keratosis<br>Cinnamon contact stomatitis |
| Smokeless tobacco keratosis | Second decade<br>Male predilection | Diffuse, white, wrinkled patch; adherent; asymptomatic; gingival recession; tooth staining | Vestibular, labial and buccal mucosa; usually mandibular site | Highly addictive habit; lesions develop after 1–5 years of use; increased risk for periodontal disease | Discontinuation of habit results in lesion reversal; biopsy of persistent lesions; low risk for malignant transformation | Leukoedema<br>Frictional keratosis<br>Cinnamon contact stomatitis |
| Leukoedema | First and second decades<br>No gender predilection | Widespread, filmy white, wrinkled mucosa; adherent; disappears when stretched | Bilateral buccal, labial mucosa and soft palate | Most common in black children; condition increases with age; more pronounced in cigarette smokers | None required; common variant of normal mucosa | Frictional keratosis<br>White sponge nevus |
| Cinnamon contact stomatitis | Second decade<br>No gender predilection | Oblong to broadly linear, white plaques with a shaggy, thickened surface; diffuse erythema; tender | Gingiva, mucosa adjacent to occlusal plane, including buccal mucosa and lateral tongue | Cinnamon flavoring in candy, chewing gum, toothpaste, mouth rinses | Identify and discontinue use of offending product | Cheek-biting keratosis<br>Hyperplastic candidiasis<br>Smokeless tobacco keratosis<br>Hairy leukoplakia |

Continued

## TABLE 2-2
### White Soft Tissue Lesions (Fig. 2-2)—cont'd

| Lesion | Pediatric Age and Gender | Clinical Findings | Location | Pediatric Significance | Treatment and Prognosis | Differential Diagnosis |
|---|---|---|---|---|---|---|
| **White Surface Thickening Lesions—cont'd** | | | | | | |
| Linea alba | Any age following the eruption of teeth<br>No gender predilection | Smooth or shaggy white line; may be scalloped; asymptomatic | Bilateral buccal mucosa, along occlusal plane | Associated with frictional irritation or sucking habit | None required; may spontaneously regress | Cinnamon contact stomatitis<br>Scar formation<br>Cheek-biting keratosis |
| Hairy tongue | Second decade<br>No gender predilection | Cream to brown discoloration; diffuse elongation of filiform papillae | Dorsal tongue | Contributes to halitosis; associated with smoking, poor oral hygiene, antibiotics | Eliminate cause; brush tongue | Frictional keratosis<br>Hyperplastic candidiasis<br>Coated tongue |
| White sponge nevus | First decade, may be present at birth<br>No gender predilection | Diffuse, symmetric, corrugated or velvety white plaques, adherent; asymptomatic | Bilateral buccal mucosa is most common; also found on labial mucosa, ventral tongue, floor of mouth and soft palate | Autosomal dominant skin disorder; reaches full expression during adolescence | None required; condition stabilizes in young adulthood | Leukoedema<br>Hereditary benign intraepithelial dyskeratosis<br>Frictional keratosis<br>Hyperplastic candidiasis<br>Syndrome-related leukoplakia |
| **White Surface Material Lesions** | | | | | | |
| Pseudomembranous candidiasis (thrush) | Any age, especially infancy<br>No gender predilection | Widespread, white spots or plaques that wipe off leaving red base; mild burning | Any mucosal site but common on buccal mucosa, tongue and palate | Caused by *Candida albicans* and other species; contributing factors are antibiotics, steroids, immune-suppression; infants may have diaper rash | Antifungal medication and proper oral hygiene; may recur if cause is not eliminated or managed | Plaque<br>Chemical burn<br>Coated tongue<br>Mucosal sloughing |

| Lesion | Pediatric Age and Gender | Clinical Findings | Location | Pediatric Significance | Treatment and Prognosis | Differential Diagnosis |
|---|---|---|---|---|---|---|
| **White Surface Material Lesions—cont'd** | | | | | | |
| Chemical burn | First and second decades<br>No gender predilection | Localized or widespread, white nonadherent plaques and erythematous erosions or ulcers; tender to painful | Any site but common on lips, tongue, buccal mucosa, and gingiva | Multiple chemicals and drugs may cause this reaction, including those used in dentistry | Identify and remove cause; symptomatic relief | Plaque<br>Pseudomembranous candidiasis<br>Coated tongue<br>Mucosal sloughing |
| Coated tongue (furred tongue) | First and second decades<br>No gender predilection | White or yellow nonadherent coating on tongue; asymptomatic; may be source of halitosis | Dorsal tongue | Common condition associated with mouth breathing, febrile illnesses, dehydration, poor oral hygiene | Brushing tongue and adequate hydration; tends to recur | Pseudomembranous candidiasis<br>Hairy tongue<br>White strawberry tongue |
| **White Subsurface Lesions** | | | | | | |
| Scar formation (Cicatrix) | First and second decades<br>No gender predilection | White or pale pink line or irregular patch with smooth surface; cross-hatch or starburst pattern; asymptomatic | Any site but common on labial mucosa, lip vermilion, tongue | History of oral trauma or surgery; may represent child abuse or self-mutilation | None required; scar revision if cosmetic concern or if restricts function | Linea alba<br>Mucosal graft<br>Lichen planus |
| Fordyce granules | Second decade<br>No gender predilection | Small, yellow-white, multifocal papules; discrete or clustered; asymptomatic | Bilateral buccal mucosa, retromolar pad and upper lip vermilion | Oral sebaceous glands occur in 20% to 30% of children; puberty stimulates development | No treatment is necessary; may increase in size | Frictional keratosis<br>Scar formation |

Continued

**TABLE 2-2**

**White Soft Tissue Lesions (Fig. 2-2)—cont'd**

| Lesion | Pediatric Age and Gender | Clinical Findings | Location | Pediatric Significance | Treatment and Prognosis | Differential Diagnosis |
|---|---|---|---|---|---|---|
| **White Subsurface Lesions—cont'd** | | | | | | |
| Oral lymphoepithelial cyst | Second decade No gender predilection | Solitary, soft, pinkish white nodule with superficial fine vascular pattern; usually nontender | Posterior lateral tongue, floor of mouth, soft palate | Mimics an abscess because it may fluctuate in size and discharge contents | Excisional biopsy; does not recur | Soft tissue abscess Lipoma Sialolithiasis Hyperplastic lymphoid aggregate |
| Sialolithiasis | Second decade No gender predilection | Solitary, hard, pinkish white nodule; episodic pain and swelling when eating | Usually floor of mouth within Wharton's duct, submandibular gland | Occlusal or panoramic radiograph may assist with diagnosis | Surgical removal or endoscopy; stone may recur | Soft tissue abscess Oral lymphoepithelial cyst Epidermoid cyst |
| Palatal cysts of the newborn | Neonates No gender predilection | Solitary or multiple, discrete or clustered papules with a smooth pearly white surface; usually 1–3 mm in size, asymptomatic | *Epstein's pearls:* median palatal raphe *Bohn's nodules:* hard palate and soft palate junction | Cysts occur in up to 85% of neonates | None required; keratin-filled cysts that spontaneously rupture within first month | Soft tissue abscess Natal/neonatal teeth Soft tissue abscess Oral lymphoepithelial cyst |
| Gingival cysts of the newborn (Dental lamina cysts) | Neonates No gender predilection | Solitary or multiple, discrete or clustered papules with a smooth translucent to pearly white surface; usually 1–3 mm in size, asymptomatic | Alveolar mucosa, especially maxillary mucosa | Cysts occur in up to 50% of neonates | None required; keratin-filled cysts that spontaneously rupture within first 3 months | Natal/neonatal teeth Soft tissue abscess |

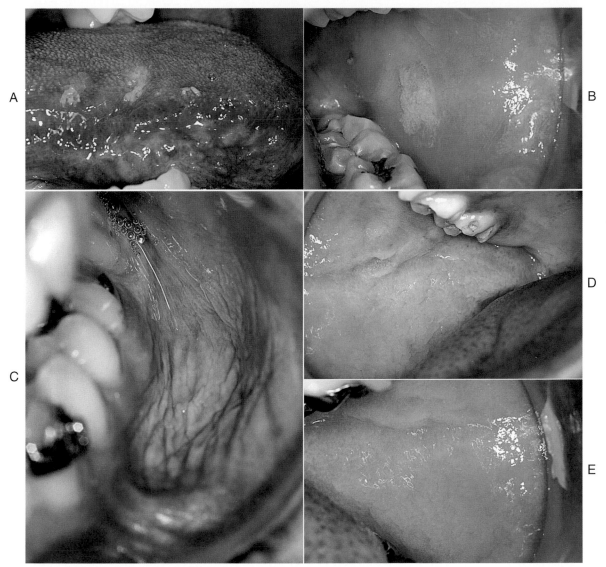

**Figure 2-2**   **White soft tissue lesions. A** and **B,** Frictional keratosis of the lateral tongue (**A**) and buccal mucosa (**B**) from chronic biting of the tissues. **C,** Smokeless tobacco keratosis of the posterior mandibular vestibule. **D** and **E,** Leukoedema of the buccal mucosa, bilaterally.                                                                     *Continued*

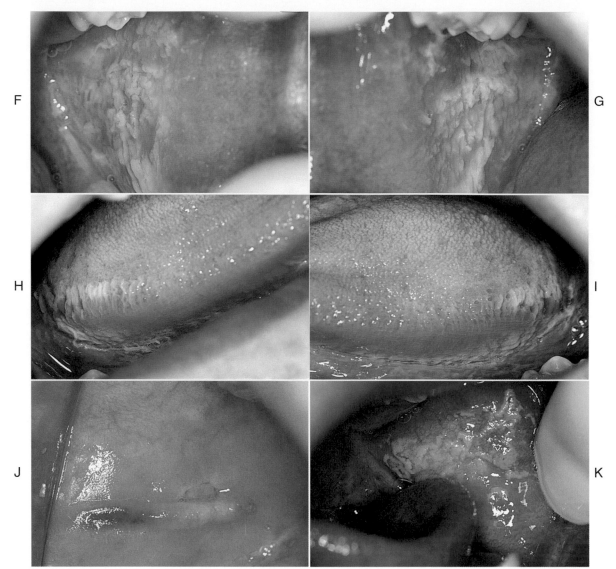

**Figure 2-2—cont'd** F to I, White sponge nevus of the buccal mucosa (F and G) and lateral tongue (H and I). J, Ulcerated linea alba from aggressive sucking habit. K, Pseudomembranous candidiasis of the buccal mucosa.

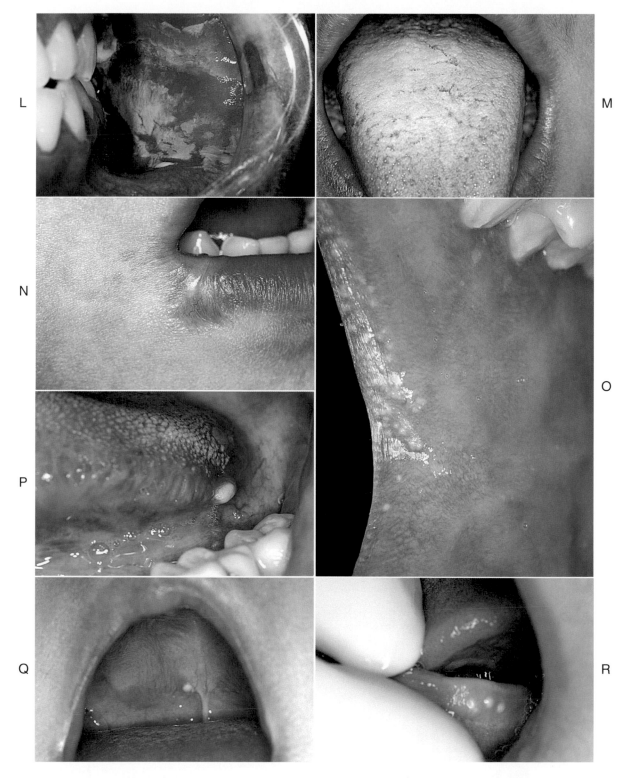

**Figure 2-2—cont'd**  L, Chemical burn from overuse of a topical anesthetic. **M,** Coated tongue in a child who is mouth breathing. **N,** Fan-shaped scar at the corners of the mouth due to an electrical burn. **O,** Cluster of Fordyce granules of the anterior buccal mucosa. **P,** Oral lymphoepithelial cyst of the posterior lateral tongue. **Q,** Single palatal cyst of the newborn on the midline hard palate. **R,** Cluster of gingival cysts of the newborn on the mandibular alveolar mucosa.

## TABLE 2-3
### Dark Soft Tissue Lesions (Fig. 2-3)

| LESION | PEDIATRIC AGE AND GENDER | CLINICAL FINDINGS | LOCATION | PEDIATRIC SIGNIFICANCE | TREATMENT AND PROGNOSIS | DIFFERENTIAL DIAGNOSIS |
|---|---|---|---|---|---|---|
| **Red or Purple-Blue Lesions** | | | | | | |
| Port wine stain (Vascular malformation) | Infancy Female predilection | Localized to diffuse, red to purple macular lesions; bleeds; blanches; grows with child | Face, along distribution of trigeminal nerve, is most common site; may have lip and oral mucosal involvement | Occurs in about 1% of newborns; may be sign of *Sturge-Weber angiomatosis*; hemorrhage is complication | Laser treatment; persistent lesion that may become darker in color and nodular with age | Hemangioma Ecchymosis |
| Petechiae, ecchymosis, hematoma | First and second decades No gender predilection | Localized to diffuse, pinpoint spots, patches or swellings with smooth surface; early lesions are red; late lesions are blue-black; may be tender | Buccal mucosa, lips, lateral tongue, and soft palate | If multiple lesions, need to exclude child abuse, bleeding disorders | No treatment; spontaneously resolve | Amalgam/graphite tattoo Blue nevus Hemangioma Blood dyscrasia |
| Erythematous candidiasis | First and second decades No gender predilection | Multiple red macules; depapillation of tongue; burning sensation | Palate, buccal mucosa, dorsal tongue | Caused by *Candida albicans* and other species; contributing factors are antibiotics, immunosuppression, xerostomia, or palatal coverage appliances | Antifungal medication and proper oral hygiene; may recur if cause is not eliminated or managed | Contact allergy Petechiae, ecchymosis, Blood dyscrasia |

Continued

| Lesion | Pediatric Age and Gender | Clinical Findings | Location | Pediatric Significance | Treatment and Prognosis | Differential Diagnosis |
|---|---|---|---|---|---|---|
| **Red or Purple-Blue Lesions—cont'd** | | | | | | |
| Median rhomboid glossitis | First and second decades. No gender predilection | Localized red, depapillated patch; oval to rhomboid in shape with smooth or lobulated surface; asymptomatic | Midline posterior dorsal tongue | Caused by candidal infection; localized palatal erythema or "kissing lesion" may be present | Antifungal medication and proper oral hygiene | Erythema migrans; Contact allergy; Hemangioma; Lingual thyroid |
| Erythema migrans (Benign migratory glossitis) | First and second decades. Female predilection | Multiple oval or circular red patches with white scalloped border; loss of filiform papillae; pattern changes; may burn | Dorsal and lateral tongue; rarely at other mucosal sites | More common in children than adults; increased risk in atopic children; may occur with fissured tongue | None required; avoidance of hot or spicy foods; topical steroids in symptomatic cases | Median rhomboid glossitis; Contact allergy; Erythematous candidiasis; Transient lingual papillitis |
| Eruption hematoma and cyst | First and second decades. No gender predilection | Localized patch or swelling; amber, red, or blue in color; overlying an erupting tooth; usually nontender | Alveolar mucosa | Eruption cyst is soft tissue counterpart of *dentigerous cyst;* infrequently delays tooth eruption; minimal bleeding may occur at this site | No treatment is usually necessary; resolves with tooth eruption; uncover tooth if symptomatic | Hemangioma; Neonatal alveolar lymphangioma; Pyogenic granuloma; Amalgam tattoo |
| **Brown-Black Lesions** | | | | | | |
| Physiologic pigmentation (Racial pigmentation) | First and second decades. No gender predilection | Gray, brown or black patches with smooth surface; patchy to generalized distribution | Any location but attached gingiva is most common | Pigmentation increases with age of child; common in dark-complexioned skin types | None required; common variant of normal mucosa | Postinflammatory pigmentation; Drug-induced pigmentation; Smoker's melanosis; Lead poisoning |

## TABLE 2-3

**Dark Soft Tissue Lesions (Fig. 2-3)—cont'd**

| LESION | PEDIATRIC AGE AND GENDER | CLINICAL FINDINGS | LOCATION | PEDIATRIC SIGNIFICANCE | TREATMENT AND PROGNOSIS | DIFFERENTIAL DIAGNOSIS |
|---|---|---|---|---|---|---|
| **Brown-Black Lesions—cont'd** | | | | | | |
| Amalgam tattoo | Second decade No gender predilection | Gray-blue, black macule with smooth surface and well-defined to irregular margins; radiographs may demonstrate opaque fragments | Gingiva, alveolar mucosa, buccal mucosa | Graphite tattoo is found on palate from self-inflicted wound; intentional tattooing usually observed on lower labial mucosa | None required unless melanocytic neoplasm cannot be excluded; permanent discoloration | Melanotic macule Graphite tattoo Melanocytic nevus Varix Late ecchymosis |
| Oral melanotic macule | First and second decades Female predilection | Brown or black, oval macule with smooth surface, well-defined margins; single or multiple | Lower lip vermilion, buccal mucosa, gingiva | Most common oral pigmentation of fair-complexioned children; multiple lip macules in *Peutz-Jeghers syndrome* | None required unless a melanocytic neoplasm cannot be excluded; no potential for malignant transformation | Amalgam/graphite tattoo Melanocytic nevus Smoker's melanosis Late ecchymosis |
| Melanocytic nevus | Second decade Female predilection | Brown, blue or black, well-defined nodule or macule with smooth surface | Lip vermilion, palate, gingiva | Oral lesions are uncommon but head and neck skin is frequently involved | Excisional biopsy; rare risk of malignant transformation | Amalgam/graphite tattoo Oral melanotic macule Melanoma |

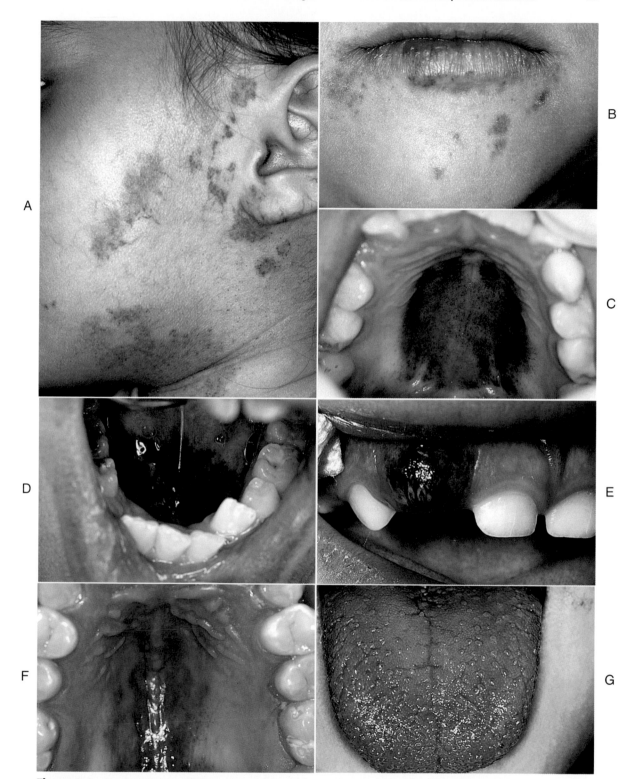

**Figure 2-3**  **Dark soft tissue lesions. A** and **B,** Vascular malformation on the side of the face (**A**) and around the lips (**B**). **C,** Ecchymosis of the hard palatal mucosa from sucking aggressively on a lollipop. **D,** Hematoma of the floor of the mouth following trauma to the chin, which is frequently associated with fracture of the condyles. **E,** Eruption hematoma of the maxillary alveolar mucosa. **F** and **G,** Erythematous candidiasis of the hard palatal mucosa (**F**) and dorsal tongue (**G**).

*Continued*

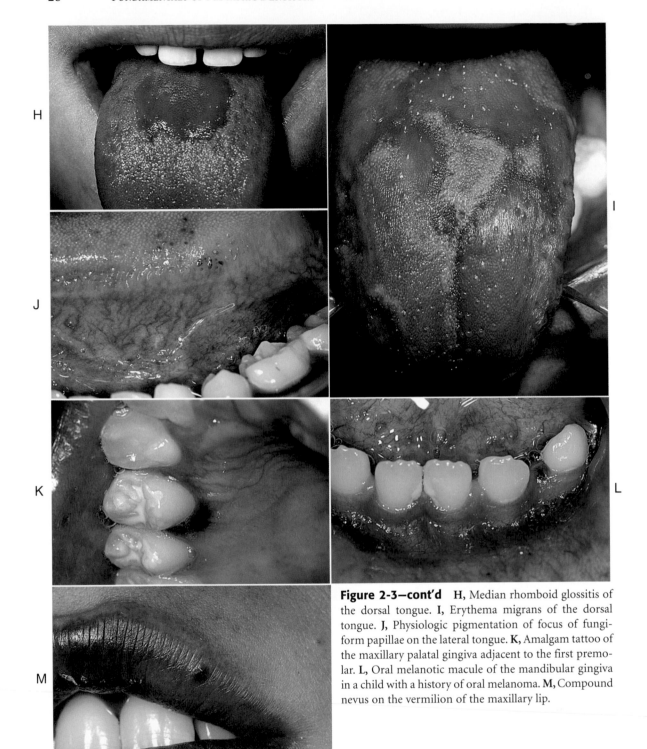

**Figure 2-3—cont'd**   **H,** Median rhomboid glossitis of the dorsal tongue. **I,** Erythema migrans of the dorsal tongue. **J,** Physiologic pigmentation of focus of fungiform papillae on the lateral tongue. **K,** Amalgam tattoo of the maxillary palatal gingiva adjacent to the first premolar. **L,** Oral melanotic macule of the mandibular gingiva in a child with a history of oral melanoma. **M,** Compound nevus on the vermilion of the maxillary lip.

## TABLE 2-4
### Ulcerative Lesions (Fig. 2-4)

| Lesion | Pediatric Age and Gender | Clinical Findings | Location | Pediatric Significance | Treatment and Prognosis | Differential Diagnosis |
|---|---|---|---|---|---|---|
| Aphthous ulcer | First and second decades Female predilection | Recurrent, painful ulcers. *Minor variant*: 1–5 superficial oval ulcers <1 cm; resolves in 7–10 days; *Major variant*: multiple, deep ulcers >1 cm; resolves in 2–6 weeks; *Herpetiform variant*: showers of multiple small ulcers | Buccal, labial mucosa are most common; occurs on nonkeratinized mucosa | Occurs in one third of children; T-cell immune dysfunction; trauma is important factor in children; genetic predisposition | Symptomatic relief, topical and systemic steroids, amlexanox, chlorhexidine oral rinse, chemical cauterizing agents, laser treatment. Major variant heals with scarring | Traumatic ulcer Secondary herpetic ulcer Crohn's disease Behçet's syndrome Celiac disease Neutropenic ulcer PFAPA syndrome |
| Secondary herpetic ulcer | First and second decades No gender predilection | Multiple, recurrent, small ulcers; painful; preceded by vesicles; clustered pattern; prodromal burning sensation; heals in 7–14 days | Herpes labialis on lip vermilion and perioral skin; intraoral herpetic ulcers on hard palate, attached gingiva; herpetic whitlow on fingers, especially with digit sucking habit | Reactivation of herpes simplex virus (HSV); occurs in one third of children; ultraviolet light, systemic diseases, trauma, stress, menses are triggering factors | Symptomatic relief; sunscreen; topical acyclovir, penciclovir, docosanol; systemic acyclovir, valacyclovir; immunocompromised children should be treated | Traumatic ulcer Aphthous ulcer Angular cheilitis Impetigo Contact allergy |

Continued

**TABLE 2-4**

**Ulcerative Lesions (Fig. 2-4)—cont'd**

| LESION | PEDIATRIC AGE AND GENDER | CLINICAL FINDINGS | LOCATION | PEDIATRIC SIGNIFICANCE | TREATMENT AND PROGNOSIS | DIFFERENTIAL DIAGNOSIS |
|---|---|---|---|---|---|---|
| Angular cheilitis | First and second decades<br>No gender predilection | Red fissures that bleed and may ulcerate; scaling and crusted surface; burning sensation; may be recurrent | Commissures of mouth; may be associated with concurrent oral candidal infection | Caused by *Candida* species and staphylococci; lip incompetence, licking of lips and drooling are aggravating factors; may be caused by contact allergy | Lubrication of lips, antifungal, antifungal/steroid or antibiotic ointments; recurring lesions may require oral antifungal treatment | Secondary herpetic ulcer<br>Impetigo<br>Exfoliative cheilitis<br>Traumatic ulcers |
| Traumatic ulcer | First and second decades<br>No gender predilection | Usually single ulcer; variable shape with irregular margins; shallow or deep; painful; typically heals in 1–3 weeks | Lateral tongue, buccal mucosa, lips and gingival; *Riga-Fede disease* occurs in infants on ventral tongue from rubbing against lower incisors | Most common oral ulcer; may indicate child abuse, neurologic impairment or factitial injuries when persistent and recurrent | Symptomatic relief; eliminate cause; factitial ulcers are diagnostic problem; may heal with scarring | Secondary herpetic ulcer<br>Aphthous ulcer<br>Contact allergy<br>Mucosal burn |
| Contact allergy | First and second decades<br>No gender predilection | Focal or widespread erythema, vesicles and ulcers; burning sensation and pain | Any mucosal site that comes in contact with allergen, especially lips, buccal mucosa and gingiva | Wide variety of allergens including foods, dental materials, oral hygiene products, topical medications, cosmetic products | Identify and eliminate allergen; patch testing helpful in older children; topical steroids to reduce symptoms; lesions recur with reexposure to allergen | Mucosal burn<br>Secondary herpetic ulcer<br>Aphthous ulcer<br>Angular cheilitis<br>Erythema multiforme |

## TABLE 2-4
### Ulcerative Lesions (Fig. 2-4)—cont'd

| LESION | PEDIATRIC AGE AND GENDER | CLINICAL FINDINGS | LOCATION | PEDIATRIC SIGNIFICANCE | TREATMENT AND PROGNOSIS | DIFFERENTIAL DIAGNOSIS |
|---|---|---|---|---|---|---|
| Erythema multiforme | Second decade Male predilection | Widespread, painful, red macules, vesicles, bullae and ulcers; blood-crusted lesions on lips; target lesions on skin; acute onset; fever, malaise | Oral lesions on lips, tongue, buccal mucosa and soft palate. Skin lesions on extremities and head and neck region | Common precipitating factors include herpes simplex virus (HSV) and medications. Severe variant is *Stevens-Johnson syndrome* | Withdrawal of medication; lubrication of lips, symptomatic relief; hospitalization if severe; recurrences are common if triggered by HSV | Primary herpetic gingivostomatitis Necrotizing ulcerative gingivitis Aphthous major ulcers Chemical burn |
| Primary herpetic gingivostomatitis | Usually first decade No gender predilection | Fever, irritability, pain, lymphadenopathy, drooling, multiple vesicles and ulcers; diffuse erythema; sudden onset; resolves in 7-10 days | Widespread oral and perioral involvement; gingival lesions are usually chief complaint | Caused by HSV; high fever and dehydration are serious complications in children; digital and ocular lesions may occur | Supportive care includes antipyretics, analgesics, palliative oral rinses, hydration; systemic acyclovir may be indicated. | Necrotizing ulcerative gingivitis Erythema multiforme Herpangina |

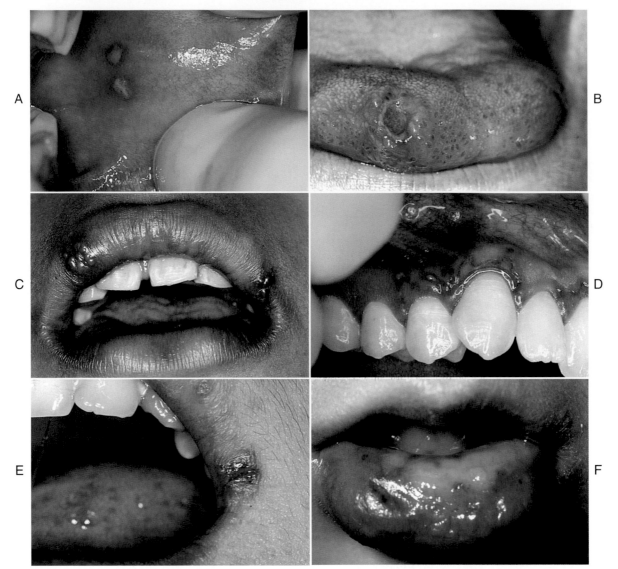

**Figure 2-4**    Ulcerative lesions. **A,** Aphthous minor ulcer of the posterior buccal mucosa. **B,** Aphthous major ulcer of the anterior dorsal tongue. **C,** Herpes labialis of the vermilion of the maxillary lip. **D,** Secondary herpetic ulcers of the maxillary attached gingiva. **E,** Angular cheilitis. **F,** Diffuse traumatic ulcer from biting the lip following local anesthesia for restorative treatment.                                                                                *Continued*

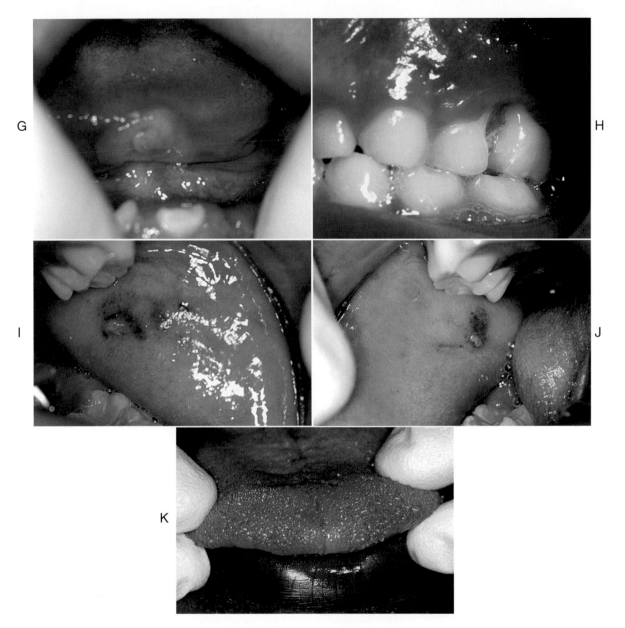

**Figure 2-4—cont'd**  G, Riga-Fede disease of the ventral tongue in a child with neonatal teeth. H, Erythema and recession of the attached gingiva between the primary first and second maxillary molars from picking the tissues with the fingernails. I to K, Bilateral erosions of the buccal mucosa (I and J) and tenderness of the fungiform papillae at the tip of the tongue (K) from a toothpaste hypersensitivity.                                        *Continued*

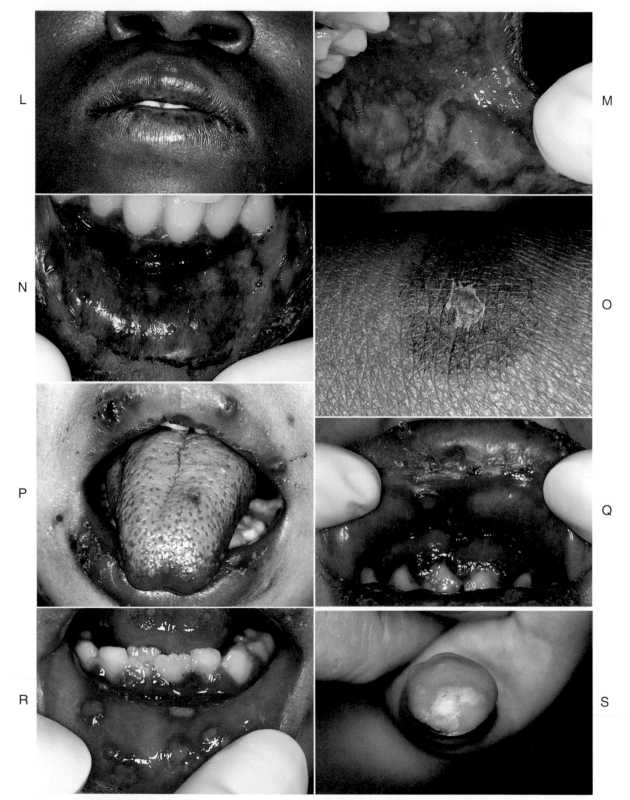

**Figure 2-4—cont'd**  L to O, Drug-induced erythema multiforme with swelling of the lips (**L**), erythema and ulcerations of the buccal mucosa (**M**) and labial mucosa (**N**), and target lesions on the skin (**O**). **P** to **S**, Primary herpetic gingivostomatitis of the tongue and lips (**P**), maxillary gingiva and labial mucosa (**Q**) and mandibular gingiva and labial mucosa (**R**), and vesicles on the thumb (**S**). *Continued*

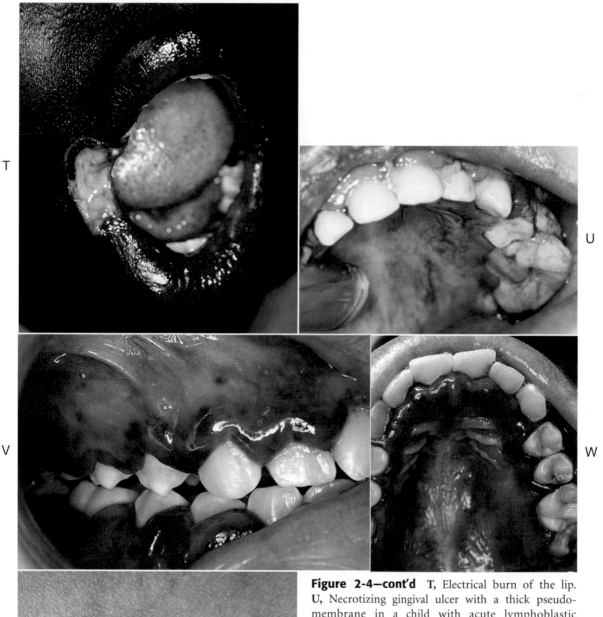

**Figure 2-4—cont'd** T, Electrical burn of the lip. U, Necrotizing gingival ulcer with a thick pseudo-membrane in a child with acute lymphoblastic leukemia. V to X, Red-purple enlargements of the buccal gingiva (V), palatal mucosa (W), and skin (X) that represent leukemic infiltrates in a child with acute myeloid leukemia.

## TABLE 2-5

### Soft Tissue Enlargements (Fig. 2-5)

| Lesion | Pediatric Age and Gender | Clinical Findings | Location | Pediatric Significance | Treatment and Prognosis | Differential Diagnosis |
|---|---|---|---|---|---|---|
| **Papillary Lesions** | | | | | | |
| Squamous papilloma | Second decade No gender predilection | Single, pedunculated nodule with finger-like projections; pink to white; soft and nontender | Any oral site but predilection for the tongue, lips, and soft palate | Caused by human papillomavirus (HPV), especially types 6, 11; low virulence and infectivity rate | Excisional biopsy; recurrence is uncommon; no evidence of malignant transformation | Verruca vulgaris Condyloma acuminatum Giant cell fibroma |
| Verruca vulgaris (Common wart) | First and second decades No gender predilection | Multiple sessile or pedunculated papules and nodules with rough, pebbly or papillary surface; white; nontender | Common on skin of hands and face; infrequently found on the lip vermilion, labial mucosa, and anterior tongue | Caused by HPV, especially types 2, 4, 6, 40; spread by autoinoculation to oral site by sucking on fingers or nail biting | Excisional biopsy of oral warts; low risk for recurrence for oral lesions; high rate of spontaneous resolution; no malignant transformation | Squamous papilloma Condyloma acuminatum Giant cell fibroma |
| Condyloma acuminatum (Venereal wart) | Second decade No gender predilection | Multiple, discrete, sessile nodules with blunted papillary surface; pink; nontender | Usually anogenital lesions; oral sites include labial mucosa, soft palate and ventral tongue | Caused by HPV, especially types 2, 6, 11, 53, 54, 16, 18; sexually transmitted disease; may indicate child abuse | Excisional biopsy, laser ablation of oral warts; highly contagious; frequently recur; malignant transformation of anogenital warts | Squamous papilloma Focal epithelial hyperplasia Inflammatory papillary hyperplasia Focal dermal hypoplasia |

| Lesion | Pediatric Age and Gender | Clinical Findings | Location | Pediatric Significance | Treatment and Prognosis | Differential Diagnosis |
|---|---|---|---|---|---|---|
| **Papillary Lesions—cont'd** | | | | | | |
| Giant cell fibroma | Second decade Female predilection | Solitary, sessile or pedunculated nodule with a pebbly surface; pink; nontender | Attached gingiva, dorsal tongue and hard palate | Reactive hyperplastic lesion that has a predilection for children | Excisional biopsy; recurrence is rare | Squamous papilloma Retrocuspid papilla Irritation fibroma |
| Focal epithelial hyperplasia (Heck's disease) | First and second decades No gender predilection | Multifocal, sessile, papules and nodules with pink grainy to stippled surface; lesions coalesce, display cobblestone appearance; nontender | Usually located on labial and buccal mucosa and tongue | Caused by HPV, types 13, 32; low infectivity rate | Excisional biopsy; laser ablation; recurrence is common; spontaneous regression may occur; no malignant transformation | Verruca vulgaris Condyloma acuminata Focal dermal hypoplasia |
| Inflammatory papillary hyperplasia | Second decade No gender predilection | Multiple, clustered papules and nodules with pink to red granular surface; cobblestone appearance; nontender | Hard palatal mucosa | Caused by continuous wear of palatal coverage appliance; other factors include mouth breathing and high palatal vault; candidal infection may be present | Remove and clean appliance; reline appliance if needed; antifungal therapy; excisional biopsy of persistent lesions | Condyloma acuminata Focal epithelial hyperplasia Erythematous candidiasis |

Continued

## TABLE 2-5
### Soft Tissue Enlargements (Fig. 2-5)—cont'd

| LESION | PEDIATRIC AGE AND GENDER | CLINICAL FINDINGS | LOCATION | PEDIATRIC SIGNIFICANCE | TREATMENT AND PROGNOSIS | DIFFERENTIAL DIAGNOSIS |
|---|---|---|---|---|---|---|
| **Acute Inflammatory Lesions** | | | | | | |
| Soft tissue abscess (Parulis) | First and second decades No gender predilection | Solitary pinkish white or deep red nodule with surrounding erythema; purulent drainage; fluctuates in size; tender to painful; may progress to cellulitis | Gingiva and alveolar mucosa are most common sites | Usually caused by odontogenic infection or entrapped foreign body; *pericoronitis* is a gingival abscess associated with erupting molars | Manage source of infection; local debridement, antibiotics may be indicated; recurs if infection is not eliminated | Gingival cysts of newborn Pyogenic granuloma Oral lymphoepithelial cyst Sialolithiasis Tonsilithiasis |
| Cellulitis | First and second decades No gender predilection | Diffuse erythematous swelling of sudden onset; soft to board-like; warm and painful tissues; fever, headache, airway obstruction and leukocytosis may be present | Upper or lower face and neck | Caused by odontogenic infection, facial or oral lacerations, insect bites, peritonsillar abscesses, jaw fractures, sialadenitis, sinusitis, and bacteremia | Manage source of infection; antibiotic therapy; incision and drainage in severe cases. *Ludwig's angina and cavernous sinus thrombosis* may be life threatening | Plunging ranula Emphysema Obstructive sialadenitis Angioedema Acute sinusitis |
| Angioedema | First and second decades No gender predilection | Diffuse swelling of sudden onset; soft and nontender; may be associated with respiratory and gastrointestinal problems | Lips, tongue, soft palate and face and other cutaneous sites | Acquired form is caused by allergic reaction to foods, plants, drugs, infections, autoimmune disease and stress; most hereditary forms are caused by C1-INH deficiency | Allergic forms are treated by antihistamines, steroids or epinephrine; hereditary forms are treated with C1-INH concentrate and esterase-inhibiting drugs; prevention with androgens; may be life threatening | Cellulitis Emphysema Traumatic edema Orofacial granulomatosis |

## TABLE 2-5
### Soft Tissue Enlargements (Fig. 2-5)—cont'd

| LESION | PEDIATRIC AGE AND GENDER | CLINICAL FINDINGS | LOCATION | PEDIATRIC SIGNIFICANCE | TREATMENT AND PROGNOSIS | DIFFERENTIAL DIAGNOSIS |
|---|---|---|---|---|---|---|
| **Acute Inflammatory Lesions—cont'd** | | | | | | |
| Mucocele | First and second decades No gender predilection | Fluid-filled nodule with a smooth, translucent, red or blue surface; sudden onset; fluctuates in size; tender if traumatized; periodically drains | Lower labial mucosa, buccal mucosa, and anterior ventral tongue | Most common lip swelling in children; may be associated with trauma and orthodontic appliances; rare cases are congenital | Excisional biopsy with removal of underlying minor salivary glands; may recur with incomplete removal or repeated trauma | Lymphangioma Hemangioma Hematoma Soft fibroma Soft tissue abscess |
| Ranula | First and second decades No gender predilection | Fluid-filled swelling with smooth, translucent to blue surface of recent onset; fluctuates in size; mildly tender; periodically drains; may elevate tongue | Floor of mouth, lateral to midline; plunging variant results in diffuse swelling of the submandibular region and neck | Usually associated with sublingual gland or aplasia of submandibular excretory duct | Excisional biopsy of sublingual gland or marsupialization; recurrences are common with marsupialization | Lymphangioma Hemangioma Mucoepidermoid carcinoma Obstructive sialadenitis Dermoid cyst |
| **Tumor and Tumor-like Lesions** | | | | | | |
| Irritation fibroma | First and second decades No gender predilection | Pedunculated or sessile nodule with pink smooth surface; firm and nontender; limited growth potential | Buccal and labial mucosa, tongue and attached gingiva | Common reactive hyperplastic lesion caused by chronic trauma and mimics a tumor | Conservative excisional biopsy; may recur if irritation continues | Fibrosing mucocele Peripheral ossifying fibroma Giant cell fibroma Benign submucosal neoplasm |

*Continued*

## TABLE 2-5

### Soft Tissue Enlargements (Fig. 2-5)—cont'd

**Tumor and Tumor-like Lesions—cont'd**

| Lesion | Pediatric Age and Gender | Clinical Findings | Location | Pediatric Significance | Treatment and Prognosis | Differential Diagnosis |
|---|---|---|---|---|---|---|
| Peripheral ossifying fibroma | Second decade Female predilection | Pedunculated or sessile nodule with pink to red surface; frequently ulcerated; firm and nontender; may resorb alveolar bone; limited growth potential | Emanates from interdental of attached gingiva; most common site is anterior region | Reactive hyperplastic lesion that contains mineralized product from cells of periosteum or periodontal ligament; may displace teeth | Excisional biopsy down to periosteum and remove local irritation; 16% recurrence rate | Irritation fibroma Peripheral giant cell granuloma Giant cell fibroma Pyogenic granuloma |
| Peripheral giant cell granuloma | Second decade Female predilection | Pedunculated or sessile nodule with red or purple-blue surface; may be ulcerated; firm and nontender; may resorb alveolar bone; limited growth potential | Attached gingiva or alveolar mucosa | Reactive hyperplastic lesion that is caused by irritation; may displace teeth | Excisional biopsy down to periosteum and remove local irritation; 10% recurrence rate | Pyogenic granuloma Irritation fibroma Peripheral ossifying fibroma Hemangioma |
| Pyogenic granuloma | First and second decades Female predilection | Pedunculated or sessile nodule with smooth to irregular, red surface; usually ulcerated; bleeds freely; soft and friable; nontender; limited growth potential | Most occur on attached gingiva; other sites include lip, tongue, and buccal mucosa | Reactive hyperplastic lesion caused by irritation and poor oral hygiene; may be associated with pregnancy (*pregnancy tumor*) | Excisional biopsy and remove local irritation; recurrence rate is low | Irritation fibroma Peripheral ossifying fibroma Peripheral giant cell granuloma Soft tissue abscess Hemangioma |

**Tumor and Tumor-like Lesions—cont'd**

| Lesion | Pediatric Age and Gender | Clinical Findings | Location | Pediatric Significance | Treatment and Prognosis | Differential Diagnosis |
|---|---|---|---|---|---|---|
| Gingival fibromatosis (Hereditary or idiopathic) | First and second decades. No gender predilection | Localized or generalized gingival enlargements; pink, smooth to stippled surfaces; firm and nontender; affects both dentitions | Attached gingiva and maxillary tuberosity | May be familial or idiopathic; associated with several syndromes; interferes with eruption of teeth; displacement of teeth | Gingivectomy and good oral hygiene; high recurrence rate | Drug-induced gingival overgrowth. Mouth breathing gingivitis. Chronic hyperplastic gingivitis. Leukemic gingival infiltrates |
| Hemangioma | Infancy. Female predilection | Localized to diffuse, red, blue or purple lesion, flat or nodular, soft and compressible, blanches; bleeds freely; 20% are multiple | 60% occur in head and neck region; lips, tongue, and buccal mucosa are most common sites; rarely occurs in jaws | Hemorrhage is potential complication; may cause malocclusion | Involution of lesion within first decade; surgery, laser ablation, corticosteroids, interferon, sclerosing agents; does not recur | Vascular malformation. Pyogenic granuloma. Lymphangioma. Eruption cyst/hematoma. Mucocele |
| Lymphangioma | Infancy; most detected by 2 years. No gender predilection | Localized to diffuse, translucent to red or purple swelling; smooth or pebbly surface; soft and compressible; crepitus may be palpated | Up to 75% occur in head and neck; common oral sites include the tongue, lip, and buccal mucosa | May cause malocclusion, dysphagia, and respiratory problems; *cystic hygroma* and *neonatal alveolar lymphangioma* are variants | Surgical excision; recurrences are common; airway obstruction and death may occur with large neck or tongue lesions | Hemangioma. Squamous papilloma. Mucocele. Plunging ranula |

*Continued*

## TABLE 2-5
### Soft Tissue Enlargements (Fig. 2-5)—cont'd

**Tumor and Tumor-like Lesions—cont'd**

| Lesion | Pediatric Age and Gender | Clinical Findings | Location | Pediatric Significance | Treatment and Prognosis | Differential Diagnosis |
|---|---|---|---|---|---|---|
| Congenital epulis (Congenital granular cell tumor) | Infancy Female predilection | Pedunculated or sessile nodule; pink to red smooth surface; may be ulcerated; 10% are multiple | Anterior alveolar ridge; usually maxilla | May cause feeding problems; usually reaches maximum size at birth | Surgical excision; occasional spontaneous regression; no recurrence | Hemangioma Pyogenic granuloma Neonatal alveolar lymphangioma Neuroectodermal tumor of infancy |
| Neurofibroma | Second decade No gender predilection | Single or multiple nodules with smooth surface; discrete or diffuse; soft to firm on palpation; nontender | Tongue, buccal mucosa, vestibule, and palate; syndrome lesions occur at any site, especially skin | *Neurofibromatosis* is autosomal dominant condition with neurofibromas, café-au-lait macules, axillary freckling, and Lisch nodules on iris | Surgical excision if solitary lesion; selective excision of syndrome type; 5% malignant transformation of syndrome type | Schwannoma Mucosal neuroma Irritation fibroma Benign submucosal neoplasm Salivary gland neoplasm |
| Mucosal neuromas (Multiple endocrine neoplasia syndrome, type 2B) | First decade No gender predilection | Multiple, pink papules and nodules; soft and nontender; marfanoid body type; narrow face with full lips | Labial and buccal mucosa, anterior tongue, gingiva; also on conjunctiva and eyelid | Autosomal dominant syndrome; other stigmata include pheochromocytoma and medullary carcinoma of thyroid gland | Surgical excision of neuromas for cosmetics; aggressive thyroid cancer develops in second decade | Neurofibromatosis Focal epithelial hyperplasia Multiple hamartoma syndrome |

## Tumor and Tumor-like Lesions—cont'd

| Lesion | Pediatric Age and Gender | Clinical Findings | Location | Pediatric Significance | Treatment and Prognosis | Differential Diagnosis |
|--------|--------------------------|-------------------|----------|------------------------|-------------------------|------------------------|
| Pleomorphic adenoma (Benign mixed tumor) | Second decade Slight female predilection | Pink, dome-shaped enlargement with smooth surface; slowly growing; firm and nontender | Parotid gland is most common site; palate is most common oral site | Most common benign salivary gland neoplasm; *mucoepidermoid carcinoma* is most common malignant salivary gland tumor in this age group | Surgical excision with adequate margins; recurrence is low; malignant transformation of 5% | Neurofibroma Schwannoma Mucoepidermoid carcinoma Irritation fibroma |
| Juvenile fibromatosis | First and second decades No gender predilection | Rapidly growing, pink, firm mass with an irregular surface; may be ulcerated; painless; large in size; facial disfigurement; destruction of adjacent bone | Head and neck region; paramandibular soft tissues are common intraoral sites | Locally aggressive and destructive lesion that mimics a malignancy | Surgical excision with wide margins; high recurrence rate | Pyogenic granuloma Fibrosarcoma Rhabdomyosarcoma Metastatic disease |

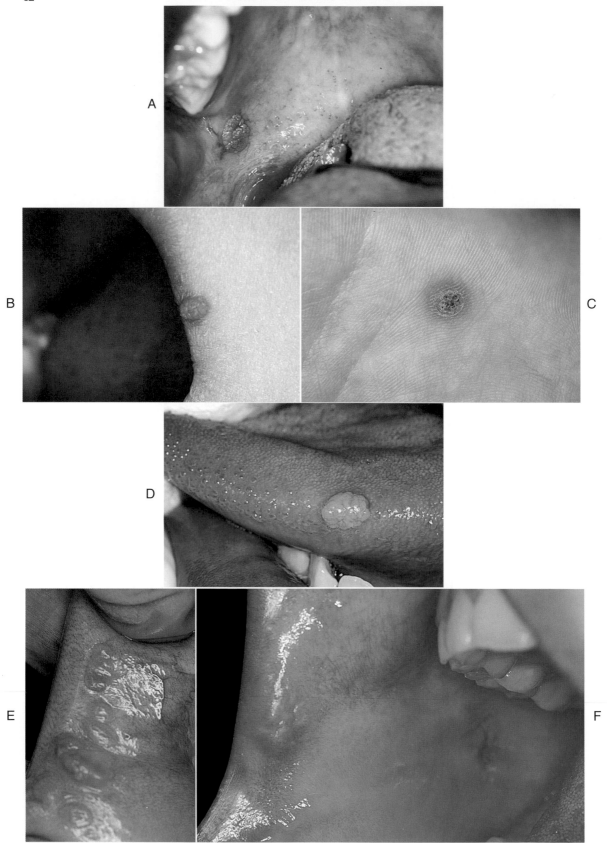

**Figure 2-5** **Soft tissue enlargements. A,** Squamous papilloma of the soft palate. **B** and **C,** Verruca vulgaris of the lip vermilion (**B**) and hand (**C**). **D,** Giant cell fibroma of the lateral tongue. **E** and **F,** Focal epithelial hyperplasia of the buccal mucosa displaying a cobblestone appearance (**E**) or a small clustered pattern (**F**). *Continued*

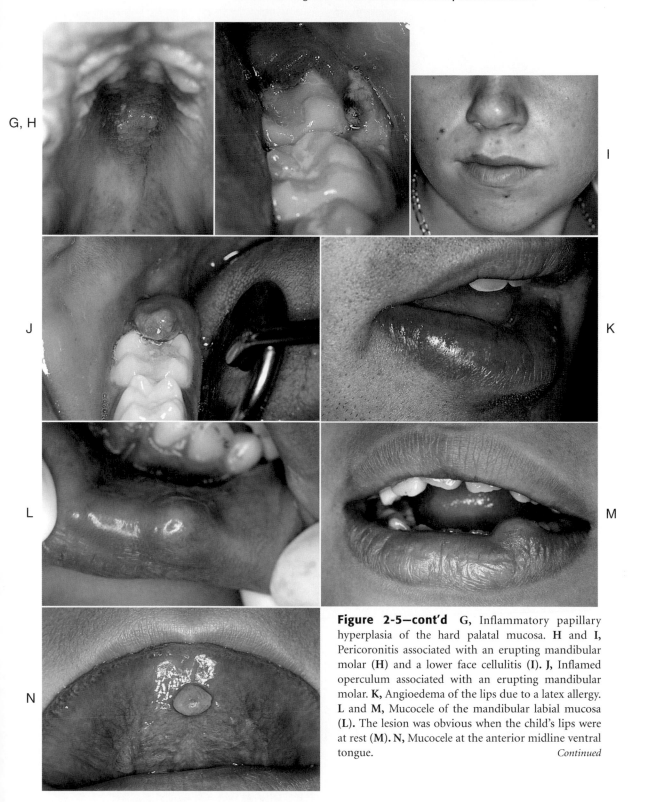

**Figure 2-5—cont'd  G,** Inflammatory papillary hyperplasia of the hard palatal mucosa. **H and I,** Pericoronitis associated with an erupting mandibular molar (**H**) and a lower face cellulitis (**I**). **J,** Inflamed operculum associated with an erupting mandibular molar. **K,** Angioedema of the lips due to a latex allergy. **L and M,** Mucocele of the mandibular labial mucosa (**L**). The lesion was obvious when the child's lips were at rest (**M**). **N,** Mucocele at the anterior midline ventral tongue.    *Continued*

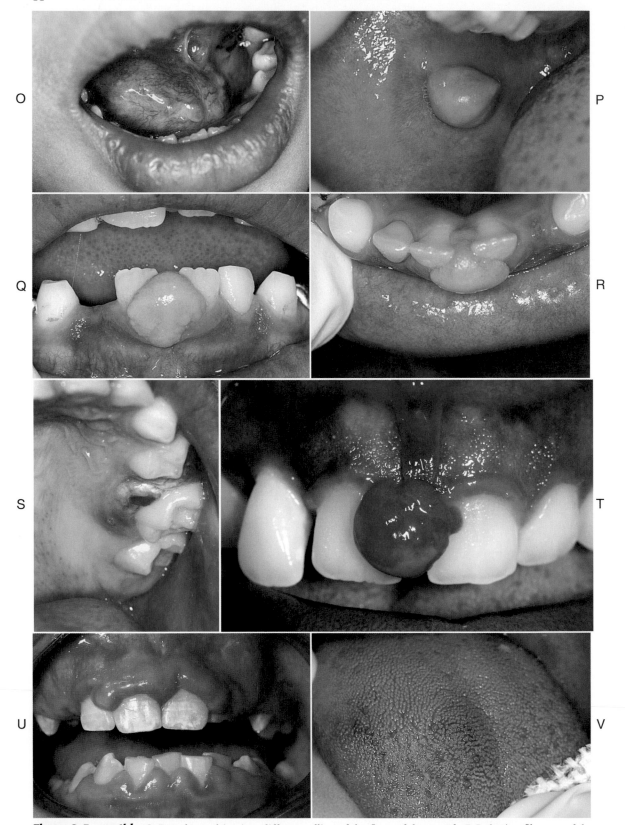

**Figure 2-5—cont'd** **O,** Ranula resulting in a diffuse swelling of the floor of the mouth. **P,** Irritation fibroma of the buccal mucosa. **Q** and **R,** Peripheral ossifying fibroma of the mandibular anterior gingival (**Q**). Note the separation of the incisors (**R**). **S,** Peripheral giant cell granuloma of the palatal gingiva between the primary molars. **T,** Pyogenic granuloma and physiologic pigmentation of the maxillary gingiva. **U,** Hereditary gingival fibromatosis. **V,** Hemangioma of the dorsal tongue.

*Continued*

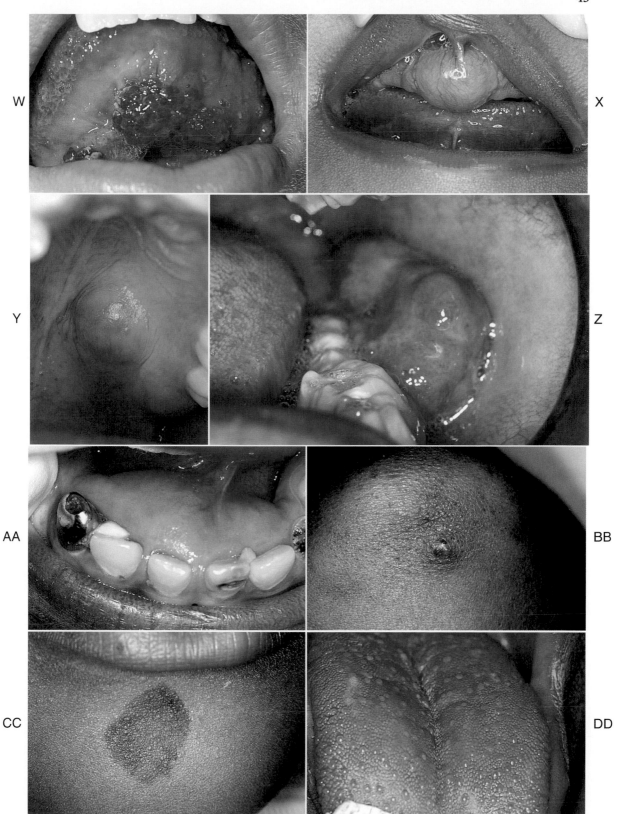

**Figure 2-5—cont'd** W, Lymphangioma of the ventral tongue. X, Congenital epulis of the anterior maxillary alveolar mucosa. Y, Pleomorphic adenoma of the posterior hard palate. Z, Juvenile fibromatosis of the posterior mandibular vestibule and gingiva. AA to DD, Child with neurofibromatosis including neurofibroma of the floor of the mouth (AA), skin of the neck (BB), café-au-lait macule on the chin (CC), and enlarged fungiform papillae (DD).

*Continued*

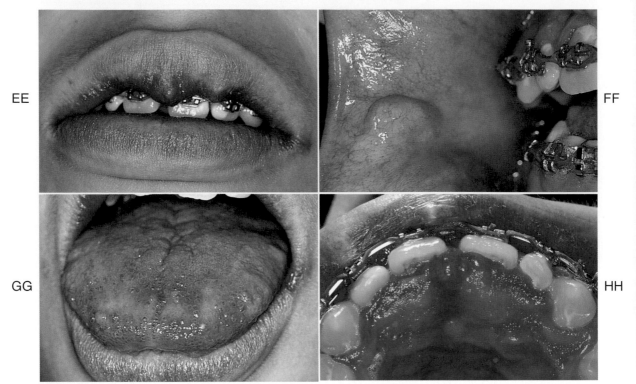

**Figure 2-5—cont'd** EE to HH, Child with multiple endocrine neoplasia syndrome, type 2B, including mucosa neuromas of the lips (EE), buccal mucosa (FF), and tongue (GG) and palatal gingiva (HH).

## TABLE 2-6
### Radiolucent Lesions of Bone (Fig. 2-6)

| LESION | PEDIATRIC AGE AND GENDER | CLINICAL AND RADIOGRAPHIC FINDINGS | LOCATION | PEDIATRIC SIGNIFICANCE | TREATMENT AND PROGNOSIS | DIFFERENTIAL DIAGNOSIS |
|---|---|---|---|---|---|---|
| Dentigerous cyst | Second decade Slight male predilection | Well-defined, unilocular, radiolucency around crown of unerupted tooth; may displace teeth, cause cortical expansion and root resorption; asymptomatic unless infected | Mandibular and maxillary third molar and canine regions | Common odontogenic cyst in children; growth may be rapid; may involve primary or supernumerary teeth; *eruption cyst* is soft tissue analogue | Enucleation; marsupialization if extensive; orthodontic treatment to assist tooth eruption; seldom recur; ameloblastoma and carcinoma are rare complications | Hyperplastic dental follicle Periapical cyst Ameloblastic fibroma Unicystic ameloblastoma Buccal bifurcation cyst |
| Odontogenic keratocyst | Second decade Male predilection | Well-defined, unilocular or multilocular radiolucency with corticated margins; expansile; 40% associated with unerupted tooth; may resorb and displace teeth; may be painful | Posterior body and ramus of mandible; maxillary third molar and canine regions | Multiple cysts are consistent with *nevoid basal cell carcinoma syndrome* and includes jaw cysts, basal cell carcinomas, palmar-plantar pits, bifid ribs, epidermal cysts and calcified falx cerebri | Surgical excision; may include peripheral ostectomy or chemical cautery; recurrence rate of 30%; malignant changes are rare | Dentigerous cyst Ameloblastic fibroma Odontogenic myxoma Ameloblastoma Central hemangioma Central giant cell granuloma |
| Ameloblastic fibroma | First and second decades Slight male predilection | Well-defined unilocular or multilocular lesion with sclerotic margins; expansile; often associated with unerupted tooth | Posterior maxilla and mandible | Rare malignant counterpart, *ameloblastic fibrosarcoma* arises de novo or from preexisting or recurrent tumor | Surgical excision; recurrences are common (18%); long-term follow-up is recommended | Dentigerous cyst Odontogenic keratocyst Central hemangioma Central giant cell granuloma Odontogenic myxoma |

*Continued*

## TABLE 2-6
### Radiolucent Lesions of Bone (Fig. 2-6)—cont'd

| Lesion | Pediatric Age and Gender | Clinical and Radiographic Findings | Location | Pediatric Significance | Treatment and Prognosis | Differential Diagnosis |
|---|---|---|---|---|---|---|
| Ameloblastoma | Second decade No gender predilection | Well-defined, unilocular or multilocular radiolucency; cortical perforation; expansile; slow growing; root displacement and resorption; usually asymptomatic | Mandibular molar and ramus areas | *Unicystic ameloblastoma* is most common variant in children; associated with unerupted molar; treatment is enucleation with 15% recurrence rate | Aggressive odontogenic tumor requires marginal or en bloc resection; 50% to 90% recurs with curettage; rarely undergoes malignant transformation | Dentigerous cyst Odontogenic keratocyst Odontogenic myxoma Central giant cell granuloma Ameloblastic fibroma |
| Melanotic neuroectodermal tumor of infancy | Infancy, may be present at birth No gender predilection | Rapidly expanding bony lesion; may exhibit blue-black pigmented surface; ill-defined, unilocular radiolucency with displacement of tooth buds; "floating tooth" appearance | Anterior maxilla | Lesion mimics malignancy with destructive, rapid growth rate; dental abnormalities due to surgery; high urinary levels of vanillylmandelic acid | Surgical excision or curettage; 15% recurrence rate; reported cases of metastasis | Metastatic sarcoma Central hemangioma Large eruption cyst Congenital epulis |
| Central giant cell granuloma | First and second decades Female predilection | Well-defined, unilocular or multilocular radiolucency with scalloped border; expansile; may displace teeth and cause root resorption; asymptomatic | Most frequently in mandible; anterior to first molar; may cross midline | Aggressive form exists; need to rule out *hyperparathyroidism, cherubism,* and other syndromes, especially with multiple lesions | Thorough curettage; experimental treatments include corticosteroids, calcitonin, interferon; recurrence rate of 20% | Odontogenic keratocyst Odontogenic myxoma Central hemangioma Aneurysmal bone cyst Ameloblastic fibroma |

Continued

| Lesion | Pediatric Age and Gender | Clinical and Radiographic Findings | Location | Pediatric Significance | Treatment and Prognosis | Differential Diagnosis |
|---|---|---|---|---|---|---|
| Cherubism | First decade; usually by 5 years<br>Male predilection | Chubby face appearance; bilateral, symmetric, painless enlargement of jaws; extensive, multiple, well-defined, multilocular radiolucencies | Maxilla and mandible; in particular, angles of mandible; all four quadrants frequently involved | Autosomal dominant condition; causes premature exfoliation of primary teeth; displacement of tooth buds, severe malocclusion, and malformed teeth | Treatment is controversial; spontaneous regression with onset of puberty; surgery may improve function and cosmetics | Nevoid basal cell carcinoma syndrome<br>Hyperparathyroidism<br>Noonan-like syndrome<br>Ramon syndrome |
| Simple bone cyst (Traumatic bone cyst) | Second decade<br>Male predilection | Well-defined, unilocular radiolucency with thin, sclerotic border; scalloping between roots of teeth; 20% are expansile; teeth are vital | Posterior and anterior body of mandible and ramus; bilateral lesions are uncommon | Cause is uncertain, but may be associated with trauma; extensive, expansile lesions may occur | Surgical exploration and curettage; persistence and recurrence are rare | Central giant cell granuloma<br>Dentigerous cyst<br>Periapical cyst<br>Odontogenic keratocyst |
| Aneurysmal bone cyst | First and second decades<br>No gender predilection | Painful swelling with rapid growth; unilocular or multilocular radiolucency with ballooning distention of buccal cortex | Posterior mandibular region | Blood-filled pseudocyst; 20% associated with preexisting lesion, including *central giant cell granuloma, fibrous dysplasia, ossifying fibroma* | Curettage or enucleation; cryosurgery may be needed to control bleeding; recurrence rate as high as 60% | Ameloblastic fibroma<br>Central giant cell granuloma<br>Central hemangioma<br>Dentigerous cyst<br>Simple bone cyst |
| Periapical abscess | First and second decades<br>No gender predilection | Nonvital, mobile tooth; tender to percussion; soft tissue swelling with purulence; painful; widening of periodontal ligament space or poorly defined radiolucency | Alveolus; primary dentition is most frequently affected in children | May progress to cellulitis; may result in aborted development or enamel hypoplasia of succedaneous tooth | Endodontic treatment or tooth extraction; antibiotics and analgesics may be needed; serious complications include *cavernous sinus thrombosis* and *Ludwig's angina* | Incomplete apexification of erupted tooth<br>Periodontal abscess<br>Periapical granuloma or cyst<br>Buccal bifurcation cyst<br>Langerhans cell histiocytosis |

## TABLE 2-6
### Radiolucent Lesions of Bone (Fig. 2-6)—cont'd

| LESION | PEDIATRIC AGE AND GENDER | CLINICAL AND RADIOGRAPHIC FINDINGS | LOCATION | PEDIATRIC SIGNIFICANCE | TREATMENT AND PROGNOSIS | DIFFERENTIAL DIAGNOSIS |
|---|---|---|---|---|---|---|
| Periapical granuloma and cyst | First and second decades No gender predilection | Nonvital tooth; usually asymptomatic unless acute exacerbation of the lesion; well or poorly defined radiolucency at the root apex; loss of lamina dura; root resorption | Alveolar bone adjacent to root apex and bifurcation | May displace succedaneous teeth and cause dental abnormalities; large lesions in primary dentition resemble a *dentigerous cyst* when a succedaneous tooth is present | Endodontic treatment or tooth extraction and gently curettage to avoid disturbing permanent tooth bud, if present | Dentigerous cyst Solitary bone cyst Central giant cell granuloma Langerhans cell histiocytosis |
| Acute osteomyelitis | First and second decades Male predilection | Diffuse radiolucency with poorly defined margins; sequestra; fever, swelling, pain, lymphadenopathy, leukocytosis, and draining sinus tracts | Posterior mandible in children; anterior maxilla in infants | Most cases are due to odontogenic infections or jaw fractures; occasionally caused by bacteremia | Incision and drainage with culture and sensitivity testing; antibiotic coverage; may develop into *chronic osteomyelitis* | Buccal bifurcation cyst Ewing's sarcoma Burkitt's lymphoma Langerhans cell histiocytosis |
| Langerhans cell histiocytosis (Histiocytosis X) | *Disseminated form:* first decade *Localized form:* second decade Male predilection | Lymphadenopathy, rash, oral pain, gingivitis, ulcers, mobile teeth, punched-out radiolucencies with "floating tooth" appearance; premature tooth loss | Skull, mandible, ribs and vertebrae are most often involved; jaws affected in 20% of cases | Neoplastic disease; chronic disseminated form includes lytic bone lesions, exophthalmos, diabetes insipidus; all forms mimic periodontal disease | Chemotherapy, low-dose radiotherapy, and surgical curettage are used, depending on form of disease; children younger than 2 years have worst prognosis | Cyclic neutropenia Burkitt's lymphoma Leukemia Aggressive periodontitis Periapical abscess or granuloma |
| Burkitt's lymphoma | First and second decades Male predilection | Lymphadenopathy, facial swelling, tenderness, tooth mobility, extrusion and premature loss; patchy loss of lamina dura, irregular radiolucencies, "floating tooth" appearance | Posterior mandible is most common site; may involve all four quadrants; African (endemic) form affects the jaws in 50% to 70% of cases | Most jaw lesions are misdiagnosed as odontogenic infection; associated with Epstein-Barr virus and chromosomal translocation | Treatment includes multiagent chemotherapy; aggressive malignancy with 5-year survival rate of 75% to 95% | Acute osteomyelitis Langerhans cell histiocytosis Periapical abscess or granuloma Acute leukemia |

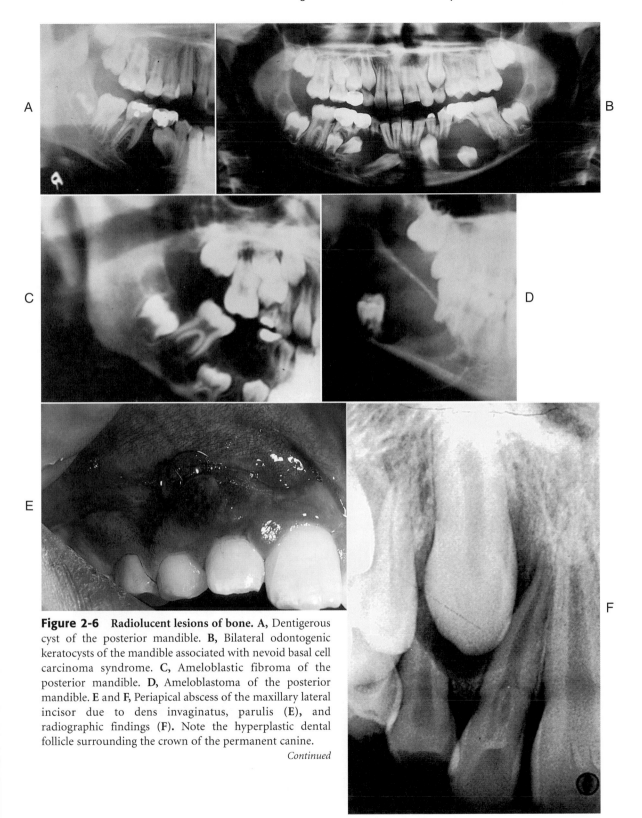

**Figure 2-6    Radiolucent lesions of bone. A,** Dentigerous cyst of the posterior mandible. **B,** Bilateral odontogenic keratocysts of the mandible associated with nevoid basal cell carcinoma syndrome. **C,** Ameloblastic fibroma of the posterior mandible. **D,** Ameloblastoma of the posterior mandible. **E** and **F,** Periapical abscess of the maxillary lateral incisor due to dens invaginatus, parulis (**E**), and radiographic findings (**F**). Note the hyperplastic dental follicle surrounding the crown of the permanent canine.

*Continued*

**TABLE 2-7**

**Mixed Radiolucent and Radiopaque Lesions of Bone (Fig. 2-7)**

| LESION | PEDIATRIC AGE AND GENDER | CLINICAL AND RADIOGRAPHIC FINDINGS | LOCATION | PEDIATRIC SIGNIFICANCE | TREATMENT AND PROGNOSIS | DIFFERENTIAL DIAGNOSIS |
|---|---|---|---|---|---|---|
| Calcifying odontogenic cyst (Gorlin's cyst) | Second decade No gender predilection | Well-defined, unilocular radiolucency with irregular calcifications or tooth-like structures; expansile; 33% associated with unerupted teeth; asymptomatic | Most develop in incisor-canine region of maxilla and mandible; may occur as gingival lesion | In this age group, this odontogenic cyst is often associated with *odontoma* | Enucleation; minimal risk of recurrence; rarely manifests aggressive or malignant behavior | Odontoma Adenomatoid odontogenic tumor Ameloblastic fibro-odontoma Calcifying epithelial odontogenic tumor |
| Adenomatoid odontogenic tumor | Second decade Female predilection | Well-defined, unilocular radiolucency with fine snowflake calcifications; most associated with unerupted tooth; root divergence; asymptomatic expansion | Anterior maxilla is most common site, followed by the anterior mandible | Most lesions occur between 10 and 20 years of age; occasionally occurs as gingival lesion | Enucleation; does not recur | Dentigerous cyst Unicystic ameloblastoma Calcifying odontogenic cyst Developing odontoma |
| Ameloblastic fibro-odontoma | First and second decades No gender predilection | Well-defined unilocular radiolucency with calcified material and tooth-like structures; expansile; often associated with unerupted tooth | Mandibular molar and premolar regions | Odontogenic tumor is frequently diagnosed because tooth fails to erupt | Conservative curettage; rarely recurs | Developing odontoma Calcifying odontogenic cyst Calcifying epithelial odontogenic tumor Central ossifying fibroma |

| Lesion | Pediatric Age and Gender | Clinical and Radiographic Findings | Location | Pediatric Significance | Treatment and Prognosis | Differential Diagnosis |
|---|---|---|---|---|---|---|
| Ossifying fibroma (Cemento-ossifying fibroma) | Second decade Female predilection | Painless swelling; circular growth pattern; well-defined, unilocular lesion with sclerotic borders; may be radiolucent, mixed, or radiopaque | Premolar and molar region; usually occurs in mandible | *Juvenile ossifying fibroma* is aggressive variant that usually occurs in maxilla and frequently recurs | Enucleation or resection; rarely recurs | Calcifying odontogenic cyst Ameloblastic fibro-odontoma Fibrous dysplasia Idiopathic osteosclerosis |
| Osteomyelitis with proliferative periostitis (Garré's osteomyelitis) | First and second decades No gender predilection | Diffuse, poorly defined, mixed radiolucent and opaque lesion; expansile; cortical bone duplication with laminated or onion skin pattern; mild tenderness | Posterior mandible; usually involves first permanent molar | Usually carious molar is noted; occlusal radiograph is helpful for demonstrating cortical laminations | Endodontic treatment or tooth extraction; if necessary, antibiotic therapy; expanded bone usually remodels without surgical recontouring | Fibrous dysplasia Fracture callus Ewing's sarcoma Infantile cortical hyperostosis Osteosarcoma |

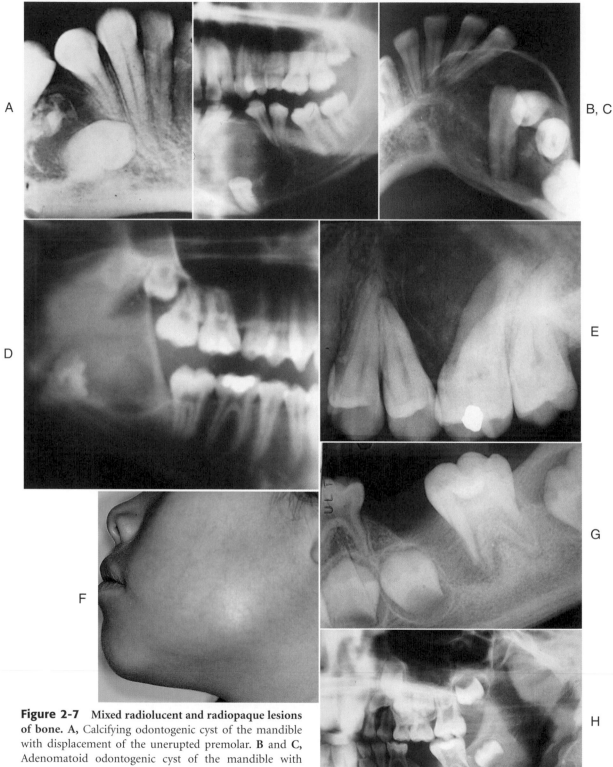

**Figure 2-7**    **Mixed radiolucent and radiopaque lesions of bone. A,** Calcifying odontogenic cyst of the mandible with displacement of the unerupted premolar. **B** and **C,** Adenomatoid odontogenic cyst of the mandible with displacement of the unerupted canine, cropped panoramic view (**B**), occlusal radiographic view (**C**). **D,** Ameloblastic fibro-odontoma of the posterior mandible and ramus. **E,** Ossifying fibroma of the posterior maxilla. **F** to **H,** Osteomyelitis with proliferative periostitis, clinical view (**F**), periapical radiographic view (**G**), and cropped panoramic view (**H**).

**TABLE 2-8**

**Radiopaque Lesions of Bone (Fig. 2-8)**

| LESION | PEDIATRIC AGE AND GENDER | CLINICAL AND RADIOGRAPHIC FINDINGS | LOCATION | PEDIATRIC SIGNIFICANCE | TREATMENT AND PROGNOSIS | DIFFERENTIAL DIAGNOSIS |
|---|---|---|---|---|---|---|
| Odontoma, compound and complex | First and second decades *Compound type:* No gender predilection *Complex type:* Female predilection | Well-defined radiopacity surrounded by narrow radiolucent rim; develop in pericoronal or radicular areas. *Compound type* resembles miniature teeth; *complex type* is amorphous opaque mass | *Compound type:* anterior maxilla *Complex type:* posterior mandible | Represents an hamartoma; most common odontogenic tumor-like lesion; frequent cause of isolated delayed tooth eruption | Local excision; recurrence is rare | Eruption sequestrum Ameloblastic fibro-odontoma Cementoblastoma Calcifying odontogenic cyst Calcifying epithelial odontogenic tumor |
| Osteoma | Second decade No gender predilection | Usually solitary, well-defined, spherical radiopacity; slow growing, may be expansile and result in facial deformity | Body of mandible and condyle are most common sites; endosteal or periosteal location | *Gardner syndrome,* autosomal dominant condition, characterized by multiple osteomas, intestinal polyposis, supernumerary teeth, and skin lesions; malignant polyps | Surgical excision; periodically evaluate small lesions; no recurrence | Torus/exostosis Complex odontoma Fibrous dysplasia Condensing osteitis Familial gigantiform cementoma Idiopathic osteosclerosis |
| Fibrous dysplasia | Second decade No gender predilection | Unilateral, fusiform enlargement; ground-glass radiopacity with ill-defined borders; may displace teeth and delay eruption; slow growing and asymptomatic; facial asymmetry | Maxilla is more frequently affected than mandible; buccal and lingual cortical expansion | *McCune-Albright syndrome* includes polyostotic fibrous dysplasia, café-au-lait macules and endocrine abnormalities | Osseous recontouring for cosmetic and functional problems; stabilizes after completion of skeletal development; rare malignant transformation | Chronic sclerosing osteomyelitis Ossifying fibroma Osteoma Segmental odontomaxillary dysplasia |

*Continued*

## Suggested Readings

Flaitz CM: Differential diagnosis of oral mucosal lesions in children and adolescents, Chapter 2, *Adv Dermatol* 16:39-79, 2000.

Flaitz CM, Coleman GC: Differential diagnosis of oral enlargements in children, *Pediatr Dent* 17:294-304, 1995.

Flaitz CM, Baker KA: Treatment approaches to common symptomatic oral lesions in children, *Dent Clin North Am* 44:671-696, 2000.

Gorlin RJ, Cohen MM Jr, Hennekam RCM: *Syndromes of the Head and Neck,* ed 4, Oxford, 2001, Oxford University Press.

Hall RK: *Pediatric Orofacial Medicine and Pathology,* London, 1994, Chapman & Hall Medical.

Laskaris G: *Color Atlas of Oral Diseases in Children and Adolescents,* Stuttgart, 2000, Thieme.

Neville BW, Damm DD, Allen CM, Bouquot JE: *Oral and Maxillofacial Pathology,* ed 2, Philadelphia, 2002, Saunders.

Neville BW, Damm DD, White DK: *Color Atlas of Clinical Oral Pathology,* ed 2, Hamilton, Ontario, 2003, BC Decker.

Scully C, Welbury R, Flaitz, C, de Almeida OP: *A Color Atlas of Orofacial Health and Disease in Children and Adolescents,* ed 2, London, 2002, Martin Dunitz Ltd.

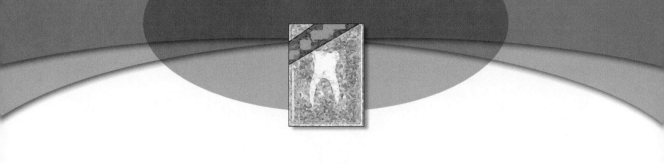

# CHAPTER 3
## Anomalies of the Developing Dentition
*Clifton O. Dummett, Jr.*

A variety of dental anomalies are associated with defects in tooth development precipitated by hereditary, systemic, traumatic, or local factors. Numerous systems have been used to classify dental anomalies, and each has merit. The one used in this text categorizes them in terms of abnormalities in tooth number, size, shape, structure, and color.[15] The advantage of this system is that the categories can be related to the stages of tooth development in which the respective anomalies are thought to originate. These stages of dental development are discussed in Chapter 12. The reader is also encouraged to review textbooks on dental histology, dental embryology, and orofacial genetics for more in-depth information.

## ANOMALIES OF NUMBER

Alterations in tooth number result from problems during the initiation or dental lamina stage of dental development. In addition to hereditary patterns producing extra or missing teeth, physical disruption of the dental lamina, overactive dental lamina, and failure of dental lamina induction by ectomesenchyme are several examples of etiologic factors that affect tooth number.[15]

### Hyperdontia

*Hyperdontia* and *supernumerary teeth* are terms describing an excess in tooth number that can occur in both the primary and permanent dentitions. Reports on the incidence of hyperdontia

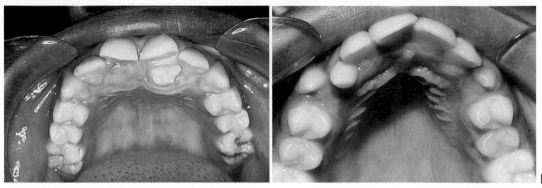

**Figure 3-1**    **A,** Supernumerary teeth: supplemental morphology. **B,** Supernumerary teeth: rudimentary, tuberculate morphology.

include values as high as 3%, with males being affected twice as frequently as females.[12] Ninety percent to 98% of supernumerary teeth occur in the maxilla, with the permanent dentition being more frequently affected than the primary dentition. The most common supernumerary tooth is the mesiodens, which occurs in the palatal midline and can assume a number of shapes and positions relative to the adjacent teeth. The majority tend to be located palatal to the central incisors.[19]

As reported by Primosch in 1981, supernumerary teeth are morphologically classified as either supplemental or rudimentary.[12] Supplemental supernumerary teeth (Fig. 3-1, *A*) duplicate the typical anatomy of posterior and anterior teeth. Rudimentary supernumerary teeth are dysmorphic and can assume conical forms, tuberculate forms (Fig. 3-1, *B*), or shapes that duplicate molar anatomy. From a clinical standpoint, the tuberculate, or barrel-shaped, supernumeraries

generate the most severe complications with respect to difficulty of removal and adverse effects on adjacent teeth, such as impaction or ectopic eruption. Additional complications associated with supernumeraries include dentigerous cyst formation, pericoronal space ossification, and crown resorption.[19] It is important in supernumerary tooth detection to rule out the presence of odontoma in light of the fact that the morphologic characteristics of a compound composite odontoma are similar to those of teeth.

*Cleft lip and palate* commonly demonstrates an excess or deficiency in the normal complement of teeth and provides a clear example of physical disruption of the dental lamina as an etiologic factor. Classic syndromes involving supernumerary teeth are summarized in Table 3-1, with *cleidocranial dysplasia* having the highest association with this dental anomaly.

## TABLE 3-1
### Syndromes Demonstrating Supernumerary Teeth

| CONDITION | CHARACTERISTICS |
| --- | --- |
| Apert syndrome | Scaphocephaly, craniosynostosis, bilateral syndactyly, midface hypoplasia |
| Cleidocranial dysplasia | Aplastic clavicles, frontal bossing, hypoplastic midface |
| Gardner syndrome | Osteomas, epidermoid cysts, odontomas, intestinal polyps |
| Down syndrome | Brachycephaly, mental retardation, epicanthal folds |
| Crouzon disease | Craniosynostosis, exophthalmos, hypoplastic midface |
| Sturge-Weber syndrome | Angiomatosis and calcification of leptomeninges, seizures, port-wine nevi of face |
| Oral-facial-digital syndrome | Hypoplastic alar cartilage, cleft tongue, clinodactyly |
| Hallermann-Streiff syndrome | Dyscephaly, mandibular hypoplasia, hypotrichosis |

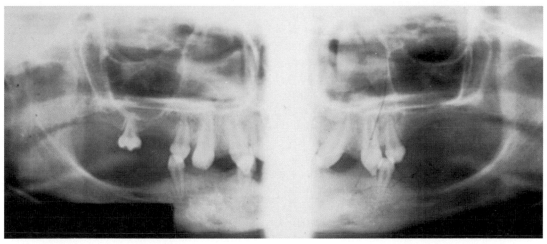

**Figure 3-2**    Hypodontia in a child with ectodermal dysplasia. Note atrophy of alveolar ridge.

| TABLE 3-2 | |
|---|---|
| **Syndromes Demonstrating Hypodontia** | |
| CONDITION | CHARACTERISTICS |
| Ectodermal dysplasia (hypohidrotic type) | Hypotrichosis, aplasia of sweat/sebaceous glands |
| Chondroectodermal dysplasia | Polydactyly, mesomelic dwarfism, hidrotic ectodermal dysplasia |
| Achondroplasia | Short-limbed dwarfism, macrocephaly, frontal bossing |
| Rieger syndrome | Iris dysplasia, midface hypoplasia, protruding umbilicus |
| Incontinentia pigmenti | Alopecia, pigmented macules, mental retardation |
| Seckel syndrome | Dwarfism, microcephaly, facial hypoplasia, low-set lobeless ears |

## Hypodontia

Hypodontia, or congenital tooth absence, is a deficiency in tooth number. Familial heredity patterns account for the largest etiologic correlation with patterns of hypodontia. Incidence reports identify a range of 1.5% to 10% excluding third molars in U.S. populations.[9] The most frequently occurring congenitally absent permanent tooth, excluding the third molar, tends to be the mandibular second bicuspid (3.4%), followed by the maxillary lateral incisor (2.2%).[17]

There is a high correlation between primary tooth absence and permanent tooth absence.[5,20] *Ectodermal dysplasia* (ED) represents a group of classic syndromes characterized by oligodontia or multiple congenitally missing teeth. The most common is hypohidrotic ED, followed in descending frequency of occurrence by hidrotic ED, ectrodactyly ED plus cleft lip and palate, Rapp-Hodgkin ED, and Robinson-type ED (Fig. 3-2). Other conditions involving hypodontia are summarized in Table 3-2 and those involving both hyperdontia and hypodontia in Box 3-1.

| BOX 3-1 |
|---|
| **Syndromes Manifesting Both Hyperdontia and Hypodontia** |
| Down syndrome<br>Oral-facial-digital syndrome type 1<br>Crouzon disease<br>Hallermann-Streiff syndrome |

## ANOMALIES OF SIZE

### Microdontia and Macrodontia

Abnormalities in tooth size are epitomized in microdontia and macrodontia. *Hemifacial microsomia* is thought to result from a hematoma of the stapedial artery during embryologic development giving rise to a deficient nutrient supply to the affected side of the face. In addition to unilateral mandibular hypoplasia and ear malformation, less growth occurs in this less vascularized area, with smaller teeth forming as a result. Peg-shaped lateral incisors are examples of microdontia and are common in *Down syndrome.* Other conditions demonstrating microdontia include *ectodermal dysplasia* and *chondroectodermal dysplasia.* These size abnormalities are thought to originate during the morphodifferentiation stage of tooth development.

*Facial hemihypertrophy* can demonstrate comparatively larger teeth on the affected side (Fig. 3-3). Of the many factors thought to cause this condition, vascular and neurogenic abnormalities are considered the most likely. In addition to an increase in crown and root size, affected teeth develop more rapidly and erupt earlier than on the uninvolved side. The *otodental syndrome,* consisting of high-frequency hearing loss and globe-shaped fused molar teeth, is another condition that involves macrodontia. Isolated teeth

with macrodontia can also result from twinning abnormalities that originate during the proliferation stage of tooth development. Fusion and gemination are the most common twinning abnormalities, and both include enlarged crowns.

## Fusion

Fusion has an incidence of 0.5% and is more common in the primary dentition.[5] The classic definition of fusion is the dentinal union of two embryologically developing teeth. Although fused teeth can contain two separate pulp chambers, many appear as large bifid crowns with one chamber, which makes them difficult to distinguish from geminated teeth.

## Gemination

Gemination has a frequency of 0.5%, which is similar to that of fusion and is more common in the primary dentition. Conceptually, a geminated tooth represents an incomplete division of a single tooth bud resulting in a bifid crown with a

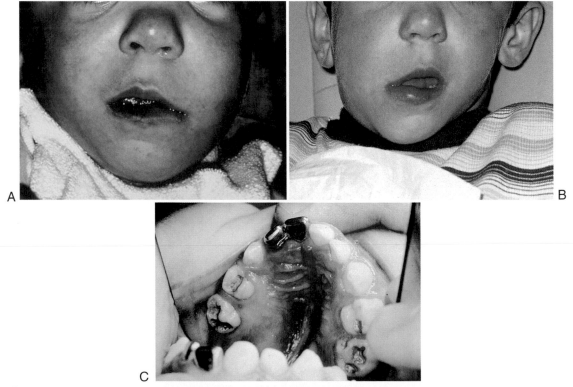

**Figure 3-3**  **A,** Hemifacial hypertrophy. Patient's affected side (right) is larger in all dimensions. **B,** Hemifacial hypertrophy. Patient's affected side (right) is larger in all dimensions. **C,** Hemifacial hypertrophy. Teeth on the patient's affected side (right) are larger in all dimensions.

single pulp chamber. Gemination tends to occur in a familial pattern, and its significance is similar to that of fusion in that both conditions may result in retarded eruption of the permanent successor. Clinically, fusion and gemination are usually distinguished by counting of teeth in the arch. If there is a deficiency in the normal complement including the bifid crown, the condition is fusion. Fusion with a supernumerary tooth must also be considered and ruled out because this would not affect the normal number of teeth.

Concrescence is a twinning anomaly involving the union of two teeth by cementum only. Its cause is thought to be trauma or adjacent tooth malposition. Because it can occur after root development, concrescence is technically not a developmental anomaly.

## ANOMALIES OF SHAPE

Abnormalities in shape originate during the morphodifferentiation stage of tooth development and are manifested as alterations in crown and root form. Modes of inheritance include both autosomal dominant and polygenic patterns.

### Dens Evaginatus

Dens evaginatus is an extra cusp, usually in the central groove or ridge of a posterior tooth and in the cingulum area of the central and lateral incisors (Fig. 3-4). In incisors, these cusps appear talon-shaped and can approach the level of the incisal edge. This extra portion contains not only enamel but dentin and pulp tissue; therefore, a pulp exposure can result from radical equilibration. It occurs with a frequency of 1% to 4% and results from the invagination of inner enamel

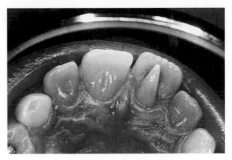

**Figure 3-4**  Dens invaginatus-talon cusp. All three elements of dental tissues are represented in the extra cusp.

epithelium cells, which are the precursors of ameloblasts.[15]

### Dens in Dente

Dens in dente is a condition resulting from invagination of the inner enamel epithelium producing the appearance of a tooth within a tooth. In 1974, Thomas reported a 7.7% prevalence, with the maxillary lateral incisors being most frequently affected.[18] The clinical significance of this anomaly results from potential carious involvement through the communication of the invaginated portion of the lingual surface of the tooth with the outside environment. The enamel and dentin in the invaginated portion can be both defective and absent, allowing direct exposure of the pulp.

### Taurodont

Taurodont teeth are characterized by a significantly elongated pulp chamber with short stunted roots, resulting from the failure of the proper level of horizontal invagination of Hertwig's epithelial root sheath (Fig. 3-5). The incidence

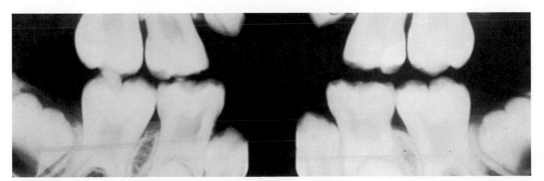

**Figure 3-5**  Taurodont teeth. Note that primary teeth as well as permanent teeth can be affected.

## TABLE 3-3
### Conditions Demonstrating Taurodontism

| CONDITION | CHARACTERISTICS |
| --- | --- |
| Klinefelter syndrome | Aspermatogenesis, mental retardation |
| Trichodentoosseous syndrome | Sclerotic bones, coarse gnarled hair, enamel defects |
| Oral-facial-digital syndrome type 2 | Dystrophic nails, hyperplastic frenum, lobed tongue |
| Ectodermal dysplasia (hypohidrotic) | Hypotrichosis, aplasia of sweat/sebaceous glands |
| Amelogenesis imperfecta type 4 | Enamel hypoplasia and hypomaturation, mottled yellow teeth |
| Down syndrome | Brachycephaly, mental retardation, epicanthal fold |

can range from 0.5% to 5%, and the condition can be classified according to the extent of the pulp chamber elongation.[10] The conditions that classically involve taurodontism are summarized in Table 3-3.

### Dilaceration

Dilaceration refers to an abnormal bend of the root during its development and is thought to result from a traumatic episode, usually to the primary dentition (Fig. 3-6). In 1971, Andreason reported a dilaceration incidence of 25% in those permanent teeth with developmental disturbances secondary to primary tooth injury.[1] Congenital ichthyosis, consisting of hyperkeratosis of the knees and elbows, fish-like scaly skin, and delayed tooth eruption, also includes root dilaceration as a consistent finding.

## ANOMALIES OF STRUCTURE

### Enamel

Tooth structure abnormalities result from disruption during the histodifferentiation, apposition, and mineralization stages of tooth development. Enamel defects are manifested as hypoplasia or hypocalcification. According to Jorgenson and Yost, they may be broadly classified as heritable defects or environmentally induced defects.[6]

#### Amelogenesis Imperfecta
Amelogenesis imperfecta (AI) is a classic example of heritable enamel defects. Estimates of the incidence of this condition include 1 in 14,000,[22] 1 in 8000,[2] and 1 in 4000.[16] Fourteen subgroup classifications of AI are listed in Box 3-2, with multiple inheritance patterns represented. It is

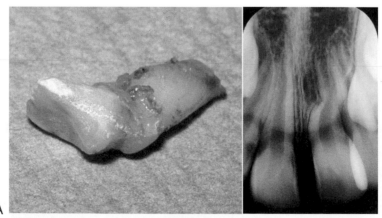

**Figure 3-6**    **A,** Dilacerated lateral incisor. **B,** Dilacerated lateral incisor.

**BOX 3-2**

## Classification of Amelogenesis Imperfecta

**Type 1  Hypoplastic**
1A  Hypoplastic, pitted autosomal dominant
1B  Hypoplastic, local autosomal dominant
1C  Hypoplastic, local autosomal recessive
1D  Hypoplastic, smooth autosomal dominant
1E  Hypoplastic, smooth X-linked dominant
1F  Hypoplastic, rough autosomal dominant
1G  Enamel agenesis, autosomal recessive

**Type 2  Hypomaturation**
2A  Hypomaturation, pigmented autosomal recessive
2B  Hypomaturation, X-linked recessive
2D  Snow-capped teeth, autosomal dominant?

**Type 3  Hypocalcified**
3A  Autosomal dominant
3B  Autosomal recessive

**Type 4  Hypomaturation, hypoplastic with taurodontism**
4A  Hypomaturation-hypoplastic with taurodontism, autosomal dominant
4B  Hypoplastic-hypomaturation with taurodontism, autosomal dominant

Adapted from Witkop CJ Jr: Amelogenesis imperfecta, dentinogenesis imperfecta and dental dysplasia revisited: problems in classification. *J Oral Pathol* 17:547-558, 1988.

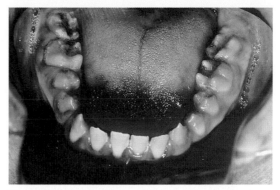

**Figure 3-7**  Amelogenesis imperfecta, hypoplastic type.

important to remember that the sole feature that distinguishes AI from other enamel defects is its confinement to distinct patterns of inheritance and its occurrence exclusive of any syndromic, metabolic, or systemic condition.[21] The four major AI categories are described according to the stages of tooth development in which each is thought to occur. Additional information on the subgroups can be obtained from more comprehensive resources.

**Hypoplastic Type.**  Heritable enamel defects occurring in the histodifferentiation stage of tooth development are exemplified by the hypoplastic type of AI wherein an insufficient quantity of enamel is formed (Fig. 3-7). This occurs because some areas of the enamel organ are devoid of inner enamel epithelium, causing a lack of cell differentiation into ameloblasts. Both primary and permanent dentitions are affected, and the condition is inherited predominantly as an autosomal dominant trait depending on the subgroup pattern. Affected teeth appear small with open contacts, and areas of the clinical crowns contain very thin or nonexistent enamel resulting in high sensitivity to thermal stimuli. Anterior open bite has been observed in 60% of reported cases.[13]

**Hypomaturation Type.**  The hypomaturation type of AI is an example of an inherited defect in enamel matrix apposition. It is characterized by teeth having normal enamel thickness but a low value of radiodensity and mineral content (Fig. 3-8). The problem is related to the persistence of organic content in the rod sheath resulting in poor calcification, low mineral content, and a porous surface that becomes stained.

**Hypoplastic/Hypomaturation Amelogenesis Imperfecta with Taurodontism.**  Hypoplastic/hypomaturation AI with taurodontism is an example of inherited defects in both apposition and histodifferentiation stages of enamel formation. The enamel appears mottled with a

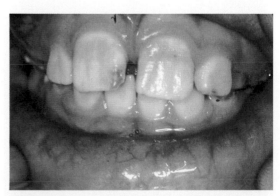

**Figure 3-8**  Amelogenesis imperfecta, hypomaturation type.

yellow-brown color and is pitted on the facial surfaces, exemplifying the features of both hypoplasia and hypomaturation previously described. Molar teeth demonstrate taurodontism, and other components of the dentition have enlarged pulp chambers.

**Hypocalcification Type.** The hypocalcification type of AI is an example of an inherited defect in the calcification stage of enamel formation. Quantitatively, the enamel is normal, but qualitatively the matrix is poorly calcified with a resultant fracturing of the enamel surface (Fig. 3-9). The hypocalcified enamel is soft and fragile, especially at the incisal regions, and is easily fractured, exposing the underlying dentin that produces an unaesthetic appearance. Increased calculus formation and marked delay in tooth eruption are consistent findings. Anterior open bite occurs in 60% of patients demonstrating this defect.[13]

### Environmental Enamel Hypoplasia

Examples of environmentally induced enamel hypoplasia can result from systemic or local causes. Examples of systemic causes producing generalized enamel hypoplasia include nutrition deficiencies, particularly in vitamins A, C, and D as well as in calcium and phosphorus.[6] Severe infection, such as exanthematous diseases and fever-producing disorders, particularly during the first year of life, can directly affect ameloblastic activity, resulting in enamel hypoplasia. *Rubella embryopathy* has a high correlation with prenatal enamel hypoplasia in the primary dentition. *Syphilis* caused by the spirochete *Treponema pallidum* produces classic patterns of hypoplastic dysmorphic permanent teeth. The tapered and notched incisal edges of anterior teeth with screwdriver shapes are called *Hutchinson's incisors,* and the crenated occlusal patterns of posterior teeth known as *mulberry molars* are classic clinical findings for prenatal syphilis infection.

Neurologic defects as exemplified in children with cerebral palsy and *Sturge-Weber syndrome* have an increased likelihood of progressing into generalized enamel hypoplasia. Children with asthma also demonstrate a higher prevalence of enamel hypoplasia than do nonafflicted children. Prematurity and excess radiation exposure can disrupt ameloblastic matrix formation or subsequent mineralization and are additional causes of systemic enamel hypoplasia. A number of syndromes involve enamel hypoplasia as a consistent dental characteristic and are listed in Box 3-3.

Excess ingestion of systemic fluoride can produce generalized enamel defects. Dental fluorosis can be manifested as a defect in the calcification of the teeth in milder forms, with significant pigmentation and ameloblastic impairment in the more severe forms. Fluorosis occurs when the concentration of ingested fluoride is above 1.8 ppm/day.[6] There is a 90% chance of some degree of dental fluorosis when the amount of ingested fluoride is greater than 6 ppm, although the severity of morphologic defects cannot be predicted from specific quantities of ingested fluoride.

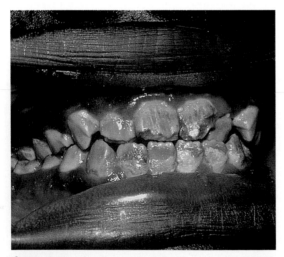

**Figure 3-9**  Amelogenesis imperfecta, hypocalcified type.

---

### BOX 3-3
#### Syndromes Demonstrating Enamel Hypoplasia

Down syndrome
Tuberous sclerosis
Epidermolysis bullosa
Hurler syndrome
Hunter syndrome
Treacher Collins syndrome
Phenylketonuria
Pseudohypoparathyroidism
Trichodento-osseous syndrome
Vitamin D–dependent rickets
Lesch-Nyhan syndrome
Fanconi syndrome
Sturge-Weber syndrome
Turner syndrome

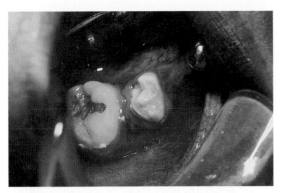

**Figure 3-10**    Turner hypoplasia. Note that cementum is formed on the crown areas that are denuded of enamel.

### Localized Enamel Hypoplasia

Causes of enamel hypoplasia affecting individual teeth include local infection, local trauma, iatrogenic surgery as occurs in cleft palate closure, and primary tooth overretention. Turner hypoplasia is a classic example of hypoplastic defects in permanent teeth resulting from local infection or trauma to the primary precursor (Fig. 3-10).

### Enamel Hypocalcification

Hypocalcification defects can be directly related to faults in the mineralization of the organic matrix in enamel formation. The same factors that cause enamel hypoplasia also cause hypocalcification. The majority of localized hypocalcific defects, as in the case of Turner hypoplasia, are subsequent to localized infection and trauma. Excess exposure to citric acid resulting from habitual sucking on citrus fruits can produce generalized erosive hypocalcified lesions that mimic the hypocalcification type of AI.

## Dentin

### Dentinogenesis Imperfecta

Dentinogenesis imperfecta is an example of an inheritable dentinal defect originating during the histodifferentiation stage of tooth development (Fig. 3-11, *A* and *B*). This anomaly involves a defect of predentin matrix that results in amorphic, disorganized, and atubular circumpulpal dentin. The mantle dentin is normal, in contrast with the previously described circumpulpal dentin, which is high in organic content and contains interglobular calcification. Its incidence is about 1 in 8000. Dentinogenesis imperfecta can be subdivided into three basic types.[14]

*Shields type 1* occurs with osteogenesis imperfecta. An inherited defect in collagen formation results in osteoporotic brittle bones, bowing of the limbs, bitemporal bossing, and blue sclera. Primary teeth tend to be more severely affected

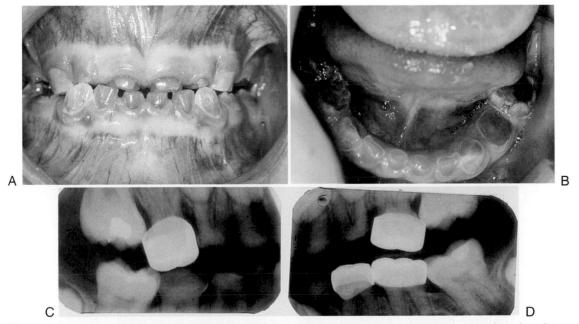

**Figure 3-11**    **A,** Dentinogenesis imperfecta, hereditary opalescent dentin. **B,** Dentinogenesis imperfecta, hereditary opalescent dentin. **C** and **D,** Dentinogenesis imperfecta, hereditary opalescent dentin.

than permanent teeth. Periapical radiolucencies, bulbous crowns, obliteration of pulp chambers, and root fractures are evident (Fig. 3-11C). An amber translucent tooth color is common.

*Shields type 2,* also known as hereditary opalescent dentin, tends to occur as a separate entity apart from osteogenesis imperfecta. In this case, both primary and permanent dentitions are equally affected and the characteristics previously described for type 1 are the same. This condition is inherited as an autosomal dominant trait.

*Shields Type 3* is rare and represents many of the features described earlier with a predominance of bell-shaped crowns, especially in the permanent dentition. Unlike types 1 and 2, type 3 involves teeth with a shell-like appearance and multiple pulp exposures. It has occurred exclusively in a triracial isolated group in Maryland known as the Brandywine population.[14] Type 3 has been proposed to be a different expression of the same Type II gene.[7]

### Dentin Dysplasia

Dentin dysplasia represents another group of inherited dentin disorders resulting in characteristic features involving the circumpulpal dentin and root morphology. In 1973, Shields and associates proposed a classification based on characteristic patterns of dentinal dysplasia.[14]

*Shields type 1* demonstrates normal primary and permanent crown morphology with an amber translucency (Fig. 3-12). The roots tend to be short and sharply constricted. Primary teeth have obliterated pulps. Both primary and permanent dentitions demonstrate multiple periapical radiolucencies and absent pulp chambers.

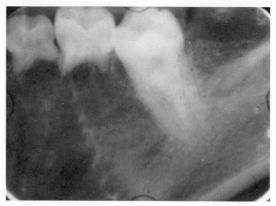

**Figure 3-12**    Dentinal dysplasia type 1. Note rootless primary teeth.

Cascading tubule patterns result from blockage of normal dentin tubules by calcified masses.

*Shields type 2* involves amber-colored primary teeth closely resembling dentinogenesis imperfecta types 1 and 2. Permanent teeth appear normal, but radiographically they demonstrate thistle-tube–shaped pulp chambers with multiple pulp stones (Fig. 3-13). No periapical radiolucencies are visible.

### Regional Odontodysplasia

Odontodysplasia is a condition representing a localized arrest in tooth development thought to result from a regional vascular developmental anomaly. Affected teeth have thin layers of poorly calcified enamel and dentin with large, diffusely calcified pulp chambers and shortened, poorly defined roots (Fig. 3-14).[3] The teeth have a ghost-like radiographic appearance with shortened roots and shell-like crowns and are dysmorphic in

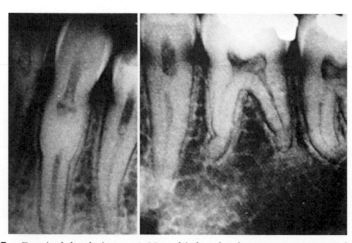

**Figure 3-13**    Dentinal dysplasia type 2. Note thistle-tube shape to permanent pulp chambers.

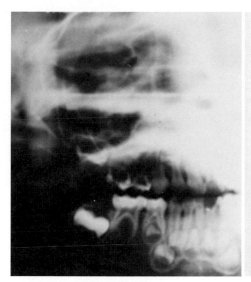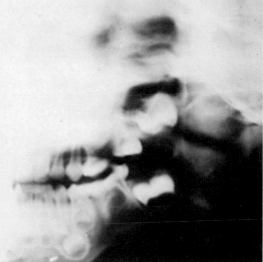

**Figure 3-14**   Odontodysplasia in the patient's upper left maxillary area.

overall appearance. No conclusive etiologic factor or inheritance pattern has been identified that can explain the reported cases.

Additional conditions involving dentin abnormalities relate to systemic abnormalities that impair normal absorption and circulating serum levels of calcium and phosphorus. *Vitamin D–resistant rickets, hypoparathyroidism,* and *pseudohypoparathyroidism* are all conditions demonstrating characteristic dentinal abnormalities that are summarized in Box 3-4.[15]

## Cementum

Developmental defects involving cementum as an exclusive entity apart from other dental structures are uncommon. It is especially difficult to identify problems in cementogenesis from diseases involving the periodontal ligament. An interesting finding in Turner hypoplasia is that in addition to coronal enamel defects of the affected permanent teeth, cementum is formed in the coronal areas denuded of enamel.[15] This underscores the protective effect that the reduced enamel epithelium has on the unerupted tooth crown. Furthermore, it represents the reciprocal inductive effect of dentin that when in direct contact with the dental follicle mesenchymal cells causes them to differentiate into cementoblasts. Areas denuded of enamel allow this phenomenon to occur.

Histologically defective cementum occurs in three noteworthy conditions. *Epidermolysis bullosa dystrophica,* an inherited vesicular and bullous

---

**BOX 3-4**

**Systemic Abnormalities Impairing Normal Absorption and Circulating Serum Levels of Calcium and Phosphorus**

**Vitamin D–resistant rickets**
- Hypomineralized dentin
- Increased width to predentin
- Odontoblastic disorganization
- Decreased alkaline phosphatase activity in tooth germ
- Enlarged pulp and pulp horns
- No enamel defect

**Hypoparathyroidism**
- Tooth defects are more severe in males
- Permanent teeth are predominantly affected
- Short, wedge-shaped roots with delayed apical closure
- Interglobular calcification in dentin, especially at apices
- Enamel hypoplasia

**Pseudohypoparathyroidism**
- Enlarged pulp chambers
- Irregular dentinal tubules
- Small crowns and short, blunted roots
- Pitted enamel surfaces

---

disease of the skin and mucous membranes, involves formation of fibrous, poorly calcified acellular cementum and overproduction of cellular cementum. Cleidocranial dysplasia also displays histologic alterations in cementum formation. Lukinmaa and associates noted that

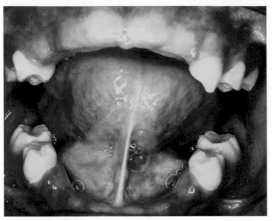

**Figure 3-15** Hypophosphatasia. Note premature exfoliation of primary anterior teeth in the upper and lower anterior areas.

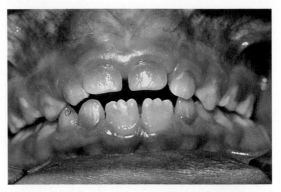

**Figure 3-16** Tetracycline staining of primary and permanent dentitions. Note darker hues to the primary teeth with more diffuse yellow stain to permanent incisors.

permanent teeth were devoid of cellular cementum and had partially hyperplastic acellular cementum.[8]

*Hypophosphatasia* is a complex condition involving the failure of bone to mineralize properly, which is associated with low serum alkaline phosphatase levels. Osteoporosis, bone fragility, and premature loss of primary incisors are classic clinical features (Fig. 3-15). The latter finding is ascribed to the failure of cementum formation on the prematurely exfoliated incisors and to a decrease in cementum formation in the retained primary teeth. The condition exerts its greatest effect prenatally and during the first year of life. Bone and dentin are affected along with cementum, so the entity is not exclusively a cementum defect.

## ANOMALIES OF COLOR

Both the primary and permanent dentitions can manifest significant color changes from extrinsic or intrinsic stains. Because of their developmental significance, only the intrinsic stains are addressed here. In 1975, Eisenberg and Bernick provided a detailed classification of the causes of tooth discolorations.[4] Causes of intrinsic stains can be due to blood-borne pigments, drug administration, and hypoplastic-hypocalcified disease states. Congenital porphyria, bile duct defects, anemias, and transfusion-reaction hemolysis are examples of blood-borne pigments.

A classic example of drug-induced intrinsic staining occurs from tetracycline antibiotics. Both dentitions can have severe discoloration from this antibiotic when given in concentrations of 21 to 26 mg/kg or greater over as brief a period as 3 days (Fig. 3-16).[11] Tetracycline hydrochloride has the greatest potential for staining among the tetracyclines. The agent forms an orthocalcium phosphate complex with dentin and enamel, which is then oxidized by ultraviolet light. The oxidation process results in pigments that stain the hard tissues. The critical period for initiation of primary and permanent tooth staining is that of intrauterine development through 8 years of age. Tetracycline administration must be especially avoided during this time.

Systemic and localized enamel hypoplasia can result in tooth discoloration. Many of the enamel and dentin dysplasias also result in tooth color changes as well as in the heritable anomalies of AI and dentinogenesis imperfecta. Excess fluoride overlaps both the drug-induced and hypoplastic categories of agents responsible for tooth discoloration. The more severe form of dental fluorosis can produce a range of discoloration, from opaque white spots with diffuse striations to a brown mottling.

## REFERENCES

1. Andreason JO: The effect of traumatic injuries to primary teeth on their permanent successor. *Scand J Dent Res* 145:229, 1971.
2. Chosack A, Edelmann E, Wisotski I, Choen T: Amelogenesis imperfecta among Israeli Jews and the description of a new type of local hypoplastic autosomal recessive amelogenesis imperfecta. *Oral Surg* 47:148, 1979.

3. Crawford PJM, Aldred MJ: Regional odontodysplasia: a bibliography. *J Oral Pathol Med* 18:251-263, 1989.

4. Eisenberg E, Bernick SM: Anomalies of the teeth with stains and discolorations. *J Prev Dent* 2:7-20, 1975.

5. Grahanen H, Granath L: Numerical variations and their correlations with the permanent dentition. *Odont Rev* 4:348-357, 1961.

6. Jorgenson RT, Yost C: Etiology of enamel dysplasias. *J Pedod* 6:316-329, 1982.

7. Levin LS et al: Dentinogenesis imperfecta in the Brandywine isolet (DI-III). *Oral Surg Oral Med Oral Pathol* 56:267, 1983.

8. Lukinmaa PL et al: Histological observations of teeth and peridental tissues in cleidocranial dysplasia imply increased activity of odontogenic epithelium and abnormal bone remodeling. *J Craniofac Genet Dev Biol* 15:212, 1995.

9. Maklin M, Dummett CO Jr, Weinberg R: A study of oligodontia in a sample of New Orleans children. *J Dent Child* 46:478, 1979.

10. Mena CA: Taurodontism. *Oral Surg Oral Pathol Oral Med* 32:812-823, 1971.

11. Moffitt JM et al: Prediction of tetracycline-induced tooth coloration. *JADA* 88:547, 1974.

12. Primosch RE: Anterior supernumerary teeth-assessment and surgical intervention in children. *J Pediatr Dent* 3:204, 1981.

13. Rowley C, Hill FJ, Winter IGB: An investigation of the association between anterior openbite and amelogenesis imperfecta. *Am J Orthod* 81:220, 1982.

14. Shields ED, Bixler D, El-Kafrawy AM: A proposed classification for heritable human dentine defects with a description of a new entity. *Arch Oral Biol* 18:543-553, 1973.

15. Stewart RE, Prescott GH: *Oral Facial Genetics.* St. Louis, Mosby, 1976.

16. Sundell S, Valentin J: Hereditary aspects of hereditary amelogenesis imperfecta. *Community Dent Oral Epidemiol* 14:211, 1986.

17. Symons AL et al: Anomalies associated with hypodontia of the permanent lateral incisor and second premolar. *J Clin Pediatr Dent* 17:109, 1993.

18. Thomas JG: A study of dens in dente. *Oral Surg Oral Pathol Oral Med* 38:653, 1974.

19. von Arx T et al: Anterior supernumerary teeth: a clinical and radiographic study. *Aust Dent J* 37:189, 1992.

20. Whittington BR, Durward CS: Survey of anomalies in primary teeth and their correlation with the permanent dentition. *N Z Dent J* 92:4, 1996.

21. Witkop CJ Jr: Amelogenesis imperfecta, dentinogenesis imperfecta and dentinal dysplasia revisited: problems in classification. *J Oral Pathol* 17:547-553, 1988.

22. Witkop CJ Jr: Genetics in dentistry. *Eugenics Q* 5:15-21, 1959.

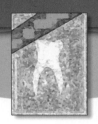

# CHAPTER 4

# Oral and Dental Care of Local and Systemic Diseases

*Marcio A. da Fonseca*

## PRIMARY HERPETIC GINGIVOSTOMATITIS

Primary herpetic gingivostomatitis (PHG) is the most common specific clinical manifestation of herpes simplex virus (HSV) type 1 infection in childhood, although the type 2 virus can also cause it.[2-4,29] The general course of the infection is 10 to 14 days, and it is self-limiting and non-scarring.[2,3] Frequently, PHG in children is a subclinical infection, but its clinical manifestations may vary from a mild illness to a severe course with hospital admission.[3] The gingiva and the lips, including the perioral region, are the most commonly affected areas with multiple crops of vesicular eruptions.[18] The oropharyngeal mucosa and the conjunctiva may also be involved.[7,29] The vesicles rupture early, leaving small vesicles covered by a pseudomembrane, surrounded by erythema.[7,29] Amir et al.[2] observed that the painful lesions lasted about 12 days (6 days to fully appear and 6 days to gradually disappear) and the mean duration of positive viral shedding was 7.1 days. Children may present with severe local pain, fever, malaise, difficulties with fluid and food intake, and lymphadenopathy.[7,18,29] Excessive drooling, halitosis, and sore throat are frequently present.[18] Diagnosis is based on the clinical findings of intraoral and extraoral lesions, the latter being pathognomonic for HG.[2] Differential diagnosis include herpangina, aphthous stomatitis, hand-foot-and-mouth disease, Stevens-Johnson syndrome, pemphigus, intraoral zoster, and erythema multiforme.[2,29,7]

Management of PHG is directed at promoting lesion healing, providing palliation, ensuring adequate hydration and nutrition, and preventing further spread of the infection.[29] Topical anesthetics and coating agents help relieve pain and facilitate food intake, with nutritional supplements added as needed.[18,29] Children who cannot expectorate should not use topical anesthetics because of the potential for aspiration.[18] Oral analgesics can be used to control fever, pain, and muscle aches.[18] Antimicrobial rinses may be beneficial when there is significant involvement of the gingiva in order to decrease the risk of secondary bacterial infection.[7] Maintenance of proper oral hygiene is important.

Early diagnosis is essential to initiate specific therapy. Treatment is done with acyclovir 200 mg/5 ml suspension every 3 hours when awake or five times a day for 10 days.[18] The dosage is 15 mg/kg, with a maximum of 80/mg/kg per day. Amir et al.[3] found that when acyclovir suspension (15 mg/kg five times a day for 7 days) was administered less than 72 hours after the onset of the symptoms, children had oral lesions for a shorter period of time and earlier disappearance of fever, extraoral lesions, eating difficulties, and drinking difficulties. Antiviral therapy with intravenous acyclovir should be considered for any case of HSV infection affecting immunocompromised patients.[29] If that fails or the patient becomes resistant to the medication, therapy with foscarnet should be initiated.

PHG is transmitted primarily by contact with infected oral secretions, but data regarding intrafamilial transmission are unclear.[2,3] Patients must be isolated to prevent cross-infection particularly during the viral shedding period. Infected children whose hands are exposed to oral secretions can be inoculated through minor abrasions on their hands.[7] Herpetic whitlow is a classic occupational hazard of dental professionals. There are no data relating to the prevention of HSV spreading by face masks.[4]

## RECURRENT HERPES SIMPLEX INFECTION

Approximately 20% to 40% of patients who experience a primary HSV infection have subsequent recurrent infections caused by reactivation of HSV that remained latent in local neuron ganglion cells after the primary infection.[18,25,29,47] Factors that may precipitate a recurrence include sun exposure, physical injury, systemic disease, menstruation, emotional stress, surgical trauma,

dental treatment, infectious febrile conditions, hyperthermia, trauma from mastication, drugs, hormonal alterations, and local, thermal, or chemical injury.[7,18,29,47]

Three forms of HSV infection are recognized: recurrent herpes labialis (RHL), intraoral recurrence, and recurrence mimicking a primary infection.[29] RHL is the most common form, typically showing clusters of vesicles affecting the vermilion border, the perioral skin, and sometimes the ala of the nose.[29] Extraoral lesions can occur anywhere along the affected sensory division of the trigeminal nerve.[47] Symptoms may range from subclinical to debilitating, depending on the host's immune response.[7,47] Signs and symptoms such as tingling, burning, soreness, and swelling precede the appearance of lesions.[7,18,47] The vesicles rupture and coalesce, forming painful ulcers.[7,18,29,47] Healing is usually complete in 7 to 14 days, and recurrences are variable.[18,47,56] The intraoral form is similar to RHL but occurs on the keratinized mucosa of the palate and gingiva without crusting.[29] Intraoral pain may interfere with eating and drinking and, in some children, may be responsible for the discomfort associated with tooth eruption.[18] Oral HSV lesions in immunocompromised patients can have a broad range of clinical presentations, involving any intraoral site including nonkeratinized areas.[7,29,56] It is recommended that all oral ulcers in immunocompromised patients be cultured for HSV regardless of their location.[56]

Lip balms and protective lotions should be used by individuals whose RHL is sun induced.[18,29] Palliative management with topical anesthetics and protective coating agents is used to relieve itching and pain. Cold fluids and ice chips can help relieve the oral discomfort, and citrus fruits, acidic foods, carbonated beverages, and mouth rinses containing alcohol should be avoided.[47] Topical antiviral medications for RHL include penciclovir cream 1% applied to the lip every 2 hours for 4 days starting when symptoms first occur.[18,29] Docosanol can be used in children older than 12 years applied five times daily to the affected area of the face and lips. The medications should be applied at the earliest sign or symptom to obtain maximal efficacy.[18] Oral valacyclovir has been shown to reduce pain and speed healing.[29] Bactroban ointment 2% is effective on secondarily infected perioral lesions.[18] Systemic acyclovir (200 mg every 3 hours while awake for 5 days) may be indicated for children with six or more episodes of recurrent HSV per year.[7,18] The safety and efficacy of most of these drugs in children have not been established.[18] Acetaminophen can be prescribed for pain relief. For immunocompromised patients, topical acyclovir 5% ointment applied at prodrome to the affected area every 2 hours until resolution can be helpful for RHL.[29] Oral famciclovir is indicated when topical therapy fails. A tertiary line of treatment is foscarnet.[29]

In cases of both PHG and recurrent HSV infections, the dental professional should address cleanliness to prevent autoinoculation and spread to others as well as proper nutrition, hydration, optimal oral hygiene, and local control of the process.[47] Hand washing and separation of eating utensils are important. Dental treatment should be avoided until healing occurs.

## OROPHARYNGEAL CANDIDIASIS

Candidiasis is an opportunistic infection caused by the overgrowth of *Candida* species due to antibiotic and/or corticosteroid use, xerostomia, diabetes mellitus, appliances covering the palate, smoking, and an immature or compromised immune system.[18,58] The most common forms in children are pseudomembranous and erythematous candidiasis. The former appears as white to yellow movable papules and patches varying in size and shape, growing in a radial pattern, and concealing the underlying erythema.[18,19,58] It typically occurs on the buccal mucosa, mucobuccal folds, dorsolateral tongue, and oropharynx.[19] The erythematous or atrophic form ranges from a diffuse to patchy redness involving mostly the palate and dorsum of the tongue.[18,19] Accumulation of saliva in deep folds of the corners of the mouth allows for colonization of fungal and bacterial organisms (angular cheilitis).[19] It is red, sometimes ulcerated and crusted, usually painful, and more common in children with a lip sucking habit, which may lead to spread of the infection to the adjacent perioral skin.[19,58] Diagnosis is reached through a consideration of patient demographic and health factors, clinical signs and symptoms, and laboratory criteria.[20,58] A thorough assessment of the patient's health and current medications is critical to assure effective antifungal therapy and to decrease the frequency of recurrences.[20] Cultures are very helpful in cases where the lesions are resistant to therapy.[19] Unexplained or frequent relapses should prompt

an evaluation for occult systemic disease or conditions that can lead to an immunocompromised state.[20]

In terms of disease management, it is important to improve the oral hygiene, control the caries, keep pacifiers and appliances clean, and replace contaminated toothbrushes.[18] Topical antifungal agents include compounded clotrimazole suspension (10 mg/ml) and nystatin oral suspension (100,000 U/ml) to swish for 2 minutes and swallow or expectorate four times daily for 2 weeks, followed by a reevaluation of the oral cavity.[18,58] The patient should not eat or drink for 30 minutes afterward. Adolescents can use one to two pastilles (200,000 U) slowly dissolved in the mouth five times daily.[19] Nystatin solution contains 30% to 50% of sucrose so oral hygiene must be reinforced. Clotrimazole troches (10 mg), also very rich in sucrose, can be used by slowly dissolving in the mouth one troche every 3 hours while awake (five per day) for 14 days.[18,58] Systemic antifungal drugs are advantageous when other topically delivered medications are administered concurrently.[20] Systemic agents include fluconazole 6 mg/kg every 12 or 24 hours for 5 to 7 days; adolescents can use a 200-mg loading dose and then 100 to 200 mg once a day for about a week.[19] Ketoconazole may also be used in children at 5 to 10 mg/kg every 12 or 24 hours and in adolescents 200 to 400 mg every 24 hours for 5 to 7 days.[19] It is highly effective and has the advantage of good patient compliance.[58] Common side effects with systemic use include nausea, vomiting, pruritus, skin rash, abdominal discomfort, headache, abnormal liver function tests, and drug-induced hepatitis.[19] Chlorhexidine gluconate 0.12% can be used as an antimicrobial rinse and is most useful for maintenance purposes rather than as a first-line antifungal agent.[18,20,58] Antifungal ointments and creams include nystatin, clotrimazole, miconazole, and ketoconazole. For chronic cases of angular cheilitis, Mycolog II is the best choice when applied to the corners of the mouth three times a day for 5 days.[18,58]

## HEMOGLOBINOPATHIES

Hereditary anemias caused by β thalassemia and sickle cell disease are autosomal recessive disorders that affect the structure and synthesis of hemoglobin, constituting the most common genetic diseases worldwide.[13,22] Treatment such as chronic lifelong transfusions and iron chelation for thalassemia, and transfusions or hydroxyurea for sickle cell disease have significantly ameliorated the clinical manifestations of the diseases, but treatment-related complications result in end-organ damage.[22,57] Allogeneic stem cell transplantation is the only cure for patients with hemoglobinopathies and should be done at a young age before the child has developed disease and complications associated with the therapies.[22] In order to provide dental care safely for the affected children, it is important to do a detailed review of their medical history and to consult with the medical team before proceeding, paying particular attention to the need for prophylactic antibiotics in cases of spleen problems and presence of a central line. Prevention of dental disease is paramount; therefore education of the child and the caretakers must be done from an early age with close follow-up.

## Sickle Cell Disease

Sickle cell anemia (SCA) is caused by a defect in chromosome 2 in which valine is substituted by glutamic acid on the sixth position of the $\beta$ chain of hemoglobin, producing distorted erythrocytes that can occlude vessels.[31,57] If only one pair of chromosomes is affected, then the child will present sickle cell trait.[53,57] Up to 40% of African, Afro-Caribbean, Asian, Southeast Asian, and Mediterranean populations are carriers.[57] In the United States, 1 in 400 African-Americans are affected by SCA. Prenatal diagnosis can be done in the first trimester by chorionic villus biopsy.[57]

Hypoxic states cause the erythrocytes to deform into sickle shapes and impede the blood flow in small vessels, leading to increased blood viscosity and tissue hypoxia, which creates a vicious cycle of sickling.[13,31] Infection, extremes of temperature, dehydration, and physical and emotional stresses may precipitate painful vaso-occlusive crises that are managed with hydration, correction of hypoxemia, use of opiate analgesia, and management of precipitating factors.[22,57] About 10% of children with SCA suffer strokes.[57] Dactylitis and hand-foot syndrome are common presentations in infancy. Splenic sequestration can be fatal, and splenectomy should be considered.[57] Acute chest syndrome, priapism, and abdominal pain episodes are other acute problems.[57] Chronic complications include leg ulcers as well as disease of the lungs, eyes, kidneys, and

joints.[13,57] Oral phenoxymethylpenicillin should be started at 3 months, and regular immunization with a pneumococcal vaccine should be offered to reduce deaths from infection in childhood.[13,22,57] Folic acid supplementation can also be given.[13,57]

### Dental Manifestations and Treatment Concerns

The same infarction process that affects other organs may also affect the oral/dental tissues.[31] Infarcts in the jaws may cause pain, which may be mistaken for toothache or osteomyelitis.[13,53] Mental nerve paresthesia and an increased risk of periapical infection and pathologic change have been reported.[31] Radiographic features include thin bone cortices, increased radiolucency of jaws, enlarged marrow spaces, and well-defined trabeculation of jaws.[13,53] Salmonella osteomyelitis is a common complication of SCA following bony infarcts.[13,53] Malocclusion is usually evident in these patients, who tend to have more permanent teeth extractions due to caries.[31]

Patients with sickle cell trait present no problems for routine dental care because they only experience sickling under extreme hypoxia.[13,53] For SCA children, routine dental treatment can be done during noncrisis periods after consultation with the physician, minimizing stress as much as possible, avoiding elective surgery, and keeping appointments short.[53] Morning visits are preferable because the patient is more rested. Odontogenic infections should be managed aggressively with the appropriate antibiotics, and salicylates should not be used because they can contribute to acidosis.[13] Use of nitrous oxide inhalation is safe when the oxygen level is kept at no lower than 50% throughout the procedure, followed by the administration of 100% oxygen for at least 5 minutes at the end of the visit.[13,53] Restoration of teeth under local anesthesia is preferable to extraction. Nonvital primary teeth, however, should only receive a pulpectomy if the dentist can be reasonably confident that they can be maintained in a noninfected state; otherwise they should be extracted.[13] General anesthesia should be avoided because of the risk of crisis induced by hypoxia; however, if it is the best alternative for treatment of a particular patient, a consultation with an experienced anesthesiologist and the patient's hematologist is warranted. Anemia should be corrected preoperatively, bringing the hemoglobin level to at least 10 g/dl.[13,53] Preoperative sedation to decrease stress, proper oxygenation, hydration, and temperature control during all phases of treatment are important considerations to prevent complications.[52]

## β Thalassemia Major

β Thalassemia major results in a failure to produce β-globin chains, impeding the synthesis of normal globin chains, leading to damage of the red cell membrane, followed by cell lysis and severe anemia.[13,26] The body responds by increasing the production of erythrocytes, causing increased marrow capacity in bones and extramedullary hematopoiesis, particularly in the spleen and liver.[13] In order to manage the organomegaly and skeletal changes, children start regular monthly blood transfusions from an early age (6 to 9 months), which continue through life if a hematopoietic cell transplant is not available.[13] Iron overload, the main cause of morbidity and mortality, is controlled by the iron-chelating drug desferrioxamine.[13] Conventional treatment–related complications include posttransfusional viral infections and multiple endocrine dysfunction, progressive liver fibrosis, and cardiac disease due to iron overload.[22]

*Dental Manifestations and Treatment Concerns*
The best known oral manifestation of β thalassemia is enlargement of the maxilla due to bony expansion ("chipmunk facies"), which leads to an increased overjet and spacing of the upper incisors.[13,26] The maxillary sinuses may be obliterated due to erythroid hyperplasia.[13] There is generalized rarefaction of alveolar bone, thinning of cortical bone, coarse trabeculae of the jaws, and a "chicken-wire" appearance of enlarged marrow spaces.[55] The lamina dura may also be thin, and the roots of the teeth may be short.[13] Usually the mandible becomes less enlarged than the maxilla apparently because the dense cortical plates of the mandible prevent the expansion.[26] The maxillary alveolar bone and the palate show a retruded position.[26] Surgical correction can be done, but relapse can be expected because of the continued marrow expansion.[26] Lateral skull radiographs show a typical "hair-on-end" calvarium.[13] Pain and swelling of the parotid glands and atrophic candidiasis have also been reported in these patients.[13,55]

Most children with the disorder can be treated normally under local anesthesia and nitrous oxide inhalation. General anesthesia should be used with care in these patients because of the cardiomyopathy, liver concerns, and endocrine complications they present. A preoperative consultation with an experienced anesthesiologist is warranted.

## HEMOPHILIA A

Hemophilia A (classic hemophilia) is an X-linked recessive disorder resulting in deficiency of plasma factor VIII coagulant activity, occurring in 1 in 5000 male births.[38,42,51] It accounts for about 85% of all hemophilias and can be classified as severe (plasma has no detectable factor VIII), moderate (only 1% to 4% of the normal factor VIII level is present), and mild (5% to 25% of the factor is present).[28,38] In mild cases there may be no history of bleeding, which may only be observed after trauma or surgery.[28,38] The condition should be suspected when a male patient presents unusual bleeding and shows a normal platelet count, bleeding time, thrombin time, and prothrombin time but a prolonged activated partial thromboplastin time.[28,38] Specific factor assays are needed to differentiate between hemophilia A and B (factor IX deficiency), which accounts for 10% to 15% of all hemophilias.[28,38,51]

The clinical hallmarks of hemophilia A are joint and muscle hemorrhages, easy bruising, and prolonged and potentially fatal hemorrhage after trauma or surgery but no excessive bleeding after minor cuts or abrasions.[28] Hemarthroses are first seen when the child begins to walk. If the joint hemorrhages go untreated, severe limitation of motion occurs and may lead to permanent disability.[28] Intramuscular hematomas can compress vital structures and may cause nerve paralysis, as well as vascular or airway obstruction.[28] Clinical management of hemophilia A is done according to the severity of the condition, type of bleeding present or anticipated, and presence of inhibitors.[38] Regular infusions of factor VIII should be used in cases of major surgery and life-threatening bleeding.[38] Vasopressin (desmopressin) increases the plasma levels of factor VIII and von Willebrand's factor and can be used in mild and moderate cases of hemophilia A if the patient responds well to a test dose administered by the hematologist a few days before the surgery.[21,28,38,42,51] Its peak effect occurs in 20 to 60 minutes, with a duration of 4 hours.[38] Less frequently used methods for management include administration of fresh frozen plasma, cryoprecipitate, and lyophilized factor VIII concentrate.[21] A challenging situation arises when the patient has developed antibodies to factor VIII, which are present in up to 15% of persons with severe hemophilia.[38,42] Gene therapy is currently being studied for the management of hemophilias.

### Dental Treatment Concerns

A careful review of the patient's medical history and recent blood tests and a consultation with the hematologist before invasive procedures are of paramount importance to restore the hemostatic system to a range of parameters deemed necessary for effective hemostasis and to support coagulation with adjunctive medications and local measure.[38] Review of the dental history is also crucial, especially in terms of previous bleeding episodes in the oral cavity, diet, and hygiene because preventive care and maintenance of a healthy oral cavity are very important for the patient with bleeding dyscrasias. No pretreatment is required for supragingival scaling in mild and moderate cases of hemophilia. However, if subgingival scaling is necessary, some pretreatment should be done.[51] Block anesthesia and certain infiltration anesthesia in severe hemophiliacs should not be done until the hemostatic problem is corrected because they can cause deep tissue bleeding and potential airway obstruction.[38,42] For patients with mild to moderate disease, the risk is low.[38,51] Use of a rubber dam with a stable clamp is important to protect the soft tissues. Wedges and matrices can be used with gentle handling, and appliances can be cemented if they are atraumatic to the tissues.[38] Pulpotomies, pulpectomies, and root canal therapy usually can be done without significant bleeding, and avoidance of instrumentation and filling beyond the apex is important.[38] Endodontic therapy may be the only option for management of dental abscesses for the high-titer or high-responder inhibitor patient.[38] The surgical technique should be atraumatic, with bony fragments and granulation tissue removed, and primary closure should be obtained to protect the blood clot.[38] Antibiotics should be considered when absorbable hemostatic agents are used or active infection exists.[38] Orthodontic treatment is not a contraindication, but particular attention should be paid to wires with sharp edges and placement of bands.[38]

Patients with moderate to severe hemophilia require factor VIII concentrate infusion before oral surgery.[38] The concentrate can be given intravenously, achieving a therapeutic level within several minutes, and should be at a 100% level after administration.[38,42] An alternative is to dose it to 50% preoperatively and 50% again 12 hours later, complemented by local hemostatics (pressure, sutures, gelatin sponge, cellulose materials, thrombin, microfibrillar collagen, fibrin glue, etc.) and oral antifibrinolytics (tranexamic acid mouthwash).[21,38,42,51] The half-life of factor VIII is 12 hours.[41] Vasopressin, ε-aminocaproic acid, and tranexamic acid can also be used systemically after dental extractions.[21,38] Patients undergoing extensive oral surgical procedures and those with inhibitors should be admitted to the hospital where close postoperative monitoring and continuous factor infusions can be done.[38]

## FETAL ALCOHOL SYNDROME

There is a wide range of expression of the teratogenic effects of alcohol. Criteria for diagnosis include a history of maternal alcohol ingestion and some component in each of the three following areas: craniofacial dysmorphism, prenatal and postnatal growth retardation, and central nervous system (CNS) dysfunction (mental retardation, learning disabilities, and behavioral difficulties).[32] More recently, alcohol exposure in utero has been linked to several other neurodevelopmental issues; thus the terms *alcohol-related neurodevelopmental disorder* and *alcohol-related birth defect* have been coined.[1] The American Academy of Pediatrics recommends abstinence from alcohol for women who are pregnant or planning to become pregnant because there is no safe amount of alcohol consumption during pregnancy.[1]

Fetal alcohol syndrome is the leading cause of mental retardation in the United States. The affected children usually come from very unstable families and present major psychosocial problems and lifelong adjustment issues.[50] School functioning is impaired, with a particular deficit in arithmetic that reflects patients' extreme difficulties with abstractions such as time and space, cause and effect, and generalizing from one situation to another. This appears to be central to their difficulty with independent living, poor judgment, and general dysfunctionality.[50]

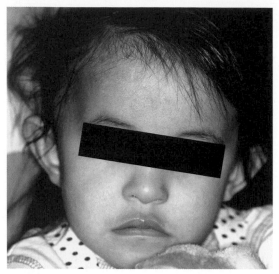

**Figure 4-1**    A 3-year-old Native American girl with fetal alcohol syndrome.

### Craniofacial Manifestations and Dental Care Considerations

The most common features of fetal alcohol syndrome are microphthalmia, short palpebral fissures, poorly developed philtrum, thin vermilion border, and/or flattening of the maxillary area (Figure 4-1). Patients with fetal alcohol syndrome can be discriminated from a sample group with 100% accuracy by only two craniofacial measurements: head circumference and bigonial breadth.[35] Affected children may also present with isolated cleft lip with or without cleft palate.[36] Short stature and microcephaly are the most prominent growth deficiencies as the children get older.[50] However, most of the physical phenotype changes, with the facies becoming normalized in adolescence because of thickening of the philtrum ridges and increased growth of the nose and chin. One study has reported mildly to moderately delayed dental development and the presence of enamel anomalies.[30] However, the number of subjects in the study was small, and further research is warranted. No studies to date have discussed the rate of dental caries in this population. In the dental office, the most challenging factor in treating children with fetal alcohol syndrome is behavior management.

## PEDIATRIC CANCER

Cancer is the leading cause of disease-related fatalities for children between 0 and 14 years of age in the United States, affecting approximately 1 in 7000 children every year.[48] The incidence is greatest in the first year of life, with a second peak at 2 to 3 years of age, followed by a decline until age 9 and then steadily increasing through adolescence.[48] The incidence is higher in boys than in girls, except during the first year of life, and white children show a 30% higher frequency than black children, particularly during the first 5 years of life.[48] Acute lymphoid leukemia (ALL) is the most common malignancy (23.5% of all childhood malignancies), followed by CNS tumors (22.1%) and sarcomas.[48] In the 1990s, 3-year survival rates exceeded 80% and 5-year survival was beyond 75%, as a result of improvement in treatment.[48]

The multimodality treatment approach uses surgery and radiotherapy to control local disease and chemotherapy to eradicate systemic disease. Chemotherapy interferes with the synthesis or function of the vital nucleic acids in all cells, whereas radiation therapy causes DNA damage in cancerous cells, with minimal harm to adjacent tissues (critical in pediatric patients).[52] Rapidly dividing cells are more sensitive and show earlier cell death than regularly dividing cells, with the nondividing ones being insensitive to radiation. Radiotherapy is given over a number of weeks in series of equally sized fractions, usually spaced by 24 hours to allow for repair of the normal tissues and to positively affect the radioresponsiveness of tumors.[51] Although improvements in chemotherapy and ionizing radiation have led to less radical and less mutilating surgical intervention, surgery may still be necessary for initial staging of a tumor, biopsies, resection, and second or third looks. Immunotherapy uses leukocytes, monoclonal antibodies, and cytokines for tumor destruction with the potential for target specificity, which may spare children from the major side effects associated with standard oncology therapies.

ALL accounts for about 75% of all childhood leukemias, with a peak incidence at age 4 years.[34] The most common signs and symptoms are anorexia, irritability, lethargy, anemia, bleeding, petechiae, fever, lymphadenopathy, splenomegaly, and hepatomegaly. Bone pain and arthralgias, caused either by leukemic infiltration of the perichondral bone or joint or by leukemic expansion of the marrow cavity, may occur, leading the child to present with a limp or refusal to walk.[34] The most common head, neck, and intraoral manifestations of ALL at the time of diagnosis are lymphadenopathy, sore throat, laryngeal pain, gingival bleeding, and oral ulceration.[27] The overall cure rate for childhood ALL is about 80%. Patients who relapse during treatment are given intensive chemotherapy followed by hematopoietic cell transplantation (HCT). Management of ALL is based on clinical risk and is usually divided into four phases:[34]

1. Remission induction: generally lasts 28 days and consists of three or four drugs (e.g., vincristine, prednisone, and L-asparaginase), with a 95% success rate. Achievement of remission is a known prerequisite for prolonged survival.
2. CNS preventive therapy/prophylaxis: the CNS can act as a sanctuary site for leukemic infiltrates because systemically administered chemotherapeutic drugs cannot cross the blood-brain barrier. Cranial irradiation and/or weekly intrathecal injection of a chemotherapeutic agent, usually methotrexate, can be used. This presymptomatic treatment can be done in each phase as well.
3. Consolidation or intensification: designed to minimize the development of drug cross-resistance through intensified treatment in an attempt to kill any remaining leukemic cells.
4. Maintenance: aimed at suppressing leukemic growth through continuous administration of methotrexate and 6-mercaptopurine. The optimal length of this phase has not been established yet, but it usually lasts 2.5 to 3 years.

The patient's blood counts normally start falling 5 to 7 days after the beginning of each treatment cycle, staying low for approximately 14 to 21 days before rising again.

### Dental and Oral Care Considerations

Oral and dental infections may complicate the oncology treatment as well as delay it, leading to morbidity and an inferior quality of life for the child. Early and radical dental intervention reduces the problem, minimizing the risk for oral and associated systemic complications (Figs. 4-2 to 4-4). Trauma associated with oral function and damage to the mucosa, such as in herpetic infections, increases the risk of bleeding.[43] Therefore, the dental consultation on a newly diagnosed patient should be done at once so that enough

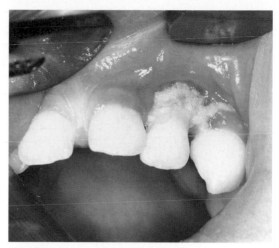

**Figure 4-2** *Pseudomonas* infection resulting in loss of primary teeth in a 2-year-old girl with acute lymphoid leukemia.

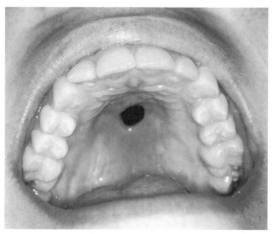

**Figure 4-3** *Aspergillus* infection in a 14-year-old girl with acute lymphoid leukemia.

time is available for care to be completed before the cancer therapy starts. Every patient should be dealt with on an individual basis, and appropriate consultations with physicians and other dental specialists should be sought before dental care is instituted.[43]

*Patient's Medical History and Hematologic Status.* A thorough review should include information about the underlying disease, time of diagnosis, modalities of treatment the patient has received since the diagnosis (chemotherapy, radiotherapy, surgeries, etc.), and complications, including relapses. Hospitalizations, emergency room visits, infections (both oral and systemic), current hematologic status, allergies, medications,

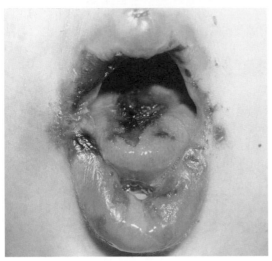

**Figure 4-4**   Moderate mucositis caused by chemotherapy in a 5-year-old girl.

| TABLE 4-1 | |
| --- | --- |
| **Blood Count Normal Reference Values**[49] | |
| **BLOOD COMPONENT** | **NORMAL VALUES** |
| Hemoglobin (g/dl) | Males: 14–18; females: 12–16 Newborn: 16–19; children: 11–16 |
| Hematocrit (%) | Males: 40–54; females: 37–47 Newborn: 49–54; children: 35–49 |
| White blood cell count | 5,000–10,000/mm$^3$ |
| Platelet count | 150,000–400,000/mm$^3$ |
| **DIFFERENTIAL** | **NORMAL VALUES** |
| Neutrophils (polymorphonuclear leukocytes) | 50–70% |
| Lymphocytes | 30–40% |
| Monocytes | 3–7% |
| Eosinophils | 0–5% |
| Basophils | 0–1% |

and a review of systems (heart, lungs, kidneys, etc.) should be noted.

Most patients are given a central line, which is an indwelling catheter inserted into the right atrium of the heart, useful for obtaining blood samples and administering chemotherapeutic agents. A central line can be partially implanted (e.g., Broviac, Hickman catheters) or subcutaneously implanted (e.g., Mediport, BardPort, Port-a-Cath), and its presence dictates the use of antibiotics against endocarditis, even if the patient is already receiving antibiotics for prevention of systemic infections.

Prolonged bleeding in childhood cancer may be caused by chemotherapy-induced myelosuppression, some medications, and disorders of clotting and platelets related to the baseline disease. Clinically significant bleeding is unlikely to occur with a level greater than 20,000/mm$^3$ in the absence of other complicating factors. Dental procedures can be done when the platelet count is greater than 40,000/mm$^3$, with attention paid to measures for controlling prolonged bleeding.[33,43] Other coagulation tests may be appropriate for patients with liver involvement and coagulopathies. See Table 4-1 for normal blood values.

Neutrophils are the body's first line of defense; therefore, the incidence and severity of infection are inversely related to their number. When the absolute neutrophil count (ANC) is less than 1000/mm$^3$, elective dental work should be deferred because the risk for development of infections increases greatly.

*Oral Hygiene, Diet, and Caries Prevention.* Regardless of the child's hematologic status, intensive oral hygiene throughout the entire oncology treatment is important to decrease oral complications.[5,14-16,33,37,39,43,49,54] Thrombocytopenia should not be the sole determinant of oral hygiene as patients are able to brush without bleeding at widely different levels of platelet count.[5] There is evidence that patients who do intensive oral care have a reduced risk of developing moderate/severe mucositis, without causing an increase in septicemia and infections in the oral cavity.[6,15,16,43] A regular soft toothbrush or an electric brush used at least twice daily is the most efficient means to reduce the risk of significant bleeding and infection in the gingiva.[5,39,43,54] Sponges, foam brushes, and supersoft brushes cannot provide effective mechanical cleansing due to their softness; therefore they should be used only in cases of severe mucositis when the patient cannot tolerate a regular brush.[5,37,39] Brushes should be air dried between uses, and a toothpaste without heavy flavoring agents should be considered because such agents can irritate the tissues.[37,44] During neutropenic periods, the use of toothpicks and water-irrigating devices should be avoided because they may break the integrity of the tissues, creating ports of entry for micro-organism colonization and bleeding. Ultrasonic brushes and dental floss can be used if the patient is properly trained.[43] Patients who present poor oral hygiene or periodontal disease can use chlorhexidine rinses daily until the gingival health has been restored or until the mucosa shows signs of the initial stages of mucositis. At that point, rinses containing alcohol and flavoring agents should be avoided because they can dehydrate and irritate the mucosa. Periodontal infection is a major concern because colonizing organisms have been shown to cause bacteremias.[42]

The child with cancer may be at high risk for dental caries from a dietary standpoint. Furthermore, many oral pediatric medications contain high amounts of sucrose (e.g., nystatin); thus they should be used in a manner that minimizes the caries risk. For example, children should not be allowed to fall asleep with a nystatin solution or with a clotrimazole troche that is not sugar free. Despite the fact that nystatin is often prescribed, it cannot be recommended for prevention of *Candida* infections in immuno-depressed patients because it is not effective.[24,43,44] Vomiting is often a side effect of the cancer therapy so the patient should rinse after emesis episodes with tap water or any bland solution to remove the gastric acid, which is irritating to the oral tissues and may cause enamel decalcification. Fluoride supplements and neutral fluoride rinses or gels are indicated for patients at risk for caries.

*Dental Procedures.* The patient's dental history should be reviewed, and a thorough examination of the head, face, neck, and intraoral soft and hard tissues should be performed, complemented by radiographs when indicated. Some patients may complain of paresthesias caused by leukemic infiltration of the peripheral nerves. Others may report dental pain mimicking irreversible pulpitis in the absence of a dental/periodontal infection. This can be a side effect of vincristine and vinblastine, two commonly used chemotherapeutic agents.[43,44] In this case, the patient should avoid situations that exacerbate the discomfort (sweets, ice, etc.), and analgesics should be prescribed for pain control. The pain disappears within a few days after the cessation of the causative chemotherapy. Patients may also complain of dental hypersensitivity usually brought on by cold or hot stimuli. The mechanism for the sensitivity is not well understood

and can be managed with topical fluoride or a desensitizing toothpaste.[43,44]

The patient's blood count usually returns to normal between the chemotherapy cycles. When time is limited for dental care before the onco-logical therapy starts, treatment priorities should be infections, extractions, periodontal care, and sources of irritation before the treatment of carious teeth, root canal therapy for permanent teeth, and replacement of faulty restorations. The risk for pulpal infection and pain should determine which carious lesions are to be treated first because a pulpal infection during immunosuppression could lead to a life-threatening situation.[44] Temporary restorations can be placed, and nonacute dental treatment can be delayed until the patient's health is stabilized.[33,43,44] Overall, routine dental care can be done when the ANC is greater than $1000/mm^3$ and the platelet count is greater than $40,000/mm^3$.[14,33,45] Some authors[33,43] recommend that endocarditis prophylaxis be prescribed when the ANC is between 1000 and $2000/mm^3$, and optional platelet transfusions be considered pre- and 24 hours postoperatively when the level is between 40,000 and $75,000/mm^3$. When the platelet level is below $40,000/mm^3$, dental care should be deferred. During immuno-suppression, all elective dental procedures should be avoided. In cases of emergency, the physician must be contacted before any dental treatment is initiated because platelet transfusions, antibiotic coverage beyond endocarditis prevention, and hospital admission may be necessary for dental management.[49]

When there is time before the initiation of cancer therapy, dental scaling and prophylaxis should be done, defective restorations should be repaired, and teeth with sharp edges should be polished. Although there have been no studies to date that address the safety of performing pulp therapy in primary teeth prior to the initiation of chemotherapy and/or radiotherapy, it is prudent to provide a more radical treatment in the form of extraction to minimize the risk for oral and systemic complications. Despite the high rate of success of pulpotomies and pulpectomies in healthy subjects, pulpal/periapical infections during immunosuppression periods can have a significant impact on cancer treatment.[43] Teeth that have already been pulpally treated and are clinically and radiographically sound present no threats. Symptomatic nonvital permanent teeth should receive root canal therapy at least one week before initiation of cancer therapy.[33] If that is not possible, extraction is indicated followed by antibiotic therapy for about 1 week.[33,43,49] Endodontic treatment of permanent teeth with asymptomatic periapical involvement can be delayed if the patient is neutropenic.[33,45] During immunosuppression, swelling and purulent exudate may not be present, masking some of the classical signs of odontogenic infections, leaving them clinically undetected.[33] In this situation, radiographs are vital to determine periapical or bifurcation pathologic processes.

Fixed orthodontic appliances and space maintainers should be removed if the patient has poor oral hygiene or the treatment protocol carries a risk for the development of moderate to severe mucositis, except for smooth appliances such as band and loops and fixed lower lingual arches.[44] Appliances can harbor food debris, compromise oral hygiene, and act as mechanical irritants, increasing the risk for secondary infection. Removable appliances and retainers that fit well may be worn as long as tolerated by the patient who shows good oral care. If band removal is not possible, mouth guards or orthodontic wax should be used to decrease tissue trauma.[44]

Partially erupted molars can become a source of infection because of pericoronitis, so the overlying gingival tissue should be excised if the dentist believes it is a potential risk.[33,44] Loose primary teeth should be left to exfoliate naturally, and the patient should be counseled to not play with them to prevent bacteremia. If the patient cannot comply with this recommendation, the teeth should be removed. Impacted teeth, root tips, partially erupted third molars, teeth with periodontal pockets greater than 6 mm, teeth with acute infections, and nonrestorable teeth should be removed ideally 2 weeks before cancer therapy starts to allow adequate healing.[33,49] If that is not possible, other authors suggest at least 4 to 7 days.[45] If a permanent tooth cannot be extracted for medical reasons at that time, the pediatric dentist can consider amputation of the crown above the gingiva, followed by initial root canal treatment with antimicrobial medicament sealed in the root canal chamber. Antibiotics should be given for 7 to 10 days after with the extraction subsequently done when the patient's hematologic status allows it.[43] Particular attention should be given to extraction of permanent teeth in patients who will receive or have received radiation to the face because of the risk of osteoradio-

necrosis. Surgical procedures must be as atraumatic as possible, with no sharp bony edges remaining and satisfactory closure of the wounds.[33,43,44,49] Local measures to control bleeding such as pressure packs, sutures, gelatin sponge, topical thrombin, or microfibrillar collagen should be readily available. If local measures fail, the physician must be contacted immediately.

When the patient is in the maintenance phase of the treatment and the overall prognosis is good, it is likely that his or her health status is close to normal. Dental procedures can be done routinely but not before checking the blood count and prescribing antibiotics for subacute bacterial endocarditis prophylaxis if a central line is in place. Orthodontic treatment may start or resume after completion of all therapy and after at least a 2-year disease-free survival.[46] By then, the risk of relapse is decreased and the patient is no longer using immunosuppressive drugs. However, the clinician must assess any dental developmental disturbances caused by the cancer therapy, especially in children treated before the age of 6 years (Figure 4-5).[10-12,17,46] A panoramic radiograph should be obtained every 12 to 18 months to monitor the dental changes and to plan dental rehabilitation accordingly. Dahllof et al.[12] described the following strategies to provide orthodontic care for patients with dental sequelae: (1) use appliances that minimize the risk of root resorption; (2) use lighter forces; (3) terminate treatment earlier than normal; (4) choose the simplest method for the treatment needs; and (5) do not treat the lower jaw. However, specific guidelines for orthodontic management, including optimal force and pace, remain undefined.[37] The role of growth hormone in the development of the craniofacial structures in pediatric cancer patients has not been fully established.

## HEMATOPOIETIC CELL TRANSPLANTATION

HCT has been used to replace the marrow of patients with hematologic disorders, congenital immunodeficiencies, lipidoses, and inborn errors of metabolism as well for marrow support to allow the administration of higher doses of chemotherapy and/or radiotherapy in patients with solid tumors.[19] The stem cells used in HCT can be obtained from multiple aspirations of bone marrow from the iliac crest and other bones, from the peripheral blood, and from the placenta

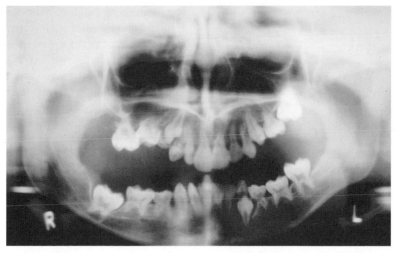

**Figure 4-5**   Long-term effects on dental development in a 14-year-old boy who received chemotherapy and total body irradiation before hematopoietic cell transplantation at age 13 months.

or umbilical cord blood. The cells can be collected from the patient's own marrow (autologous transplant), from a donor related to the recipient or from an unrelated person (allogeneic transplant), from an identical twin (syngeneic transplant), and from a different species (xenogeneic transplant).[41] Human leukocyte antigen (HLA) tissue typing is done to identify antigens on the short arm of chromosome 6 of potential donors to match as closely as possible those of the recipient (full or partial match).[41] A few days prior to transplantation, the patient is admitted to receive high-dose chemotherapy alone or in combination with total body irradiation (TBI). Evidence of engraftment should be indicated between days 20 and 30, sometimes earlier, by increased peripheral white cell and platelet counts and is substantiated by the presence of donor cells on marrow aspirations.

*Dental and Oral Care Considerations*
Most of the principles of dental and oral care for the pediatric patient undergoing HCT are similar to those discussed in the section on pediatric cancer. The two major differences are as follows: (1) in HCT, there are no cycles of chemotherapy with periods of rest in-between when the blood counts return to normal as it occurs in the management of cancer, and (2) there will be prolonged immunosuppression following transplantation, with most immune functions probably fully restored by 1 year if chronic graft versus host disease or other complication is not present. Therefore, all dental treatment must be com-

pleted before the child is admitted in order to eliminate disease that could lead to complications during and after transplantation.

In the long term, the frequency of oral examinations will vary depending on the severity of oral problems, compliance with oral hygiene, and the patient's overall state of health.[44] Regular dental examinations with radiography can be done routinely but elective dental work, including prophylaxis, should be avoided in patients with profound impairment of immune function.[44] If a dental emergency arises during that period, the patient's physician must be consulted before any treatment is instituted. Orthodontic treatment considerations are the same as discussed in the previous section.

## ACUTE AND CHRONIC ORAL COMPLICATIONS OF CHEMOTHERAPY AND RADIOTHERAPY

Cancer therapy can cause much morbidity in the oral cavity (Box 4-1), compromising the child's quality of life and increasing treatment costs. Among all complications, mucositis (see Figure 4-4) is the most common cause of oral pain in cancer treatment and the most common complication in HCT.[15,16] The agents used in the preparative regimen can largely affect tissues of the gastrointestinal mucosa, inhibiting its basal layers to replace the superficial cells leading to a generalized mucosal inflammation. The occurrence and severity of mucositis show great

## BOX 4-1

### Oral and Craniofacial Complications of Cancer Therapy[43]

**Acute Complications from Chemotherapy and Radiotherapy**
  Mucositis
  Salivary gland dysfunction
  Sialadenitis (radiation only)
  Xerostomia
  Neurotoxicity
  Taste dysfunction
  Dentinal hypersensitivity
  Temporomandibular dysfunction
  Oral bleeding
  Opportunistic infections (viral, fungal, bacterial)

**Long-Term Complications of Radiotherapy to the Face**
  Mucosal fibrosis and atrophy
  Xerostomia
  Dental caries
  Osteoradionecrosis
  Taste dysfunction
  Muscular/cutaneous fibrosis
  Fungal and bacterial infections
  Dental and craniofacial developmental problems (also with chemotherapy)

individual variability, with tissue changes noticeable between 4 and 7 days after the initiation of therapy and generally lasting from 10 to 14 days.[15,16,45] Its management is directed at symptom management and prevention of infection and trauma. Mucositis and all other acute and long-term complications of chemotherapy and radiotherapy have been extensively reviewed elsewhere.*

A long-term issue of particular interest for pediatric dentists is the development of dental and/or craniofacial abnormalities (see Figure 4-5). The younger the child is at the beginning of therapy (especially before 6 years of age), the greater the risks for craniofacial and dental disturbances such as tooth agenesis, complete or partial arrest of root development with thin, tapered roots, early apical closure, globular and conical crowns, dentin and enamel opacities and defects, microdontia, enlarged pulp chambers, taurodontism, and abnormal occlusion.[8,11,12,23,46] Delayed eruption of permanent teeth can be observed,

*References 5,8,9,15,16,37,40, 43,48.

although some children with hematologic malignancies who received chemotherapy alone do not have abnormalities in dental maturity or eruption of their permanent dentition.[44] Vertical growth of the condyles, and the alveolar and molar heights are adversely affected by pre-HCT conditioning.[11]

Patients who have experienced chronic or severe mucositis are at risk for malignant transformation of the oral mucosa and thus should be followed closely.[17] Careful monitoring of chronic xerostomia and oral graft versus host disease are also very important issues.

## REFERENCES

1. American Academy of Pediatrics Committee on Substance Abuse and Committee on Children with Disabilities: Fetal Alcohol Syndrome and Alcohol-Related Neurodevelopmental Disorders. *Pediatrics* 106:358, 2000.
2. Amir J, Harel L, Smetana Z, Varsano I: The natural history of primary herpes simplex type 1 gingivostomatitis in children. *Pediatr Dermatol* 16:259-263, 1999.
3. Amir J, Harel L, Smetana Z, Varsano I: Treatment of herpes simplex gingivostomatitis with acyclovir in children: a randomised double blind placebo controlled study. *BMJ* 314:1800-1803, 1997.
4. Amir J, Nussinovitch M, Kleper R et al: Primary herpes simplex virus type 1 gingivostomatitis in pediatric personnel. *Infection* 25:310-312, 1997.
5. Bavier AR: Nursing management of acute oral complications of cancer. Consensus Development Conference on Oral Complications of Cancer Therapies: Diagnosis, Prevention and Treatment. *NCI Monogr* 9:123, 1990.
6. Borowski B, Benhamou E, Pico JL et al: Prevention of oral mucositis in patients treated with high-dose chemotherapy and bone marrow transplantation: a randomised controlled trial comparing two protocols of dental care. *Oral Oncol Eur J Cancer* 30B:93, 1994.
7. Briek C: Herpesvirus-induced diseases: oral manifestations and current treatment options. *J Cal Dent Assoc* 28:911-921, 2000.
8. da Fonseca MA: Long-term oral and craniofacial complications following pediatric bone marrow transplantation. *Pediatr Dent* 22:57, 2000.
9. da Fonseca MA: Pediatric bone marrow transplantation: oral complications and recommendations for care. *Pediatr Dent* 20:386, 1998.
10. Dahllof G: Craniofacial growth in children treated for malignant diseases. *Acta Odontol Scand* 56:378, 1998.
11. Dahllöf G, Forsberg CM, Ringdén O et al: Facial growth and morphology in long-term survivors

after bone marrow transplantation. *Eur J Orthod* 11:33, 1989.

12. Dahllof G, Jonsson A, Ulmner M, Huggare J: Orthodontic treatment in long-term survivors after bone marrow transplantation. *Am J Orthod Dentofac Orthop* 120:459, 2001.

13. Duggal MS, Bedi R, Kinsey SE, Williams SA: The dental management of children with sickle cell disease and beta-thalassemia: a review. *Int J Paediatr Dent* 1996; 6:227-234, 1996.

14. Epstein JB: Infection prevention in bone marrow transplantation and radiation patients. Consensus Development Conference on Oral Complications of Cancer Therapies: Diagnosis, Prevention and Treatment. *NCI Monogr* 9:73, 1990.

15. Epstein JB, Schubert MM: Oral mucositis in myelosuppressive cancer therapy. *Oral Surg Oral Med Oral Pathol Oral Radiol Endod* 88:273, 1999.

16. Epstein JB, Schubert MM: Oropharyngeal mucositis in cancer therapy - review of pathogenesis, diagnosis, and management. *Oncology* 17:1767, 2003.

17. Euvrard S, Kanitakis J, Claudy A: Skin cancers after organ transplantation. *N Engl J Med* 348:1681, 2003.

18. Flaitz CM, Baker KA: Treatment approaches to common symptomatic oral lesions in children. *Dent Clin North Am* 44:671-696, 2000.

19. Flaitz CM, Hicks MJ: Oral candidiasis in children with immune suppression: clinical appearance and therapeutic considerations. *J Dent Child* 66:161-166, 1999.

20. Fotos PG, Vincent SD, Hellstein JW: Oral candidosis: clinical, historical and therapeutic features of 100 cases. *Oral Surg Oral Med Oral Pathol* 74:41-49, 1992.

21. Garfunkel AA, Galili D, Findler M, Lubliner J: Bleeding tendency: a practical approach in dentistry. *Compend Contin Educ Dent* 20:836-852, 1999.

22. Gaziev J, Lucarelli G: Stem cell transplantation for hemoglobinopathies. *Curr Opin Pediatr* 15:24-31, 2003.

23. Goho C: Chemoradiation therapy: effect on dental development. *Pediatr Dent* 15:6, 1993.

24. Gotzche PC, Johansen HK: Nystatin prophylaxis and treatment in severely immunocompromised patients. *Cochrane Database Syst Rev* (2):CD002033, 2002.

25. Greenberg MS: Herpesvirus infections. *Dent Clin North Am* 40:359-368, 1996.

26. Hes J, van der Waal I, de Man K: Bimaxillary hyperplasia: the facial expression of homozygous beta-thalassemia. *Oral Surg Oral Med Oral Pathol* 69:185-190, 1990.

27. Hou G-L, Huang J-S, Tsai C-C: Analysis of oral manifestations of leukemia: a retrospective study. *Oral Dis* 3:31, 1997.

28. Hoyer LW: Hemophilia A. *N Engl J Med* 330:38-47, 1994.

29. Huber MA: Herpes simplex type-1 virus infection. *Quintessence Int* 34:453-467, 2003.

30. Jackson IT, Hussain K: Craniofacial and oral manifestations of fetal alcohol syndrome. *Plast Reconstr Surg* 85:505, 1990.

31. Laurence B, Reid BC, Katz RV: Sickle cell anemia and dental caries: a literature review and pilot study. *Spec Care Dent* 22:70-74, 2002.

32. Leppert M, Hofman K: Fetal alcohol syndrome. In: Capute AJ, Accardo PJ, editors. *Developmental Disabilities in Infancy and Childhood,* 2nd ed. Baltimore, Brookes, 1996.

33. Little JW, Falace DA, Miller CS, Rhodus NL: *Dental Management of the Medically Compromised Patient,* 6th ed. St. Louis, Mosby, 2002.

34. Margolin JF, Steuber CP, Poplack DG: Acute lymphoblastic leukemia. In: Pizzo PA, Poplack DG, editors. *Principles and Practice of Pediatric Oncology,* 4th ed. Philadelphia, Lippincott Williams & Wilkins, 2002.

35. Moore ES, Ward RE, Jamison PL et al: The subtle facial signs of prenatal exposure to alcohol: an anthropometric study. *J Pediatr* 139:215, 2001.

36. Munger RG, Romitti PA, Daack-Hirsch S et al: Maternal alcohol use and risk of orofacial cleft birth defects. *Teratology* 54:27, 1996.

37. National Cancer Institute: Oral complications of chemotherapy and head/neck radiation. Available at www.nci.nih.gov/cancerinfo/pdq/supportivecare/oralcomplications/healthprofessional/#Section_28.

38. Patton LL, Ship JA: Treatment of patients with bleeding disorders. *Dent Clin North Am* 38:465-482, 1994.

39. Ransier A, Epstein JB, Lunn R, Spinelli J: A combined analysis of a toothbrush, foam brush, and a chlorhexidine-soaked foam brush in maintaining oral hygiene. *Cancer Nurs* 18:393, 1995.

40. Rubenstein EB, Peterson DE, Schubert M, et al: Clinical practice guidelines for the prevention and treatment of cancer therapy–induced oral and gastrointestinal mucositis. *Cancer* 100 (9 suppl): 2026-2046, 2004.

41. Sanders JE: Bone marrow transplantation for pediatric malignancies. *Pediatr Clin North Am* 44:1005, 1997.

42. Schardt-Sacco D: Update on coagulopathies. *Oral Surg Oral Med Oral Pathol Oral Radiol Endod* 2000; 90:559-63.

43. Schubert MM, Epstein JB, Peterson DE: Oral complications of cancer therapy. In: Yagiela JA, Neidle EA, Dowd FJ, editors. *Pharmacology and Therapeutics for Dentistry,* 4th ed. St. Louis, Mosby–Year Book, 1998.

44. Schubert MM, Peterson DE, Lloid ME: Oral complications. In: Thomas ED, Blume KG, Forman SJ, editors. *Hematopoietic Cell Transplantation,* 2nd ed. Malden, Mass, Blackwell, 1999.

45. Semba SE, Mealy BL, Hallmon WW: Dentistry and

the cancer patient. 2. Oral health management of the chemotherapy patient. *Compend Contin Educ Dent* 15:1378, 1994.

46. Sheller B, Williams B: Orthodontic management of patients with hematologic malignancies. *Am J Orthod Dentofac Orthop*109:575, 1996.

47. Siegel MA: Diagnosis and management of recurrent herpes simplex infections. *JADA* 133: 1245-1249, 2002.

48. Smith MA, Ries LAG: Childhood cancer: incidence, survival, and mortality. In: Pizzo PA, Poplack DG, editors. *Principles and Practice of Pediatric Oncology,* 4th ed. Philadelphia, Lippincott Williams & Wilkins, 2002.

49. Sonis S, Fazio RC, Fang L: *Principles and Practice of Oral Medicine,* 2nd ed. Philadelphia, Saunders, 1995.

50. Streissguth AP, Aase JM, Clarren SK, et al: Fetal alcohol syndrome in adolescents and adults. *JAMA* 265:1961, 1991.

51. Stubbs M, Lloyd J: A protocol for the dental management of von Willebrand's disease, haemophilia A and haemophilia B. *Austr Dent J* 46:37-40, 2001.

52. Tarbell NJ, Kooy HM: General principles of radiation oncology. In: Pizzo PA, Poplack DG, editors. *Principles and Practice of Pediatric Oncology,* 4th ed. Philadelphia, Lippincott Williams & Wilkins, 2002.

53. Taylor LB, Nowak AJ, Giller RH, Casamassimo PS: Sickle cell anemia: a review of the dental concerns and a retrospective study of dental and bony changes. *Spec Care Dent* 15:38-42, 1995.

54. Toth BB, Martin JW, Fleming TJ: Oral and dental care associated with cancer therapy. *Cancer Bull* 43:397, 1991.

55. Van Dis ML, Langlais RP: The thalassemias: oral manifestations and complications. *Oral Surg Oral Med Oral Pathol* 62:229-233, 1986.

56. Woo S-B, Lee SF-K: Oral recrudescent herpes simplex virus infection. *Oral Surg Oral Med Oral Pathol Oral Radiol Endod* 83:239-243, 1997.

57. Yardumian A, Crawley C: Sickle cell disease. *Clin Med* 1:441-446, 2001.

58. Zegarelli DJ: Fungal infections of the oral cavity. *Otolaryngol Clin North Am* 26:1069-1089, 1993.

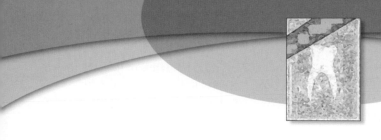

# CHAPTER 5
## Topics in Pediatric Physiology

*Dianne M. McBrien*

The treatment of children presents particular challenges to the health care professional.

The body of the pediatric patient is not simply a miniaturized version of his or her adult counterpart; child physiology and anatomy significantly differ from that of adults. Pediatric dentists must consider these differences when making therapeutic choices about young patients, especially when treatment includes drug therapy. Route and rate of drug administration, dosage, onset and duration of action, and possibility of toxicity all are influenced by the unique physiology of childhood.

This chapter will review basic principles of pediatric physiology—including pharmacokinetic characteristics of the child—and anatomy. For the sake of simplicity, the material will be presented by organ system. Because a comprehensive review of these subjects is beyond the scope of this chapter, the text stresses only the principles that differ significantly from those of the adult patient. Wherever possible, clinical applications to pediatric dentistry are made.

## RESPIRATORY SYSTEM

### Anatomy

Several anatomic features of the pediatric respiratory tract predispose the young patient to obstruction and collapse of both large and small airways. A child's upper respiratory tract is prone to obstruction at several sites. The narrow nasal passages, tongue/oral cavity disproportion, and decreased airway diameter characteristic of infants and young children predispose this patient population to partial or complete upper airway obstruction.[5] Additional risk may be generated by routine office procedures: a tightly clamped mask over the nares, a mouth pack depressing the oral cavity floor, or a retractor posteriorly displacing the tongue all may increase the likelihood of upper airway obstruction. The secretions and edema associated with upper respiratory infections also can compromise the pediatric airway and should be kept in mind when an acutely ill child reports for an elective procedure. Bronchospasm, laryngospasm, acute subglottic edema with stridor, intraoperative and perioperative hypoxia, atelectasis, and postextubation croup are among the complications of anesthesia that are reported after the child with respiratory infection has surgery, particularly involving intubation. In the past, most clinicians recommended postponement of an elective procedure until the child had been free of symptoms for 1 week. Recently, however, workers in pediatric anesthesia who examined data from mildly ill children undergoing elective procedures concluded that the criteria for canceling elective procedures without endotracheal intubation should include signs and symptoms of lower tract involvement such as fever of 38.5° C or greater, chills, productive cough, wheezing, or tachypnea.[8]

Anatomic differences in the child's chest cage can also contribute to respiratory problems. The child's chest wall is more elastic than that of an adult, which means that lower ventilation pressures are needed to expand the lungs. The sternum is less rigid, which means that ribs and intercostal muscles have less support. In a resting position, the child's ribs are more horizontally placed than those of the adult; this positional difference makes intercostal muscle retraction inefficient. Thus the diaphragm becomes the primary breathing muscle in the pediatric patient. Anything that limits diaphragmatic excursion should therefore be avoided, including the supine position, which promotes gastric organ pressure on the diaphragm. Instead, a 20- to 30-degree head-up position is recommended by many authors to avoid such pressure and thereby minimize risk of regurgitation and aspiration.[5]

Lung infrastructure is different in the pediatric population as well. The majority of alveoli are formed after birth; indeed, the adult number of alveoli is generally present only at about the sixth year of life. And although ratios of lung volume to body size are similar throughout the life span, children have a greater proportion of alveolar surface area to lung size.

## Physiology

Because of this relative difference in alveolar surface area, children have a greater rate of *alveolar ventilation* (AV) per unit of area (a proportionally greater exchange of gas across the alveoli). However, the total volume of gas exchanged is less than that of adults, as is the *functional residual capacity* (FRC). FRC is defined as the volume of gas remaining in the lungs at the end of a normal expiration.

## Drug Considerations

The AV/FRC ratio helps to determine the rate at which changes in inspired gas concentration effect a clinical response. While AV supports transport of inhaled gas through the bloodstream and to the brain, FRC determines how much gas remains in the lungs during normal breathing. Thus as the AV/FRC ratio increases, the body reacts more quickly to changes in inhaled gas concentration.

Given the child's high AV and low FRC, the pediatric AV/FRC ratio is almost five times that of an adult. This ratio difference means that children react more rapidly to inhaled gases such as nitrous oxide and halothane, and can be adequately anesthetized with lower gas concentrations than those required for adult patients. For this reason and also because of some unique aspects of the pediatric heart discussed later in this chapter, children are at higher risk of overdose effects from inhalants, including hypotension, bradycardia, and hypoventilation. Careful monitoring of vital signs is therefore essential in children undergoing inhalant anesthesia for dental procedures.

# CARDIOVASCULAR SYSTEM

## Physiology

Immediately after birth, the infant's cardiovascular system begins a series of complex changes that will continue for the next decade. After umbilical cord clamping and the first extrauterine breaths, pulmonary vascular resistance falls and

## TABLE 5-1
### Changes in Heart Rate During Development

| Age | Mean Heart Rate |
|---|---|
| Newborn | 115–170 |
| 6 mo | 100–150 |
| 1 yr | 90–135 |
| 3 yr | 80–125 |
| 5 yr | 80–120 |
| 10 yr | 75–110 |
| 15 yr | 700–110 |
| Adult | 70 |

## TABLE 5-2
### Changes in Blood Pressure During Development

| Age | Mean Systolic Blood Pressure (mm Hg) |
|---|---|
| Newborn | 60–75 |
| 6 mo | 80–90 |
| 1 yr | 96 |
| 3 yr | 100 |
| 5 yr | 100 |
| 10 yr | 110 |
| 15 yr | 120 |
| Adult | 125 |

the heart itself undergoes several changes including closure of the ductus arteriosus and foramen ovale.

Other physiologic changes continue throughout infancy and childhood. The heart rate, which averages about 120 in the newborn, decreases throughout childhood: by 4 years of age, rates are less than 100. Adult heart rates are generally reached by 10 to 12 years of age (Table 5-1).

*Cardiac output*, defined as the product of heart rate and *stroke volume* (the amount of blood pumped by one contraction of the left ventricle), is influenced by several variables in the child. The infant heart is relatively inelastic and cannot make rapid changes in stroke volume. Thus, the heart rate is a much more important determinant of cardiac output in infants and young children than it is in adults; a significant drop in heart rate can result in decreased cardiac output and hypotension. At the same time, parasympathetic tone is more marked in the immature nervous system, which means that this age group is more prone to significant bradycardias with vagal stimulation. Examples of maneuvers producing vagal stimulation include defecation, bladder distention, pressure on the eyeballs, application of throat packs, and tracheal intubation. Because of the potential for vagally induced bradycardia with intubation, children undergoing manipulation of the airway are frequently premedicated with atropine or a similar parasympathetic blocking agent.[8,9]

Blood pressure, in contrast, tends to rise throughout childhood. Mean systolic blood pressure in newborns ranges from 75 to 85 mm Hg; there is a 5 to 10 mm Hg increase over the first several weeks of life. Adult blood pressure values are generally reached by early adolescence. Table 5-2 displays average blood pressures for children.

Cardiac output also changes with age. Cardiac output per kilogram of body weight is highest in the newborn and gradually declines in the first several weeks of life. The relatively noncompliant infant myocardium adapts poorly to sudden changes in afterload; fluid overload and systemic hypertension produce cardiac failure more quickly in young children.

### Drug Considerations

Changes in cardiac output can have a dramatic impact on the uptake of inhaled anesthetic agents. A sudden decrease in heart rate results in decreased cardiac output, which in turn increases the rate of inhaled anesthetic uptake. Since 40% of a child's cardiac output perfuses the brain, increases in inhaled anesthetic uptake associated with decreased cardiac output can significantly depress the central nervous system. These depressant effects can include central reduction in vasomotor tone and peripheral vasodilation, which can worsen the hypotension associated with significant bradycardia.

Because of these potential adverse effects, inhaled anesthetics should be used carefully in the pediatric population. These agents act more rapidly in children than adults, and children are adequately sedated by lower gas concentrations than those required for adults.

To minimize the hypotensive response associated with potential drops in heart rate, pediatric patients should be well hydrated prior to procedures requiring inhaled or intravenous sedation. Recurrent vomiting, diarrhea, or poor oral intake in the days prior to the procedure are appropriate indications to reschedule.

## GASTROINTESTINAL SYSTEM

The gastrointestinal tract undergoes continuous developmental change from birth to old age. Since many drugs are absorbed and metabolized by the gut, these changes must be considered when administering medications to children. There are several important physiologic differences in the child's gastrointestinal system. These are as follows:

**Decreased acidity.** In infants and young children, immature gastric mucosa secretes low levels of acid; adult levels of gastric acidity are generally not reached until 3 years of age. Before this time, the low acidity of the infant gut favors absorption of weakly acidic drugs such as penicillins and cephalosporins, whereas the absorption of weakly basic drugs such as the benzodiazepines is delayed.[4,6,7]

**Altered motility.** Gastric emptying times are significantly longer during infancy. Average emptying times in the young infant can reach 8 hours, and only reach adult values—2 to 3 hours—between 6 and 8 months of age. Longer emptying times combined with the irregular peristalsis of infancy generally result in slower gastric drug absorption.[4]

**Altered hepatic metabolism.** Many drugs are metabolized by the liver. Hepatic enzymes may act to detoxify a drug or to alter it to a more potent form. Because infants and young children are relatively deficient in these enzymes, they are at high risk for toxicity if not dosed correctly. Low levels of cytochrome P-450 enzymes are associated with sluggish oxidation of diazepam, phenytoin, and phenobarbital in the neonate; all of these drugs thus have prolonged clinical effects in this age group. Glucuronyltransferase, which conjugates drugs into excretable form, is also deficient in the neonate but reaches adult levels after the first month of life. Morphine, acetaminophen, steroids, and sulfa antibiotics all are conjugated by glucuronyltransferase and thus are used with caution in the neonate.

The infant liver is also deficient in pseudocholinesterase; enzyme levels are at 60% of adult levels for the first several months of life. Even when calculated on an adjusted body weight scale, succinylcholine doses do not reach adult levels until after 2 years of age. Succinylcholine is therefore administered with caution to infant patients, who may respond with prolonged apnea.[7]

## RENAL SYSTEM

While drugs can be excreted by a number of physiologic routes, such as sweat, bile, and feces, the vast majority undergo renal excretion. Because of its immature capacity, the young kidney is less competent to excrete drug. Most renally excreted drugs are cleared by glomerular filtration, tubular transport, or a combination of both processes.

The *glomerular filtration rate* (GFR)—the volume of fluid filtered by the kidney per unit of time—doubles its newborn value by 2 months of age; adult levels are roughly five times the newborn level and are approached at about 12 months of age. GFR participates in the excretion of such commonly used pediatric drugs as the penicillins, short-acting barbiturates, and phenobarbital; recommended dosages of these agents for infants and toddlers are calculated to consider the low infant GFR.[1]

*Tubular transport* describes a group of mechanisms that transfer drug and drug metabolites across renal tubular epithelium. Drugs in which tubular transport plays an excretory role include morphine, atropine, and sulfa antibiotics. Many such drugs have decreased tubular transport rates in young infants and thus have narrower margins of toxicity in this patient population.[1,7]

## BLOOD AND BODY FLUIDS

### Terminology

Drug metabolism and excretion are profoundly affected by the size of various body fluid compartments. Fluid distribution among these compartments is significantly different in infancy and childhood, which in turn alters the action of certain drugs in this age group.

A brief review of body fluid nomenclature may be helpful at this point. The *total body water* space consists of *intracellular fluid* (ICF) and *extracellular fluid* (ECF) compartments. The *volume of distribution* ($V_d$) is that volume into which a drug distributes in the body at equilibrium. While $V_d$ is usually measured in plasma (the volume of plasma at a given drug concentration that is required to account for all drug in the body), many drugs distribute into body tissues as well. Thus, $V_d$ may be estimated at many times the total plasma volume.

## Physiology

### Alterations in Body Fluids

As the child grows, changes in body mass are accompanied by changes in body fluid compartments. While total body water equals 80% of the infant's weight, it makes up only 50% to 60% of normal adult body weight (Table 5-3). Much of this volume loss comes from the ECF compartment. Because so much of infant weight is water, any water-soluble drug must be administered at higher levels per unit of body weight to attain therapeutic concentration in this age group. [12]

### Plasma Protein Differences

A number of plasma proteins function to bind drug in the bloodstream. Plasma proteins both transport drug and render it less physiologically active while bound. Several of these proteins, including serum albumin and plasma globulin, are deficient in the newborn and young infant. Certain drugs that are highly protein bound (e.g., warfarin and digoxin) must be given at relatively low levels per unit of body weight in these patients. [12]

## BODY HABITUS AND INTEGUMENT

Children are obviously smaller than adults. It makes intuitive sense that they need smaller drug doses to maintain therapeutic drug concen-

trations and that smaller doses are needed to produce toxicity. The "maximal safe dose" listed in standard drug reference manuals is frequently enough to overdose a pediatric patient; weight-based formulas are much safer in the pediatric population and are appropriate in all but the smallest neonates.

Not only is the pediatric patient smaller, but his proportions are also different from those of the adult. Because a child's height triples from birth to adulthood but his weight increases 20-fold during that same period, many professionals feel that *body surface area* (BSA) is a more accurate parameter on which to base drug dosage. [2] Measured in square meters, BSA is estimated by plotting the child's height and weight on a nomogram. The BSA method should not be used in patients weighing less than 10 kg. The ratio of BSA to body weight is highest in the neonate and falls to about one-sixth of this level when adult proportions are reached just before puberty. While BSA is rarely used in the clinical setting—it is inconvenient to calculate and unwieldy to use—it has been shown to be proportional to multiple physiologic variables such as fluid requirements, oxygen consumption, metabolic rate, and cardiac output. [2,3]

The tissue composition of infants and children differs as well, depending on developmental stage. Fat makes up 10% to 15% of full-term newborn weight, increases to 20% to 25% during the first several months of life, and then declines during the toddler and preschool years as the child becomes more active. Some commonly used dental sedatives (benzodiazepines and barbiturates) are lipid soluble and are extensively bound by fatty tissue, thus decreasing serum drug levels. It follows that children with lower percentages of body fat may be more sensitive to these agents.

## SPECIAL PHARMACOLOGY TOPICS FOR THE PEDIATRIC DENTIST

Some of the medications routinely used in dental procedures are discussed below, with emphasis on their use in the pediatric population and potential problems associated with their administration.

### Benzodiazepines

Benzodiazepines have been used as premedication in the pediatric population for decades. Of this

### TABLE 5-3

### Differences in Distribution of Body Fluids Between Infants and Adults (%)

| Fluid | Infants | Adults |
| --- | --- | --- |
| Total body water | 80 | 50 (males), 60 (females) |
| Extracellular fluid | 35–40 | 20 |
| Intracellular fluid | 40–45 | 40 |

class, the two most commonly used agents are midazolam (Versed) and diazepam (Valium). Both can be administered via oral, intravenous, intramuscular, and rectal routes. There is an intranasal preparation of midazolam as well.

Midazolam has a relatively rapid onset and brief duration of action. Onset of action occurs in about 2 to 3 minutes by parenteral routes and 20 to 30 minutes from enteral routes; half-life ranges from 1 to 4 hours. In addition, it creates profound, if brief, amnesia. Midazolam causes no burning on intramuscular injection, in contrast to diazepam. Standard oral dosage is 0.5 to 0.75 mg/kg. Profound respiratory depression has been associated with midazolam use, especially when administered intravenously in combination with fentanyl. No significant morbidity has been reported in association with oral midazolam, but some transient emotional lability, vomiting, and poor head control have been reported.[7,8]

Diazepam is typically administered at 0.2 mg/kg for conscious sedation in children, but dosage requirements can vary widely even among young patients. The half-life of diazepam is about 18 hours in children and adults, but it can last up to 54 hours in preterm infants. Absorption from the intramuscular route can be delayed and thus prolong the half-life; oral administration is usually preferred.[7,8,10]

Flumazenil is used to reverse benzodiazepine sedation in cases of overdose. The dosage is 0.01 mg/kg IV; because its half-life is brief at 30 minutes, the effect of flumazenil may wear off sooner than that of benzodiazepine. Doses may be repeated in 20 minutes up to a maximum of 3 mg in 1 hour. Flumazenil may precipitate seizures in patients with tricyclic antidepressant ingestion or in those on long-term benzodiazepine therapy.[3]

### Chloral Hydrate

Commonly used in dental and radiologic settings, chloral hydrate is a sedative hypnotic agent that has no analgesic properties. It is formulated in oral and rectal preparations, and it has no antidote. Initial dosage is 50 to 75 mg/kg with maximal dose not to exceed 100 mg/kg or 2.0 g, whichever is less. If no clinical effect is observed, the dose can be repeated after 30 minutes as long as the total dose does not exceed the clinical guidelines.[3,7,11] Chloral hydrate has a fairly long onset of action (about 40 minutes) and a duration of 1 to 2 hours. Only modest depressions in respiratory rate and blood pressure are observed with therapeutic doses. Adverse effects associated with chloral hydrate include nausea, vomiting, and bradyarrhythmias. Chloral hydrate has been implicated as a potential hepatic carcinogen, but a 1993 statement from the American Academy of Pediatrics Committee on Drugs recommended its continued use as there were insufficient data to warrant concern.

## SUMMARY

Child anatomy and physiology differ significantly from that of adults. A working knowledge of those differences is essential for the pediatric dental care provider, who assesses and treats children at every developmental stage. Careful consideration of the unique needs of this patient population will promote safe and efficacious dental care. Resources available to the pediatric dentist include reference books such as the *Harriet Lane Handbook*, the internet and other computer resources, and pediatricians in the community.

## REFERENCES

1. Coulthard MG: Maturation of glomerular filtration in preterm and mature babies. *Early Hum Dev* 11:281-293, 1985.
2. Crawford JD et al: Simplification of drug dosage calculation by applications of the surface area principle. *Pediatrics* 5:783-789, 1950.
3. Gunn VL, Nechyba C, editors: *The Harriet Lane Handbook: A Manual for Pediatric House Officers*, 16th ed. Philadelphia, Mosby, 2002.
4. James LP: Pharmacology for the gastrointestinal tract. *Clin Perinatol* 29(1):115-133, 2002.
5. Johnson TR, Moore WM, Jeffries JE: *Children are Different: Developmental Physiology*. Columbus, OH, Ross Laboratories, 1978.
6. Kearns GL: Impact of developmental pharmacology on pediatric study design: overcoming the challenges. *J Allergy Clin Immunol* 106(3 suppl): S128-S138, 2000.
7. Lerman J: Anesthesia. In: Radde I, Macleod S, editors. *Pediatric Pharmacology and Therapeutics*. St Louis, Mosby, 1993, pp 476-479.
8. Maxwell LG: Perioperative management issues in pediatric patients. *Anesthesiol Clin North Am* 18(3):601-632, 2000.

9. McAllister JD: Rapid sequence intubation of the pediatric patient: fundamentals of practice. *Pediatr Clin North Am* 46(6):1249-1284, 1999.

10. Morselli PL, Principli N, Tognono G et al: Diazepam elimination in premature and full term infants and children. *J Perinat Med* 1:133-141, 1973.

11. Radde IC, Kalow W: Drug biotransformation and its development. In: Radde IC, Macleod S, editors. *Pediatric Pharmacology and Therapeutics.* St Louis, Mosby, 1993, pp 60-65.

12. Radde IC: Drugs and protein binding. In Radde I, Macleod S, editors. *Pediatric Pharmacology and Therapeutics,* St Louis, Mosby, 1993, pp 31-36.

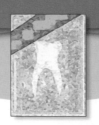

# CHAPTER 6

## Nonpharmacologic Issues in Pain Perception and Control

*Stephen Wilson*

The English word *pain* is derived from an ancient Greek word meaning "penalty" and a Latin word that meant "punishment" as well as "penalty." When the term pain is used in clinical dentistry or medicine, it is synonymous with strong discomfort. It is important to realize that despite the distress experienced by the person in pain, pain has a uniquely purposeful and necessary function. Pain signals real or apparent tissue damage that thereby energizes the organism to take action in relieving or alleviating its presence. In this sense, it is a desirable experience for maintaining and guiding the activities in life.

It is important to understand that pain is more than just a sensation and a consequential response. It is a highly complex, multifaceted interaction of physical, chemical, humoral, affective (emotional), cognitive, psychological, behavioral, and social elements. Certainly, the determinants of how an individual interprets and reacts to pain are not clearly understood. However, the body of knowledge surrounding the understanding of pain recently has begun to evolve and is accelerating rapidly into a scientific and useful discipline.

An interesting and clinically relevant parallel experience to pain is the presence of anticipatory responses secondarily acquired from the pain experience. These are conceptualized and broadly referred to as "stress" and "fear." Children and adults can be profoundly influenced by the processes attending many events perceived as fearsome, stressful, or both, including various dental procedures. For example, the 2-year-old child who presents with painful, abscessed maxillary anterior teeth due to nursing bottle caries and poorly endures the injection of local anesthesia and extractions while restrained in a papoose board will most likely develop strong disruptive and avoidance behaviors. Such behaviors may include crying with or without tears, placing hands over the mouth, refusing to open the mouth, kicking, screaming, shaking the head, spitting, and biting. These may manifest during subsequent dental appointments.

Likewise, adult patients who have been hurt either as a child or as an adult by a dentist who was not considerate or empathetic may have difficulty making and keeping appointments.

## DEFINITION OF PAIN

Pain is a highly personalized state attending tissue damage that is either real (e.g., skin laceration) or apparent (e.g., excess bowel distention) as a result of an adequate stimulus. Under normal circumstances, the state of pain implies that there is a simultaneous activation of cognitive, emotional, and behavioral consequences that provides both motivation and a direction to action.

Pain can fluctuate in intensity and quality as a consequence of the passage of time. This may be as significant to the individual as the original insult. For instance, the intensely sharp, shooting pain in the lower back of a person who used an improper weight-lifting technique may change over time (and therapies) to an intermittent deadening, dull ache that may significantly interfere with a routine life-style.

Physiologically, pain involves neural signals that are transmitted over a multitude of pathways involving neurons that are specialized in space, biochemistry, size, and shape. These signals induce a host of secondary responses that may become organized in a hierarchy of systems involving portions of the central nervous system (CNS). At the physiologic level, some of these responses involve further transmission of neural signals and the release of neurochemicals and humorally active chemicals (e.g., $\gamma$-aminobutyric acid and endogenous opioids). Other systems within this response hierarchy include those that activate motor activities for purposeful escape; still others result in emotional and cognitive appreciation of the pain experience.

Research is showing that the emotional and cognitive elements in the pain process have critical roles in the degree of pain awareness and,

possibly more importantly, in the individual's ability to induce self-control while enduring the suffering or its consequences.[29] For instance, cognitive mechanisms (e.g., cognitive dissociation) that reduce the *perceived* quality and quantity of discomfort can be effectively taught to a patient prior to the experience of clinical or laboratory-induced pain. Children, through the process of suggestion, can be taught (to varying degrees) to ignore or to inhibit responsiveness to painful stimuli during cancer therapies.[28,34]

## THEORIES OF PAIN PERCEPTION: WHY AND HOW IT IS EXPERIENCED

### Specificity

In the late $19^{th}$ century, it was believed that the pain experience was merely a function of activating a particular set of neurons that resulted, metaphorically speaking, in a "ringing of the bell" at higher levels of the CNS signifying discomfort.[21,26] The neural receptors (i.e., free nerve endings) and their pathways were considered to be specialized for the process of pain, just as other elements and pathways were rigidly designed as passages for other sensory information (i.e., pressure sensation).

Portions of this theory are reasonably accurate descriptions and therefore remain prominent in our understanding of the pain mechanism, but the simplicity of the theory is inadequate to explain the multifaceted nature of the pain experience (e.g., the phantom pain experienced by an amputee in the missing limb).

### Pattern

A slightly more sophisticated model of pain mechanisms arose as a consequence of the technological ability to record stimulus-induced activity within neural pathways. Neural activity recorded and amplified on an oscilloscope allowed some appreciation of the changes in timing and grouping of nerve action potentials as a consequence of modification in stimulus parameters. A light stroking across a patch of skin may provoke one or two isolated action potentials in large-diameter neurons servicing the area, whereas a hot thermistor (warming element) may cause an initial burst followed by a steady discharge of action potentials in smaller neurons.

It was theorized that the recognition of painful stimuli by the individual was based primarily on the pattern of nervous activity that entered the CNS. Again, this theory was inadequate to explain the complexity of the pain experience, but it contributed significantly to the advancement of knowledge about pain mechanisms.[21,26]

## Gate Control Theory

The gate control theory of pain was developed by Melzack and Wall in 1965 and has been the most influential, comprehensive, and adaptive conceptualization of pain and its consequences to date. The essence of the theory proposes that various "gates" controlling the level of noxious input via small-fiber neurons to the spinal cord can be modulated by other sensory, large-fiber neurons, higher CNS input, or both. Postulated mechanisms for the gates include presynaptic inhibitory effects on secondary transmission cells in the spinal cord. In essence, this implies that large fibers (e.g., those for touch) can cause partial depolarization of the nerve terminals of small fibers (e.g., for pain) that innervate transmission cells in the spinal cord. This results in the release of fewer "packets" of neurotransmitter molecules and a decreased likelihood that transmission cells will summate and fire.

A simplistic example would be the ameliorative inhibitory effect of the parent's rubbing a "bumped" area of the knee immediately following a toddler's fall. The light rubbing disproportionately activates greater numbers of large fibers that inhibit previously activated small fibers. In dentistry, a shaking of the lip during insertion of the needle and delivery of local anesthesia is commonly believed by many to distract or lessen the associated discomfort.

Transcutaneous electrical nerve stimulation (TENS), or the use of low-intensity electrical stimulation at peripheral sites, has been shown to provide pain relief.[31] Although the mechanism for TENS is not known, it has been suggested that its segmental effects may be due to activation of large-diameter, primary afferent fibers that in turn inhibit small-fiber transmission as predicted by the gate theory. A similar mechanism may account for the effects of acupuncture. TENS has been shown to produce partial analgesia to electrical tooth pulp stimulation in school-aged children.[2]

Proportionately more emphasis has been placed on the role and influence of higher CNS modulation of pain perception and reactivity.[18,19,29] This reorientation is partially the result of more sophisticated studies suggesting the need for a more comprehensive explanation of cognitive, behavioral, and emotional influences in pain perception and control.[23] Discoveries of endogenous opioids, widespread locations of opioid receptors throughout the CNS, and unnatural (i.e., electrical) stimulation of CNS sites resulting in pain threshold elevations also have sparked renewed interest in pain research.

In addition, animal studies have documented the presence and influence of descending supraspinal mechanisms on modulating painful input at the level of the spinal cord.[13] Interestingly, a phenomenon called stimulation-produced analgesia (SPA) has been demonstrated in both humans and animals. SPA results in specific inhibition of pain or avoidance behaviors during electrical stimulation of discrete brain sites (e.g., periaqueductal gray area of the medulla) and has few side effects. SPA of the periaqueductal gray area has been shown to inhibit jaw-opening reflexes due to tooth pulp stimulation in cats.[22]

## CENTRAL NERVOUS SYSTEM EFFECTS ON PAIN PERCEPTION AND CONTROL

An endogenous opioid system that is both complex in function and widespread throughout the mammalian CNS has been partially characterized and described.[11] Endogenous opioids are peptides that are naturally synthesized in the body and cause effects similar to those of opiates (e.g., morphine). β-Endorphin is one of the most potent peptides and has an N terminal identical to that of metenkephalin, which was one of the first opioid peptides isolated.

The active opioid peptides are cleaved from larger precursors and act at various CNS opioid receptor sites, including the spinal cord. The peptides are not equally potent, but all are inactivated by naloxone, a narcotic antagonist, and each may contribute to selective and specialized mechanisms underlying the pain perception process.

Correspondingly, there have been at least three opiate receptors characterized (μ, δ, and κ) throughout the CNS. However, the contribution of each in producing analgesia is not clear. Opioid ligands that bind to μ receptors produce potent analgesia when injected into the periaqueductal gray (PAG) area of the medulla. Other sites, extending from the hypothalamus to the rostral ventromedial medulla including the PAG, produce analgesia when properly stimulated electrically or by opiates. Curiously, the analgesic effects of nitrous oxide are believed to be partially mediated by endogenous opioid ligands or capable of directly activating opiate receptors.[10]

Theoretically, this system could mediate changes in the appreciation, motivation, and reactive processes of pain perception at higher levels of the CNS. In addition, spinal cord influences in terms of either synaptic effectiveness or neuronal sensitivity are possible.

There is evidence to suggest that this system develops early in the CNS and thus should be functional in younger children. The extent of its influence and the conditions necessary for its activation are not understood. Future studies probably will underscore the means and usefulness of activating this system in addressing clinical pain states.

## COGNITIVE ELEMENTS OF PAIN PERCEPTION

Cognition is a complex process resulting in an appreciation and often subsequent recognition of potential consequences as a function of "knowing." Knowing involves a multitude of processes including, but not limited to, perceiving, organizing, judging, meaning, reasoning, and responding.

Cognition implies an awareness of internal and external environmental influences on oneself. It also insinuates that steps can be taken to gain or command control over those influences and use the control to alter one's response (e.g., coping). For instance, one may be experiencing some discomfort but can possibly diminish the degree of discomfort by practicing mental processes (e.g., imagining pleasant events or counting holes in a ceiling tile).

A person can cope with a variety of conditions, including stressful environments, depending on his or her perception of the situation. Factors such as consequences and repercussions of the situation, its timing, and individual resources apparently are important to the outcome of coping strategies. Coping, whether realized or not, is a statement of personal success that is most rewarding.

Coping strategies may include hypnosis and relaxation techniques, imagery, modeling, distraction, and reconceptualization. Typically, thera-peutic coping strategies of pain management have a number of common elements, including (1) an assessment of the problem, (2) reconceptualization of the patient's viewpoint, (3) development of appropriate skills (e.g., breathing and relaxation), (4) generalization and maintenance of those skills in preventing relapse, and (5) measurement of therapeutic success.[27]

Evidence supports the notion that coping skills in the context of pain and anxiety can be taught even to children, and the effectiveness of cognitive training can be evaluated through self-report, physiologic, or behavioral measures. In one study, children who were undergoing restorative procedures were taught distraction and self-support techniques prior to undergoing dental procedures and subsequently compared with a group of children who were read stories. Self-report of anxiety for specific procedures (e.g., the injection) was less in those who received the cognitive training than in those who did not.[25] This lends credence to the idea that school-aged children who have had opportunities to exercise self-control in anxiety-provoking circumstances may do better if they know that they are to receive an injection as part of their treatment rather than to proceed without any forewarning. This forewarning permits the child to invoke his or her own personalized coping skills in preparation for the "dreaded event."

However, knowing ahead of time about impending discomfort can have a detrimental effect under certain conditions. For instance, the less time between informing a young child who cognitively is incapable of significant coping strategies (i.e., 3 years or less) of a procedurally related painful stimulus (i.e., injection) and doing it allows correspondingly less time for interference behaviors to occur. It is even possible that the length of emotional outburst prior to and following the procedure may be reduced under these circumstances.

Some studies indicate that adults who are led to believe that they have some control over impending discomfort do exhibit more tolerance of painful stimuli.[29] However, a strong *belief* in their ability to gain self-control is apparently an important factor in modulating the degree of discomfort. Those who lack this ability may place more trust in others (e.g., physician) and "suffer less" under their care.

Cognitive development and maturation are keys to the success of cognitive strategies. There is evidence that anxiety reduction can be attained in the medical and dental environment as a function of age in school-aged cohorts. The extent to which these strategies can be successfully applied to preschoolers is yet to be determined. However, younger children are capable of significant pain modulation through processes resembling cognitive strategies. In one study, play therapy with needles and dolls prior to venipuncture resulted in a significantly more rapid return of heart rate and less body movement within 5 minutes of blood drawing compared with controls. This finding was interpreted as evidence of reduced anxiety in the children.[32]

## EMOTIONAL ELEMENTS OF PAIN PERCEPTION

Although pain and the anticipation of painful stimuli (i.e., anxiety) invoke a personalized emotional experience, most humans have a common understanding of the attendant emotions of such experiences. Certainly, we are adept at recognizing another's suffering and possibly even better attuned to appreciating another person's anticipation of discomfort.

The expression of emotional content during or preceding painful experiences is most likely a complex combination of a partially inherited yet learning-tempered phenomenon that occurs early in life. An infant's expression of discomfort resulting from inoculations changes with aging from a more diffuse, crying, and reflexive response to one of anticipation, attentiveness toward the noxious object, and sometimes expression of anger.[7,16]

An injured child may not be overly upset until she or he notices an adult's emotional outpouring over her or his condition. This is an important consideration when allowing parents to observe injections, extractions, and other treatment procedures. Careful assessment by the practitioner of the parent's concerns and likely response mode is most important. If one anticipates that the parent will not be stoic or supportive of the procedure, it may be advisable for the parent to leave the area or have the "more stoic" parent stay with the child.

The social response to pain can be a commanding and attention-gathering entity.[12] For example, the toddler who skins a knee during a fall initially may not react as if in pain until the parent secondarily reacts to the injury. Depending on the parental response, the child may burst into tears if the parent looks upset or "toughen up" with the support of the parent's verbal encouragement.

Although one might conceive of the emotional elements of pain as being secondary to the pain itself, the emotional overtones may act in concert to modulate painful experiences. Indirect and anecdotal evidence suggests that certain pharmacologic agents (i.e., nitrous oxide and benzodiazepines) act on areas of the CNS responsible for emotional influence. A person feels the pain but is not particularly annoyed by it.

In contrast, emotional distress in anticipation of discomfort is known to lower pain thresholds and increase reactivity. Cognitive strategies designed to elicit positive emotional states can be effective in reducing anxiety and the degree of responsiveness to painful stimuli.

## CHILDREN AND PAIN

Surprisingly little is known about children and pain. Studies suggest that the developmental changes in response to painful stimuli occur early in infancy. In fact, anticipatory fears of sharp objects can be seen in children around 1 year of age.[4] As a child matures, develops a broader vocabulary, and witnesses a variety of environments, his or her ability to communicate feelings becomes increasingly sophisticated. Paralleling and reflecting the child's cognitive development are signs manifesting the evolution of coping skills.[5] In general, the pain threshold tends to decline and the self-management of pain becomes more effective with increasing age.[17] Similar self-management trends are noteworthy in the young dental patient.[33] This phenomenon undoubtedly results from the interactions of multiple factors, including the maturation of coping skills, appreciation of self-control, and social influences.

The pain associated with dental or other medically imposed procedures might be instrumental in invoking the opportunity for the development and testing of certain self-control and coping mechanisms.[6] Many children are efficient with their coping skills and tolerate mild discomfort with little overt expression. A few lack good coping skills and display hysterical behaviors (i.e., extreme panic, screaming, and struggling) in anticipation of or during minor discomforts. Consequently, any assessment of a child's behav-

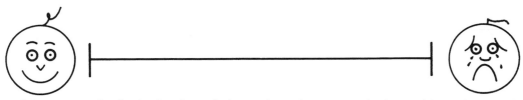

**Figure 6-1**    An example of a visual analog scale that can be used to measure the degree of discomfort in children. Note that the line is 100 mm long and is anchored at either end by happy-sad faces. The child is instructed to make a mark on the line that best describes how much pain he or she is having. The distance from the left end bar to the mark made by the child is the measure of discomfort for the child.

ioral and cognitive responses to the dental environment should be considered in light of age-appropriate expressions, specific procedures, and the use of cognitive probes.

It may appear difficult to measure the degree of pain or discomfort in a young child, especially preschool children, because of their level of cognitive and language development. Several tools have been developed for this purpose, including nonverbal self-report techniques. Thus, the intensity of pain may be represented by the number of poker chips selected, the ranking of variable expressions on happy-sad faces, the rating along a "pain thermometer" scale, and color selections.

An accumulation of evidence indicates that the visual analog scale (VAS) is one of the most reliable and valid measurement tools for self-report of pain in children. Typically, a VAS is a line approximately 100 mm in length with each end anchored by extreme descriptors (e.g., "no pain" versus "worst pain imaginable") or happy-sad faces. The patient indicates the degree of perceived pain by making a mark on the line. The length of the line from the left-hand margin to the mark determines the magnitude of pain for that individual (Fig. 6-1). Certain physiologic measurements, especially heart rate, in conjunction with self-report of discomfort are thought to add another important dimension to the characterization of response specificity to painful stimuli.[30]

Family and cultural elements are apparent in the mediation of pain-related expressions and their effects. An infant's cry may elicit protective and indulging types of behavior or, sadly, abusive behaviors in adult caretakers. Family members may respond differentially to a child's painful expressions, with females being more supportive and soothing and males more coarse and distracting. Some societies are highly sensitive to infant distress whereas others are less sensitive.

In summary, many factors may contribute to a child's perception of pain. McGrath and col-

---

**BOX 6-1**

**Factors Exacerbating Children's Pain**

**Intrinsic Factors**
  Child's anxiety, depression, and fear
  Previous experience with inadequately managed pain
  Child's lack of control
  Experience of other aversive symptoms (nausea, fatigue, and dyspnea)
  Child's negative interpretation of situation

**Extrinsic Factors**
  Anxiety and fears of parents and siblings
  Poor prognosis
  Invasiveness of treatment regimen
  Parental reinforcement of extreme underreaction (stoicism) or overreaction to pain
  Inadequate pain management practices of health care staff
  Boring or age-inappropriate environment

From McGrath PJ, Beyer J, Cleeland C et al: Report of the Subcommittee on Assessment and Methodologic Issues in the Management of Pain in Childhood Cancer. *Pediatrics* 86:814-817, 1990.

leagues[20] have listed factors that tend to exacerbate the pain in children with cancer and suggest developmental considerations for quantification of pain (Box 6-1 and Table 6-1).

## BEHAVIOR MANAGEMENT TECHNIQUES

A variety of techniques can be used to manage the behavior of a child in the dental environment. The establishment of communication combined with a caring attitude is the key building block for developing sound rapport with any patient. Consequently, the great majority of children require minimal management efforts other than

## TABLE 6-1
### Age and Measures of Pain Intensity

| AGE | SELF-REPORT MEASURES | BEHAVIOR MEASURES | PHYSIOLOGIC MEASURES |
|---|---|---|---|
| Birth to 3 years | Not available | Of primary importance | Of secondary importance |
| 3 to 6 years | Specialized, developmentally appropriate scales available | Primary if self-report not available | Of secondary importance |
| >6 years | Of primary importance | Of secondary importance | Of secondary importance |

From McGrath PJ, Beyer J, Cleeland C et al: Report of the Subcommittee on Assessment and Methodologic Issues in the Management of Pain in Childhood Cancer. *Pediatrics* 86:814-817, 1990.

providing information on what is going to happen (e.g., tell, show, and do). An important caveat is that every child responds to his or her environment with an individualized style. Practitioners must be perceptive and flexible with the use of their management techniques and optimize the likelihood of a successful encounter by matching their selection of techniques to that of the patient's style of interaction.

The American Academy of Pediatric Dentistry[1] has published guidelines on the clinical management of children and special patients. That publication includes definitions, rationales, and descriptions of techniques that are commonly used to manage the behavior of these patients (Table 6-2). The list of techniques is not exhaustive but represents the major body of empirically and scientifically derived knowledge presently available on patient management. It is probable that newer techniques as well as refinements of those presently in existence will be developed with the goal of providing both a pleasant experience and positive learning. Some of these techniques are discussed further in Chapter 23.

Behavioral and physiologic findings suggest that the three most feared or anxiety-producing stimuli in the dental operatory are the injection of local anesthesia, application of the rubber dam, and initiation of tooth preparation with the high-speed handpiece.[3,8,9,15] Knowledge of these findings should prepare the dentist and staff to anticipate and manage disruptive behaviors that may accompany these procedures. For instance, the dental assistant should passively place his or her arms slightly above the torso and arms of the patient during the injection. In this fashion, assistants are prepared to intercept the child's hands if she or he attempts to grab the dentist's hands. Otherwise, the patient may inadvertently cause trauma to themselves or the dental staff. (See Chapter 28, Figure 28-2, for an example of this procedure.)

Natural fears of bright lights, loud noises, sudden movements, and strange environments are easily aroused in and produce the most overt expressions of anxiety during the first 3 years of a child's life. These stimuli are found in every dental operatory! Consequently, the dentist and assistant should anticipate disruptive behaviors in very young children. Taking time for development of rapport and trust, using instruments that are familiar to these patients (e.g., toothbrush), and allowing a child to use them initially is a fairly successful method for gaining a young child's confidence.

Nitrous oxide/oxygen ($N_2O/O_2$) can be effective for children who are mildly to moderately anxious, can respond to guidance, and have no medical contraindications to $N_2O/O_2$ administration. In sedative concentrations (30% to 45%), the patient can derive from $N_2O/O_2$ both a calming effect and some analgesia (although local anesthesia is usually required). Key elements to improve the effectiveness of $N_2O/O_2$ include proper patient selection, maximizing nasal breathing, minimizing oral shunting of air during crying episodes, snug fit of the nasal hood over the nose, soft flexible rubber hoods that adapt to the young child's face, adequate titration, and clinical monitoring.

Nitrous oxide is not without its perils. Results of laboratory studies as well as prolonged continuous clinical exposure or recreational abuse have been associated with significant sequelae, including bone marrow depression; teratogenic, mutagenic, and carcinogenic effects; spontaneous abortions; and neuropathies.[10]

The immediate and long-term goals for the use of any behavioral management technique are

## TABLE 6-2
### American Academy of Pediatric Dentistry's Standards of Care for Behavior Management

| MANAGEMENT TYPE | DESCRIPTION | OBJECTIVES | INDICATIONS | CONTRAINDICATIONS |
|---|---|---|---|---|
| 1. Communications management | | | | |
| (a) Tell-show-do | Explanations tailored to cognitive level; followed by demonstration; followed by actual procedure | a. Allay fears<br>b. Shape patient's responses<br>c. Give expectations of behavior | All patients who can communicate regardless of communication | None |
| (b) Voice control | Modulation in voice volume, tone, or pace to influence and direct patient's behavior | a. Gain patient's attention<br>b. Avert negative or avoidance behaviors<br>c. Establish authority | Uncooperative or inattentive, but communicative child | Children who are unable to understand due to age, disability, medication, or emotional immaturity |
| (c) Positive reinforcement | Process of shaping patient's behavior through appropriately timed feedback (e.g., praise, facial expression) | a. Reinforce desired behavior | Any patient | None |
| (d) Distraction | Diverting patient's attention from perceived unpleasant procedure | a. Decrease likelihood of unpleasantness perception/threshold | Any patient | None |
| (e) Nonverbal communication | Conveying reinforcement and guiding behavior through contact, posture, and facial expressions | a. Enhance effectiveness of other communicative management techniques<br>b. Gain and/or maintain patient's attention and compliance | Any patient | None |
| 2. Conscious sedation | Pre- or intraoperative administration of sedative agents | a. Reduce or eliminate anxiety<br>b. Reduce untoward movement/reaction<br>c. Enhance communication<br>d. Increase tolerance for longer periods | Any ASA class I or II patients who cannot cooperate due to lack of psychological/emotional maturity; mental, physical, or medical disability | a. Patient with minimal dental needs<br>b. Medical contraindication to sedation |

The information in this table was taken with the permission and encouragement of the American Academy of Pediatric Dentistry: Clinical guideline on behavior management. *Pediatr Dent* 25:69-74, 2003.

*Continued*

## TABLE 6-2
### American Academy of Pediatric Dentistry's Standards of Care for Behavior Management—cont'd

| MANAGEMENT TYPE | DESCRIPTION | OBJECTIVES | INDICATIONS | CONTRAINDICATIONS |
|---|---|---|---|---|
| 2. Conscious sedation—cont'd | | e. Aid treatment of mentally, physically, or medically compromised patient | | |
| 3. General anesthesia* | Use of general anesthetics (intravenous, intramuscular, inhalation) for intraoperative care | a. Provide safe, efficient, and effective dental care | Patients with certain physical, mental, or medically compromising conditions; local anesthesia is ineffective because of acute infection, allergy; extremely uncooperative, fearful, anxious, or uncommunicative child or adolescent in whom dental care cannot be deferred; extensive orofacial/dental trauma; protection of developing psyche | a. Healthy, cooperative patient with minimal dental needs<br>b. Medical contraindication to general anesthesia |
| 4. Hand-over-mouth (HOM)* | Placement of hand over mouth while explaining behavioral expectations; removing hand when appropriate behavior is to be reinforced; reapplication if necessary | a. Gain child's attention for establishing communication<br>b. Eliminate inappropriate avoidance responses<br>c. Enhance child's self-confidence in coping during treatment<br>d. Ensure child's safety during delivery of care | A healthy child who is able to understand and cooperate, but elects to display defiant, obstreperous, or hysterical avoidance behaviors | Children who are unable to understand due to age, disability, medications, or emotional immaturity |

*Requires informed consent.

## TABLE 6-2

**American Academy of Pediatric Dentistry's Standards of Care for Behavior Management—cont'd**

| MANAGEMENT TYPE | DESCRIPTION | OBJECTIVES | INDICATIONS | CONTRAINDICATIONS |
|---|---|---|---|---|
| 5. Nitrous oxide-oxygen inhalation* | Inhalation of nitrous oxide/oxygen through nasal hood | a. Reduce or eliminate anxiety<br>b. Reduce untoward movement/reaction<br>c. Enhance communication<br>d. Increase tolerance for longer periods<br>e. Aid treatment of mentally, physically, or medically compromised patient | Fearful, anxious, or obstreperous patients; certain mentally, physically, or medically compromised patients; gag reflex is hyperactive; profound local anesthesia cannot be obtained | Chronic obstructive pulmonary disease; severe emotional disturbances; first trimester of pregnancy; drug- or disease-induced pulmonary fibrosis |
| 6. Physical restraint* | Partial or complete immobilization of patient's body or portions thereof | a. Reduce or eliminate untoward movement<br>b. Protect patient/staff from injury<br>c. Facilitate delivery of care | Cannot cooperate due to immaturity; mental or physical disability; failure of other management techniques; safety of patient/practitioner would be at risk | Cooperative patient; those who have medical or systemic conditions contraindicating restraint |

to provide as pleasant an experience as possible for the patient, instill the understanding of the attainment and maintenance of a positive oral health attitude, and promote and foster lifelong care-seeking and preventive behaviors. Hence, the dentist's attitudes and demeanor toward his or her patients are most critical to the development of a positive attitude about dentistry in those patients.

## SHORT- AND LONG-TERM CONSEQUENCES OF BEHAVIOR MANAGEMENT

Unfortunately, few well-controlled studies have addressed the impact of behavioral management techniques used in childhood on behaviors later exhibited in the adult patient. Anecdotally, it has been noted that some aggressive techniques do not interfere with a patient's seeking of future care, especially if the child was relatively young when the technique was used. On the other hand, more aggressive techniques applied in childhood have been implicated as being prominent factors in the behavior of adult phobic dental patients. Frankly, there is not enough information available to satisfactorily define this issue, but considerations of life-style, personality development, and extenuating circumstances should be addressed before any significant conclusions are drawn.

In one study, the use of hand-over-mouth in preschool children judged successful on a short-term basis by the practitioner was not found to be a significant deterrent to the development of positive attitudes of the children toward dental care.[14]

As for short-term effects, positive reinforcement has been shown to produce decreased disruptive behavior within a treatment session in children who have variable levels of baseline disruptive behaviors. Positive reinforcement may include patient praise, tokens or "stickers," and privileged socially related events (e.g., gaining the opportunity to watch a sibling or friend undergo dental treatment).

Time out (i.e., the separating of the child from the social environment or procedure that provokes disruptive behavior) appears to decrease patient disruptiveness in selected cases. The degree of success of time out varies, and factors such as the time-out period and the frequency of applied time-out episodes are important considerations. Apparently, if time out is to be effective,

it should be short and only used once or twice in attempts to gain the acceptable behavior. Longer periods and numerous uses on any given child doom the technique to failure.

Variables such as parenting style, personality, temperament, and sociability have not been studied systematically. Nonetheless, it is recognized that each child is unique in "how" he or she responds and has a distinguishable background; thus future studies will no doubt prove the importance of these variables in the child's behavior.[24]

It should be emphasized that the great majority of pediatric dental patients can be managed with simple, nonaggressive techniques. However, even the use of tell-show-do, which is perceived as the most innocuous technique, is no guarantee that the patient will not become a dental phobic or that the parent won't react strongly to its use on their child if described as a "technique." It is the wise and competent practitioner who knows children's behaviors and parents' expectations.

Chapter 23 discusses behavior management in terms of verbal and nonverbal techniques, predictors of child misbehavior, and related themes.

## REFERENCES

1. American Academy of Pediatric Dentistry: Clinical guideline on behavior management. *Pediatr Dent* 25:69-74, 2003.
2. Abdulhameed SM, Feigal RJ, Rudney JD, Kajander KC: Effect of peripheral electrical stimulation on measures of tooth pain threshold and oral soft tissue comfort in children. *Anesthesia Progr* 36:52-57, 1989.
3. Badalaty MM., Houpt MI, Koenigsberg SR et al: A comparison of chloral hydrate and diazepam sedation in young children. *Pediatr Dent* 12:33-37, 1990.
4. Barr RG: Pain in children. In: Wall PD, Melzack R, editors. *Textbook of Pain*. New York, Churchill Livingstone, 1989.
5. Brown JM, Okefe Saunders SH, Baker B: Developmental changes and children's cognition of stressful and painful situations. *Pediatr Psychol* 11:343-357, 1986.
6. Corah NL: Effect of perceived control on stress reduction and pedodontic patients. *J Dent Res* 52:1261-1264, 1973.
7. Craig KD, McMahon RJ, Morison JD, Zaskow C: Developmental changes in infant pain expressions during immunization injections. *Soc Sci Med* 19:1331-1337, 1984.

8. Currie WR, Biery KA, Campbell RL, Mourino AP: Narcotic sedation: an evaluation of cardiopulmonary parameters and behavior modification in pediatric dental patients. *J Pedodont* 12:230-249, 1988.

9. Doring KR: Evaluation of an alphaprodine-hydroxyzine combination as a sedative agent in the treatment of the pediatric dental patient. *JADA* 111:567-576, 1985.

10. Eger EI. *Nitrous Oxide.* New York, Elsevier, 1985.

11. Fields HL, Basbaum AI: Endogenous pain control mechanisms. In: Wall PD, Melzack R, editors. *Textbook of Pain.* New York, Churchill Livingstone, 1989.

12. Frodi AM, Lamb ME: Sex differences and responsiveness to infants: a developmental study of psychophysiological and behavioral responses. *Child Dev* 49:1182-1188, 1978.

13. Guilbaud G, Peschanski M, Besson JM: Experimental data related to nociception and pain at the supraspinal level. In: Wall PD, Melzack R, editors. *Textbook of Pain.* New York, Churchill Livingstone, 1989.

14. Hartmann C, Pruhs RJ, Taft TBJ: Hand-over-mouth behavior management technique in a solo pedodontic practice: a study. *J Dent Child* 52:293-296, 1985.

15. Houpt MI, Koenigsberg SR, Weiss NJ, Desjardins PJ: Comparison of chloral hydrate with and without promethazine in the sedation of young children. *Pediatr Dent* 7:292-296, 1985.

16. Izard CE, Hembree EA, Heubner RR: Infants' emotion expressions to acute pain: developmental change and stability to individual differences. *Dev Psychol* 23:105-113, 1987.

17. Katz ER, Kellerman J, Seagle SE: Behavioral distress in children with cancer undergoing medical procedures: developmental considerations. *J Consult Clin Psychol* 48:356-365, 1980.

18. Lavigne JV, Schulein MJ, Hahn YS: Psychological aspects of painful medical conditions in children: I. Developmental aspects and assessment. *Pain* 27:133-146, 1986.

19. Lavigne JV, Schulein MJ, Hahn YS: Psychological aspects of painful medical conditions in children: II. Personality factors, family characteristics and treatment. *Pain* 27:147-169, 1986.

20. McGrath PJ, Beyer J, Cleeland C et al: Report of the subcommittee on assessment and methodologic issues in the management of pain in childhood cancer. *Pediatrics* 86:814-817, 1990.

21. Melzack R, Wall PD: Pain mechanisms: a new theory. *Science* 150:971-979, 1965.

22. Oliveras JL, Woda A, Guilbaud G, Besson JM: Inhibition of the jaw-opening reflex by electrical stimulation of the periaqueductal gray matter in the awake, unrestrained cat. *Brain Res* 72:328-331, 1974.

23. Rasnake LK, Linscheid TR: Anxiety reduction in children receiving medical care: developmental considerations. *J Dev Behav Pediatr* 10:169-175, 1989.

24. Schechter NL, Bernstein BA, Beck A et al: Individual differences in children's response to pain: Role of temperament and parental characteristics. *Pediatrics* 87:171-177, 1991.

25. Siegel LJ, Peterson L: Stress reduction in young dental patients through coping skills and sensory information. *J Consult Clin Psychol* 48:785-787, 1980.

26. Sternbach RA: *Pain: A Psychophysiological Analysis.* New York, Academic Press, 1968.

27. Turk DC, Meichenbaum DH: A cognitive-behavioural approach to pain management. In: Wall PD, Melzack R, editors. *Textbook of Pain.* New York, Churchill Livingstone, 1989.

28. Weisenberg M: Pain and pain control. *Psychol Bull* 84:1008-1041, 1977.

29. Weisenberg M: Cognitive aspects of pain. In: Wall PD, Melzack R, editors. *Textbook of Pain.* New York, Churchill Livingstone, 1989.

30. Winer GA: A review and analysis of children's fearful behavior in dental settings. *Child Dev* 53:1111-1133, 1982.

31. Woolf CF: Segmental afferent fibre-induced analgesia: transcutaneous electrical nerve stimulation (TENS) and vibration. In: Wall PD, Melzack R, editors. *Textbook of Pain.* New York, Churchill Livingstone, 1989.

32. Young MR, Fu VR: Influence of plan and temperament on the young child's response to pain. *Child Health Care* 18:209-215, 1988.

33. Zachary RA, Friedlander S, Huang LN et al: Effects of stress-relevant and -irrelevant filmed modeling on children's responses to dental treatment. *J Pediatr Psychol* 10:383-401, 1985.

34. Zeltzer L, LeBaron S: Hypnosis and nonhypnotic techniques for reduction of pain and anxiety during painful procedures in children and adolescents with cancer. *J Pediatr* 101:1032-1035, 1982.

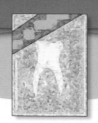

# CHAPTER 7

## Pain Perception Control

*Stephen Wilson, Diane C. Dilley, and William F. Vann, Jr.*

Pain is a complex, multidimensional phenomenon mediated by physicochemical processes in the peripheral and central nervous system (CNS). Perception of pain can be significantly modified by any of a host of mechanisms, including drugs, environmental stimuli, cognitive and emotional processes, and social and cultural conditions. In terms of a conceptual context, pain may be thought of as a continuum whose boundaries are limited yet variable for each individual. On the lower end of the continuum is the pain perception threshold. The pain perception threshold can be defined as the least amount of stimulation applied to tissue that an individual can barely detect as being unpleasant. The pain tolerance threshold is a notable point of intensely noxious stimulation on the pain continuum above which the individual cannot reasonably endure and will seek definitive measures to relieve the pain. Determination of the pain perception threshold usually is associated with experimental conditions; however, more intense stimulation approaching or exceeding the pain tolerance threshold is more characteristic of clinical conditions.

The overwhelming majority of pharmacologic agents used in dentistry are administered to control anxiety and pain. Generally the elimination of pain sensation in the dental setting requires blocking of pain perception either peripherally using local anesthesia or centrally with general anesthesia. Anxiety is controlled, in part or completely, by using sedation that may involve pharmacologic or nonpharmacologic techniques or both. Anxiety and pain control in actual clinical practice overlap to a significant degree.

There is no *best* technique for control of anxiety and pain. A practitioner may have a favorite technique, but one technique is not useful for all dental patients in all situations. The prudent and wise dentist has a working knowledge of several techniques and selects, on an individual basis, the one that appears to be the most appropriate for a particular patient. In some cases, this may necessitate referral.

## GENERAL ANESTHESIA

General anesthesia renders the patient unconscious through depression of the CNS, thus eliminating patient cooperation as a factor.

There are categories of patients in whom the only reasonable anesthetic alternative for safe treatment is general anesthesia. Examples may include very young, precooperative children and mentally retarded children who are unable to cooperate during complicated or extensive dental procedures.

General anesthesia should be administered under the direction and supervision of an individual who has completed an American Medical Association– or American Dental Association–accredited training program, usually at the postdoctoral level, which provides comprehensive and appropriate training necessary to manage general anesthesia cases. Such individuals must be licensed by the state to administer general anesthesia.

## LOCAL ANESTHESIA

### Mechanisms of Action

Pain perception may be altered at the peripheral level by blocking propagation of nerve impulses using local anesthesia. One dimension of the process of pain perception involves production of nerve impulses, or action potentials, by a noxious stimulus that activates specific receptors (nociceptors) at nerve endings. The nerve impulses travel along the nerve fibers via a physiochemical process involving ion transport across the neuronal membrane. The primary effect of local anesthetic agents is to penetrate the nerve cell membrane and block receptor sites that control the influx of sodium ions associated with membrane depolarization.[4] Current thinking holds that the sequence of events involved in a local

anesthetic block consists of (1) binding of the local anesthetic to a receptor site that exists on the inside of the cell membrane, (2) blockade of the sodium channels through which the sodium ions would normally enter during depolarization, (3) decrease in sodium conductance, (4) depression of the rate of electrical depolarization, (5) failure to achieve threshold potential, and (6) lack of development of a propagated action potential and thus blockade of conduction of the nerve impulse.[2] In general, small nerve fibers are more susceptible to the onset of action of local anesthetics than large fibers. Accordingly, the sensation of pain is one of the first modalities blocked, followed by cold, warmth, touch, and pressure.

Local anesthetic agents are weak chemical bases and are supplied generally as salts, such as lidocaine hydrochloride. The salts may exist in one of two forms: either the uncharged free base or the charged cation. The free-base form, which is lipid soluble, is capable of penetrating the nerve cell membrane. Penetration of the tissue and cell membrane is necessary for the local anesthetic to have an effect because the receptor sites are located on the inside of the cell membrane. This explains in part why local anesthetic agents are not as effective in areas of an acute infection where the local tissues are acidic. Once the free base has penetrated the cell, it re-equilibrates, and the cation is thought to be the form that then interacts with the receptors to prevent sodium conductance.

### Local Anesthetic Agents

*Esters*
Discovered in 1860, cocaine was the first local anesthetic. Because of the number of adverse side effects associated with cocaine, attempts were made to develop alternatives that retained the local anesthetic properties of cocaine while eliminating the side effects. Several other benzoic acid ester derivatives were developed, including benzocaine, procaine (Novocain), tetracaine (Pontocaine), and chloroprocaine (Nesacaine). The major problem with the ester class of local anesthetics is their propensity for producing allergic reactions.

*Amides*
The amides, a relatively new class of local anesthetics, were introduced with the synthesis of lidocaine in 1943. These compounds are amide

derivatives of diethylaminoacetic acid. They are relatively free from sensitizing reactions. Since lidocaine was synthesized, several other local anesthetics have been introduced. All are amides and include mepivacaine (Carbocaine), prilocaine (Citanest), bupivacaine (Marcaine), and etidocaine (Duranest).

## Local Anesthetic Properties

Individual local anesthetic agents differ from each other in their pharmacologic profiles (Table 7-1). They vary in their potency, toxicity, onset time, and duration. All these characteristics may be clinically important, and all vary as a function of the intrinsic properties of the anesthetic agent itself and the regional anesthetic procedure employed. Furthermore, these characteristics may be modified by the addition of vasoconstrictors.

### Potency

The intrinsic potency of a local anesthetic is the concentration required to achieve the desired effect of nerve blockade. Procaine has the lowest intrinsic potency; lidocaine, prilocaine, and mepivacaine have intermediate potency; and tetracaine, bupivacaine, and etidocaine are of high potency. It is important to note that these types of local anesthetics do not necessarily come in the same percent concentration; hence, caution is needed to prevent exceeding toxic doses of local anesthesia, especially when used in combination with other agents affecting the cardiovascular and CNS (e.g., sedatives).

### Onset Time

Onset time is the time required for the local anesthetic solution to penetrate the nerve fiber and cause complete conduction blockade. Clinically, it must be understood that conduction blockade requires time for onset; otherwise, unnecessary pain may result from beginning a procedure too soon.

### Duration

Duration of anesthesia is one of the most important clinical properties considered when choosing an appropriate local anesthetic agent for a given procedure. A local anesthetic with increased protein binding capacity and a vasoconstrictor will have a longer duration than an agent with decreased protein binding and no vasoconstrictor. Generally, procaine and chloro-

procaine, which are used primarily for spinal anesthesia, are considered of short duration. Lidocaine, mepivacaine, and prilocaine have an intermediate duration, whereas bupivacaine and etidocaine have a long duration.

### Regional Technique

A major factor that determines drug characteristics is the type of regional (local) anesthetic procedure employed. Depending on whether topical, infiltration, or a major or minor nerve block is employed, onset and duration of the various agents will vary. Potency is not affected.

**Onset.** Local anesthesia of the soft tissues by the infiltration technique occurs almost immediately with all of the local anesthetics. As more tissue penetration becomes necessary, the intrinsic latency of onset previously discussed plays a greater role. Generally, in dentistry, for any given drug the onset time required is shortest with an infiltration block, longer with a peripheral (minor) nerve block, and longest for topical anesthesia.

**Duration.** Duration of anesthesia varies greatly with the regional technique performed. This profile may differ for different agents, depending on their intrinsic pharmacologic properties. For example, lidocaine (1%) with epinephrine (1:200,000) has a duration of 416 minutes with infiltration, 178 minutes with ulnar nerve block, 156 minutes with epidural anesthesia, and 94 minutes with spinal block.[2]

### Other Factors

**Dose.** The quality, onset time, and duration of a local anesthetic block may be improved by increasing the dose of the agent by using a higher concentration or greater volume. Increases in dosage must be limited by anesthetic toxicity; however, for consistently effective local anesthetic block, an adequate concentration and volume must be administered as close to the target nerve(s) as possible.

**Vasoconstrictors.** Onset time, duration, and quality of block are also affected by the addition of vasoconstrictor agents to the local anesthetic solution. Vasoconstrictor agents such as epinephrine decrease the rate of drug absorption by decreasing blood flow to the tissues, prolonging the duration of the anesthesia produced, and increasing the frequency with which adequate anesthesia is attained and maintained. Toxic effects of local anesthetics are reduced as a result

## TABLE 7-1

### Properties of Common Dental Local Anesthetics

| Generic Name | Brand Name | Type | Concentration | Vasoconstrictor | Max. Rec. Dose (mg/kg) | Absolute Max. (mg) | Av. Duration Pulpal Tissue (min) | Av. Duration Soft Tissue (hr) |
|---|---|---|---|---|---|---|---|---|
| Propoxycaine with procaine | Ravocaine / Novocain | Ester / Ester | 0.4% / 2% | 1:20,000 levonordefrin (Neo-Cobefrin) | 6.6 | 400 | 30–60 | 2.3 |
| Lidocaine | Xylocaine | Amide | 2% | 1:100,000 epinephrine | 4.4 | 300 | 60 | 3–5 |
| Mepivacaine | Carbocaine | Amide | 3% | | 4.4 | 300 | 60–90 | 2–3 |
| Mepivacaine | Carbocaine | Amide | 2% | 1:20,000 levonordefrin (Neo-Cobefrin) | 4.4 | 300 | 60–90 | 3–5 |
| Prilocaine | Citanest | Amide | 4% | | 6.0 | 400 | 10 (infil) 60 (block) | 1½–2 2–4 |
| Prilocaine | Citanest Forte | Amide | 4% | 1:200,000 epinephrine | 6.0 | 400 | 60–90 | 3–8 |
| Bupivacaine | Marcaine | Amide | 0.5% | 1:200,000 epinephrine | 1.3 | 90 | 90–180 | 4–12 |
| Etidocaine | Duranest | Amide | 1.5% | 1:200,000 epinephrine | 8.0 | 400 | 90–180 | 4–9 |
| Articaine* | Ultracaine D-S | Amide | 4% | 1:200,000 epinephrine | 7.0 (adult) 5.0 (child) | 500 | Infil: 220 (adult) 150 (child) Block: 270 (adult) 225 (child) | NA |
| Articaine* | Ultracaine D-S Forte | Amide | 4% | 1:100,000 epinephrine | 7.0 (adult) 5.0 (child) | 500 | Infil: 180 (adult) 150 (child) Block: 285 (adult) 230 (child) | NA |

*Available in Europe and Canada.

NA, Not available

of delay in absorption into the circulation. Onset time of anesthesia is sometimes shortened as well.

In pediatric dental patients, a vasoconstrictor is needed because the higher cardiac output, tissue perfusion, and basal metabolic rate tend to remove the local anesthetic solution from the tissues and carry it into the systemic circulation more quickly, thus producing a shorter duration of action and a more rapid accumulation of toxic levels in the blood. Finally, vasoconstrictors produce local hemostasis following local anesthetic infiltration into the operating field. This assists in postoperative hemorrhage control, an advantage in the management of young children undergoing dental extractions.

Vasoconstrictors are all sympathomimetic agents that carry their own intrinsic toxic effects. These include tachycardia, hypertension, headache, anxiety, tremor, and arrhythmias. It has been shown that 2% lidocaine containing a concentration of 1:250,000 epinephrine is as effective in increasing the depth and duration of local anesthesia block as higher concentrations of epinephrine such as 1:100,000 or 1:50,000.[3] To avoid vasoconstriction toxicity in children, a concentration of 1:100,000 epinephrine should not be exceeded. The pharmacologic properties of the local anesthetics commonly used in dentistry are summarized in Table 7-1.

## Toxicity

The use of local anesthetics is so common in dentistry that the potential for toxicity with these agents can be easily overlooked. Dentists who treat children should always be mindful of local anesthetic toxicity. Toxic reactions to local anesthetics may be due to overdose, accidental intravascular injection, idiosyncratic response, allergic reaction, or interactive effects with other agents (e.g., sedatives).

The dental practitioner should be familiar with the maximal recommended dose for all local anesthetic agents that are used on a dose-per-body-weight basis (i.e., milligrams per kilogram). Simply knowing a total milligram for the average adult is not adequate and may lead to overdose in pediatric patients. Maximal safe doses for local anesthetics are listed in Table 7-1.

### Central Nervous System Reactions
Local anesthetic agents cause a biphasic reaction in the CNS as blood levels increase. Although local anesthetics have depressant effects in general, they are thought to selectively depress inhibitory neurons initially, producing a net effect of CNS excitation. Subjective signs and symptoms of early anesthetic toxicity include circumoral numbness or tingling, dizziness, tinnitus (often described as a buzzing or humming sound), cycloplegia (difficulty in focusing), and disorientation. Depressant effects may be evident immediately. These include drowsiness or even transient loss of consciousness. Objective signs may include muscle twitching, tremors, slurred speech, and shivering followed by overt seizure activity. Generalized CNS depression characterizes the second phase of local anesthetic toxicity, accompanied sometimes by respiratory depression.

### Cardiovascular System Reactions
The cardiovascular response to local anesthetic toxicity is also biphasic. During the period of CNS stimulation, the heart rate and blood pressure may increase. When plasma levels of the anesthetic increase, vasodilatation followed by myocardial depression occurs, with a subsequent fall in blood pressure. Bradycardia, cardiovascular collapse, and cardiac arrest may occur at higher levels of the agents. Most local anesthetics used in dentistry cause little cardiovascular alteration even at levels associated with seizure activity. The depressant effect on the myocardium is essentially proportional to the inherent potency of the local anesthetic, with procaine being least toxic, lidocaine and mepivacaine of intermediate toxicity, and bupivacaine and etidocaine the most cardiotoxic.

The use of local anesthetic in pediatric dentistry has changed the quality and quantity of procedures possible as much as any other advances in the field. In children who are properly prepared psychologically, high-quality local anesthesia is usually all that is necessary to eliminate pain completely. One must be ever mindful of the pharmacokinetics of the agents used with children. Because of the higher cardiac output, higher basal metabolic rate, and higher degree of tissue perfusion in children, the agents tend to be absorbed more rapidly from the tissues. The less mature liver enzyme systems in young children may detoxify these chemicals at a slower rate than in adults. Also, the immature central nervous and cardiovascular systems probably are more susceptible to toxicity at lower drug levels than in adults. For these reasons, a precise local anesthetic technique should be used, aspiration techniques should be practiced, a vasoconstrictor is necessary, and a thorough knowledge of the intrinsic properties of local anesthetic agents is essential. *Above all, the recommended maximal safe dose of local anesthetic should be calculated precisely for each patient and must never be exceeded.*

## ANALGESICS

Occasionally pharmacologic relief of pain may be necessary for the child dental patient. The agents used for pain relief are termed analgesics. Ideally, analgesic drugs should relieve pain without significantly altering consciousness. Analgesics act either in the peripheral tissues or centrally in the brain and spinal cord. Narcotic analgesics are thought to act primarily in the CNS. Nonnarcotic analgesics, such as aspirin, are thought to act in the periphery at the nerve endings. The great majority of dental pain in pediatric patients can be managed using nonnarcotic agents of relatively low potency. However, children of all ages are capable of experiencing pain, and recently some investigators have expressed concern that younger children and infants may be undermedicated following certain clinical procedures.

### Nonnarcotic Analgesics

Generally, the nonnarcotic analgesics are useful for mild to moderate pain, which includes 90% of the pain of dental origin. The nonnarcotic analgesics differ from the narcotics in their site of action, their lesser degree of toxicity and side effects, and their absence of drug dependence. These drugs exert their effects primarily at the peripheral nerve endings. The standard prototype drugs in this class are aspirin, acetaminophen, and nonsteroidal antiinflammatory drugs (NSAIDs).

#### Aspirin
Since its introduction in 1899, aspirin, a salicylate (acetylsalicylic acid), has found widespread use for its analgesic, antipyretic, and antiinflammatory properties. Despite the advent of many newer drugs, aspirin remains a standard drug of choice for management of mild pain.

The most significant side effects of aspirin include alterations of coagulation by inhibition of platelet aggregation, gastric distress and dyspepsia, occult blood loss, and, very rarely, sensitivity

reactions such as urticaria, angioneurotic edema, asthma, or anaphylaxis. The anticoagulant properties of aspirin are rarely a problem in children; however, because a single dose of aspirin can increase bleeding time, aspirin should not be used prior to surgery. Aspirin should be avoided in patients with bleeding or platelet disorders and in those taking warfarin (Coumadin) or similar drugs.

The gastrointestinal effects of aspirin are the problems most commonly encountered and may be modulated by administering the drug with food or by using a buffered or enteric-coated preparation, although absorption may be affected. The more severe allergic-type reactions have been shown to occur more often in patients with preexisting asthma, atopy, or nasal polyps, and aspirin should probably be avoided in patients with such a history. The possible association of aspirin with certain viral illnesses and the development of Reye syndrome has resulted in many practitioners opting for aspirin substitutes.

**Dosage.** The recommended dosage for analgesia and antipyretic purposes in children is 10 to 15 mg given at 4-hour intervals up to a total of 60 to 80 mg/kg per day, with a maximal limit of 3.6 g/day.

#### Acetaminophen
Acetaminophen (e.g., Tylenol, Tempra, Datril) is the most common analgesic used in pediatrics in the United States today. It is an effective analgesic and antipyretic that is as potent as aspirin for management of mild pain. Unlike aspirin, acetaminophen does not inhibit platelet function.[5] It also causes less gastric upset and has not been implicated in Reye syndrome. The primary disadvantage of acetaminophen is that it has no clinically significant antiinflammatory properties.

Toxicity as a result of overdosage may result in acute liver failure with serious or fatal hepatic necrosis. It is estimated that 15 g of acetaminophen is required in an adult to produce liver damage, or more than 3 g for a child under 2 years of age. Allergic reactions are very rare. Acetaminophen is a good alternative analgesic in patients who do not require an antiinflammatory effect.

**Dosage.** The recommended dosage for acetaminophen is

Adult: 300 to 650 mg every 4 hours
Children: 10 to 15 mg/kg/dose every 4 to 6
  hours
Maximal dose: 1000 mg every 6 hours

*Nonsteroidal Antiinflammatory Drugs*

There is now available a series of drugs called nonsteroidal antiinflammatory agents, principally derivatives of phenylalkanoic acid. They exert their analgesic effects peripherally by inhibiting prostaglandin synthetase. These agents possess analgesic and antiinflammatory properties that are superior to those of aspirin, especially for arthritis, and are effective for the management of acute pain following minor surgery or trauma. The NSAIDs produce fewer bleeding problems than aspirin because their inhibition of platelet aggregation is reversible as soon as they have been excreted fully. Other side effects reported include gastrointestinal upset, rash, headache, dizziness, eye problems, hepatic dysfunction, and renal dysfunction. There are relatively few clinical drug trials evaluating NSAIDs in children, but common agents approved by the Food and Drug Administration (FDA) for children are ibuprofen (PediaProfen, Children's Advil) 4 to 10 mg/kg every 6 hours; naproxen (Naprosyn) 5 to 7 mg/kg two to three times per day; and tolmetin (Tolectin) 5 to 7 mg/kg three to four times per day. Both ibuprofen and naproxen are available in oral suspension form.

## Narcotic Analgesics

The narcotics or opioids have been shown to interact with opioid receptors in the CNS.[6] These interactions result in the pharmacologic effects characteristic of the narcotics, including analgesia, sedation, and cough suppression. Narcotics are significantly more effective against severe and acute pain than the nonnarcotic analgesics. However, they carry the serious drawbacks of a much greater incidence of adverse effects such as sedation, respiratory depression, and dependence and abuse. There are many narcotic analgesics available, including morphine, meperidine (Demerol), fentanyl (Sublimaze), codeine, oxycodone (Percodan), and hydromorphone (Dilaudid). Most of these drugs must be administered parenterally. Meperidine, oxycodone, and codeine are available in an oral form. Only codeine will be discussed in this section.

*Codeine*

Codeine is the standard of comparison for oral narcotics and is the most commonly prescribed narcotic for moderate to severe pain. It is absorbed well when given orally and may be used for more severe pain that is not responsive to aspirin, acetaminophen, or NSAIDs. Codeine is much less potent than its relative morphine. It has far less addictive potential because it does not alter mood significantly. Side effects include nausea, sedation, dizziness, constipation, and cramps. When given in low doses, its antitussive effect makes it an important drug for the management of cough. If given in high doses or over prolonged periods, codeine may produce the more serious side effects of respiratory depression and dependence seen with the other, more potent narcotics.

Codeine may be given alone or in combination with another analgesic. Because the narcotics act at a central site and the nonnarcotic analgesics act at a separate peripheral site, it is prudent to combine the two types of analgesics for enhanced activity. An example is acetaminophen with codeine (Tylenol No. 3).

**Dosage.**   It is recommended that codeine be given in combination with acetaminophen when it is given orally for pediatric analgesia. The recommended dosage is

Children:  0.5 to 1.0 mg/kg given every 4 to 6 hours as needed

Adults:  30 to 60 mg given every 4 to 6 hours as needed.

It has been reported that 17% of children undergoing invasive restorative treatment and 22% of children needing tooth extraction require postoperative analgesia.[1] When choosing an analgesic agent, it is rare that the recommended doses of acetaminophen or NSAIDs will not control dental pain. Should this situation occur, codeine in combination with acetaminophen usually provides the needed relief. In the very rare situation in which dental pain is refractory to these modalities, a more potent agent such as meperidine may be used. The duration of such drug usage should always be very brief and embarked on with great care. Definitive dental therapy must be provided expediently.

## REFERENCES

1. Acs G, Drazner E: The incidence of postoperative pain and analgesic usage in children. *ASDC J Dent Child* 59:48-52, 1992.
2. Covino BG: *Local Anesthetics: Mechanism of Action*

*and Clinical Use.* New York, Grune and Stratton, 1976.

3. Keesling GR, Hinds EC: Optimal concentration of epinephrine in lidocaine solutions. *JADA* 66:337, 1963.

4. Malamed SF: *Handbook of Local Anesthesia,* 3rd ed. St Louis, Mosby, 1990.

5. Shannon M, Berde CB: Pharmacologic management of pain in children and adolescents. *Pediatr Clin North Am* 36(4):855-871, 1989.

6. Tyler DC: Pharmacology of pain management. *Pediatr Clin North Am* 47:59-71, 1994.

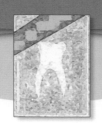

# CHAPTER 8

## Pain Reaction Control: Sedation

*Stephen Wilson, William F. Vann, Jr., and Diane C. Dilley*

The majority of pediatric dental patients can be treated in the conventional dental environment. By establishing good rapport with the patient and parent and by relying on sound behavior management techniques (see Chapter 23), the anxiety and pain of many pediatric dental patients can be managed effectively using only local anesthesia. In a few children who are unable to tolerate dental procedures comfortably despite gentle encouragement and adequate local anesthesia, anxiety and pain control will have to go beyond communicative behavioral modification and physiochemical blockade of the anatomic pathways. For such patients additional steps must be taken to control anxiety. Pharmacologic management is indicated for children who cannot be managed with traditional behavioral management techniques and local anesthesia.

The primary purpose of pharmacologic management of young patients is to minimize or eliminate anxiety. General anesthesia, to our knowledge, totally eliminates anxiety and the pain reaction threshold. Sedation, depending on its depth, produces a relative reduction in anxiety facilitating (1) the opportunity to invite the patient to use learned coping skills and (2) the raising of the pain reaction threshold. However, sedation and general anesthesia are not without significant risks against which the benefits of these techniques must be measured. The degree of sedation depends on a host of factors with the more prominent being dose, rate, and route of drug administered and patient metabolic rate, surface area, age, and general health. Thus and importantly, sedation represents a continuum whose effects vary from very mild anxiolysis to a deep sedation indistinguishable from general anesthesia. Traditionally, this continuum has been divided into the broad classes of "conscious sedation" and "deep sedation" based on conventional wisdom. In recent years the term "conscious sedation" has received considerable scrutiny; hence the term "minimal and moderate sedation" has replaced "conscious sedation" and is now the standard terminology in medical settings. For the purposes of this textbook, the new terminology of minimal and moderate sedation will be adopted and replace conscious sedation found in previous editions. For the practitioner who uses sedation, education and training beyond most dental school curricula involving sedation techniques is necessary for deep sedation and some levels of minimal and moderate sedation.

In 1985, the American Academy of Pediatric Dentistry and the American Academy of Pediatrics jointly endorsed "Guidelines for the Elective Use of Conscious Sedation, Deep Sedation, and General Anesthesia in Pediatric Patients."[2] These guidelines set the current standard of care for those who practice these sedation techniques for pediatric patients. The American Academy of Pediatric Dentistry has revised the guidelines, with the latest revision appearing in 2004. The revised guidelines are unique in the sense that they use descriptive levels of sedation, based on behavioral and clinical indices, to refine the traditional concepts and definitions of minimal, moderate, and deep sedation[1] (Table 8-1).

The guidelines emphasize that the goals of sedation are to (1) facilitate the provision of quality care; (2) minimize the extremes of disruptive behavior; (3) promote a positive psychological response to treatment; (4) promote patient welfare and safety; and (5) return the patient to a physiologic state in which safe discharge, as determined by recognized criteria, is possible.

The purpose of this chapter is to focus on minimal and moderate sedation and its use, as an adjunct, in the management of anxiety and pain control in pediatric patients. Because of the potential overlap of minimal and moderate sedation with deep sedation and general anesthesia, the latter modalities must be discussed and clarified in the context of defining what minimal and moderate sedation is and, more important, what it is not.

Before discussing minimal and moderate sedation, several key definitions will be spelled out, and the fundamental differences between minimal and moderate sedation, deep sedation, and general anesthesia will be delineated. These terms are defined clearly in the guidelines as follows.

## MINIMAL AND MODERATE SEDATION

Minimal and moderate sedation is a depressed level of consciousness in which the patient retains the ability to maintain a patent airway independently and continuously and to respond appropriately to light physical stimulation or verbal command, such as "Open your eyes." For the very young or handicapped individual who is incapable of giving the usually expected verbal responses, a minimally depressed level of consciousness for that individual should be maintained. Unfortunately, this is contrasted usually with the need to overcome more primal and emotional responses often associated with such an individual and thus requires deeper levels of sedation. Ideally, the caveat that loss of consciousness should be unlikely is a particularly important part of the definition of minimal and moderate sedation, and the drugs and techniques used should carry a margin of safety wide enough to render unintended loss of consciousness unlikely. Note that moderate sedation suggests that a child may be in a state wherein eyes are temporarily closed; however, the child is arousable following a verbal prompt (i.e., opens his or her eyes) or responds to the degree that crying *and* withdrawal reflexes occur following mildly painful stimulus such as an injection of local anesthetic. Crying and withdrawal reflexes are prominent at this level of sedation, whereas deeper levels of sedation may result only in moaning *or* withdrawal reflexes. If arousal, as described above, does not occur, especially following a repeated moderately painful stimulus (e.g., trapezius muscle pinch), then the child is in a state of deep sedation and must be monitored accordingly. Currently, the minimal monitoring requirement for most levels of minimal and moderate sedation is the use of a pulse oximeter, blood pressure cuff, and a precordial stethoscope. Future guidelines may require capnography for moderate levels of sedation.

## DEEP SEDATION

Deep sedation is a controlled state of depressed consciousness or unconsciousness from which the

## TABLE 8-1
### Definitions and Characteristics for Levels of Sedation

| LEVEL | MINIMAL SEDATION | MODERATE SEDATION | DEEP SEDATION | GENERAL ANESTHESIA |
|---|---|---|---|---|
| Goal | Decrease or eliminate anxiety; facilitate coping skills. | Decrease or eliminate anxiety, facilitate coping skills. Younger patients show age-appropriate behaviors including crying; older patients demonstrate interactive state. | Eliminate anxiety; coping skills unaffected and overridden. Patient uneasily aroused but may respond to purposeful stimulation. | Eliminate sensory and skeletal motor activity, autonomic activity depressed. |
| Patient responsiveness | Subjectively, the patient may sense and/or express less anxiety about the clinical procedure compared to presedation periods. Objectively, the patient may appear calmer and less overtly responsive to clinical stimuli, and purposefully interactive with the clinician compared to presedation periods. | Subjectively, the patient may sense and/or express less anxiety about the clinical procedure compared to presedation periods. Objectively, the patient may appear less tense, cognizant of, but less overtly to, clinical stimuli, responsive and purposefully interactive with the clinician compared to presedation periods. The patient, if behaviorally and cognitively cooperative, should be able independently to move his/her head and/or mandible, as directed by the clinician, and to assist in maintaining optimal airway patency. | Subjectively, the patient may sense and/or express limited or no feelings of anxiety associated with the clinical procedure. Objectively, the patient may appear very relaxed, not cognizant of and minimally or nonresponsive to clinical stimuli, and noninteractive with the clinician at any time. The patient would not be able independently to move his/her head and/or mandible to maintain optimal airway patency consistent with the clinical situation and under these circumstances, requires continuous monitoring of the airway and continual assistance of the clinician (e.g., head tilt, chin lift procedure). | Unconscious and unresponsive to surgical stimuli. |

*BP*, Blood pressure; *BPC*, blood pressure cuff/sphygmomanometer; *PO*, pulse oximetry; *PC*, precordial/pretracheal stethoscope; *Capno*, capnograph/end-tidal carbon dioxide monitor; *ECG*, electrocardiogram.

**TABLE 8-1**

**Definitions and Characteristics for Levels of Sedation—cont'd**

| Level | Minimal Sedation | Moderate Sedation | Deep Sedation | General Anesthesia |
|---|---|---|---|---|
| Physiologic changes | Patient remains stable and within age-appropriate and health status norms for parameters involving hemodynamic, ventilation, and oxygenation functions. No loss of protective reflexes. | Patient remains stable and within age-appropriate and health status norms for parameters involving hemodynamic, ventilation, and oxygenation functions. No loss of protective reflexes. | Patient remains stable and either minimally or moderately below the patient's age and health status norms for hemodynamic, ventilation, and oxygenation functions. Accompanied by partial or complete loss of protective reflexes. | Partial or complete loss of protective reflexes including the airway; does not respond purposefully to verbal command or physical stimulus |
| Personnel needed | 2 | 2 | 3 | 3 |
| Monitoring equipment | Clinical observation unless patient becomes moderately sedated, then appropriate monitoring needed. | BPC, PO, PC, or Capno. | BPC, PO, PC/Capno, ECG.  AU: ECG as meant? | BPC, PO, PC/Capno, ECG, Temp. |
| Monitoring info and frequency | Skin color, respiratory effort. | HR, RR, BP, Sao₂. | HR, RR, BP, Sao₂, ETco₂, ECG. | HR, RR, BP, Sao₂, ETco₂, Temp, ECG. |
| | (Continual) | (q15m) | (q5m) | (q5m) |

patient is not aroused easily. Deep sedation may be accompanied by a partial or complete loss of protective reflexes, including the ability to maintain a patent airway independently and to respond purposefully to physical stimulation or verbal command. Young patients who are in deep sedation may respond with only a reflex withdrawal to an intensely painful stimulus, if at all. Monitoring requirements for deep sedation require a minimum of a pulse oximeter, capnograph, precordial stethoscope, electrocardiograph, and blood pressure cuff.

## GENERAL ANESTHESIA

General anesthesia is a controlled state of unconsciousness accompanied by a loss of protective reflexes, including the inability to maintain an airway independently and respond purposefully to physical stimulation or verbal command.

## MINIMAL AND MODERATE VERSUS DEEP SEDATION: A CRITICAL QUESTION

The difference between minimal and moderate versus deep sedation is a concept that must be comprehended thoroughly by those who sedate pediatric dental patients. Practitioners must realize that the goal of minimal and moderate sedation is a level of sedation that does not render the patient unconscious or unresponsive to verbal prompting or, at the most, to repetitive but minimally painful stimuli. A reflex withdrawal response alone to repeated minimal or moderately painful stimuli is not appropriate for minimal and moderate sedation and is indicative of deeper levels of sedation. The patient under minimal and moderate sedation can respond appropriately to verbal commands or minimally noxious stimuli and is able to maintain a patent airway at all times. If sedation techniques are practiced in this manner, the patient's cardiovascular and respiratory functions should always be within normal limits for the age of the child and well maintained.

Why is it a problem for the practitioner to move from the threshold of minimal and moderate sedation to deep sedation? The answer is simple: The patient has a much more frequent and serious risk of respiratory or cardiovascular misadventures during deeper levels of sedation.

When the patient has a partial or complete loss of protective reflexes and cannot maintain an airway independently, laryngospasms, apnea, or hypoxemia may be serious or life-threatening outcomes.[4] Because the separation between moderate and deep sedation can sometimes be difficult to discern, it is the wise practitioner who obtains proper training in sedation and monitoring techniques before routinely using pharmacologic management for children. Furthermore, the current guidelines indicate that the practitioner should be sufficiently trained to "rescue" the child should he or she become compromised. Although it is appropriate to call 911 in an emergency, the practitioner must not rely solely on the arrival and intervention of the emergency management system (EMS) personnel. In other words, active intervention using basic or advanced life support must be accomplished by the practitioner and his or her staff while awaiting arrival of the EMS team. Since the depth of sedation levels is not always predictable, especially with oral routes of administration, the practitioner needs to be trained and able to rescue a child who enters a deeper level of sedation than originally intended or planned for the procedure.

For those practitioners who choose to practice deep sedation for pediatric patients, the guidelines are specific about requirements for a higher level of personnel training as well as a higher level of vigilance in monitoring the patient's vital signs and level of sedation. They spell out requirements for personnel, the operating facility, intravenous access, monitoring procedures, and recovery care that carry a higher level of expectation and training than is the case with the use of minimal or moderate sedation.[3] In short, for practitioners who choose to use deep sedation, the standard of care specified in the guidelines is nothing less than stringent, and it is doubtful that many general practitioners or pediatric dentists currently have the training or facilities to undertake deep sedation in an office-based setting.

## RELIANCE ON THE GUIDELINES AS THE STANDARD OF CARE FOR MINIMAL AND MODERATE SEDATION

The guidelines have established a new standard of care for minimal and moderate sedation of pediatric patients. Because they were initially promulgated relatively recently (1985), it is instructive to examine those areas that have been affected most dramatically. In considering presedation events, the guidelines focus on parental instructions, dietary precautions, and a preoperative health evaluation. Essentially, the guidelines intensify the presedation activities with a keen eye toward eliminating the possibility of sedation misadventures. They call also for documentation and recording of events during treatment (i.e., vital signs, medications given, and patient response).

The three standards in the guidelines that have most dramatically changed the manner in which pediatric sedation is practiced in the office setting relate to (1) personnel, (2) patient monitoring, and (3) preprocedural prescriptions. Relative to personnel, the guidelines specify that an assistant other than the dental operator must participate in the sedation procedure and that this assistant must be trained to monitor appropriate physiologic parameters and assist in any support or resuscitation measures required. Relative to intraoperative monitoring procedures during sedation, the guidelines specify continuous monitoring by a trained individual. A precordial stethoscope, blood pressure cuff, and pulse oximeter are considered the minimal equipment needed for obtaining continuous information on heart rate and respiratory rate. Based on recent research in this area, the pulse oximeter is currently considered the standard of care for monitoring pediatric patients under moderate and deeper levels of sedation.[4,14,15]

Preprocedural prescriptions refer to the practitioner writing a script for the parent to administer an agent outside of the treatment facility. Preprocedural prescriptions for antianxiety (i.e., diazepam [Valium]) for older children who are extremely anxious may be helpful, although no strong evidence is available to support this notion. For younger children (i.e., pre-school age), use of prescriptions outside of the treatment facility and without professional supervision is not appropriate. Any sedative that causes the child to become sleepy or lose consciousness should never be administered at home by parents or guardians on the night before or during the day prior to transporting a child to a facility where a procedure will be performed (e.g., chloral hydrate, meperidine [Demerol], or high-dose benzodiazepines). Again, chloral hydrate and meperidine are not considered minor tranquilizers or antianxiety agents and thus should not be administered to a child outside of the dental office.

In summary, the guidelines have had a major impact on how the practitioner must approach the sedation of children. There are no systematic evaluations of the impact of the guidelines on safety in pediatric sedation; however, it is our opinion that these guidelines are having a dramatic impact in improving the safety of sedation in the dental office environment. Unfortunately, significant morbidity and mortality have occurred [6-9]; however, no deaths have occurred, to our knowledge, when the guidelines have been faithfully followed by the practitioner.

## ROUTES OF ADMINISTRATION

The primary routes of administration for minimal and moderate sedation are (1) inhalational, (2) enteral (e.g., oral or rectal), (3) and parenteral (e.g., intramuscular, subcutaneous, submucosal, intranasal, or intravenous). In reviewing these techniques, only the primary advantages and disadvantages will be discussed briefly.

### Inhalational Route (Nitrous Oxide)

*Advantages*
The primary advantages of nitrous oxide for sedation in pediatric dentistry are discussed in the following sections.

**Rapid Onset and Recovery Time.** Because nitrous oxide has very low plasma solubility, it reaches a therapeutic level in the blood rapidly; conversely, blood levels decrease rapidly when nitrous oxide is discontinued.

**Ease of Dose Control (Titration).** There are two ways to initially administer nitrous oxide to children. One is the standard titration technique used on adults, and the other is the rapid induction technique. For the standard titration technique, nitrous oxide should be started at 10% concentration and administered in increments of concentration, ranging from 5% to 10%, until the patient becomes comfortable and some clinical signs of optimal sedation are noted. The signs of optimal sedation include slight relaxation of the limbs and jaw muscles; ptosis of the eyelids; a blank stare as if looking up at a star-filled evening sky; palms open, warm, and slightly moist; slight change in the pitch of the patient's voice; and patient reports of being comfortable and relaxed.

Each time the clinician increases the concentration, he or she should wait approximately 30 seconds while talking with the child and watch for classic signs of optimal sedation before deciding to increase the concentration again. The end point in terms of maximal concentration of nitrous oxide usually should not exceed 50% for children. Most children seem comfortable and demonstrate optimal signs of sedation in the concentration range of 35% to 50% nitrous oxide. The standard titration technique is primarily used for mildly anxious but cooperative children.

A second option to the standard titration technique of nitrous oxide administration is the rapid induction technique. This technique is usually indicated for the mild to moderately anxious, potentially cooperative child who may be on the edge of losing coping abilities and needs to be controlled quickly by the clinician. The technique involves administering 50% nitrous oxide immediately to the patient without any titration steps.

In either technique, nitrous oxide should be discontinued if the child becomes disruptive and no longer breathes through the nitrous oxide hood or if the child becomes nauseated, vomits, or both. Also, good nitrous oxide hygiene is always indicated and includes the use of a scavenging system, large operatories, rapid room-air exchanges, supplemental movement of air (i.e., fans), and a nasal hood that adapts closely to the nose area of the face.

**Lack of Serious Adverse Effects.** Nitrous oxide is considered to be inert and nontoxic when it is administered with adequate oxygen. The most commonly encountered side effect is nausea, which should be very rare unless high concentrations of nitrous oxide are used. Poor technique with high concentrations may also result in an excitement phase, in which the patient may become uncomfortable, uncooperative, and delirious.

### Disadvantages

The use of nitrous oxide in pediatric dentistry also has several disadvantages.

**Weak Agent.**  Attempts to increase the concentration of nitrous oxide in order to control *moderately or severely* anxious patients will be fraught with failure and will not be pleasant for the operator or the patient.

**Lack of Patient Acceptance.**  There are some patients (adults and children) who do not find the effects of nitrous oxide pleasant. These patients may become overtly noncompliant, removing the nasal mask or becoming otherwise uncooperative.

**Inconvenience.**  In some areas, such as the maxillary anterior teeth, the use of a nitrous oxide nasal mask may hinder exposure of the area. This may be a problem especially in small children.

**Potential Chronic Toxicity.**  Retrospective survey studies of dental office personnel who were exposed to trace levels of nitrous oxide suggest a possible association with an increased incidence of spontaneous abortions, congenital malformations, certain cancers, liver disease, kidney disease, and neurologic disease.[5,13] These results underscore the necessity of scavenging (removing) waste gases adequately from the dental operatory. It should be noted that it can be difficult to scavenge nitrous oxide adequately in the uncooperative child because gases that are exhaled through the mouth cannot be scavenged effectively.

**Potentiation.**  Although nitrous oxide is a weak and very safe agent when used with oxygen, deep sedation or general anesthesia may be easily produced if nitrous oxide is added to the effects of other sedative drugs given by another route. The combination of nitrous oxide with any other sedation agents must be undertaken with extreme care and by an individual who has the proper training and experience.

**Equipment.**  Equipment must be purchased, installed, tested for proper function, and maintained. The level of nitrous oxide may be adjusted in small increments to produce the desired effect.

### Practical Utilization of Inhalation Sedation Techniques

Nitrous oxide analgesia is relatively safe and effective for the treatment of children in the dental office. It is useful for decreasing minimal levels of anxiety and is indicated for patients who have the capacity to be compliant and follow instructions during nitrous oxide administration. Children who have nasal obstructions or are uncooperative when directed to breathe through the nose are poor candidates for nitrous oxide administration. The analgesic properties of nitrous oxide help to raise the pain threshold and may be used to lessen the discomfort during a local anesthetic injection. However, nitrous oxide will not eliminate the need for local anesthetic pain control in most children except for very minor dental procedures (e.g., small class V preparations).

Nitrous oxide changes the patient's perception of the environment and the passage of time and is therefore helpful in managing children with short attention spans. This minimal dissociation may be perceived by some children as unpleasant, in which case the level of nitrous oxide concentration should be decreased or the administration discontinued.

A total liter flow rate per minute of gases should be established first with 100% oxygen. An adult will require 5 to 7 L/min, whereas a 3- to 4-year-old will require 3 to 5 L/min. While adjusting the controls, the dentist should use the "tell-show-do" technique with terminology appropriate for the age level of the child (e.g., "smell the happy air"). The nosepiece should be introduced with instructions to breathe nasally. Minimal finger pressure under the lower lip to produce an oral seal and gentle tapping of the nosepiece can be helpful to encourage nasal breathing in the young child.

After stabilization of the nosepiece and delivery of 100% oxygen for 3 to 5 minutes, the nitrous oxide level should be increased to 30% to 35% and administered for 3 to 5 minutes for the induction period. While administering the nitrous oxide, the dentist should talk gently to the child to promote relaxation and reinforce cooperative behavior. Although asking older children and adults if they feel tingling sensations in the fingers and toes is appropriate for verification of early signs of central nervous system (CNS) effects from the nitrous oxide, these suggestive questions to the young child may lead to undesirable body movements. An indication of such CNS effects would be minimal or continual movements of the fingers and toes in the young child.

Most dentists prefer to increase the level of nitrous oxide to 50% for 3 to 5 minutes to provide maximum analgesia for the local anesthetic injection; however, concentrations of nitrous oxide in excess of 50% are usually contraindicated for dental office sedation. When the dental injection is completed, the nitrous oxide level should be reduced to 30% to 35% for a maintenance dose during the dental treatment; alternatively, 100% oxygen may be administered when the nitrous oxide is only needed for behavior management related to the dental injection.

Upon termination of nitrous oxide administration, inhalation of 100% oxygen for not less than 3 to 5 minutes is recommended. This allows rapid diffusion of nitrous oxide from the venous blood into the alveolus while maintaining oxygenation, enabling the patient to return without incident to pretreatment activities. Inadequate oxygenation may produce such postoperative side effects as nausea, light-headedness, or dizziness, all of which can be reversed with continued oxygen administration.

It is important for the dentist to recognize that nitrous oxide analgesia should not be used as a substitute for the traditional nonpharmacologic approach to child management problems in the dental office. Nitrous oxide should be considered an adjunct to aid in management of minimal anxiety in the child who is capable of cooperating in the dental chair.

## Oral Route

A route of administration used commonly for minimal and moderate sedation in pediatric dentistry is oral premedication.

### Advantages

**Convenience.**   Usually oral drug administration is easy and convenient, especially if the medication tastes good and can be delivered in low volume. Usually it is best to administer oral premedications in a separate, quiet room in the office where induction of sedation can be facilitated by the parent in a conducive environment.

**Economy.**   To administer oral premedications, no special office equipment needs to be purchased or maintained. However, special equipment is needed to monitor patients' vital signs and level of sedation as specified in the guidelines.

**Lack of Toxicity.**   If therapeutic doses are calculated for each patient (keeping the previous discussion on pharmacokinetics in mind) and single drugs are used in single doses, the oral route of sedation is extremely safe. However, if drug combinations are used or if two routes are combined (e.g., oral premedication followed by intravenous or inhalational medications), the chance of adverse side effects increases dramatically.

### Disadvantages

**Variability of Effect.**   The biggest disadvantage of oral premedication is the fact that a standard dose must be used for all patients on a weight or body surface area (BSA) basis. However, individuals of the same weight (or BSA) may respond quite differently to the same dose of drug, depending on many variables. Absorption of the drug from the gastrointestinal tract can be altered by several factors, such as the presence of food, autonomic tone, fear, emotional makeup, fatigue, medications, and gastric emptying time. The patient may not cooperate in ingesting the medication or may vomit, making estimation of the dose actually received impossible. In some cases, a paradoxical response may be seen, which may be due to a direct effect or loss of emotional inhibitions. The patient may become agitated and more uncooperative rather than sedated and cooperative. These factors make the oral route of administration least dependable as far as certainty of effect is concerned. A second dose of oral medication to offset a presumably inadequate dose should never be given. Titration is not possible or safe with oral medication. If absorption of the initial dose has been delayed for any reason and a second dose is subsequently given on the assumption that the first dose was ineffective, both doses will eventually be absorbed, possibly resulting in a high serum level of the CNS-depressant drug and leading to possible serious consequences such as respiratory arrest, cardiovascular collapse, and death.

**Onset Time.**    Oral drug administration has the longest time of onset of any route used for sedation. The lag time varies from 15 to 90 minutes depending on the drug and should be allowed from the time of administration until treatment is attempted.

Oral premedication is very useful in pediatric dentistry, but its limitations must be clearly understood. An adequate dose must be given, and enough time must be allowed to elapse for absorption to take place before the desired effect can be expected.

## Intramuscular Route

The intramuscular route of drug administration involves injection of the sedative agent into a skeletal muscle mass. It also involves certain advantages and disadvantages when used in pediatric dentistry.

*Advantages*
**Absorption.**    Absorption from an injection deep into a large muscle is much faster and more dependable than absorption from the oral route.

**Technical Advantages.**    Technically, the intramuscular route of administration might be considered the easiest of all routes. It requires no special equipment except a syringe and needle.

Patient cooperation is required for the oral route of administration, sometimes making it very difficult to give a full dose of a bitter-tasting medication to an uncooperative child. When intramuscular medications are administered, little or no patient cooperation is required, and the full calculated dose is given with a high degree of certainty. Even when a child requires restraint, intramuscular injections are easier to accomplish technically than placement of an intravenous cannula.

*Disadvantages*
**Onset.**    Absorption of the injected drug can be decreased or delayed by several factors. A patient who is cold or very anxious may experience peripheral vasoconstriction in the area of the injection, significantly decreasing the rate of absorption. Perhaps the biggest variable in onset is related to where the drug is actually deposited. If the drug is deposited deep into a large muscle mass, the high degree of vascularity there will allow quite rapid uptake. If, however, some or the entire drug is deposited between muscle layers, on the surface of the muscle, or not in the muscle at all (all distinct possibilities in small, struggling children), absorption may be quite unpredictable.

**Effect.**    As with the oral route, a standardized dose is used, calculated on the patient's weight or BSA. Drug effect cannot be titrated safely by administering additional doses for much the same reason as that described for the oral route, that is, the possibility of cumulative overdose. A standard dose may have little or no effect in some children, whereas it may sedate others heavily.

**Trauma.**    Injection sites that are devoid of large nerves and vessels are used for intramuscular injections, such as the mid-deltoid region, the vastus lateralis muscle of the thigh, and the gluteus medius muscle. Proper selection of the injection site and proper technique should minimize the possibility of tissue trauma.

**Intravenous Access.**    The potential for more rapid side effects and toxicity is higher with the intramuscular route than with the inhalational or oral route. Compared with the intravenous route, a major disadvantage of this route is the lack of a patent intravascular means of access (an intravenous catheter) in the event of a medical emergency.

**Liability Costs.**    Malpractice insurance carriers charge a higher premium for dentists who administer parenteral sedatives in the dental office. In addition, many state dental practice acts have established requirements for permits for dentists who administer parenteral medications.

## Subcutaneous Route

Occasionally, the subcutaneous route of administration is used in pediatric dentistry for sedation. In this situation, the drug is injected into the subcutaneous or submucosal space, not into the muscle. Generally, similar advantages and disadvantages apply to this route as to the intramuscular route with the following exceptions.

### Advantages

**Site.**    For dental procedures, some drugs may be injected submucosally within the oral cavity, usually into the buccal vestibule. This may be less objectionable to some patients and parents than multiple injection sites, and the dentist may find it more comfortable and convenient to perform.

### Disadvantages

**Technical Disadvantages.**    The rate of absorption is slower with the subcutaneous route than with the other parenteral routes. Blood supply to the subcutaneous tissue often is sparse compared with muscle. However, submucosal injections in the oral cavity have a relatively rapid effect because the vascularity is abundant.

**Tissue Slough.**    Because the drug is deposited close to the surface of the skin or mucosa, the possibility of tissue sloughing is present. For this reason, only nonirritating substances should be given subcutaneously, and large volumes of solution should not be injected.

**Liability Costs.**    Administration of parenteral medications increases the costs of malpractice coverage and may be subject to state dental laws that require permits for the use of parenteral sedation.

## Intravenous Route

The intravenous route is the optimal and ideal route for administration of sedative agents.

### Advantages

**Titration.**    Among the parenteral routes, only the intravenous route allows exact titration to a desired drug effect. Because the drug is injected directly into the bloodstream, absorption is not a factor. Within a few circulation times, the intravenous drug will exert its maximal effect. Small, incremental doses may be given over a relatively short period until the desired level of sedation is achieved, thus avoiding under- or overdosing with a standardized single-bolus dose, as is necessary with oral, intramuscular, or subcutaneous injections.

**Test Dose.**    With the intravenous route, a very small initial test dose can be administered, and a short time is allowed to pass to observe for an allergic reaction or extreme patient sensitivity to the agent.

**Intravenous Access.**    In the event of a medical emergency, administration of emergency drugs is almost always best accomplished through the intravenous route. Establishing intravenous access after an emergency has occurred can be very difficult and can consume precious time.

### Disadvantages

The intravenous route would be used for all patients requiring sedation if it did not involve some disadvantages.

**Technical Disadvantages.**    Establishment of intravenous access (venipuncture) is technically the most difficult skill that must be mastered in the practice of minimal and moderate sedation. Placing and maintaining an intravenous catheter in children can be difficult even for a seasoned clinician. The procedure requires both training and extensive practice.

**Potential Complications.**    Because potent drugs are injected directly into the bloodstream, the intravenous route carries an increased potential for complications. Extravasation of drug into the tissues, hematoma formation, and inadvertent intraarterial injections are possible complications of a misplaced intravenous catheter. If the medication is injected too rapidly, exaggerated effects may be produced. An immediate anaphylactic allergic reaction will become life threatening more rapidly if it is due to an intravenous bolus of a drug than if it is due to an oral or intramuscular dose. All of these complications should be avoidable by using a test dose and a proper, careful technique. Thrombophlebitis is a rare complication that is attributable directly to the intravenous cannula.

**Patient Monitoring.**    Because of the previously discussed increased potential of developing complications rapidly, the patient receiving intravenous sedation requires the highest level of monitoring.

**Liability Costs.** Again, because the intravenous route is a parenteral route, the liability costs are considerably higher than for oral administration. With the additional monitoring and the armamentarium required, intravenous sedation is considered by many to be cost prohibitive for the routine practice of general dentistry.

## PHARMACOLOGIC AGENTS FOR SEDATION

A large number of drugs are available for use in sedation and anesthesia. In this text individual drugs or techniques will be put into perspective rather than discussed in detail. Three primary groups of drugs are used for sedation in pediatric dentistry: the sedative-hypnotics, the antianxiety agents, and the narcotic analgesics (Table 8-2). Each group acts primarily in a different area of the brain and should be expected to produce a distinctive primary effect. The wise practitioner will understand which specific effect to expect from a given drug and will use the drug principally to achieve that effect.

### Sedative-Hypnotics

The sedative-hypnotics are drugs whose principal effect is sedation or sleepiness. As the dose of a sedative-hypnotic drug is increased, the patient will become increasingly drowsy until sleep (hypnosis) is produced. Further increasing the dose can produce general anesthesia, coma, and even death. It is important to note that the primary effect of these drugs is not to decrease anxiety or to raise the pain threshold (analgesia). In fact, a sedative-hypnotic used alone may lower the pain reaction threshold in some cases by removing inhibitions, and at inadequate dosages it may simply produce a patient who is more responsive to pain stimulation. The principal action of the sedative-hypnotics results from the initial primary effect of these drugs on the retic-ular activating system, an area of the brain involved in maintaining consciousness. Further increases in dose will affect other brain areas, especially the cortex.

The sedative-hypnotic drugs fall into two categories: barbiturates, such as pentobarbital, secobarbital, and methohexital; and nonbarbiturates, such as chloral hydrate and paraldehyde.

Oral chloral hydrate, alone or in combination with other drugs, is a common sedative agent used in pediatric dentistry. When used in low doses (25 to 40 mg/kg), chloral hydrate can produce minimal and moderate sedation, or it can have the opposite effect, producing a resistive and agitated patient, as occurs also with barbiturate sedation in children. Higher doses (50 to 60 mg/kg), especially in combination with other premedications such as hydroxyzine (Atarax or Vistaril) or meperidine can produce deeper levels of sedation; therefore, patients' vital signs and level of consciousness must be monitored closely, according to the guidelines, because of the increased risk of respiratory depression and loss of consciousness.[11] Chloral hydrate is bitter tasting, which can produce management problems during administration. A final disadvantage is that chloral hydrate can induce nausea and vomiting secondary to gastric irritability.

### Antianxiety Agents

Previously the antianxiety agents were called minor tranquilizers (the major tranquilizers are the antipsychotic drugs). These drugs have the primary effect of removing or decreasing anxiety. The primary site of action of these agents is the limbic system, which is the "seat of the emotions." Theoretically, a dose exists for each antianxiety agent at which anxiety will be decreased without producing significant sedation. As doses are increased, however, the reticular activating system and then the cortex are affected, producing sedation and sleep as well. Because anxiety is often the

---

**TABLE 8-2**

**Minimal and Moderate Sedation: Pharmacologic Agents**

| GROUP | SITE OF PRIMARY EFFECT | EFFECT |
|---|---|---|
| Sedative hypnotics | Reticular activating system | Sedation/sleep |
| Antianxiety agents | Limbic system | Decrease in anxiety |
| Narcotics | Opioid receptors | Analgesia |

primary problem in people with dental phobias, a primary effect against anxiety appears to be desirable, especially in reasonably cooperative adults. Antianxiety drugs possess a flatter dose-response curve pharmacologically than many of the sedative-hypnotics (especially barbiturates), allowing for a safer therapeutic index. This means that for most antianxiety drugs (e.g., diazepam), a larger difference exists between the dose that will produce loss of consciousness than is the case with a rapid-acting sedative-hypnotic (e.g., methohexital [Brevital]), which has a steep dose-response curve; that is, the difference between a minimally sedating dose and general anesthesia is quite small. Drugs such as methohexital should not be used for sedation for this reason. The antianxiety agents produce no analgesia.

The antianxiety agents consist primarily of the benzodiazepines, such as diazepam (Valium), midazolam (Versed), and triazolam (Halcion). This group of agents is the one principally used for minimal and moderate sedation in adults. Unfortunately, there is a lack of extensive clinical experience and research on these agents in children, but clinical evidence is increasing for the potential of these drugs in pediatric patients.[10] Midazolam has become the most popular benzodiazepine for pediatric sedation in the medical and dental settings primarily because of its rapid onset, decreased likelihood of inducing loss of consciousness, and reversibility with a benzodiazepine antagonist (i.e., flumazenil). However, midazolam has some characteristics that are not always beneficial to the practitioner for some operative procedures (e.g., short acting and increased patient irritability primarily after local anesthetic administration).

Some of the antihistamines, such as hydroxyzine (Atarax, Vistaril) and diphenhydramine (Benadryl) possess both antianxiety and sedative-hypnotic properties. They are often classified with the antianxiety agents. These drugs are not very useful for sedation when used alone but are useful in combination with other drugs, such as the sedative-hypnotics, at potentiating agents. They may be also used as comedicaments because of their antiemetic properties.

## Narcotics

The narcotics were discussed previously in the section on analgesics. These drugs are used also in sedation for their primary action of analgesia.

The site of action of the narcotics is the opioid receptors of the CNS. These drugs modify the interpretation of the pain stimulus in the CNS and therefore raise the pain threshold. As the dose of the narcotic is increased, other effects such as sedation will occur. It should be recognized that sedation per se is not the principal end point sought from a narcotic. If narcotic dosage is pushed to achieve sedation, serious side effects will be encountered, the most common of which are respiratory depression and apnea, which can lead to hypoxia. If sedation is desired, the narcotic should be accompanied by a drug that produces sedation as its primary effect.

Narcotics may produce nausea and vomiting, especially when used alone. In high doses, narcotics may also produce cardiovascular depression. Narcotics are potent potentiators of other CNS depressant drugs. Therefore the principal use of narcotics in minimal and moderate sedation should be to augment the effects of the sedative-hypnotic or antianxiety agents and to contribute some degree of analgesia that other agents do not provide. It should be noted, however, that the analgesia obtained with narcotics cannot be used as a substitute for adequate local anesthesia.

Narcotics used in sedation techniques include morphine, meperidine, and fentanyl (Sublimaze). Alphaprodine (Nisentil) was formerly a popular synthetic narcotic for pediatric sedation but was withdrawn from the U.S. market in 1986 owing to multiple adverse reactions resulting in death or severe morbidity. When considering the use of narcotics in pediatric dentistry, it is wise to remember the definition of minimal and moderate sedation as spelled out in the guidelines. To reiterate, the caveat that loss of consciousness should be unlikely is a particularly important part of the definition of minimal and moderate sedation. The drugs and techniques used should carry a margin of safety wide enough to render unintentional loss of consciousness unlikely.[3] Narcotics have steep dose-response curves. They must be used with extreme caution for minimal and moderate sedation because they carry a high risk of producing respiratory depression and loss of consciousness, especially if they are combined with other agents such as nitrous oxide.

## Ketamine

The dissociative agent ketamine has had periods of popularity in pediatric dental practice. It produces a cataleptic state with profound analgesia and amnesia. Because ketamine acts primarily on the thalamus and cortex, not on the reticular activating system, the patient does not appear to be asleep but rather dissociated from the environment. Respirations usually are not depressed with proper dosages. Profound stimulatory cardiovascular changes usually are produced, so tachycardia and increased blood pressure can be expected.

Ketamine is mentioned primarily to point out that it is classified as a general anesthetic because the patient under its influence is incapable of making appropriate responses to verbal commands or stimulation. It may cause respiratory depression and arrest in some patients as well as delirium and hallucinations. Ketamine should be used only by practitioners qualified to administer general anesthesia.

## Monitors

There are a host of monitors used during sedation and general anesthesia.[15] The most common are pulse oximeters, capnographs, blood pressure cuffs, precordial stethoscopes, electrocardiographs, temperature probes, and defibrillators. The mix of monitors required for any sedation will depend on the final depth of sedation. The most common monitors for minimal and moderate sedation are pulse oximeters, precordial stethoscopes, and blood pressure cuffs. These will be briefly outlined.

### Pulse Oximeter

A pulse oximeter is a self-contained instrument that noninvasively monitors the degree of oxygen saturation of hemoglobin molecules in the patient's blood and the patient's heart rate. Oxygen sensors placed across perfused tissue beds in which a pulse can be detected (e.g., the fingertip) determine oxygen saturation by measuring differences in the absorption of red and infrared light that is emitted by the sensors. Normally, the hemoglobin in arteries of healthy children and adults is 97% saturated (but is read as 100% by pulse oximeters). However, several factors can cause "false alarms" or indications of desaturation when, in fact, the hemoglobin molecule is completely saturated with oxygen. Such factors may include patient movement artifacts, cold tissue beds, poor perfusion of tissue beds, and crying.

### Precordial Stethoscope

Precordial stethoscopes are essentially stethoscopes whose bell is temporarily attached to the chest wall. By listening through the stethoscope, the clinician can determine the quality and relative quantity of air movement during breathing as well as the heart sounds. The closer the bell of the stethoscope is placed to the precordial notch (i.e., in the soft tissue area immediately above the manubrium of the chest), the louder are the breathing sounds in comparison with the heart sounds. Partially occluded airways or restrictive airways have different qualities of sounds, including wheezing, stridor, and crowing. The precordial stethoscope is especially sensitive to competing operatory sounds (e.g., the pitch of the high-speed handpiece), and the operator must rely frequently on other clinical signs or physiologic monitors (e.g., capnographs) to determine the stability and condition of the patient.

## THE FUTURE

The level of training required for a dentist to administer sedation or anesthesia safely is currently under debate and is changing throughout the United States. In many states special permits are required to practice certain anesthetic techniques.

Deep sedation and general anesthesia are grouped together for training requirements, medicolegal reasons, and purposes of malpractice insurance. *The clinician should remember that a sedation technique from which a patient is not easily aroused and may not respond purposefully to verbal commands at all times is, by definition, deep sedation.* The suggested educational requirements for administration of deep sedation or general anesthesia is a minimum of 2 years of advanced study or its equivalent as described in Part II of the American Dental Association's "Guidelines for Teaching the Comprehensive Control of Pain and Anxiety in Dentistry."[12] Many states have adopted requirements for deep sedation and general anesthesia.

In summary, a pharmacologic approach to managing the behavior of uncooperative children in the dental office with sedation is very complex and requires additional training beyond the scope of this textbook. An undersedated child may continue to pose a management problem, whereas oversedation of a child may quickly become a life-threatening emergency in the dental office.

# REFERENCES

1. American Academy of Pediatric Dentistry: Elective use of minimal, moderate, and deep sedation and general anesthesia in pediatric dental patients. *Pediatr Dent* 24:90-98, 2004.

2. American Academy of Pediatric Dentistry: Guidelines for the elective use of conscious sedation, deep sedation, and general anesthesia in pediatric patients. *Pediatr Dent* 7:334-337, 1985.

3. American Academy of Pediatric Dentistry: Guidelines on the elective use of conscious sedation, deep sedation, and general anesthesia in pediatric dental patients. *Pediatr Dent* 24:74-80, 2002.

4. Anderson JA, Vann WF Jr: Respiratory monitoring during pediatric sedation: pulse oximetry and capnography. *Pediatr Dent* 10(2):94-101, 1988.

5. Cohen EN, Gift HC, Brown BW et al: Occupational disease in dentistry and chronic exposure to trace anesthetic gases. *JADA* 101(1):21-31, 1980.

6. Cote CJ, Karl HW, Notterman DA et al: Adverse sedation events in pediatrics: analysis of medications used for sedation. *Pediatrics* 106(4):633-644, 2000.

7. Cote CJ, Notterman DA, Karl HW et al: Adverse sedation events in pediatrics: a critical incident analysis of contributing factors. *Pediatrics* 105(4 Pt 1):805-814, 2000.

8. Jastak JT, Peskin RM: Major morbidity or mortality from office anesthetic procedures: a closed-claim analysis of 13 cases. *Anesth Prog* 38(2):39-44, 1991.

9. Krippaehne JA, Montgomery MT: Morbidity and mortality from pharmacosedation and general anesthesia in the dental office. *J Oral Maxillofac Surg* 50(7):691-698; discussion 698-699, 1992.

10. Moore PA: Monitoring and management: adult vs. pediatric patients (scientific abstract). *Anesth Prog* 32:168-169, 1985.

11. Nathan JE, West MS: Comparison of chloral hydrate-hydroxyzine with and without meperidine for management of the difficult pediatric patient. *ASDC J Dent Child* 54(6):437-444, 1987.

12. National Institutes of Health: Consensus development conference statement on anesthesia and sedation in the dental office. *JADA* 111:90-93, 1985.

13. Rowland AS, Baird DD, Weinberg CR, et al: Reduced fertility among women employed as dental assistants exposed to high levels of nitrous oxide. *N Engl J Med* 327(14): 993-997, 1992.

14. Wilson S: Conscious sedation and pulse oximetry: false alarms? *Pediatr Dent* 12:228-232, 1990.

15. Wilson: Review of monitors and monitoring during sedation with emphasis on clinical applications. *Pediatr Dent* 17:413-418, 1995.

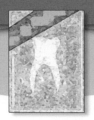

# CHAPTER 9
## Antimicrobials in Pediatric Dentistry

*Michael W. Roberts and Thomas H. Belhorn*

The second most commonly prescribed group of drugs for use in dentistry after the local anesthetics are the antibiotics. Infections involving the teeth and oral cavity can become quite severe and even life threatening if not properly managed. The management of infections usually involves a definitive dental or surgical procedure and often requires the use of antibiotics. Antimicrobials are substances that kill or suppress the growth or multiplication of microorganisms, either bacteria, viruses, fungi, or parasites. Antibiotics are substances produced by microorganisms or by synthetic chemical methods that have the capability to produce an antibacterial action. Antibiotics are indicated for diseases in which a specific bacterial pathogen has been identified, for clinical situations likely caused by a bacterial agent, and for use as a lifesaving measure in a severely ill patient. Prophylactic use of antibiotics is indicated in some specific instances, such as prophylaxis against bacterial endocarditis for patients with congenital heart disease. Antibiotic therapy is maximally successful if the causative pathogen is identified by culture or serologic testing and the therapeutic agent most active against that pathogen (confirmed by susceptibility testing) is administered in appropriate doses.

## ANTIMICROBIAL CLASSIFICATION

A large number of antimicrobial agents are available for use in pediatric dentistry. There are multiple classification schemes for these agents, including differentiation by microbial target, mode of action, and effect on the bacterial pathogen.

## Microbial Target

Antimicrobial agents are often categorized according to microbial target group. The principal emphasis of this chapter is on antibacterial agents, i.e., antibiotics. Antibiotics are considered to be either of narrow or wide spectrum. Narrow-spectrum antibiotics are effective primarily against either gram-positive or gram-negative organisms. Broad-spectrum drugs are effective against a wider range of organisms (Table 9-1).

## TABLE 9-1
### Antimicrobial Spectrum and Preferred Therapeutic Agents

| MICROBIAL SPECTRUM | CLASS OF PREFERRED ANTIMICROBIAL | EXAMPLES |
|---|---|---|
| Gram-positive aerobic bacteria | Natural penicillins | Penicillin G, Penicillin V K |
| | Penicillinase-resistant penicillins | Oxacillin, nafcillin, methicillin, dicloxacillin |
| | Aminopenicillins | Ampicillin, amoxicillin |
| | Macrolides | Erythromycin, clarithromycin, azithromycin |
| | Glycopeptides | Vancomycin, teicoplanin |
| | Cephalosporins | Cefazolin, cephalothin, cephalexin, cefaclor |
| | Lincosamides | Clindamycin |
| | Oxazolidinones | Linezolid |
| | Streptogramins | Quinupristin:dalfopristin |
| | Topicals | Bacitracin, mupirocin |
| Gram-negative aerobic bacteria | Aminoglycosides | Gentamicin, tobramycin, amikacin |
| | Extended-spectrum penicillins | Azlocillin, mezlocillin, piperacillin |
| | Antipseudomonal penicillins | Carbenicillin, ticarcillin |
| | Monobactams | Aztreonam |
| | Carbapenems | Imipenem, meropenem |
| | Cephalosporins | Ceftazidime |
| | Sulfonamides | Trimethoprim-sulfamethoxazole |
| Broad-spectrum antibacterial | Third-/ fourth-generation cephalosporins | Cefotaxime, ceftriaxone, cefepime, cefdinir, ceftibuten, cefpodoxime |
| | β-lactam + β-lactamase Inhibitor combinations | Ampicillin + sulbactam |
| | | Amoxicillin + clavulanate |
| | | Ticarcillin + clavulanate |
| | | Piperacillin + tazobactam |
| | Quinolones | Ciprofloxacin, ofloxacin, sparfloxacin, norfloxacin |
| | Carbapenems | Imipenem + cilastin, ertapenem |
| | Tetracyclines | Tetracycline |
| | Chloramphenicol | Doxycycline, minocycline |
| Anaerobic bacteria | Penicillins | Penicillin G |
| | Cephalosporins | Cefotetan, cefoxitin |
| | Carbapenems | Imipenem + cilastin, ertapenem |
| | Lincosamides | Clindamycin |
| | Chloramphenicol | Chloramphenicol |
| | Metronidazole | Metronidazole |
| Fungal infections | Polyenes | Amphotericin B |
| | Azoles | Fluconazole, itraconazole, voriconazole |
| | Echinocandins | Caspofungin |
| | Topical antifungal agents | Nystatin, clotrimazole, miconazole, tolnaftate |
| Viral infections | Anti-herpesvirus agents | Acyclovir, ganciclovir, foscarnet, famciclovir |
| | Topical anti-herpes agents | Trifluridine, idoxuridine |

Considerable overlap in effectiveness can exist with the broad-spectrum drugs. Efficacy against a particular microorganism is ideally determined by testing the susceptibility of the actual causative pathogen (obtained by culture) to specific antibiotics. Unfortunately, culture and susceptibility results may take 24 hours to several days and would delay initiation of antimicrobial therapy. This requires that a best guess be made for specific clinical situations as to which pathogen is most likely the causative agent and which antibiotic is usually most effective against it. This antibiotic, or combination of antibiotics, is used until culture and sensitivity results are available. Dental and periodontal infections are most commonly caused by bacteria that normally colonize the mouth, throat, and upper alimentary canal, e.g., aerobic and anaerobic streptococci, *Micrococcus* species, anaerobic gram-negative bacteria (*Bacteroides*, *Fusobacterium*, and *Veillonella* species), and occasionally staphylococci or spirochetes.[5] Many of these organisms are sensitive to penicillins; hence, penicillins remain the single most useful class of antibiotics for dental and periodontal infections. Occasionally, dental infections are caused by aerobic gram-negative bacteria, *Actinomycetes*, or fungi. In these cases, other antimicrobials are needed for optimal therapy.

Convenient tables listing antimicrobial treatment recommended for various medical and dental clinical syndromes and sites of infection are published and updated periodically. *Nelson's Pocket Book of Pediatric Antimicrobial Therapy*[2] and the *Sanford Guide to Antimicrobial Therapy*[6] are two publications containing such guidelines. Data from local clinical microbiology laboratories can be consulted for information on local antibiotic susceptibility patterns of common pathogens.

---

## BOX 9-1

### Antimicrobials: Mode of Action

**Inhibition of Cell Wall Synthesis**
  Penicillins
  Cephalosporins
  Monobactams
  Carbapenems
  Glycopeptides
  Azole antifungals
  Echinocandins

**Inhibition of Protein Synthesis**
*Bind 50s ribosome*
  Macrolides
  Chloramphenicol
  Lincosamides
  Oxazolidinones
  Streptogramins

*Bind 30s ribosome*
  Aminoglycosides
  Tetracyclines

**Antimetabolites**
  Sulfonamides

**Alteration of Cell Membrane Permeability**
  Polymyxins
  Clotrimazole (antifungal)
  Polyene antifungals

**Inhibition of Nucleic Acid Synthesis**
  Rifampin
  Griseofulvin
  Nucleoside antivirals

**Topoisomerase Inhibitors**
  Nalidixic acid
  Quinolones

**Inhibition of Cytochrome Sterol**
  Azoles (antifungal)

---

## Mode of Action

Antimicrobials may also be categorized according to their mode or site of action.[8] Common modes of action for antimicrobial agents are described in Box 9-1 and as follows: (1) inhibition of synthesis of the bacterial cell wall, a structure required for bacterial survival; (2) inhibition of protein synthesis, occurring at one of several possible steps; (3) interference with folic acid metabolism, thereby inhibiting bacterial growth; (4) interference with cell membrane permeability; (5) inhibition of nucleic acid synthesis; (6) inhibition of bacterial topoisomerase enzymes; and (7) inhibition of cytochrome P-450 sterol. By these mechanisms of action, the antimicrobial agents produce toxic effects that selectively interfere with the life cycle of the microbial agent while minimizing significant alterations in the cells of the human host.

## BOX 9-2

### Bactericidal and Bacteriostatic Antibiotics

**Bactericidal**
  Penicillins
  Cephalosporins
  Glycopeptides
  Carbapenems
  Monobactams
  Aminoglycosides
  Quinolones

**Bacteriostatic**
  Macrolides
  Tetracyclines
  Chloramphenicol
  Sulfonamides
  Lincosamides
  Rifampin
  Oxazolidinones
  Streptogramins

## Bactericidal Versus Bacteriostatic Antibiotics

Antibiotics may also be classified as bactericidal or bacteriostatic. Bactericidal antibiotics actually kill the microorganisms, whereas bacteriostatic antimicrobials inhibit bacterial growth or multiplication and depend on the normal host defense mechanisms (immune system) to eliminate the microorganism. The same antibiotic may be bactericidal for some pathogens but bacteriostatic for others, or the activity may be concentration dependent. Bactericidal agents are preferable in most situations. Bacteriostatic agents should be avoided if possible in immunocompromised patients as a compromised immune system may be unable to facilitate clearance of the offending microorganisms. Box 9-2 lists the agents in these categories.

## ANTIBIOTIC RESISTANCE

Bacterial resistance to antibiotics is one of the most significant challenges in the management of infectious diseases. It has been exacerbated by widespread indiscriminate use of antibiotics in veterinary, medical, and dental applications. Some of the most common current mechanisms of bacterial resistance to antibiotics are summarized in Table 9-2.

Current issues in bacterial resistance include increasing resistance of staphylococci to penicillinase-resistant penicillins (e.g., methicillin, oxacillin), resistance of pneumococci to penicillins by alteration of bacterial penicillin-binding proteins, resistance of enterococci to glycopeptide antibiotics (i.e., vancomycin), and multidrug resistance among gram-negative bacteria due to bacterial modifying enzymes and extended-spectrum β-lactamases. The oral flora causing dental and periodontal infections may be affected by the growing problem of antibiotic resistance.

The development of resistant bacterial strains may be minimized by consistently using an appropriate antibiotic dosage for an adequate period of time. For gram-negative infections, especially *Pseudomonas* infections, or infections with enterococci, treatment with combinations of antibiotics (e.g., a β-lactam and aminoglycoside) may help to prevent the emergence of resistant strains. Antibiotic combinations may also be necessary for infections with mixed types of bacteria. When planning combination drug therapy, it is important to select antibacterial agents that have synergistic or additive activity. Use of drugs that are antagonistic in combination may result in suboptimal clinical outcomes and an increased likelihood of the emergence of resistant strains.[7]

## TABLE 9-2

### Mechanisms of Bacterial Resistance

| ANTIBIOTIC CLASS | COMMON MECHANISMS OF RESISTANCE |
| --- | --- |
| Penicillin | Hydrolysis by bacterial β-lactamases, altered bacterial binding proteins |
| Cephalosporins | Hydrolysis by extended-spectrum β-lactamases, cephalosporinases |
| Macrolides | Alteration of target sites, active efflux pump |
| Aminoglycosides | Alteration in uptake, modification by bacterial enzymes |
| Glycopeptides | Modification of bacterial cell wall precursors, with decreased binding |
| Trimethoprim-sulfamethoxazole | Resistant bacterial enzymes in folate pathway |

In most university-related clinical settings, the use of antibiotics is increasingly scrutinized by formulary committees and antibiotic review panels. Multiple guidelines have been developed to provide recommendations for the appropriate use, and discourage inappropriate use, of antibiotics in various clinical situations. Hopefully, such efforts will promote an increase in the rational and appropriate use of antibiotics to minimize the spread of bacterial resistance.

## ANTIBIOTIC AGENTS

The antibiotic agents that are used most commonly in pediatric dentistry include penicillins, clindamycin, macrolides, and cephalosporins.

### Penicillins

Sir Alexander Fleming in 1928 discovered that penicillin mold lysed gram-positive microorganisms. This observation did not gain clinical usefulness until the 1940s, when the antibiotic era began. The penicillins are a group of antibiotics that differ in their pharmacologic properties. They are primarily active against gram-positive aerobic and anaerobic bacteria, but their spectrums of coverage can vary. As a group, they are the most allergenic antibiotics, and all exhibit cross-allergenicity.

#### Penicillin G
Penicillin G was the prototype of this group of antibiotic agents and continues to be the drug of choice for many infections. Its coverage is limited primarily to gram-positive organisms and selective gram-negative cocci. Penicillin G has two primary unfortunate properties. First, it is poorly absorbed orally, owing to its destruction by gastric acid, so that it is best given by the intramuscular or intravenous route. Second, it is readily destroyed by penicillinase-producing microorganisms. Semisynthetic penicillins have been developed to expand coverage and to overcome some of these disadvantages.

#### Penicillin V
The primary advantage of penicillin V is that it is stable at gastric pH, allowing for much improved absorption when it is administered orally. Its spectrum of coverage is the same as for penicillin G except for slightly less efficacy against *Neisseria gonorrhoeae* and some anaerobes. However, it is also inactivated by penicillinase. Penicillin V is the primary oral antibiotic used to manage dental infections.

#### Ampicillin and Amoxicillin
Ampicillin has a broader spectrum of coverage than penicillin G or V, covering more gram-negative organisms, including some strains of *Escherichia coli*, *Haemophilus influenzae*, and *Salmonella*. It is, however, less effective against some gram-positive organisms. Although ampicillin is absorbed better orally than penicillin G, significant degradation occurs in the gut, and diarrhea or gastrointestinal upset is common. Nine percent of children develop a maculopapular rash after receiving ampicillin. Amoxicillin has the same spectrum of coverage as ampicillin, but it is absorbed better orally and causes less diarrhea. Despite the usefulness of these drugs in pediatrics, they are not indicated over penicillin G or penicillin V for management of dental infection. Development of resistance to these agents, especially by *H. influenzae*, is becoming increasingly problematic.

#### Penicillinase-Resistant Penicillins
Most strains of staphylococci produce an enzyme, penicillinase, which destroys penicillins, resulting in drug resistance. Several penicillins have been developed that are resistant to destruction by penicillinase, including oxacillin, methicillin, nafcillin, cloxacillin, and dicloxacillin. These drugs should be reserved for infections involving penicillinase-producing staphylococci and are not indicated in common dental infections.

### Clindamycin

Clindamycin has continued to gain favor as a useful antibiotic in the management of dental infections. It possesses good activity against most gram-positive bacteria as well as most anaerobic bacterial species associated with oral infections. The development of resistance to clindamycin has not been as common as resistance to the macrolides and other classes of antibiotics. Gastrointestinal upset, including diarrhea associated with *Clostridium difficile* toxin, is occasionally associated with this drug. However, the spectrum of activity, as well as the availability of oral and intravenous formulations, has made clindamycin a good option for management of oral infections.

## Macrolides: Erythromycin, Azithromycin, and Clarithromycin

Erythromycin is a macrolide antibiotic that was introduced in 1952. Its spectrum of coverage is similar to penicillin's, with the addition of some penicillinase-producing staphylococci, chlamydiae, *Legionella*, mycoplasma, and others. It is well absorbed orally. However, the free-base form is unstable at gastric pH, so it is administered with an enteric coating or in a salt form (stearate or estolate). Gastrointestinal upset in the form of diarrhea is a major disadvantage of erythromycin. Azithromycin and clarithromycin are structural derivatives of erythromycin that possess a broader spectrum of activity and improved bioavailability. The improved tolerability, specifically with less gastrointestinal upset, has resulted in greater use of these two agents compared with erythromycin. Macrolides are usually bacteriostatic rather than bactericidal. In addition, increasing resistance to macrolides has been a concern and presents another drawback to the routine use of these agents.

## Cephalosporins

The cephalosporins are a varied group of bactericidal antibiotics that are chemically related to penicillin. They are broad spectrum in coverage and are divided into four "generations" by coverage. Many cephalosporins are similar to penicillins in their activity against gram-positive organisms (except *Streptococcus faecalis*) and are resistant to penicillinase. First-generation cephalosporins have limited activity against gram-negative enterobacteria, but the newer drugs have increasing activity against these agents. The cephalosporins exhibit some cross-sensitivity in patients who are allergic to penicillin. The oral cephalosporins include cephalexin, cefadroxil, cefaclor, and multiple other agents. They have fewer adverse effects than penicillins and taste less bitter when given orally. The cephalosporins are effective against oral pathogens, but they generally have less anaerobic activity than penicillins and at best similar activity against aerobic oral floral. Therefore, cephalosporins generally offer no advantage over penicillins for most dental infections and are usually more expensive. Cephalosporins should be reserved for severe infections involving gram-negative organisms or mixed infections.

## Summary

Most dental and periodontal bacterial infections are caused by gram-positive aerobes, facultative streptococci, and, occasionally, staphylococci. Other occasional pathogens include anaerobic gram-negative organisms such as *Bacteroides, Veillonella, Fusobacterium,* gram-negative aerobes, and diphtheroids. Penicillins, clindamycin, and perhaps azithromycin are considered good choices for initial empirical therapy. Owing to the bactericidal action and narrow spectrum of activity, penicillin V (oral) or penicillin G (intramuscular) is often recommended as the primary drug of choice for dental and periodontal infections. Resistance to antibiotic agents presents an increasing threat to effective management of bacterial infections. Current editions of publications such as the *Drug Information Handbook for Dentistry*[4] and the *American Academy of Pediatric Dentistry Reference Manual*[1] can be consulted for updated recommendations on optimal therapy of infections in the oral cavity.

# ANTIBIOTIC PROPHYLAXIS

## Endocarditis Prophylaxis

Bacterial endocarditis is a microbial infection of the endocardium (inner layer of the cardiac muscle). Certain patients with congenital cardiac lesions or acquired cardiac defects are believed to be at high risk for developing this condition if a procedure or manipulation causes a transient bacteremia. The blood-borne bacteria may lodge on the abnormal endocardium or heart valves and cause serious endocardial infection. Recommended prophylactic antibiotic regimens are based on in vitro studies, clinical experience, animal models, and assessment of the bacteria common to a particular site and those most commonly identified with endocarditis.[9]

In 1997, an ad hoc writing group appointed by the American Heart Association for their expertise in endocarditis and treatment published updated recommendations regarding antibiotic prophylaxis of bacterial endocarditis.[3] The cardiac conditions for which antibiotic prophylaxis is, and is not, recommended to prevent bacterial endocarditis are listed in Box 9-3. Antibiotic prophylaxis is recommended for *all* dental procedures likely to cause significant bleeding from soft and hard tissues, including professional oral

---

## BOX 9-3

### Cardiac Conditions Associated with Endocarditis

**Endocarditis Prophylaxis Recommended**
  High-risk category
  Prosthetic cardiac valves, including bioprosthetic and homograft valves
  Previous bacterial endocarditis
  Complex cyanotic congenital heart disease (e.g., single ventricle states, transposition of the great arteries, tetralogy of Fallot)
  Surgically constructed systemic pulmonary shunts or conduits
  Moderate-risk category
  Most other congenital cardiac malformations (other than above and below)
  Acquired valvar dysfunction (e.g., rheumatic heart disease)
  Hypertrophic cardiomyopathy
  Mitral valve prolapse with valvar regurgitation and/or thickened leaflets

**Endocarditis Prophylaxis Not Recommended**
  Negligible-risk category (no greater risk than that of the general population)
  Isolated secundum atrial septal defect
  Surgical repair of atrial septal defect, ventricular septal defect, or patent ductus arteriosus (without residua beyond 6 months)
  Previous coronary artery bypass grafting
  Mitral valve prolapse without valvar regurgitation
  Physiologic, functional, or innocent heart murmurs
  Previous Kawasaki disease without valvar dysfunction
  Previous rheumatic fever without valvar dysfunction
  Cardiac pacemakers (intravascular and epicardial) and implanted defibrillators

From Dajani AS et al: Prevention of bacterial endocarditis. *JAMA* 277:1794-1801, 1997. Copyright 1997, American Medical Association.

---

prophylaxis and initial placement of orthodontic bands (but not bracket placement), in at-risk patients. Simple orthodontic adjustments that are unlikely to cause bleeding and spontaneous shedding of deciduous teeth are felt not to present a significant risk of endocarditis; therefore, prophylaxis is not recommended in these situations.

Bacterial endocarditis after dental manipulations is most commonly caused by α-hemolytic streptococci. Therefore prophylaxis is specifically directed against these organisms. Gingivitis, periodontitis, and periapical infections can be the source of a bacteremia. Excellent oral hygiene and maintenance of dental health are important to reduce the potential for bacterial seeding in the bloodstream of at risk patients.

The dental procedures for which antibiotic prophylaxis is, and is not, recommended are listed in Box 9-4. The antibiotic prophylaxis regimens for dental, oral, or respiratory treatment or esophageal procedures are described in Table 9-3.

Additional guidelines have also been provided, including those listed in Box 9-5.

### Prophylaxis for Other High-Risk Patients

Children with a compromised immune system may be at increased risk of developing focal or systemic infection following transient bacteremia associated with dental procedures. Therefore antibiotic prophylaxis may be considered for patients with significant primary or acquired immune deficiency. Bacteremia in children with any form of indwelling hardware, including vascular shunt, ventricular shunt, central venous line, various orthopedic devices, and the like, may also provide a source of infection for the hardware. In addition to consulting current guidelines regarding prophylaxis, consulting with the child's physician is recommended for optimizing patient treatment.

## ANTIFUNGAL AGENTS

*Candida* species, and especially *C. albicans*, can often be found on the healthy mucous membranes of the body. However, multiplication of the *Candida* species and invasion of the tissues rarely occur unless the immunity of the host is compromised. Candidiasis is common in children receiving oncology treatment, particularly during periods of severe immunosuppression and neu-

## BOX 9-4

**Dental Procedures and Endocarditis Prophylaxis**

| Endocarditis Prophylaxis Recommended* | Endocarditis Prophylaxis Not Recommended |
|---|---|
| Dental extractions | Restorative dentistry[†] (operative and prostho- |
| Periodontal procedures including surgery, scaling and root planing, probing, and recall maintenance | dontic) with or without retraction cord[‡] |
| | Local anesthetic injections (nonintraligamentary) |
| Dental implant placement and reimplantation of avulsed teeth | Intracanal endodontic treatment; post placement and buildup |
| Endodontic (root canal) instrumentation or surgery only beyond the apex | Placement of rubber dams |
| | Postoperative suture removal |
| Subgingival placement of antibiotic fibers or strips | Placement of removable prosthodontic or orthodontic appliances |
| Initial placement of orthodontic bands but not brackets | Taking of oral impressions |
| | Fluoride treatments |
| Intraligamentary local anesthetic injections | Taking of oral radiographs |
| Prophylactic cleaning of teeth or implants where bleeding is anticipated | Orthodontic appliance adjustment |
| | Shedding of primary teeth |

From Dajani AS et al: Prevention of bacterial endocarditis. *JAMA* 277:1794-1801, 1997. Copyright 1997, American Medical Association.

*Prophylaxis is recommended for patients with high- and moderate-risk cardiac conditions.

[†]This includes restoration of decayed teeth (filling cavities) and replacement of missing teeth.

[‡]Clinical judgment may indicate antibiotic use in selected circumstances that may create significant bleeding.

## TABLE 9-3

**Prophylaxis Regimens for Dental, Oral, Respiratory Tract, or Esophageal Procedures**

| SITUATION | AGENT | REGIMEN* |
|---|---|---|
| Standard general prophylaxis | Amoxicillin | Adults: 2.0 g; children: 50 mg/kg orally 1 h before |
| Unable to take oral medications | Ampicillin | Adults: 2.0 g intramuscularly (IM) or intravenously (IV); children: 50 mg/kg IM or IV within 30 min before procedure |
| Allergic to penicillin | Clindamycin | Adults: 600 mg; children: 20 mg/kg orally 1 h before procedure |
| | *or* Cephalexin[†] or cefadroxil[†] | Adults: 2.0 g; children: 50 mg/kg orally 1 h before procedure |
| | *or* Azithromycin or clarithromycin | Adults: 500 mg; children: 15 mg/kg orally 1 h before procedure |
| Allergic to penicillin and unable to take oral medications | Clindamycin *or* Cefazolin[†] | Adults: 600 mg; children: 20 mg/kg IV within 30 min before procedure — Adults: 1.0 g; children: 25 mg/kg IM or IV within 30 min before procedure |

From Dajani AS, et al: *JAMA* 277:1794-1801, 1997. Copyright 1997, American Medical Association.

*Total children's dose should not exceed adult dose.

[†]Cephalosporins should not be used in persons with immediate-type hypersensitivity reaction (urticaria, angioedema, or anaphylaxis) to penicillins.

**BOX 9-5**

**Additional Guidelines for Antibiotic Prophylaxis**

1. In the case of delayed healing or of a procedure that involves infected tissue, additional doses of antibiotics may be needed, even though bacteremia rarely persists longer than 15 minutes after completion of the procedure.
2. Amoxicillin is the preferred oral antibiotic because it is better absorbed from the gastrointestinal tract and provides higher and more sustained serum levels.
3. If a patient is taking amoxicillin on a long-term basis for some reason (e.g., rheumatic fever prevention), a different class of antibiotic, such as oral clindamycin, azithromycin, clarithromycin, or one of the other parenteral regimens, should be used for antibiotic therapy.
4. If a high-risk patient (e.g., a patient with a prosthetic valve) has maintained a "high level" of oral health, oral antibiotic prophylaxis may be used for simple dental procedures rather than the parenteral regimen. However, some physicians may still prefer parenteral antibiotic administration for these high-risk patients. The patient's physician should be consulted when planning dental care for high-risk individuals. Clindamycin phosphate is recommended for parenteral administration in individuals known to be allergic to amoxicillin or ampicillin.

tropenia. The extensive use of broad-spectrum antibiotics, steroids, chemotherapy-associated immunosuppression, and inadequate oral hygiene and nutrition alter the balance of the oral microflora and place children at risk for candidiasis.

The clinical management of oral candidiasis in children is similar to that in adults and consists principally of antifungal agents. Suspected *Candida* infections should be confirmed by culture and/or potassium hydroxide smear prior to initiating prompt and aggressive therapy in immunosuppressed patients. The medicament and route of administration is determined by the severity of the infection. Oral and esophageal candidiasis is usually treated with topical suspensions or troches of antifungal agents, e.g., nystatin or clotrimazole. All antifungal agents formulated for oral topical use contain sweet-eners, which can promote caries if used for an extended period. Daily use of topical fluorides is recommended to reduce the caries potential.

### Nystatin

Nystatin is the most common topical agent used for treatment of oral candidiasis in children. The drug is available as an oral suspension (100,000 U/ml), tablet (500,000 U), and pastille/troche (200,000 U). A dose of 1 million to 3 million units per day in three to five divided doses for 10 to 14 days is recommended.

### Clotrimazole

Clotrimazole is a fungicidal agent that is available only as a 10-mg troche for intraoral application. However, an oral suspension can be compounded from the vaginal tablets. The recommended dose is one troche dissolved slowly in the mouth five times a day for 14 days to achieve maximal effectiveness. The child must be of age and maturity to comprehend and follow instructions to use the troche vehicle. Liver toxicity has been reported in patients using clotrimazole, and clinical studies have not been conducted to establish the safety of the drug for children younger than 3 years.

### Fluconazole and Other Azoles

Systemic antifungal therapy in oral candidiasis is usually reserved for children either not tolerating or failing topical treatment or those at risk of systemic infection. Fluconazole is a commonly used agent in these circumstances. The drug is available for oral or intravenous administration, and it achieves high levels in saliva. It has proved efficacious for the management of a variety of candidal species, although some species are resistant to the drug. Fluconazole is generally preferred over ketoconazole, which has a greater risk of associated hepatotoxicity. Itraconazole and voriconazole are two additional azoles with excellent activity against *Candida* and may eventually have a role in the management of infections associated with more resistant strains.

### Amphotericin B and Caspofungin

Amphotericin has long been the primary drug of choice for systemic management of severe fungal infections. Efficacy of amphotericin has been demonstrated for infection caused by the majority of fungal pathogens. Adverse effects such as nephrotoxicity, metabolic disorders, and fever with administration are not uncommon. Caspofungin, a newer fungal cell wall inhibitor, has a narrow spectrum of activity but demonstrated efficacy in severe disease caused by certain fungal pathogens. This agent will likely have an increasing role in systemic antifungal therapy.

## ANTIVIRAL AGENTS

Primary herpetic gingivostomatitis is the most commonly recognized manifestation of the herpes simplex virus type 1 (HSV). It is an acute illness often with concomitant fever, malaise, irritability, cervical lymphadenopathy, together with the characteristic oral and perioral ulcerative lesions involving the gingiva and mucous membranes of the mouth. HSV gingivostomatitis in healthy children resolves spontaneously within 10 to 14 days and requires only supportive therapy. However, primary or reactivation of latent HSV infections in immunosuppressed patients requires more aggressive therapy. Ulcerated herpetic lesions may be a portal for bacteria and fungi, resulting in serious disseminated infection.

### Antiherpetic Agents

Effective agents for the management of HSV infection in immunocompromised patients include acyclovir, valacyclovir, and famciclovir. Drugs often used for management of cytomegalovirus are also efficacious for HSV but exhibit more toxicity. The route of therapy (e.g., oral versus intravenous acyclovir) is dependent on the host and site and severity of disease. Prophylactic therapy may be considered in patients seropositive for

the HSV and at high risk for reactivation. Acyclovir is not indicated for patients at low risk for clinically significant disease or reactivation. Adverse effects on the central nervous system or kidneys may uncommonly be seen with intravenous acyclovir, whereas oral administration may be associated with headache, nausea, or neutropenia (the latter in infants). The likelihood of developing resistance to acyclovir is low but is more likely in immunocompromised hosts.

## REFERENCES

1. *American Academy of Pediatric Dentistry Reference Manual 2002–03, Pediatr Dent* 24 (suppl):105-122, 2002.
2. Bradley JS, Nelson JD: *Nelson's Pocket Book of Pediatric Antimicrobial Therapy,* 15th ed. Baltimore, Lippincott Williams & Wilkins, 2002-2003.
3. Dajani AS, Taubert KA, Wilson W et al: Prevention of bacterial endocarditis. *JAMA* 277:1794-1801, 1997.
4. Wynn RL, Meiller TF, Crossley HL, editors: *Drug Information Handbook for Dentistry,* 9th ed. Hudson, Ohio, Lexi-Comp, 2003.
5. Flynn TR, Piecuch JF, Toparian RG: Infections of the oral cavity. In: Feigin RD, Cherry JD, editors: *Textbook of Pediatric Infectious Diseases.* Philadelphia, Saunders, 1998.
6. Gilbert DN, Sande MA, Moellering RC: *The Sanford Guide to Antimicrobial Therapy,* 33rd ed. Hyde Park, NY, Antimicrobial Therapy, 2003.
7. Gold HS, Moellering RC: Antimicrobial-drug resistance. *N Engl J Med* 335:1445-1453, 1996.
8. Hickey SM, McCracken GH: Antibacterial therapeutic agents. In: Feigin RD, Cherry JD, editors: *Textbook of Pediatric Infectious Diseases.* Philadelphia, Saunders, 1998.
9. American Academy of Pediatrics: *Report of the Committee on Infectious Diseases,* 26th ed. Elk Grove, Ill., The Academy, 2003.

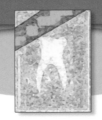

# CHAPTER 10
## Medical Emergencies
### *Kaaren G. Vargas*

Dentistry is an invasive, surgical specialty that is often associated with high levels of patient anxiety. These factors combine to produce a situation that may be conducive to medical emergencies, especially those that are induced or aggravated by stress. Also, pharmacologic agents are used routinely in the dental office. All drugs, whether local anesthetics, antibiotics, sedatives, or analgesics, carry the potential for producing toxicity or allergy.

The specter of medical emergencies is often frightening and bewildering to dental students because of the implication that they will be called on to diagnose and manage medical conditions that they are not trained or equipped to handle. It may be comforting to realize that the dentist is not expected to diagnose the underlying cause of all emergencies accurately and immediately render curative treatment. The accurate diagnosis of a medical condition often, in fact, requires hours to days to determine in the hospital setting. The primary responsibilities of the dentist in the area of medical emergencies fall into the area of prevention, preparation, basic life support, and procurement of help and transport.

## PREVENTION OF MEDICAL EMERGENCIES

Perhaps the most important aspect of dealing with medical emergencies is preventing their occurrence. Prevention of medical emergencies can generally be accomplished, as much as possible, by an adequate history and physical examination, medical consultation (when indicated), and vigilant patient monitoring.

### History and Physical Examination

A thorough knowledge of all existing medical conditions, physical or psychological, that may predispose the patient to development of a problem will prevent the vast majority of emergency situations. This knowledge is gained through the medical history and physical examination. The easiest way to obtain a medical history is to have the patient complete a simple medical history questionnaire, such as the short form available through the American Dental Association (ADA). Included are questions pertaining to any present or past medical conditions, allergies, hospitalizations, medications, and so forth. The dentist reviews this form, notes positive findings, and conducts a brief interview with the patient to clarify any questions and expand on the questionnaire.

The physical examination should include baseline vital signs (heart rate, respiratory rate and character, and blood pressure in older children), a thorough head and neck examination, and observation of general appearance (gait, mental status, skin tone and color, etc.). Further physical evaluation should be dictated by the dentist's training and expertise. If a practitioner uses sedation techniques that may depress the patient's cardiovascular or respiratory function, it is recommended that the practitioner possess skills in the physical diagnosis of the cardiovascular and pulmonary systems (e.g., chest and heart auscultation).

A thorough history and physical examination should make the dentist aware of any preexisting conditions that may lead to a medical emergency.

This knowledge should allow the development of a treatment protocol for the patient that will make such an event highly unlikely. This may involve the use of conscious sedation for stress-induced conditions such as asthmatic attacks or epileptic seizures, proper timing of appointments, bacterial endocarditis prophylaxis, or even performing the needed procedures in the hospital operating room if necessary.

### Medical Consultation

If any questions arise regarding the management of a medically compromised child, it is highly desirable to contact the patient's physician by telephone for guidance.

### Patient Monitoring

The level of monitoring that is necessary to treat a pediatric dental patient safely will vary, depending on the patient's condition and the patient management technique being used. Patient monitoring involves the observation of physiologic parameters over time in order to detect any change and deal with it before a potentially dangerous situation develops. The dentist should always monitor (observe) the general appearance of the patient, including the level of consciousness, level of comfort, muscle tone, color of the skin and mucosa, and respiratory pattern. For the majority of healthy patients being treated with local anesthesia alone, this is all the monitoring that is necessary.

When conscious sedation is used, especially in children, in whom a much narrower margin of safety often exists because of smaller degrees of respiratory and cardiovascular reserve, additional monitoring should be routinely employed. The primary systems to be monitored during dental treatment with conscious sedation or deep sedation are the central nervous system (CNS), respiratory system, and cardiovascular system. Presedation vital signs, including heart rate, respiratory rate, blood pressure, and temperature, must always be obtained. The heart sounds and breath sounds should be continuously monitored using a precordial stethoscope in all patients undergoing conscious sedation (Fig. 10-1). This allows the dentist to perform continuous auscultation of the patient's heart rate and rhythm and respiratory pattern without having to look consciously at a monitor screen for data.

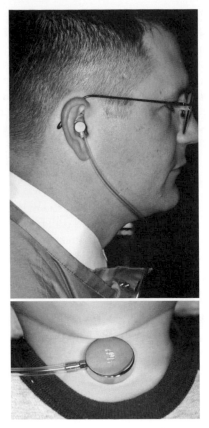

**Figure 10-1**    Use of a precordial stethoscope.

In addition to these essential monitors, several other devices are available that further enhance one's ability to monitor the patient's vital functions. For cardiovascular monitoring, blood pressure and heart rate may be conveniently monitored utilizing noninvasive blood pressure devices that measure systolic, diastolic, and mean blood pressure and heart rate at predetermined intervals and display the data digitally. Several devices have been advocated for respiratory monitoring, including the capnograph, pulse oximeter, ear oximeter, impedance plethysmograph, and transcutaneous oxygen and carbon dioxide monitors. Of these devices, the pulse oximeter is the most useful and accurate for detecting developing hypoxia, and the capnograph is the most sensitive and accurate system for assessing whether the patient is breathing. The pulse oximeter measures oxyhemoglobin saturation instantaneously and provides immediate feedback on the status of the patient's oxygenation. The capnograph continuously analyzes the carbon dioxide content of respired gases, providing a breath-to-breath representation of the presence or absence of air flow.

Whenever deep sedation or general anesthesia is used, more sophisticated monitoring is essential. In addition to the essential observations, precordial stethoscope, and use of pulse oximetry, monitoring during deep sedation should include recording of vital signs at a minimum of 5-minute intervals (including blood pressure), continuous temperature monitoring, and electrocardiography. Placement of an intravenous catheter is also highly recommended. The use of restraining devices in small children makes monitoring especially difficult. When these devices are used, the dentist should observe at least one extremity and the face for color, check head position frequently to ensure a patent airway, and monitor heart and breath sounds continuously with a precordial stethoscope. The use of a pulse oximeter and capnograph should be standard.

## PREPARATION FOR EMERGENCIES

Despite preventive measures, medical emergencies occasionally occur. The dental practitioner must be adequately prepared for such events. Preparation involves personal, staff, and office preparation.

### Personal Preparation

As previously stated, it cannot be expected that the practicing dentist will be able to diagnose and manage every possible medical emergency. However, it is possible to anticipate with some certainty which emergency situations are most likely to arise in the dental office and be well prepared to deal with them. Examples include syncope, hyperventilation, seizures, hypoglycemia, postural hypotension, asthma, allergic reactions, and airway obstruction. Certainly, any emergency situation that might logically occur as a direct result of medications or techniques being used must be anticipated, well understood, and prepared for. Examples include local anesthetic reactions and respiratory depression secondary to sedation. Personal preparation for the dentist should include, as a minimum, a good working knowledge of the signs, symptoms, course, and therapy for these common treatable conditions. Training in basic life support (cardiopulmonary resuscitation; CPR) should be considered essential for any practicing health professional. If conscious sedation techniques are to be used, advanced cardiac life support (ACLS) training is desirable.

## Staff Preparation

Office personnel should be trained in the recognition and management of common medical emergencies. It is desirable to require that all office staff members be certified in basic cardiac life support (CPR). A team approach to medical emergencies will provide for organized management of emergency situations. Each staff member should have a preassigned role in case of an emergency so that emergency equipment will be brought (and maintained) by an assigned person, emergency drugs will be prepared by another, and all tasks will be performed in an organized fashion. Because medical emergencies, fortunately, occur relatively rarely in the dental office, it is desirable to run mock medical emergency drills on a regular basis in order to keep the team protocol running smoothly and to reduce panic in an actual emergency.

## Office Preparation

Every dental office contains a great deal of equipment and supplies. There is a minimum of additional equipment that is essential for every office to be properly prepared for medical emergencies. These essentials can be divided into emergency equipment and emergency drugs.

## EMERGENCY EQUIPMENT

Keeping in mind the dentist's primary responsibilities of basic life support and transport in most situations, it should be apparent that very little equipment is necessary to deal with medical emergencies. First of all, oxygen must be readily available. An oxygen source capable of delivering greater than 90% oxygen at flows in excess of 5 L/min for a minimum of 1 hour must be available. This means that an "E" cylinder is the minimal size required. The initial primary goal of basic life support is establishment and maintenance of proper respiratory function. Hypoxemia (low oxygen content in the arterial blood) is the final common pathway leading to morbidity and mortality in the majority of severe medical emergency situations. Adequate oxygenation must be ensured by the administration of supple-

mental oxygen. If the patient is breathing adequately spontaneously, oxygen may be delivered by way of a face mask, nasal mask, or nasal prongs. However, the patient may cease breathing during an emergency situation, making artificial ventilation necessary. Therefore a positive-pressure oxygen delivery system (bag-valve-mask) is also considered essential equipment in order to deliver oxygen to the apneic patient.

A high-volume suction device is the third piece of equipment that is considered essential for the management of medical emergencies. Emergency situations, especially those involving an obtunded patient, often induce vomiting. The aspiration of vomitus can be disastrous. This can usually be prevented by proper positioning and suctioning. Of course, most dental offices contain high-volume suction equipment for restorative purposes.

Other emergency equipment items that are desirable and recommended include syringes and needles, the armamentarium for establishing an intravenous line; cricothyrotomy equipment; oral and nasal airways; a laryngoscope; and endotracheal tubes.

## EMERGENCY DRUGS

Most medical emergencies in the dental office do not require the use of drugs. The practitioner's thought process should be primarily directed to basic life support measures and should turn to drug therapy only when clearly indicated. The contents of an appropriate emergency drug kit may be quite different for individual dentists, depending on the drugs used in the office, the dentist's individual level of training, and the level of medical support immediately available. It is expected that pharmacologic agents be available to definitively manage any medical emergency that may be expected to arise as a direct result of any drug that is used to treat patients. This includes the use of local anesthetics, which may produce toxic or allergic reactions.

The dentist should be very familiar with each drug in the emergency kit. Commercially available emergency kits are not only very expensive, they are also almost never optimal as far as which drugs are included for any individual practitioner's purposes. One of the biggest dangers of owning a commercially available emergency kit is gaining a false sense of security simply by purchasing it. If the practitioner does not know the uses, dosages, and probable side effects of each drug in the kit and keep them up to date, the kit may be more dangerous than potentially beneficial. A good drug kit should contain as few drugs as possible and should be simple, neat, and readily available. The dentist should be familiar with every drug, including its recommended dosage, indications, and side effects.

The following list is the author's recommendation for drugs that might be included in a basic emergency drug kit for the dentist who treats children. The list contains only superficial information and must be expanded on as recommended previously.

## Drugs to Manage Allergy

### Epinephrine

**Use.**    Epinephrine is the most important drug in any emergency kit. It is the treatment of choice for life-threatening anaphylactic reactions and for severe asthmatic reactions, and it is a basic cardiac life support drug. If a dentist is administering any drugs to patients, including local anesthetics, epinephrine must be available in case of allergy.

**Action.**    Epinephrine is a sympathomimetic that stimulates both $\alpha$ and $\beta$ receptors. Epinephrine increases heart rate and blood pressure, relaxes bronchial smooth muscle, and has an antihistaminic action.

**How Supplied.**    1:1000 ampule (1 mg/ml) or 1:10,000 preloaded syringe (0.1 mg/ml).

**Dosage.**    0.01 mg/kg (0.1 ml/kg of 1:10,000 IV), (0.01 ml/kg of 1:1000 IM); may need to repeat after 5 to 10 minutes as needed. Single pediatric doses should not exceed 0.3 mg. Administration of the agent is either subcutaneous or intramuscular/intralingual.

**Side Effects.**    Side effects of epinephrine include hypertension, cardiac arrhythmias, anxiety, and headache.

### Diphenhydramine (Benadryl)

**Use.**    Diphenhydramine is used for allergic reactions of slower onset or less severity than anaphylaxis and as an adjunct to epinephrine in severe allergic reactions.

**Action.**    Diphenhydramine is a histamine ($H_1$) antagonist that blocks the response of the $H_1$ receptor to histamine.

**How Supplied.**    50 mg in 1-ml ampule or 10 mg/ml vial.

**Dosage.**    1 to 2 mg/kg, IV or IM.

**Side Effects.**    Sedation, anticholinergic.

## Anticonvulsant

### Diazepam (Valium)

**Use.**    Diazepam is used for management of status epilepticus (recurrent seizures).

**Action.**    Anticonvulsant.

**How Supplied.**    5 mg/ml vials or preloaded syringe.

**Dosage.**    <5 years: 0.3 mg/kg, with initial dose not exceeding 0.25 mg/kg to a maximum of 0.75 mg/kg total dose for episode, slow IV (or deep IM);* maximal total dose, 5 mg; >5 years: 1 mg/dose, slow IV;* maximal total dose, 10 mg.

**Adults.**    5 to 10 mg/dose, slow IV;* maximal total dose, 30 mg.

**Side Effects.**    Sedation, respiratory depression.

## Benzodiazepine Antagonist

### Flumazenil (Anexate, Romazicon)

**Use.**    Flumazenil is used to reverse the respiratory depression or other undesirable effects of several benzodiazepines, including methylclonazepam, diazepam, flunitrazepam, and midazolam.

**Action.**    Benzodiazepine receptor antagonist.

**How Supplied.**    Flumazenil injection is supplied in multiple-dose vials of 5 ml and 10 ml.

**Dosage.**    The recommended initial dose is 0.2 mg administered intravenously over 15 seconds. If the desired level of consciousness is not obtained within 60 seconds, an additional dose of 0.1 mg can be injected and repeated at 60-second intervals, up to a maximal total dose of 1 mg. The usual dose is between 0.3 and 0.6 mg.

**Side Effects.**    Very rarely, the following side effects can be seen: agitation, anxiety, dizziness, hypertension, tachycardia, nausea, and vomiting.

## Narcotic Antagonist

### Naloxone (Narcan)

**Use.**    Naloxone is used to reverse respiratory depression or other undesirable effects of narcotic analgesics. This drug is essential if any narcotics are administered.

**Action.**    Narcotic antagonist.

---

*May repeat dose every 15 minutes as needed, to maximal dose.

**How Supplied.** 0.4 mg/ml ampule.

**Dosage.** 0.01 mg/kg, IV or IM; may repeat with a subsequent dose of 0.1 mg/kg if needed.

**Side Effects.** Very rarely, cardiac arrest has been reported with the use of naloxone.

## Steroid

*Hydrocortisone Sodium Succinate (Solu-Cortef)*

**Use.** The inclusion of a corticosteroid is recommended for the management of acute adrenal insufficiency if it should occur in a steroid-dependent patient, or as an adjunctive treatment for a severe anaphylactic reaction or asthmatic attack.

**Action.** An adrenal corticosteroid: antiinflammatory and membrane stabilization.

**How Supplied.** 50 mg/ml in 2-ml Mix-O-Vial.

**Dosage.** 0.2 to 1 mg/kg. Higher doses may be needed for acutely life-threatening situations.

## Antihypoglycemics

*50% Dextrose*

**Use.** If loss of consciousness or obtundation occurs as a result of hypoglycemia, the treatment of choice is to obtain intravenous access and administer 50% dextrose to raise serum glucose levels.

**Action.** Directly raises serum glucose levels (immediately).

**How Supplied.** Dextrose 50% in sterile water, 50-ml bottle (1 ml = 0.5 g).

**Dosage.** 0.5 to 1 g/kg (1 to 2 ml/kg), IV, until patient regains consciousness.

*Glucagon*

**Use.** If intravenous access cannot be established, the hormone glucagon may be used. It must be kept in mind that restoration of consciousness may require a delay of 10 to 20 minutes.

**Action.** Raises serum glucose levels by encouraging glycogenolysis.

**How Supplied.** 1 mg/ml solution.

**Dosage.** 0.5 to 1 mg, IM (0.025 to 0.1 mg/kg), may repeat dosing after 20 minutes if needed. Maximal single dose is 1 mg.

## Vasopressors

Especially if intravenous sedation techniques are being utilized, a drug to raise blood pressure in case of severe hypotension is advisable. If hypotension should occur, the situation must be assessed before any drug is given. If hypotension is due to a cardiac arrhythmia, the arrhythmia must first be treated with appropriate therapy. If hypotension is due to a drug effect (vasodilatation), appropriate fluid therapy with or without a vasopressor is indicated. Two possible alternative vasopressors are given.

*Ephedrine*

**Use.** Ephedrine is used to raise blood pressure and heart rate from shock levels.

**Action.** Indirect $\alpha$ and $\beta$ sympathomimetic actions by release of endogenous catecholamines.

**How Supplied.** 25 or 50 mg/ml ampule.

**Dosage.** 0.5 mg/kg, IV or IM.

**Side Effects.** Hypertension, tachycardia, arrhythmias, headache.

*Methoxamine (Vasoxyl)*

**Use.** Methoxamine is used to raise blood pressure from shock levels.

**Action.** Methoxamine has a direct $\alpha$ sympathomimetic effect only. The drug produces an increase in blood pressure by peripheral vasoconstriction, without direct cardiac effects. Reflex bradycardia can be produced by methoxamine.

**How Supplied.** 10 mg/ml vial or 20 mg/ml ampule.

**Dosage.** 0.25 mg/kg, IM, or 0.08 mg/kg, slow IV.

**Side Effects.** Bradycardia, hypertension, headache.

## Analgesic

For acute emergencies in which the presence of pain and anxiety may significantly worsen the clinical situation, a narcotic analgesic may be indicated. This situation is primarily the case with acute myocardial infarction, which is obviously principally a problem of elderly patients. Morphine, meperidine (Demerol), or many other narcotics may be used.

## ACLS Drugs

If the dentist has training in ACLS, or if he or she performs deep sedation or general anesthesia, basic ACLS drugs may be included in the emergency kit. An electrocardiography monitor and a defibrillator should be available when these drugs are used.

*Atropine*

**Use.**    Atropine is used in the management of bradycardia.

**Action.**    Atropine is a parasympathetic (vagal) blocking agent; therefore, it increases the patient's heart rate.

**How Supplied.**    0.4 mg/ml ampules or vials.

**Dosage.**    0.01 mg/kg, IV or IM. For ACLS, 0.02 mg/kg, IV or IM.

**Side Effects.**    Tachycardia, arrhythmia, dry mouth.

*Sodium Bicarbonate*

**Use.**    Acidosis, cardiac arrest.

**Action.**    Raises blood pH directly.

**How Supplied.**    1 mEq/ml.

**Dosage.**    1 mEq/kg, slow IV at 10-minute intervals, as needed during resuscitation.

**Side Effects.**    Alkalosis, hypernatremia.

*Calcium Chloride*

**Use.**    Asystole, hypotension, electromechanical dissociation.

**Action.**    Increased cardiac contractility.

**How Supplied.**    10% solution (100 mg/ml).

**Dosage.**    0.2 ml/kg of 10% calcium chloride IV will provide 20 mg/kg, every 10 minutes as needed.

**Side Effects.**    Phlebitis.

*Lidocaine (Xylocaine)*

**Use.**    Lidocaine is used to manage ventricular arrhythmias (ventricular extrasystoles and ventricular tachycardia).

*Note: Only "cardiac lidocaine" may be used for this purpose. Dental lidocaine should not be injected intravenously.*

**Action.**    Lidocaine depresses automaticity and suppresses ectopic ventricular pacemakers.

**How Supplied.**    1% (10 mg/ml) or 2% (20 mg/ml) vials or prefilled syringe.

**Dosage.**    1 mg/kg, IV.

**Side Effects.**    Sedation, local anesthetic toxicity in high doses (seizures).

## Other Drugs

Other agents that are not injectable drugs but that might be included as part of the emergency drug kit include (1) a respiratory stimulant, such as aromatic ammonia inhalants; (2) sugar (to manage hypoglycemia in an awake patient); (3) a vasodilator such as nitroglycerin; and (4) a "Medihaler" of metaproterenol (Metaprel), albuterol (Ventolin, Proventil), or isoetharine (Bronkosol) to manage an asthmatic attack.

## Backup Medical Assistance

The final essential component of office preparation for medical emergencies involves securing backup medical assistance in advance. This involves having the current telephone numbers of the nearest rescue squad and emergency room facility conveniently displayed where they will be immediately available if needed. When feasible, arrangements should be made with a physician whose office is nearby for immediate assistance should an emergency arise. Such a relationship must be prearranged, not assumed.

## MANAGEMENT OF MEDICAL EMERGENCIES

The management of basically all medical emergencies, especially those involving a change in the state of consciousness, should be approached in a similar fashion, keeping certain priorities in mind (Box 10-1). Not only will this approach make patient management more efficient and effective, it will also make it less anxiety provoking and confusing for the dentist.

## Position

For emergencies involving obtundation of consciousness or hypotension, the best position for managing the situation is to place the patient lying flat on his or her back with the feet raised slightly above the level of the heart. This will minimize the work of the heart, increase return of pooled blood from the extremities, and increase vital blood flow to the brain. Fortunately, this position is easily accomplished in the dental chair. For medical emergencies in the conscious patient involving respiratory distress (e.g., asthmatic

---

**BOX 10-1**

**Management of Medical Emergencies**

Position
Airway
Breathing
Circulation
Definitive therapy

attack) or chest pain (angina), the semisitting position is generally preferred by the patient.

## Airway ("A")

The first priority in the management of all medical emergencies is the establishment of a patent, functioning airway. If the supply of oxygen to the lungs is cut off for even a short period, especially in a child, rapid neurologic and cardiovascular deterioration will ensue, leading to cardiac arrest, brain cell damage, and death. The airway may be obstructed by progressive swelling, trauma, a foreign body, or other factor.

However, by far the most common cause of airway obstruction is the tongue. When a patient becomes obtunded or unconscious, the musculature supporting the mandible and tongue becomes lax, allowing the base of the tongue to fall back against the posterior pharynx, thus blocking the airway between the oral and nasal cavities and the trachea. Extending the head on the neck and thrusting the jaw forward while opening the patient's mouth (head tilt-chin lift or jaw thrust maneuver) is usually adequate to open the airway that is obstructed by the tongue. An oral or nasal airway device may be useful in keeping the tongue forward in the unconscious or deeply obtunded patient. However, these devices should not be used in conscious patients owing to their propensity to produce laryngospasm, gagging, and vomiting.

If the airway is obstructed by a foreign body, such as a cotton roll or dental restoration, management depends on the patient's condition. In the conscious patient, the initial step should be to deliver four sharp blows with the heel of the hand to the patient's back, between the scapulae, over the spine. Sharp back blows will rapidly raise intrathoracic pressure, causing a burst of air to be expelled through the larynx, hopefully dislodging the obstruction. The four back blows should be delivered in rapid succession and should immediately be stopped if the patient begins to cough up the foreign body. If the back blows are not successful, the abdominal thrust (Heimlich maneuver) should be attempted. In the sitting or standing position, the operator positions himself behind the patient, places one fist below the xiphoid process over the mid-upper abdomen, clenches it with the other hand, and pulls up and back forcefully. This maneuver pushes the diaphragm up and produces a more sustained and

forceful increase in intrathoracic pressure, expelling air through the larynx and hopefully dislodging the obstruction. Four abdominal thrusts are performed in rapid succession. The abdominal thrust may be modified for the patient who is lying down (as in the dental chair) in that the rescuer delivers the thrust with the heel of the hand from the side or front of the patient.

The abdominal thrust should not be performed with small children because of their relatively large abdominal organs (especially the liver), which could be damaged. In these cases, a chest thrust maneuver should be delivered instead, with the heel of the hand positioned over the child's midsternum, as would be the position for chest compressions during CPR. Chest thrusts are also used with pregnant females and the obese. The sequence of four back blows followed by four abdominal thrusts is repeated until success in dislodging the obstruction is attained or the patient loses consciousness.

In the unconscious patient with an obstructed airway, the patient is positioned supine (face up), the airway is positioned by tilting the head back and elevating the chin, and an attempt is made to ventilate the patient manually utilizing either mouth-to-mouth resuscitation or a bag-valve-mask system. Although back blows and abdominal thrusts may have been unsuccessful in dislodging an obstruction up to this point, the mechanism of positive-pressure breathing is quite different because the air flow is in the opposite direction and may dislodge the obstruction. If the attempt to ventilate manually is unsuccessful, the sequence of four back blows (accomplished by rolling the patient toward the rescuer temporarily) and four abdominal or chest thrusts (from the side or front) is delivered. With an unconscious patient, these maneuvers are followed by sweeping a finger from the side of the patient's mouth deep into the oropharynx in order to remove any foreign body that may have been dislodged. An attempt at positive-pressure ventilation is again made. This sequence is repeated until a patent airway is obtained or until an invasive technique is deemed necessary.

### Invasive Techniques
In children, total airway obstruction leads to cardiac arrest and brain dysfunction quite rapidly. In most small children, total airway obstruction is not tolerated for longer than 1 minute. If the above sequences do not result in rapid opening of

the airway rapidly and the patient is displaying signs and symptoms of hypoxia (cyanosis, arrhythmias), an invasive technique for opening the airway must be used.

The initial invasive tool in the dentist's armamentarium for dealing with airway obstruction should be direct laryngoscopy utilizing the laryngoscope. Use of the laryngoscope requires a certain amount of training and skill. With the laryngoscope, the larynx may be exposed so that any foreign body may be removed under direct vision. The trachea may then be intubated with an appropriate endotracheal tube for manual ventilation as needed.

Opening of the airway using cricothyrotomy is the last-resort method of airway control. The cricothyroid membrane between the thyroid cartilage and the cricoid bone is either incised with a scalpel or punctured with a large-bore needle in order to ventilate the trachea with a flow of oxygen or allow respiration to be assisted. This technique, along with the critical anatomic landmarks, should be thoroughly understood by every dentist.

## Breathing ("B")

The second priority in dealing with medical emergencies, once a patent airway is established, is to ensure that adequate breathing is present. The chest should be observed for expansion and the nose and mouth observed for air flow during respiration by feeling and listening. If the patient is not breathing, rescue breathing should be initiated immediately. Initially, four rapid breaths are given in order to expand the lungs, followed by one breath every 3 seconds for children or one breath every 5 seconds for adults, until spontaneous respiration resumes.

Rescue breathing may be accomplished by the mouth-to-mouth or the bag-valve-mask technique. Mouth-to-mouth ventilation is sometimes necessary in the emergency situation, but its efficacy is severely limited by the fact that exhaled air, containing a maximum of 15% to 18% oxygen, is delivered to the hypoxic patient's lungs.

Use of a positive-pressure breathing system (bag-valve-mask), which can deliver close to 100% oxygen, is highly preferable. A mask is used, which fits tightly over the patient's mouth and nose. The mask is attached to a one-way valve, which allows oxygen to enter the patient when the reservoir bag is squeezed forcibly. The empty bag then refills with oxygen only. The technique entails securing a tight mask fit on the patient's face and opening the airway with one hand and compressing the bag with the other, forcing oxygen by positive pressure into the patient's lungs. Exhalation is passive. This technique of rescue breathing is much more efficient than mouth-to-mouth resuscitation and should be mastered by all dentists. A bag-valve-mask system, such as an Ambu bag, is considered essential emergency equipment for every dental office.

## Circulation ("C")

Once the airway and breathing have been established, the condition of the patient's circulatory system should be established. The most rapid, convenient, and accurate method for assessing circulation is palpation of the carotid pulse. The carotid artery should be felt just under the sternocleidomastoid muscle in the neck. One should never palpate both carotid arteries simultaneously, since pressure on the baroreceptors of the carotid sinuses may precipitate reflex bradycardia. The quality, rate, and rhythm of the pulses should be noted. If the pulse is absent, CPR should be initiated immediately. If the pulse is present, a more accurate assessment of cardiovascular status should be obtained by measuring blood pressure and heart rate.

## Definitive Therapy ("D")

Only after the "A," "B," and "C" of emergency management have been satisfied should one consider definitive drug therapy. Whether or not definitive drug therapy should be embarked on by the dentist depends on several factors, including his or her training and expertise, the availability of medical assistance, and the situation that the dentist is presented with. If the emergency is acute and life threatening, especially if the cause is clear or was precipitated by treatment or a drug that was administered, definitive therapy may be indicated and essential. Some common medical emergencies for which definitive therapy is indicated will be briefly discussed.

### Syncope

Vasodepressor syncope, or the simple faint, is probably the most common cause of loss of consciousness in the dental office. It is, however, much less common in children than in young adults. Syncope is a maladaptive stress reaction that is usually triggered by anxiety. As the patient becomes anxious, the fight-or-flight response of the sympathetic nervous system is triggered, and endogenous epinephrine and norepinephrine are released into the circulation. This response involves a large increase in blood flow to the muscles of the body. If the muscles are contracting, as would be the case if the individual is running, blood flow is maintained. However, in the dental chair little or no muscle contraction is occurring and so the blood pools in the muscles, especially in the lower extremities, effectively decreasing the relative blood volume available to the central circulation and, therefore, the brain. The heart rate will reflexively increase in an attempt to maintain the blood pressure, and the blood vessels in the periphery will constrict, producing the typical cold, pale, and sweaty skin. As blood flow to the brain decreases in the upright position, the patient feels dizzy or faint. This phase of the condition is called presyncope. It may begin rapidly and last a few minutes.

If presyncope is recognized in a susceptible patient and dealt with quickly, loss of consciousness may be avoided. Management of presyncope consists of positioning the patient flat on the back, lowering the head, and raising the feet to augment blood flow to the brain by gravity. Encouraging the patient to contract muscles, especially in the legs, will also augment return of pooled venous blood from the musculature. Administration of oxygen is appropriate in any emergency involving a decrease in brain perfusion. The use of an ammonia inhalant to stimulate the patient may be of some benefit.

If the process of syncope continues, the sympathetic nervous system will fatigue, and the parasympathetic nervous system will suddenly become dominant. This vagal response results in a sudden, severe decrease in heart rate and blood pressure, often to startlingly low levels. Blood flow to the brain is decreased, and consciousness is lost. Breathing becomes irregular, the pupils dilate, and convulsive movements are often noted. The muscles relax, and the airway may become obstructed. Loss of consciousness from syncope is usually rapidly responsive to positioning as previously mentioned. Oxygen should be administered; airway, breathing, and circulation maintained; tight and constrictive clothing loosened; and vital signs monitored.

Consciousness is usually regained fairly quickly, but recovery of heart rate and blood pressure may be quite slow. If recovery of consciousness is delayed beyond 5 minutes or is incomplete after 15 to 20 minutes, medical assistance should be sought. Drug therapy is usually not indicated with syncope unless the heart rate or blood pressure remain dangerously depressed after positioning. In such a case, atropine to increase heart rate or a vasopressor to increase blood pressure may be necessary.

### Allergic Reaction

Allergic reactions involve hypersensitivity responses by the immune system to antigens that are recognized as foreign, with subsequent antibody formation. There are several different types of allergic responses, ranging from mild, delayed rashes to severe, sudden, life-threatening anaphylaxis. The primary agents employed in pediatric dentistry that might provoke an allergic reaction are the penicillins, intravenous sedative agents, and the ester-type local anesthetics.

The anaphylactic reaction is mediated primarily by the release of histamine from sensitized mast cells. Histamine is a potent toxic agent that produces inflammation and vascular effects. The body systems primarily involved in a clinical allergic reaction are the skin, respiratory system, and cardiovascular system. Skin involvement is the most common reaction and may range from a mild erythematous rash, to urticaria (hives), to angioedema (severe swelling).

In general, the more rapid the onset and the more intense the symptoms, the more severe the generalized reaction can be expected to become. Angioedema that involves the face and neck may be rapidly progressive, leading to airway obstruction and death. The respiratory system is usually involved after the skin reaction starts in generalized anaphylaxis. The primary problem is constriction of bronchial smooth muscle producing respiratory distress owing to airway obstruction, primarily expiratory in nature. The principal recognizable sign is wheezing, a distinctive breathing sound associated with bronchoconstriction. As the obstruction worsens, the patient has increasing difficulty in exchanging adequate volumes of air, usually becomes panicked, which worsens the situation, and may become severely hypoxic. Other smooth muscles also contract and may produce symptoms of abdominal cramps, nausea and vomiting, or incontinence. As anaphylaxis progresses, the cardiovascular system is affected. Hypotension is produced by the vaso-dilating effect of histamine and other mediators of the response. Reflex tachycardia, arrhythmias, and eventually cardiac arrest may follow.

Management of allergic reactions depends on the time course and severity of the symptoms. If symptoms are immediate or severe, epinephrine at 0.01 mg/kg should be administered, preferably intravenously in the 1:10,000 dilution or intra-muscularly in the 1:1000 dilution. Epinephrine counteracts most of the effects of histamine. It produces bronchodilation (countering broncho-constriction) and raises blood pressure and heart rate by its $\alpha$ and $\beta$ effects. It also counters skin rash, urticaria, and angioedema by an unknown mechanism.

Diphenhydramine, a histamine receptor blocker, should also be administered. This antihistamine will not reverse to any great extent histaminic effects that have already occurred, but it may prevent further progression or recurrence of symptoms. If the reaction is delayed or mild, diphenhydramine may be all that is necessary to prevent progression of the allergic reaction. Diphenhydramine should also be administered orally at 6-hour intervals for 24 to 48 hours fol-lowing any allergic reaction. Oxygen should always be administered if any respiratory symptoms are present. Use of an aerosolized sympathomimetic agent such as epinephrine, isoproterenol, or metaproterenol to manage bronchospasm may also be of benefit. If the reaction is severe, the patient should be transported to the hospital, and supplemental use of a corticosteroid, such as hydrocortisone sodium succinate, should be considered. Ideally, the steroid preparation should be given early in the course of the reaction.

## Seizures

Of the multiple types of seizures, the tonic-clonic (grand mal) type is the most frightening and the one that most often requires treatment. Only this type will be considered here. Grand mal seizures are manifested in four phases: the prodromal phase, the aura, the convulsive (ictal) phase, and the postictal phase.

The prodromal phase consists of subtle changes that may occur over minutes to hours. It is usually not clinically evident to the practitioner or the patient. The aura is a neurologic experience that the patient goes through immediately prior to the seizure. It is specifically related to the trigger areas

of the brain in which the seizure activity begins. It may consist of a taste, a smell, a hallucination, motor activity, or other symptoms. A given patient's aura is often the same for all seizures. As the CNS discharge becomes generalized, the ictal phase begins. The patient loses consciousness, falls to the floor, and tonic, rigid skeletal muscle contraction ensues. As the chest wall musculature contracts, air is expelled through the larynx, producing vocalization called the epileptic cry. Clonic movements then begin, producing rapid jerking of the extremities and trunk. Breathing may be labored during this period, and patients may injure themselves. This clonic phase usually lasts 1 to 3 minutes. As the clonic phase ends, the muscles relax and movement stops. A significant degree of CNS depression is usually present during this postictal phase, and it may result in respiratory depression. The patient has amnesia from the prodromal phase throughout the entire seizure.

Management of a seizure consists of gentle restraint and positioning of the patient in order to prevent self-injury, ensuring adequate ventilation, and supportive care, as indicated, in the postictal phase, especially airway management. Single seizures do not require drug therapy because they are self-limiting. Should the ictal phase last longer than 5 minutes or if seizures continue to develop with little time between them, a condition called status epilepticus has developed. This may be a life-threatening medical emergency, since the uncontrolled muscle activity can result in hyper-thermia, increased oxygen consumption, tachycar-dia, hypertension, impaired ventilation, and cardiac arrhythmias. This condition is best man-aged with intravenous diazepam, and transport should be arranged to take the patient to the hospital.

## Hyperventilation

Hyperventilation syndrome, like syncope, is a maladaptive anxiety reaction that primarily occurs in apprehensive young females who attempt to hide their anxiety. It is much less common in males and is rare in young children. The syndrome is often triggered by an anxiety-provoking event such as the local anesthetic injection. The patient is usually unaware of the fact that she is beginning to hyperventilate. The respiratory rate may increase to 25–30 breaths per minute, with an increase in tidal volume as well. The patient may complain of difficulty in getting her breath. The increased ventilation causes carbon dioxide to be eliminated from the blood. The decrease in the arterial partial pressure of carbon dioxide ($PaCO_2$), referred to as hypocarbia, causes a physiologic vasoconstriction of the arteries supplying the brain with a consequent decrease in blood flow to the brain. The patient will begin to feel dizzy and light-headed, which further enhances the anxiety, worsening the condition in a vicious cycle. Other symptoms that may occur include numbness and tingling of the extremities and perioral area, muscle twitching and cramping, seizures, and loss of consciousness.

Management of hyperventilation involves early recognition of the patient's anxiety and discussing it openly with the patient. Reassurance, patient rapport, and calmly coaching the patient to breathe slowly may be sufficient to stop the process. Oxygen should not be administered. If the cycle cannot be broken, steps should be taken to increase the $PaCO_2$. This can be accomplished simply by having the patient breathe into a paper bag, which causes rebreathing of exhaled $CO_2$-containing air, thus raising the $PaCO_2$ and reversing the process. Of course, this should not be done for an extended period because of the possibility of producing hypoxia. Occasionally, use of an antianxiety agent (e.g., intravenous diazepam) is helpful.

## Asthma

The primary type of asthma that occurs in children is allergic or extrinsic asthma, which is immunoglobulin E (IgE) antibody mediated. This type of asthma is usually outgrown by the late teens or early twenties. The asthma attack in this case is usually triggered by specific allergens such as pollens, dust, and molds. The tracheobronchial tree is hyperreactive in asthma and contains increased amounts of tenacious secretions. During an acute asthmatic attack, constriction of the smooth muscle in the bronchial walls causes bronchospasm and the characteristic wheezing. Thick secretions are produced, which can plug the small airways, and bronchial wall edema may develop rapidly, further compromising the airway. This process may produce various signs and symptoms varying from mild wheezing and coughing to severe dyspnea, cyanosis, and death.

In adults, the primary type of asthma is termed extrinsic asthma. With extrinsic asthma, attacks may be precipitated by infections, irritants,

exercise, and, importantly, stress. Some overlap in these asthma types certainly occurs. With any asthmatic patient, a thorough history should be taken, including how often attacks occur and how severe they have become (if hospitalization has been required, what triggers attacks, and what medications are being taken). All attempts should be made to avoid precipitating factors. If the patient is taking medications, he or she should be instructed to continue taking them prior to the dental appointment. If patients use a Medihaler to self-administer aerosolized medications (isoproterenol [Isuprel], metaproterenol [Metaprel]), they should bring it to their appointment.

If patients with asthma begin to wheeze and develop any respiratory distress in the dental chair, they should be given oxygen and allowed to sit up (if they are more comfortable sitting). If they have a Medihaler, they should utilize it, which will usually abort the attack. If aerosolized adrenergic agents fail to reverse the bronchospasm, 0.01 mg/kg (maximal dose, 0.5 mg) of epinephrine (1:1000) should be injected subcutaneously. This should reverse the attack in most cases. If no relief has been afforded after two doses of epinephrine, emergency transport to the hospital should be arranged. If the attack becomes very severe, intravenous aminophylline may be initiated in an attempt to relieve bronchospasm. A loading dose of 5.6 mg/kg is infused over 10 minutes, followed by a continuous intravenous infusion of 1 mg/kg per hour. Any patient requiring parenteral drug administration to control an asthma attack should be transported to the hospital. Early administration of a corticosteroid (hydrocortisone or dexamethasone) may also be helpful in severe attacks.

## Diabetes Mellitus

Diabetes mellitus is a disorder involving poor insulin production and, consequently, disorders of carbohydrate, fat, and protein metabolism. It is characterized by hyperglycemia if it is untreated. Diabetes mellitus occurring in children is termed juvenile-onset diabetes mellitus and usually carries the worst prognosis. These patients have little or no pancreatic β cell function and therefore require parenteral insulin daily. Blood glucose levels may be very difficult to control. The principal emergencies that develop are due to either hypoglycemia or hyperglycemia. If plasma insulin levels remain low or absent for a prolonged period, blood glucose levels will become extremely elevated. However, the glucose cannot enter the cells due to the lack of insulin, and as a result the cells metabolize fat and proteins to produce more glucose as well as ketones and other metabolic acids. A condition known as diabetic ketoacidosis occurs, which may lead to coma and death if the patient is not treated. The important fact to realize concerning ketoacidosis is that it requires several days to develop, during which time the patient is ill. It does not occur suddenly in a previously alert and well patient.

If a diabetic patient who is doing well has a sudden deterioration in the dental office, the condition is far more likely to be due to acute hypoglycemia, or insulin shock. The usual scenario involves a patient who has taken his or her morning insulin and has forgotten to eat a meal or has ingested inadequate carbohydrate. Exercise and stress may also increase carbohydrate utilization and lower blood glucose concentrations. Glucose and oxygen are the primary metabolites for brain cells. As the serum glucose level begins to decrease, neurologic symptoms may appear. Most diabetic patients are well attuned to this phenomenon and carry a carbohydrate source to be ingested in this event. If carbohydrate is not ingested and the blood glucose concentration continues to decrease, evidence of deteriorating cerebral function will ensue. The patient may become lethargic, have a change in mood, act strangely, or become nauseated. The sympathetic nervous system becomes hyperactive in an attempt to raise the blood glucose level, producing symptoms of tachycardia, hypertension, anxiety, and sweating. The patient develops slurred speech, ataxia, mental obtundation, and eventually loss of consciousness. Seizures may occur.

Management of hypoglycemia involves the administration of glucose. The oral route is used only if the patient is fully conscious and is experiencing early symptoms. Sugar dissolved in juice or a sugar-containing soft drink may be used. If the patient has become mentally obtunded, an intravenous catheter should be established and 50% dextrose administered until consciousness is regained. Alternatively, glucagon may be administered intramuscularly if establishment of intravenous access is not possible. It must be remembered that consciousness will be regained more slowly when glucagon is utilized. The dentist should never attempt to administer glucose orally to a mentally obtunded or unconscious patient.

It is recommended that the dental practitioner further expand on this material, becoming familiar with other medical emergency situations that may occur in the dental office, especially those drug-related emergencies that may result from pharmacologic agents being utilized in daily practice.

## BIBLIOGRAPHY

Goodson JM, Moore RA: Life-threatening reactions after pediatric sedation: an assessment of narcotic, local anesthetic, and anti-anxiety drug interaction. *JADA* 107:239-245, 1983.

Malamed SF: *Medical Emergencies in the Dental Office*, 5th ed. St Louis, Mosby, 2000.

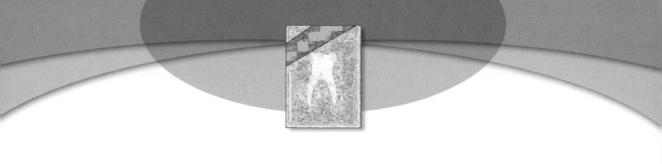

# CHAPTER 11

# Dental Public Health Issues in Pediatric Dentistry

*Michael J. Kanellis, John J. Warren, and Peter C. Damiano*

Increasingly, one of the primary challenges facing the dental profession is ensuring that all children and adults enjoy the benefits of good oral health. While treatment of children in an office setting is the cornerstone of pediatric dental practice, it cannot address all the needs of all children because of limited access to dental care and limited capacity. Thus, to optimize the oral health of all children, community-based, public health approaches are necessary. This chapter provides an overview of dental public health and outlines ways in which the oral health of children is enhanced by various public health activities.

## DEFINITION OF DENTAL PUBLIC HEALTH

Dental public health is defined as "the science and art of preventing and controlling dental diseases and promoting dental health through organized community efforts."[1] A common misconception about dental public health is that its primary objective is the delivery of dental care to low-income persons. Although this is important, the actual delivery of dental care is only one aspect of dental public health.

The three major core functions of public health, as identified by the 1988 Institute of Medicine study, are assessment, policy development, and assurance.[27] The major activities of dental public health can be divided into these same categories. Examples of core dental public health activities that affect the oral health of children are given in Box 11-1.

## BOX 11-1

### Examples of Dental Public Health Activities Affecting Children

**Assessment**

1. Documenting the oral health status of children through epidemiologic surveys
2. Assessing the supply and availability of dentists to meet the needs of children
3. Assessing the status of water fluoridation in communities
4. Assessing the need for dental care for children with special health care needs
5. Identifying barriers to dental access
6. Screening children before entering school

**Policy Development**

1. Developing policies and advocating for legislative action to ensure access to oral health services for low-income, underserved, hard-to-reach, and vulnerable children
2. Developing programs that focus on primary and secondary prevention
3. Developing programs to provide dental care to children with special health needs or without access to adequate dental care
4. Adopting state rules mandating oral health screening for children entering school for the first time

**Assurance**

1. Encouraging and coordinating efforts to provide oral health education and promotion in schools, clinics, community settings, and other settings
2. Expanding or establishing new dental clinical sites (e.g. CHC expansions)
3. Developing promotional activities by the State Health Agency to meet the oral health needs of a specific target group or community
4. Targeting topical and systemic fluoride programs to areas with nonfluoridated water supplies and high-risk populations
5. Including an oral health component in all school health initiatives
6. Establishing school-based prevention programs and school-based or school-linked dental clinics as components of comprehensive school health
7. Establishing programs to train medical professionals and other health related workers to recognize oral health problems, including early childhood caries
8. Integrating oral health services into appropriate health, education, and social service programs (e.g., Maternal and Child Health, nutrition, WIC, health promotion, PATCH program, school health)

Adapted from Association of State and Territorial Dental Directors' Guidelines for State and Territorial Dental/Oral Health Programs: *Essential Public Health Services to Promote Oral Health in the United States.* January 3, 1997.

## ROLE OF THE INDIVIDUAL PRACTITIONER

It is important for the individual practitioner to understand that the oral health status and needs of children receiving care in a private practice setting may not represent the status and needs of *all* children in the community. The challenge for dentists, therefore, is to look beyond the individual dental office and make a broad assessment of their community's needs while assessing their own role in enhancing the oral health of the entire community.

In 1995 the Association of State and Territorial Dental Directors (ASTDD) developed and disseminated a needs assessment model designed to help communities identify and address their oral health needs.[3,23] This model is known as the ASTDD Seven-Step Model (Fig. 11-1). It provides a straightforward approach for identifying the oral health needs of a community and for designing a program to meet these needs based on

available resources. Historically, needs assessments have relied on findings from intraoral examinations, which are typically expensive and time consuming to conduct. The ASTDD model provides an alternative for assessing needs that is more economical and utilizes existing resources and existing data when available. A community-based needs assessment will also provide an excellent opportunity to educate a community about the importance of oral health.[23]

In addition to participating in needs assessment activities, practitioners are often called on to participate in other public health activities, including advocating fluoridation of community water supplies, participating in school and community health promotion activities, and advising policy makers regarding dental care programs including Medicaid. Support and guidance for the individual practitioner becoming involved in dental public health activities can be sought from a variety of sources, including the oral health

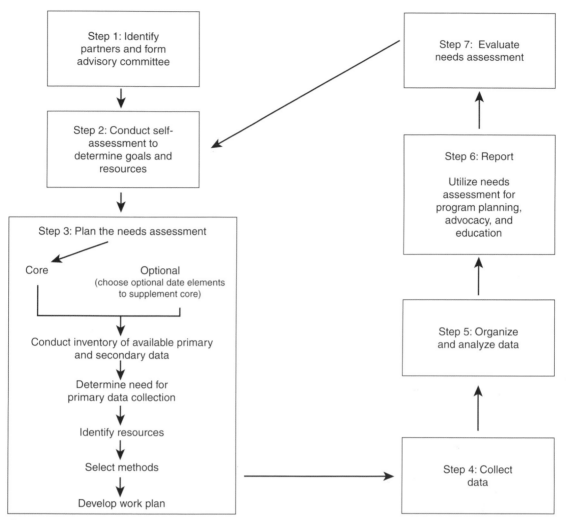

**Figure 11-1** Association of State and Territorial Dental Directors Seven-Step Needs Assessment Model. (From Kuthy RA, Siegal MD: Assessing oral health needs: ASTDD Seven-Step Model. Available at http://www.astdd.org/index.php?template=seven_steps.html.)

components of state public health agencies, county boards of health, and various community boards and organizations.

One important issue practitioners often find themselves involved with is enhancing access to dental care for members of their communities. This topic is discussed in the following sections.

## ACCESS TO CARE

Although regular dental care contributes substantially to healthy mouths for millions of children, a significant number of children and adults have serious problems receiving the care they need. These children are most often from low-income or minority families, and unfortunately these groups tend to experience more oral disease than other children.[8,21,29] Some of the factors that can limit access to dental care for these children are (1) lack of finances (including lack of third-party coverage), (2) lack of transportation, (3) language and cultural barriers, and (4) lack of perceived need for care.

### Dental Participation in Medicaid

Historically, financial limitations have been among the most formidable barriers for low-income children in receiving health care. In 1965, the federal government attempted to reduce these financial barriers by creating the Medicaid program (Title 19), which pays for medical and dental care for eligible low-income people. Adult dental coverage under Medicaid is optional, and covered services vary widely from state to state. However, coverage for child dental services is mandatory because of a 1968 amendment to the Medicaid program creating the Early and Periodic Screening, Diagnostic and Treatment (EPSDT) program.[35] The purpose of the EPSDT program is to identify the health problems of children as early as possible and to provide comprehensive preventive and remedial care.

Since 1965, the Medicaid program has been the primary public insurance program for the financing of dental services for low-income children in the United States. Most children below the poverty level who receive dental care do so through the Medicaid (Title 19) program.[34] In 1997, the State Children's Health Insurance Program (SCHIP) was started to expand public insurance to children in families with incomes too high to qualify for Medicaid.[32] SCHIP and Medicaid are linked in 37 states that have chosen to cover children in their SCHIP program either through an expansion of their existing Medicaid program (19 states) or through a program that is part private and part Medicaid expansion (18 states; usually Medicaid covers the lower income children eligible through SCHIP).

While Medicaid and SCHIP have been successful in improving access to dental services for some, a report from the Inspector General of the U.S. Department of Health and Human Services indicated that only one in five Medicaid-eligible children receive any dental services annually.[37] One of the biggest barriers to dental care is the lack of dentists willing to accept Medicaid-enrolled children. Rates of participation vary by state and by the definition of participation. For example, in California in 1990, only 16% of general and pediatric dentists accepted a new Medicaid-enrolled child into their practice.[12] In Connecticut in 1994, 66% of dentists reported having Medicaid-enrolled children in their practice and 52% were accepting new Medicaid-enrolled children.[26] A study in Iowa in 1995 found that 42% of dentists reported that they were accepting all new Medicaid patients into their practice, a decline of almost 50% from 1992.[13] Twenty-nine percent of dentists in Missouri had accepted a Medicaid patient into their practice in 1998.[25]

The most common reason cited by dentists for their lack of participation in Medicaid was the low reimbursement rates. Other nonfinancial issues, however, were important as well. For example, in the Iowa study, although dentists were more likely to rank low fees as the most important problem, more dentists said that broken appointments were a *more important* problem in their practice than low fees. Dentists who were less busy and those who believed that dentists have an ethical obligation to treat Medicaid enrollees were most likely to be accepting all new Medicaid patients in their practice. A number of states, including Indiana in 1998 and Iowa in 2000, have increased reimbursement rates to try and improve dentists' acceptance of Medicaid enrollees. Several other states, including California and Texas, were forced to increase their Medicaid reimbursement rates after being successfully sued because of poor access to dental care. Michigan chose a different approach and improved dentist participation in Medicaid by "carving out" the dental portion of their Medicaid program in 39 counties to Delta Dental of Michigan to remove the stigma that Medicaid has among dentists and increase reimbursement rates. While all solutions come with a financial cost, finding ways to improve access to dental care for Medicaid and SCHIP enrollees by encouraging dentists to participate in the program is critically important to improve the oral health of these children in need.

## Community Health Centers

As part of his "Great Society" plan to eliminate poverty, President Lyndon Johnson funded eight neighborhood health centers in 1965. This neighborhood health center concept has continued to develop and expand through the years and has evolved into a nationwide network of more than 1000 community health centers (CHCs) and migrant health centers. The mission of these centers is to increase access to affordable health care services for low-income families. CHCs are located throughout the country in areas where barriers limit access to primary health care for a significant portion of the population. These barriers can be economic, geographic, and/or cultural in nature. CHCs provide primary and preventive health care services including dental care in many centers.

Fiscal year (FY) 2002 appropriations for CHCs were $1.3 billion. Program statistics from the 2000 Uniform Data System (UDS) for that same year were as follows:[6]

- Total users: 9.6 million (of that 3.9 million are uninsured)
- Total physicians: 4803 (19,220,237 encounters)
- Total nurse practitioners/physician assistants: 2367 (6,657,449 encounters)
- Total dentists: 977 (2,606,326 encounters)
- Total hygienists: 283 (401,946 encounters)

In 2002, President George W. Bush launched a 5-year initiative to expand the existing network of CHCs with a goal of adding 1200 new and expanded health center sites and increasing the number of people served by CHCs annually from approximately 10 million in 2001 to more than 16 million by 2006. In August 2003 the Bush administration announced a $7 million expansion of oral health services through establishment of new and expanded oral health services in CHCs in 28 states.

The role of CHCs in the provision of oral health care for individuals who would otherwise not be able to access or afford care will likely increase in years to come.

## CHILDREN AND DENTAL PUBLIC HEALTH

This textbook is organized by children's developmental stages. It works well to discuss dental public health issues within this same developmental context. The remainder of this chapter is devoted to introducing some dental public health issues as they relate to children of different age groups.

### Barriers to Care for Infants and Toddlers from Low-Income Families

Dental care for infants and toddlers from low-income families presents a dilemma for several reasons. These children often (1) lack financial access to care, (2) have caregivers who fail to recognize the importance of early dental visits, (3) have difficulty finding a dentist who accepts Medicaid, and (4) have difficulty finding a dentist who will treat children younger than 3 years.

As stated elsewhere in this text, dental care for children should begin in infancy. This is especially true for low-income children who are at higher risk for disease. Although it is true that many children never experience decay in their primary dentition, others experience severe decay. For young children, particularly those under age 3, such treatment often requires hospitalization and general anesthesia. Thus, for low-income children with severe decay, the costs of treatment can be very high and present a major barrier to patients, parents, and practitioners.

Despite EPSDT program requirements that eligible children visit a dentist by age 3 (or younger in some states), the use of dental services by low-income children ages 0 to 3 remains extremely low.[13] Continuing efforts are needed to convey the importance of early dental visits for this group of children. In addition, oral health screening and counseling should be a part of existing public health programs where young children appear for other services. Successful integration of oral health activities, including prevention, education, and screening, has already occurred in many public health programs, including Maternal Child Health Clinics and Women, Infants, and Children (WIC) Clinics.

Although dental components are often an integral part of public health programs, rarely are public health clinics established solely to meet the needs of low-income infants. However, at least one international model exists for a clinic designed specifically for the oral health care of infants. In Brazil, a state-sponsored infant oral health clinic has existed since 1986.

### Project Head Start

Prior to beginning kindergarten or first grade, large numbers of children in the United States participate in formal preschool programs. Preschools provide a unique opportunity to study the oral health status of children in the 3- to 6-year-old group[15] and for increasing access to services for low-income children.

The largest preschool program in the country is Head Start, which primarily serves children from low-income families and children with disabilities. Head Start, established in 1965, is administered by the Department of Health and Human Services (DHHS). Head Start is a comprehensive child development program that serves children

# Iowa's Infant Oral Health Program at WIC
*Karin Weber*

The American Academy of Pediatric Dentistry recommends that children have a first dental visit within 6 months of the eruption of their first tooth or no later than 1 year of age.[1] The rationale for recommending early dental visits centers on the importance of preventive education, anticipatory guidance, screening and risk assessment, and establishing a dental home for the child. Despite the many benefits of early dental visits, dental utilization among children less than 3 years of age is low. This is especially true for children from low-income families and at highest risk for tooth decay. In a review of Medicaid claims data for Iowa children younger than 6 years, fewer than 4% of children received any dental services during the year.[2]

The University of Iowa has had a long tradition of recommending preventive dental visits for infants, but it has historically relied on patients presenting to the College of Dentistry's pediatric dental clinic to receive care. In 1998 the University of Iowa's Department of Pediatric Dentistry established an Infant Oral Health Clinic (IOHC) at the Johnson County Health Department. The primary objectives of the clinic were (1) to improve access and utilization of infant/toddler dental care by providing oral health services in an environment where high-risk children were already presenting; (2) to prevent and intercept early childhood caries in a high-risk population; and (3) to provide an opportunity for senior dental students to receive hands-on experience with infant/toddler patients.

The IOHC operates in conjunction with Johnson County's "Women, Infants and Children" (WIC) program and is available to children ages 0 to 5 who are enrolled in WIC. WIC is a special supplemental nutrition program funded by the U.S. Department of Agriculture, Food and Consumer Service, and available throughout the United States. To qualify for WIC, children must (1) live in the United States; (2) have a nutritional risk (this can include dietary habits that place a child at risk for tooth decay); and (3) have an income of 185% or less of federal poverty guidelines.

Senior dental students at the University of Iowa rotate weekly through the clinic under the supervision of faculty members from the Department of Pediatric Dentistry. By May 2003, 263 senior dental students had rotated through the IOHC. Dental services provided at the clinic include examinations, preventive services, limited restorative treatment, parental education, and referral. Oral examination of children is done either in the knee-to-knee position or on an examining table available at the WIC clinic. For infants, the oral examination can also be done using a Macri. The Macri is a piece of equipment used to facilitate clinical examination of very young children that was developed at the State University of Londrina, Brazil. This sling/chair-like device does not require the child's cooperation but provides a comfortable position with minimal restraint as well as excellent visualization of the oral cavity. Because of the young age of children attending the IOHC (0 to 3 years), parents are always welcome to remain near the child during the appointments to provide encouragement and support.

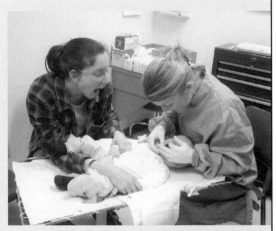

A young child being examined in a Macri.

The dental education provided at the IOHC is facilitated and reinforced using different materials and approaches. Parental education is generally done on an individual basis through one-on-one counseling. At the first visit, all parents watch a videotape called "Lift-the-Lip" developed by the University of Washington in Seattle. This video helps instruct parents how to examine their child's oral cavity and recognize early signs of early childhood caries. At the end of each dental appointment, parents are given a list of findings and recommendations that contains all pertinent information about their child's oral health discussed during the appointment.

Preventive services provided at the IOHP include application of fluoride varnish, as well as sealants for primary molars with incipient pit and fissure decay. Limited restorative treatment (atraumatic restorative treatment) using glass-ionomer materials is provided when indicated. At each

## Iowa's Infant Oral Health Program at WIC—cont'd

appointment a caries risk assessment is performed. Based on the caries risk, children are classified as either low risk or high risk for dental decay. Children classified as low risk are seen on a 6-month recall basis, and those classified as high risk are seen at least every 3 months. Appropriate referral for children with more complex dental needs is also done. By age 3, all children are referred to a dentist in the community in order to establish routine dental care throughout childhood.

The IOHP has been successful in providing dental care to high-risk children in a public health setting and in providing learning opportunities for dental students.

### REFERENCES

1. American Academy of Pediatric Dentists: Reference manual and guidelines. *Infant Oral Health Care* 24(7; special issue):47, 2002-2003.
2. Kanellis MJ, Damiano PC, Momany ET: Utilization of dental services by Iowa Medicaid-enrolled children younger than 6 years old. *J Pediatr Dent* 19(5):310-314, 1997.

from birth to age 5, pregnant women, and their families. They are child-focused programs and have the overall goal of increasing the school readiness of young children in low-income families.

For 30 years, Head Start provided services to preschoolers (3 to 5 years) only. In 1994, Congress approved the development of Early Head Start, serving pregnant women, infants, and toddlers. Whereas the preschool program serves children in a classroom setting, Early Head Start mostly serves pregnant women, infants, and toddlers through weekly home visits of 90 minutes each.

Also in 1994, Head Start and Early Head Start began providing services through community child care centers; many grantees now have formal partnership agreements that extend Head Start program performance standards to these community organizations.

In 2003, the total budget for Head Start and Early Head Start was $6,667,533,000, and the number of children enrolled topped 1 million. Early Head Start programs served more than 62,000 children under the age of 3.

Head Start operates in all 50 states, Puerto Rico, Virgin Islands, and Outer Pacific Islands. In addition, Head Start provides child development services to migrant children and families and Indian tribal nations. Head Start is organized by "grantees"; in 2003, there were 1570 grantees and 49,000 classrooms. Some grantees serve a large city; others might serve as many as 13 counties across rural areas of a state.

Head Start has historically maintained a strong commitment to the health of children and their families enrolled in its programs. This commitment reflects the documented connection between school readiness and good health, including good oral health. "Early tooth loss caused by dental decay can result in failure to thrive, impaired speech development, absence from and inability to concentrate in school, and reduced self-esteem" (MCH Fact Sheet: Oral Health and Learning). Head Start and Early Head Start have a mandatory dental component that requires that all enrolled children receive a dental examination complete with prophylaxis as well as follow-up care for necessary restorative treatment. Head Start programs establish and maintain dental records for children enrolled in their program, but the necessary dental treatment is usually provided by dental professionals in the community or with public health clinics. Head Start programs are the payor of last resort for necessary dental treatment for children enrolled in their program who are not eligible for funding from Medicaid or other sources. This unique public-private partnership has been instrumental in helping ensure access to care for low-income preschool children nationwide. One of the stated goals of Head Start is to attempt to link families to an ongoing health care system to ensure that the child continues to receive comprehensive health care even after leaving the Head Start program.[36]

All Head Start grantees have a health services manager, who must ensure that families, staff, and community resources are coordinated for the delivery of quality health services to children. This work includes training families and staff to conduct ongoing observations to spot signs of health problems, including "lift the lip" techniques. The health services manager and staff recruit and build professional relationships with community health and dental professionals to work toward good health for all children.

## School-Based Dental Care

The attainment of school age presents another unique opportunity for enhancing the oral health of children. Schools are a logical site for promoting oral health through educational and prevention programs and delivering dental services to school-aged children because they provide a high concentration of children at the same location.[24] The United States has enjoyed a long tradition of successfully implementing oral health activities in school settings. Examples of services that can be provided in a school-based setting include oral health education, fluoride mouth rinsing, sealant placement, oral health screenings and referrals, and comprehensive restorative care.

Health education, including oral health education, has long been considered an important part of school curricula in the United States. Dentists and other dental health professionals often have the opportunity to contribute to these activities by visiting classrooms and participating in health fairs or other special events. Oral health information presented in these forums can generate interest and stimulate changes in knowledge and attitudes. However, it is important for the oral health professional to understand that these changes are commonly short-lived and that desired behavioral changes require regular, long-term follow-up.[7]

School-based fluoride mouth rinsing programs in the United States have been a common public health prevention strategy for nearly 30 years. In 1988, an estimated 3.25 million children were participating in school-based fluoride mouth rinsing programs in 11,683 schools.[7] Historically, school-based fluoride mouth rinsing programs have been most commonly targeted at schools where the majority of children do not have access to fluoridated drinking water, regardless of the socioeconomic level of the students. The general decline in the caries rate among children has caused researchers to question the cost-effectiveness of these programs.[5] These programs are most likely to be cost-effective when targeted at schools with additional risk factors

besides a lack of water fluoridation (e.g., low-income status, high caries rate, lack of access to primary care). Typically, children participating in school-based fluoride mouth rinsing programs rinse once a week with 10 ml of a 0.2% neutral sodium fluoride solution. Alternatively, children may rinse daily with 0.05% sodium fluoride. Mouth rinsing activities are generally supervised by a classroom teacher, a school nurse, or other persons with appropriate training.

School-based sealant programs have become increasingly popular as a means of increasing the prevalence of sealants among low-income children.[4,10,22,30] Although pit and fissure sealants have been known to be effective in preventing dental decay for more than 25 years,[31] only 11% of U.S. school children had dental sealants on their teeth in 1989[38] with sealant use even lower for children from low-income families (4.3% for children from families with incomes of less than $10,000).[38] In 1995, 109 school-based/school-linked dental sealant programs were identified in 27 states.[2] These programs usually target schools with a high percentage of low-income children (based on eligibility for free and reduced meal programs). Certain grades are usually chosen to participate, based on the eruption patterns of the permanent molars. Because of the timing of eruption for first permanent molars, second grade is a common age to initiate sealant programs. The majority of sealant programs use a four-handed approach, with each sealant team generally providing sealants to 10 to 15 children a day (Fig. 11-2).

Oral health screenings are carried out in schools under a number of different circumstances. Often, oral health screenings are provided as part of health fairs, or in combination with other educational/promotional activities. The purpose of these screenings is generally to identify gross problems and to refer children for dental care. A minimum of equipment is needed for this level of screening, with a pen light and tongue blade often sufficing. When screenings are performed in conjunction with school-based sealant programs or as part of surveys gathering data on the oral health status of children, the mirror and explorer examination is often more complete.

Following school-based oral health screenings, referrals for follow-up care are generally made to area dentists, public health agencies, or school-based clinics. Only rarely are school-based screenings or examinations intended to take the place of complete dental examinations by dentists outside

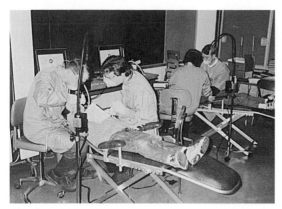

**Figure 11-2** Third-year dental students placing sealants in a school-based sealant program.

the school. This information should be communicated to parents and guardians of children who are screened in school-based settings in order that they understand the intent of the school-based screening and the limitations of the procedures provided (e.g., no radiographs).

Comprehensive school-based dental care is not common in the United States, although some school-based programs providing a wide range of services have been in existence for more than 75 years. In Virginia, comprehensive school-based dental programs were first introduced in 1921, with ongoing programs in existence ever since.[14] Although examples of school-based programs offering comprehensive care can be found in the

## School-Based Sealant Programs
*Mark Siegal*

School dental sealant programs seek to assure that children receive a highly effective but underutilized dental prevention service through a proven community-based approach. School sealant programs generally are designed to maximize effectiveness by targeting high-risk children. High-risk children include vulnerable populations less likely to receive private dental care, such as children eligible for free or reduced-cost lunch programs. Children and their parents are made aware of dental sealants in terms of their value and their availability through the school program. Once signed parental consent forms have been returned, children are evaluated for their sealant needs and sealants are placed by dental professionals (usually dental hygienists).

There are variations in how school sealant programs are designed:

- School-based programs are conducted completely within the school setting, usually with teams of dental hygienists and dental assistants utilizing portable dental equipment.
- School-linked programs are connected with schools in some manner but deliver the sealants at a site other than the school (i.e., clinic, private dental office). For example, school-linked programs may make informational presentations, distribute consent forms, and conduct dental screening at school.
- Hybrid programs incorporate school-based and school-linked components (some

schools may have school-based and others school-linked approaches).

School sealant programs are faced with the issues of how to deal with the restorative dental care needs of the children they see and how to assure quality by providing follow-up evaluation and repair, as necessary, of the sealants placed through the program.

In its systematic review of the literature, the Task Force on Community Preventive Services (2002) found that school-based sealant programs are effective in preventing tooth decay and issued a strong recommendation that school sealant programs be included as part of a comprehensive population-based strategy to prevent or control tooth decay in communities.[1]

An effective school dental sealant program will have the following attributes:

- Delivers sealants to large numbers of high-risk children with susceptible permanent molar teeth
- Maximizes program efficiency
- Reexamines children within 1 year of initial sealant placement. At this time, newly erupted teeth may be sealed, and previously placed sealants may be repaired or reapplied as necessary
- Maintains a quality assurance system
- Identifies children with treatment needs and assures that they receive appropriate dental care
- Maintains descriptive program data
- Is sustainable

*Continued*

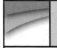

## School-Based Sealant Programs—cont'd

Ohio leads the nation in the number of children who receive sealants through its network of 21 local school-based programs[2] and has documented the reduction of disparity in sealant prevalence according to race and income.[3] Perhaps the nation's best example of a model school-based sealant program can be found in the city of Cincinnati. The Cincinnati program targets children in second and sixth grades in schools with at least 50% of children eligible for the free/reduced-cost lunch program. All children in those grades are eligible for the program, with parental consent.

Individual arrangements are made with each school for two dental teams to set up a portable dental office in the schools. The equipment and supplies are delivered in a van and take about 45 minutes to set up. The portable dental office includes all of the infection control considerations necessary to meet state and Occupational Safety and Health Administration requirements. Depending on the enrollment and participation, the sealant program's stay ranges from a day to more than a week. After a dentist has evaluated each child's need for sealants and determined which teeth are to be sealed, the sealants are placed by a dental hygienist–dental assistant team. In Ohio, as in most states with sealant programs, a dentist need not be present while the sealants are placed. However, some state dental practice acts require a dentist's presence. On a typical school day, each team places sealants on 18 to 20 children in the Cincinnati program. The Cincinnati program has been a model for other Ohio programs and the nation.

### REFERENCES

1. Truman BI, Gooch BF, Sulemana I et al: Reviews of evidence regarding interventions to prevent dental caries, oral and pharyngeal cancers, and sports-related craniofacial injuries. *Am J Prev Med* 23(suppl 1):21-54, 2002.
2. Available at http://www2.cdc.gov/nccdphp/doh/synopses/index.asp.
3. Impact of targeted, school-based dental sealant programs in reducing racial and economic disparities in sealant prevalence among schoolchildren, Ohio, 1998–1999. *MMWR Morb Mortal Wkly Rep* 50(34):736-738, 2001.

United States, perhaps the best known model for comprehensive school-based dentistry is the School Dental Service of New Zealand, which has been in existence for more than 60 years.[20]

School-based dental care can provide a means for increasing both access and use of dental services for children who do not or cannot receive care in the private sector. School-based dental programs, regardless of scope, should have careful planning in order to optimize chances for success. The most fundamental aspect of planning involves a careful assessment of the need for school-based dental services and ongoing evaluation of such programs. School-based programs should not attempt to replace services provided in the private sector, nor should they compete for patients who are adequately served by existing resources.

### The Challenge of Adolescence

Providing oral health care to adolescents can be a rewarding experience for the practitioner. This is generally a very "teachable" age, with most adolescents acutely interested in their appearance and their health. For some adolescents, however, daily life challenges may make dental care a very low priority. Adolescence is a period of life typically associated with increased risks in the areas of health and education[19] and, in some estimations, adolescents today face greater risks to their current and future health than ever before.[17] Consider a few of the following statistics from 1995 concerning life for American teenagers:[11]

1. Every 22 seconds, an American teenager becomes pregnant.
2. Every 47 seconds, an American child is abused or neglected. About half of these children are teens.
3. Every 67 seconds, an American teenager has a baby.
4. On any given day, 40,000 American teens are in jails or detention facilities.
5. Every day, 6 teenagers commit suicide.

Needless to say, the oral health needs of adolescents are often overshadowed by other pressing concerns.

The term "at risk" has become a general term used to describe people in trouble[34] and is often used to categorize adolescents who are not likely to succeed in school or in life because of one or more factors.[9] Factors that can place an adolescent at risk may include, but are not limited to, chemical dependency, teenage pregnancy, poverty, disaffection with school and society, emotional and physical abuse, physical and emotional disabilities, and learning disabilities.[39]

Many of these same factors can affect an adolescent's oral health and ability or willingness to seek dental care. Low-income adolescents experience more decay than other adolescents,[28] and adolescents with risk factors of poverty, teenage pregnancy, low grades, or disaffection with school are less likely to use or receive dental care than other adolescents.[18]

As with other age groups, lack of finances is a significant barrier to oral health care for at-risk adolescents. It is estimated that one in five American teenagers lives in poverty[11] and that one-third of American teenagers living in poverty are not covered by Medicaid.[11] Nonfinancial barriers to care also exist and may include (1) low priority given to oral health, (2) no perceived need for dental care, (3) a "dislike" for going to the dentist, (4) lack of office hours that do not interfere with school and other activities, and (5) lack of transportation.

Addressing the oral health needs of at-risk teens is a relatively newly recognized problem, and strategies for dealing with this problem have not been as well developed as for other age groups. Possible strategies that may offer solutions include integrating oral health services into comprehensive school-based health centers, offering screening and referral programs in community settings frequented by teens, and maximizing the participation of adolescents in the EPSDT program.[16]

# REFERENCES

1. American Board of Dental Public Health: Informational brochure. Gainesville, Fla, The Board, 1992.
2. Amini H, Bouchard J, Farquehar C et al: Assessment of school-based/linked sealant programs in the U.S. *J Dent Res* 74 (AADR Abstract 267):45, 1995.
3. Association of State and Territorial Dental Directors' Guidelines for State and Territorial Dental/Oral Health Programs: *Essential Public Health Services to Promote Oral Health in the United States.* January 3, 1997.
4. Bohannan HM, Disney JA, Graves RC et al: Indications for sealant use in a community-based preventive dentistry program. *J Dent Educ* 48(2):45-55, 1984.
5. Bohannan HM, Stamm JW, Graves RC et al: Fluoride mouthrinse programs in fluoridated communities. *JADA* 111:783-789, 1985.
6. Bureau of Primary Care: http://www.bphc.hrsa. gov/chc/. Last accessed 5/16/04.
7. Burt BA, Eklund SA: *Dentistry, Dental Practice, and the Community,* 6th ed. St. Louis, Saunders, 2005.
8. Call RL: Effects of poverty on children's dental health. *Pediatrician* 16:200-206, 1989.
9. Capuzzi D, Gross D: *Youth at Risk.* Alexandria, Va, American Association for Counseling and Development, 1989.
10. Cohen LA, Horowitz AM: Community-based sealant programs in the United States: results of a survey. *J Public Health Dent* 53(4):241-245, 1993.
11. Cohen MI: Great transitions, preparing adolescents for a new century: a commentary on the health component of the concluding report of the Carnegie Council on Adolescent Development. *J Adolesc Health* 19:2-5, 1996.
12. Damiano PC et al: Factors affecting dentist participation in a state Medicaid program. *J Dent Educ* 54(11):638-643, 1990.
13. Damiano PC, Kanellis MJ, Willard JC, Momany ET: *A Report on the Iowa Title XIX Dental Program: Final Report to the Iowa Department of Human Services.* Iowa City, University of Iowa Public Policy Center and College of Dentistry, 1996.
14. Day KC, Doherty J: Celebrating 75 years of dental public health in Virginia. *Virginia Dent J* 73(3), 1996.
15. Edelstein BL, Douglass CW: Dispelling the myth that 50 percent of U.S. schoolchildren have never had a cavity. *Public Health Rep* 110:522-530, 1995.
16. English A: Early and periodic screening, diagnosis, and treatment program (EPSDT): a model for improving adolescents' access to healthcare. *J Adolesc Health* 14:524-526, 1993.
17. Gans JE, Blyth DA: *America's Adolescents: How Healthy Are They?* AMA Profiles of Adolescent Health Series. Chicago, American Medical Association, 1990.
18. Harvey HL: Factors affecting the utilization of dental services by adolescents. Thesis, University of Iowa, 1996.
19. Hechinger FM: *Fateful Choices: Healthy Youth for the 21st Century.* Washington, DC, Carnegie Council on Adolescent Development, 1992.
20. Jones R: The school-based dental care systems of New Zealand and South Australia: a decade of change. *J Publ Health Dent* 44(3):120-124 1984.

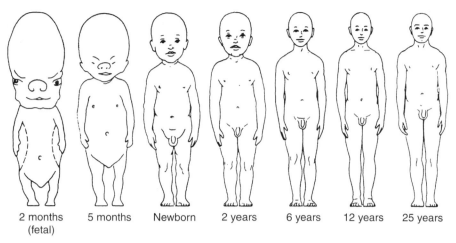

| 2 months (fetal) | 5 months | Newborn | 2 years | 6 years | 12 years | 25 years |

**Figure 12-1** The changing proportions of the human body from 2 months in utero to adulthood. (From Jackson CM: Some aspects of form and growth. In: Robbins WJ, Brody S, Hogan AF et al, editors. *Growth.* New Haven, Yale University Press, 1929, p 118.)

during maturation. No year is more dramatic in terms of growth than the first year of life, during which most children undergo a 50% increase in length and almost a 200% increase in weight. Toward the end of the first year of life, the growth rate slows. After the first birthday, the growth rate stays very stable and the height and weight increments of the child remain relatively predictable all the way to adolescence.

There are no accurate predictors of the child's final height before age 3. At age 3, however, correlations between the child's height and weight at maturity are fairly strong. The process of a newborn changing into an adult is one of elongation. The legs, at first shorter than the trunk, become longer. Also, the length of the child's trunk, compared with his or her breadth, becomes considerably greater.

As the body changes and matures, the infant is afforded increasingly sophisticated postural and locomotive actions. Table 12-1 shows some of the physical and cognitive developmental hallmarks of a child during his or her first 18 months of life. (Piagetian psychology as well as object permanency and causality is discussed in this chapter's section on cognitive development.)

By age 2, a child has the gross motor skills to run, climb, walk up and down steps, and kick a ball. His fine motor skills allow him to stack blocks (up to six), make parallel crayon strokes, and turn the pages of a book one page at a time. Table 12-2 shows a variety of motor skills and the mean age at which they are acquired.

### TABLE 12-2

**Median Age and Range in Acquisition of Motor Skills**

| MOTOR SKILL | AGE IN MONTHS | |
| --- | --- | --- |
| | MEDIAN | RANGE* |
| Transfers objects hand to hand | 5.5 | 4-8 |
| Sits alone 30 seconds or more | 6.0 | 5-8 |
| Rolls from back to stomach | 6.4 | 4-10 |
| Has neat pincer grasp | 8.9 | 7-12 |
| Stands alone | 11.0 | 9-16 |
| Holds crayon adaptively | 11.2 | 8-15 |
| Walks alone | 11.7 | 9-17 |
| Walks up stairs with help | 16.1 | 12-23 |
| Walks up stairs both feet on each step | 25.8 | 19-30 |

Adapted from Bayley N: Manual for the Bayley Scales of Infant Development. New York, Psychological Corporation (1969). From Zuckerman BS, Frank DA: Infancy. In Levine MD et al (eds): *Developmental-Behavioral Pediatrics*, Philadelphia, WB Saunders, 1983, p 89.
*5th to 95th percentile.

The nervous system of the child grows dramatically from birth until age 3. In fact, by the end of the second year the child's brain has attained 75% of its adult weight.[1]

# REFERENCES

1. Hurlock EB: *Child Development.* New York, McGraw-Hill, 1950.

## Craniofacial Changes

*Jerry Walker*

### Intrauterine Growth and Development

The organization and complexity of growth and development are nowhere more evident than in the changes that take place in the head and face (Table 12-3). The human face begins its first observable growth during the fourth week of intrauterine life with the development of the branchial apparatus. The branchial apparatus is first seen as a series of ridges on the lateral aspect of the cephalic end of the embryo at approximately the third week of intrauterine life. A 1-month-old embryo has no real face but the key primordia have already begun to gather. These slight swellings, depressions, and thickenings then rapidly undergo a series of mergers, rearrangements, and enlargements that transform them from a cluster of separate masses into a face (Fig. 12-2).[7]

Sperber[6] described the presomite stage of development (21 to 31 days), during which the 3-mm embryo develops at its cranial end five mesenchymal elevations or processes. The five mesenchymal elevations constitute the initial features of the face. These include the frontonasal process, two maxillary processes, and two mandibular arches. These processes grow differentially, and by obliterating the ectodermal grooves between them, they eventually contour the features of the face.

The oral cavity of the embryo is bounded by the frontonasal process and by the maxillary and mandibular processes of the first branchial arch (Fig. 12-3). Each maxillary process moves toward the midline and joins with the lateral nasal fold of the frontonasal process. As this is happening, a shelf-like process (the palatal process) develops on the medial side of each maxillary process. These two palatal processes move toward the midline, where they fuse. This palatal fusion is normally completed by the eighth intrauterine week. The mandibular processes fuse at the midline somewhat before the maxillary and nasal processes (Fig. 12-4). The palate grows more

rapidly in width than in length during the fetal period as a result of midpalatal sutural growth and appositional growth of the lateral alveolar margins. A failure in the fusion of the processes gives rise to oral or facial clefts or both. In the mandible, the cartilaginous skeleton of the first branchial arch, known as Meckel's cartilage, provides a form for the development of the mandible.

The muscles of mastication, that is, the temporalis, the masseter, and the medial and lateral pterygoids, and the trigeminal nerve also are derived from the first branchial arch. At approximately 60 days of gestation, the embryo has acquired all of its basic morphologic characteristics and enters the fetal period, which is marked by osseous development.

Rapid orofacial development is characteristic of the advanced development of the cranial portion of the embryo compared with its caudal portion. The different rates of growth result in a pear-shaped embryonic disk, with the head region

## TABLE 12-3
### Developing Structures of the Head and Face

| DEVELOPING STRUCTURES | INITIATION (WEEKS IN UTERO) |
|---|---|
| Neural plate | 2 |
| Buccopharyngeal membrane | 2 |
| Mandibular arch initiation | 3 |
| Hypoglossal muscles (tongue) | 5 |
| Medial and lateral nasal processes | 5 |
| Lens of the eye | 5 |
| Retina | 5 |
| External carotid artery | 6 |
| Eustachian tube | 6 |
| Larynx | 6 |
| Maxillary process | 6 |
| External auditory meatus | 7 |
| Nasal septum | 8 |
| Two palatal shelves fuse together | 8 |
| Palatal shelves fuse with nasal septum | 10 |
| Ossification of craniofacial skeleton | 10 |
| Eyelids completely formed and closed | 10 |
| Eyelids open | 28 |

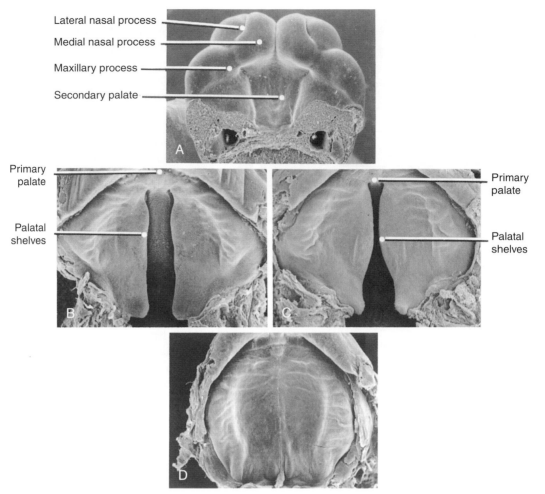

Lateral nasal process
Medial nasal process
Maxillary process
Secondary palate

Primary palate
Palatal shelves

Primary palate
Palatal shelves

**Figure 12-4** These scanning electron micrographs of human specimens (except **A**, which is a mouse specimen) show several stages of palate closure from 53 to 59 days after conception. **A**, At the completion of primary palate closure. B, Palatal shelves during elevation. **C**, Just prior to fusion of the shelves. **D**, The secondary palate following fusion. (Courtesy Dr. K. Sulik. A reproduced with permission from Proffit WR: *Contemporary Orthodontics,* 3<sup>rd</sup> ed. St Louis, Mosby, 2000.)

width of the mandible. By the second year, the symphysis is closed and growth becomes localized in the mandible as well as in the nasomaxillary complex. An enormous metamorphosis has taken place, but many more changes need to occur before the child's adult appearance is realized.

## REFERENCES

1. Caffey J: *Pediatric X-Ray Diagnosis.* Chicago, Year Book, 1950.
2. Enlow DH: *Handbook of Facial Growth.* Philadelphia, Saunders, 1982.
3. Fields HW: Craniofacial growth from infancy through adulthood. *Pediatr Clin North Am* 38:1053-1088, 1991.
4. Proffit WR: *Contemporary Orthodontics.* St Louis, Mosby, 1986.
5. Ranly DM: *A Synopsis of Craniofacial Growth.* New York, Appleton-Century-Crofts, 1980.
6. Sperber GH: *Craniofacial Embryology.* Bristol, UK, John Wright and Sons, 1978.
7. Stewart RE, Barber TK, Troutman KC et al: *Pediatric Dentistry: Scientific Foundations and Clinical Practice.* St Louis, Mosby, 1982.

### Dental Changes

*Clemons A. Full*

The purpose of this section is to address the growth, development, and eruption of each tooth unit from its initiation to complete eruption. By definition, *growth* signifies an increase, expansion,

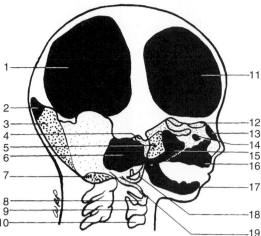

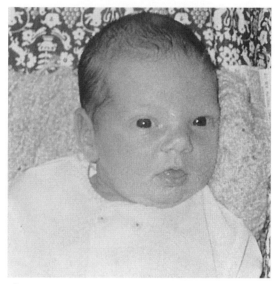

**Figure 12-5** Human skull at about 3 months. Intramembranous bones are shown in black. Cartilage is represented by light stippling, and bones developing by endochondral ossification are indicated by darker stippling. Approximate time of appearance for each bone is indicated in parentheses. 1, Parietal bone (10 weeks). 2, Interparietal bone (8 weeks). 3, Supraoccipital (8 weeks). 4, Dorsum sellae (still cartilaginous). 5, Temporal wing of sphenoid (2 to 3 months; the basisphenoid appears at 12 to 13 weeks, orbitosphenoid at 12 weeks, and presphenoid at 5 months). 6, Squamous part of temporal bone (2 to 3 months). 7, Basioccipital (2 to 3 months). 8, Hyoid (still cartilaginous). 9, Thyroid (still cartilaginous). 10, Cricoid (still cartilaginous). 11, Frontal bone ($7\frac{1}{2}$ weeks). 12, Crista galli (still cartilaginous; inferiorly, the middle concha begins ossification at 16 weeks, the superior and inferior conchae at 18 weeks; the perpendicular plate of ethmoid begins ossification during the first postnatal year, the cribriform plate during the second postnatal year, the vomer at 8 fetal weeks). 13, Nasal bone (8 weeks). 14, Lacrimal bone ($8\frac{1}{2}$ weeks). 15, Malar (8 weeks). 16, Maxilla (end of sixth week; premaxilla, 7 weeks). 17, Mandible (6 to 8 weeks). 18, Tympanic ring (begins at 9 weeks, with complete ring at 12 weeks; petrous bone, 5 to 6 months). 19, Styloid process, still cartilaginous. (From Enlow DH: *Handbook of Facial Growth.* Philadelphia, Saunders, 1982. Modified from Patten BM: *Human Embryology,* 3rd ed. New York, McGraw-Hill, 1968.)

**Figure 12-6** The small nose, lips, jaws, ears, and chin of this 3-week-old girl are shared with other young babies. Babies have a uniformity of appearance. With growth, of course, the subtle differences among young babies' faces become explicit and easily recognized.

or extension of any given tissue. For example, a tooth grows as more enamel is deposited by ameloblasts. *Development* addresses the progressive evolution of a tissue. A tooth develops as the ameloblasts develop from less specific ectodermal tissue and as the dentinoblasts develop from unspecialized mesoderm.

Teeth are formed by tissues originating from both ectoderm and mesoderm. At approximately 6 weeks of age, the basal layer of the oral epithelium of the fetus shows areas of increased activity and enlargement in the areas of the future dental arches. This increase and expansion give rise to the dental lamina of the future tooth germ. As the tooth bud continues to develop, it reaches a point at which it is recognized as the cap stage. At this time, it will begin to incorporate mesoderm into its structure. Therefore, the tooth-forming organ is initially formed from ectoderm but shortly thereafter includes mesoderm.

The expansion of tissue on the epithelial borders represents the beginning of the life cycle of the tooth. The ectoderm will become responsible for the future enamel, and the mesoderm will become primarily responsible for pulp and dentin. The tooth germ is accountable for the development of the following three formative tissues:

1. Dental organ (epithelial)
2. Dental papilla
3. Dental sac

The 6-week-old fetus demonstrates ten sites of epithelial activity on the occlusal (soft tissue) border of both the developing maxilla and the mandible.[1] These sites are lined next to each other and ultimately predict the position of the future 10 primary teeth in both the maxilla and the mandible (Fig. 12-8).

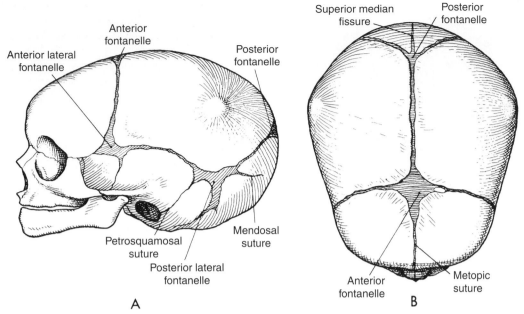

Figure 12-7   The cranium at birth. Note the fontanelles, one at each corner of the parietal bones. (From Kuhn JP, Slovis TL, Haller JO: *Caffey's Pediatric Diagnostic Imaging,* 10th ed. St Louis, Mosby, 2004.)

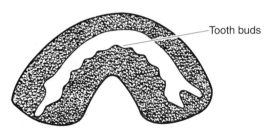

Figure 12-8   Diagrammatic representation of the tooth buds in an approximately 8-week-old fetus.

In addition to developing 20 primary teeth, each unit also develops a dental lamina that is responsible for the development of the future permanent tooth.[3] Therefore, the primary centrals, laterals, and cuspids produce a dental lamina for the future permanent centrals, laterals, and cuspids. The first and second primary molars produce a dental lamina for the future first and second permanent premolars. The unaccounted-for permanent molars develop from and on three successive locations on one dental lamina extend-

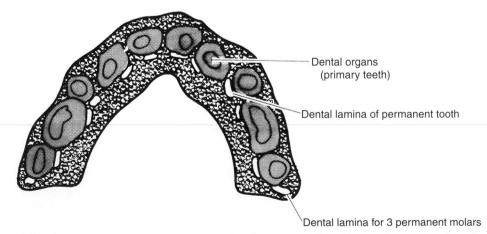

Figure 12-9   Diagrammatic representation of the dental organs and dental lamina in an approximately 4-month-old fetus.

ing distally from each of the second primary molars (Fig. 12-9).[3]

An analysis of the successive periods of growth of the tooth germ can be organized by the following stages of the life cycle of the tooth:[3]

Growth
    Initiation
    Proliferation
    Histodifferentiation
    Morphodifferentiation
    Apposition
Calcification
Eruption
Attrition

## Growth

**Initiation.**   The initiation stage is first noticed in the 6-week-old fetus (Fig. 12-10). As the word *initiation* suggests, this stage is recognized by the initial formation of an expansion of the basal layer of the oral cavity immediately above the basement membrane. The basal layer is a row of organized cells lined up on the basement membrane, which is a tissue division line between the ectoderm (epithelium) and the mesoderm (Fig. 12-11). The cells of the basal layer are the innermost cells of the oral epithelium (ectoderm) adjacent to the basement membrane.

At 10 specific intermittent locations along the basement membrane, the cells of the basal layer multiply at a much faster rate than the surrounding cells.[4] This development occurs at that point on the oral epithelium that is the tooth bud

and is responsible for the initial growth of that tooth (Fig.12-12).

It can be noted that the times of initiation of the various teeth differ.[1] This period of tooth development is also recognized as the bud stage. Such a description assists in visually understanding the developmental process of the immature tooth.

**Proliferation.**   Proliferation is really only a further multiplication of the cells of the initiation stage and an expansion of the tooth bud, resulting in the formation of the tooth germ (Fig. 12-13). The tooth germ is a result of the prolific epithelial cells forming a cap-like appearance with the subsequent incorporation of the mesoderm. This incorporation of mesodermal tissue below and within the cap gives rise to the dental papilla.

The mesenchyme (mesoderm) surrounding the dental organ and dental papilla is the tissue that will form the dental sac. The dental sac ultimately gives rise to the supporting structures of the tooth. These structures are the cementum and periodontal ligament.

As the tooth germ continues to proliferate in an irregular fashion, it produces a cap-like appearance. This stage is called the cap stage because the structure takes on the form of a cap (Fig. 12-14). Like the bud stage, it is so referenced for visual identification. As the cap begins to form, the mesenchyme changes within the cap to initiate the development of the dental papilla.

The dental papilla evolves from the mesenchyme invaginating the inner dental epithelium

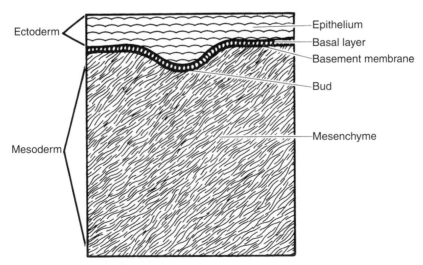

**Figure 12-10**   Diagrammatic representation of the initiation stage of the life cycle of the tooth in an approximately 5- to 6-week-old fetus.

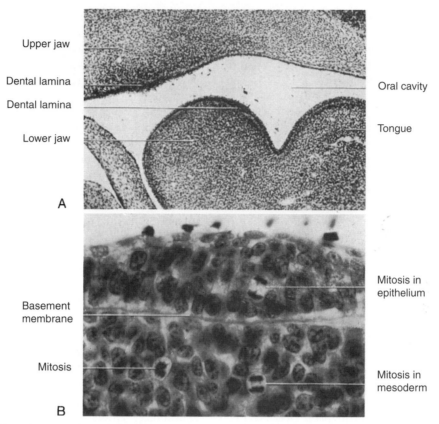

Upper jaw

Dental lamina

Dental lamina

Lower jaw

Oral cavity

Tongue

A

Basement membrane

Mitosis

Mitosis in epithelium

Mitosis in mesoderm

B

**Figure 12-11**    Initiation of tooth development. Human embryo 13.5 mm long, fifth week. **A,** Sagittal section through upper and lower jaws. **B,** High magnification of thickened oral epithelium. (From Orban B: *Dental Histology and Embryology,* 2nd ed. New York, McGraw-Hill, 1929.)

and specializes to form the pulp and dentin. The dental sac also comes into being by a marginal condensation in the mesenchyme surrounding the dental organ and dental papilla. The stellate (star-like) reticulum (network) is an organization of cells within the descending portion of the dental organ that is enamel-forming tissue and is called the enamel pulp. Therefore, the tooth germ during this stage has all the necessary formative tissues to embrace the development of a tooth and its periodontal ligament.[3]

In summary, the tooth germ consists of all the necessary elements for the development of the complete tooth. The germ is composed of the following three distinct parts: (1) dental organ, (2) dental papilla, and (3) dental sac. The dental organ produces the enamel. The dental papilla generates the dentin and pulp. The dental sac gives rise to the cementum and periodontal ligament.[3]

**Histodifferentiation.**    The histodifferentiation stage is marked by the histologic difference in the appearance of the cells of the tooth germ

because they are now beginning to specialize (Fig. 12-15). The cap continues to grow and takes more of the appearance of a bell. The image of a bell is registered because the extensions of the cap grow deeper into the mesoderm. This part of development is appropriately called the bell stage. The tissue within the bell is the tissue that gives rise to the dental papilla.

The dental organ is now completely surrounded by the basement membrane and is divided into an inner and outer dental epithelium. The dental organ ultimately becomes enamel.

The condensation of the tissue (mesoderm) adjacent to the outside of the bell is responsible for the dental sac. The dental sac ultimately gives rise to the cementum, which is the covering of the tooth's root, and to the periodontal ligament, which attaches the tooth to the bone around the tooth roots.

The dental lamina continues to shrink with the result that it looks more like a cord. The dental lamina for the permanent successor becomes

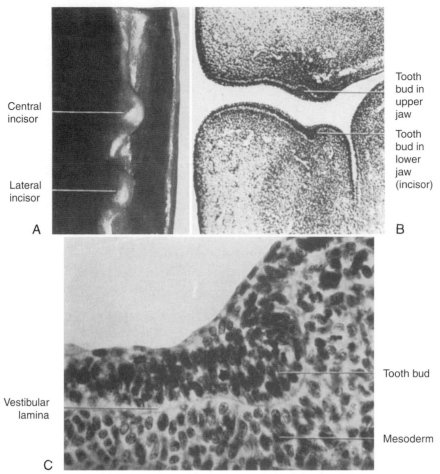

**Central incisor**

**Lateral incisor**

A

**Tooth bud in upper jaw**

**Tooth bud in lower jaw (incisor)**

B

**Vestibular lamina**

**Tooth bud**

**Mesoderm**

C

**Figure 12-12**   Bud stage of tooth development (proliferation stage). Human embryo 16 mm long, sixth week. **A,** Wax reconstruction of the germs of the central and lateral lower incisors. **B,** Sagittal section through upper and lower jaws. **C,** High-magnification view of the tooth germ of the lower incisor in bud stage. (From Orban B: *Dental Histology and Embryology,* 2nd ed. New York, McGraw-Hill, 1929.)

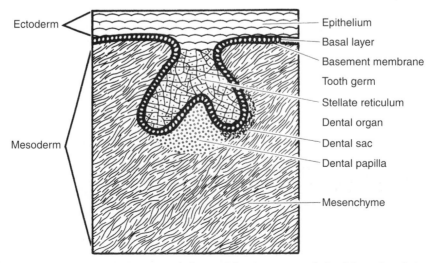

**Ectoderm**

**Mesoderm**

**Epithelium**

**Basal layer**

**Basement membrane**

**Tooth germ**

**Stellate reticulum**

**Dental organ**

**Dental sac**

**Dental papilla**

**Mesenchyme**

**Figure 12-13**   Diagrammatic representation of the proliferation stage of the life cycle of the tooth in an approximately 9- to 11-week-old fetus.

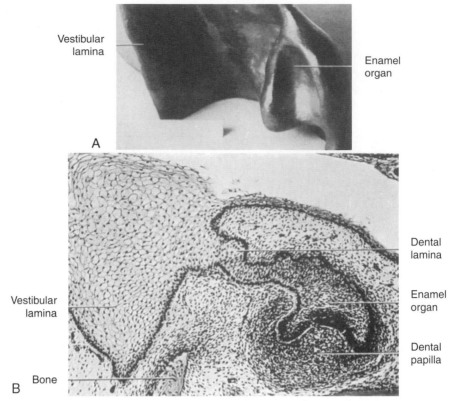

Vestibular lamina

Enamel organ

A

Dental lamina

Vestibular lamina

Enamel organ

Dental papilla

Bone

B

**Figure 12-14** Cap stage of tooth development. Human embryo 60 mm long, 11th week. **A,** Wax reconstruction of the dental organ of the lower lateral incisor. **B,** Labiolingual section through the same tooth. (From Orban B: *Dental Histology and Embryology,* 2nd ed. New York, McGraw-Hill, 1929.)

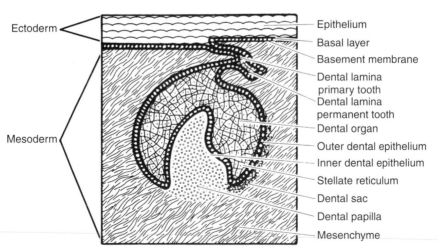

Ectoderm

Epithelium

Basal layer

Basement membrane

Dental lamina primary tooth

Dental lamina permanent tooth

Dental organ

Outer dental epithelium

Inner dental epithelium

Stellate reticulum

Dental sac

Dental papilla

Mesenchyme

Mesoderm

**Figure 12-15** Diagram of the histodifferentiation stage of the life cycle of the tooth. Approximately 14-week-old fetus.

obvious as an extension of the dental lamina of the primary tooth. The basal layer continues to exist and is now divided into an inner and an outer dental epithelium. The stellate reticulum expands and organizes to incorporate more intercellular fluid in preparation for the formation of enamel (Figs. 12-16 to 12-18).

**Morphodifferentiation.** The morphodifferentiation stage, as the name implies, is the stage at which the cells find an arrangement that ultimately dictates the final size and shape of the tooth (Fig. 12-19).[1] This stage is called the advanced bell stage (see Fig. 12-19). The cells of the inner dental epithelium become the ameloblasts, which produce the enamel matrix. As the ameloblasts begin their formation, the tissue of the dental papilla immediately adjacent to the basement membrane begins to differentiate into odontoblasts (Figs. 12-20 and 12-21). The odontoblasts and the ameloblasts are responsible for the formation of dentin and enamel, respectively.

Although the development of dentin is not clearly understood, structures have been identified that show progressive changes. The first change

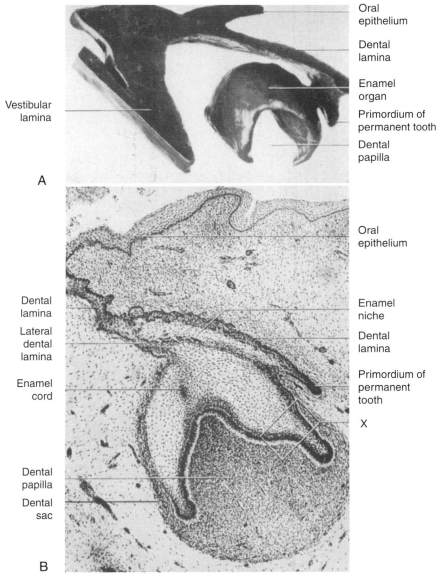

Oral epithelium

Dental lamina

Enamel organ

Primordium of permanent tooth

Dental papilla

Vestibular lamina

A

Oral epithelium

Dental lamina

Lateral dental lamina

Enamel cord

Enamel niche

Dental lamina

Primordium of permanent tooth

X

Dental papilla

Dental sac

B

**Figure 12-16**    Bell stage of tooth development. Human embryo 105 mm long, 14th week. **A,** Wax reconstruction of lower central incisor. **B,** Labiolingual section of the same tooth. "X" designates inset (see Fig. 12-17). (From Orban B: *Dental Histology and Embryology,* 2nd ed. New York, McGraw-Hill, 1929.)

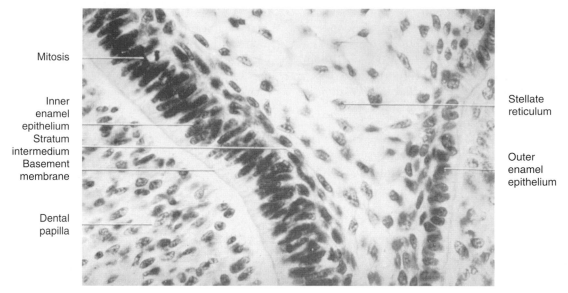

**Figure 12-17**    The four layers of the epithelial dental organ in high magnification (area "X" of Fig. 12-16). (From Orban B: *Dental Histology and Embryology,* 2ⁿᵈ ed. New York, McGraw-Hill, 1929.)

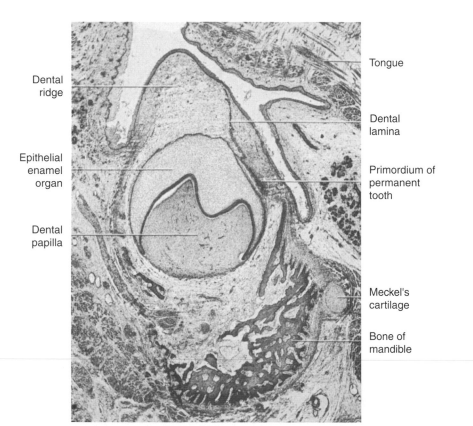

**Figure 12-18**    Advanced bell stage of tooth development. Human embryo 200 mm long, age about 18 weeks. Labiolingual section through the first primary lower molar. (From Bhaskar S: *Synopsis of Oral Histology.* St. Louis, Mosby, 1962, p 44.)

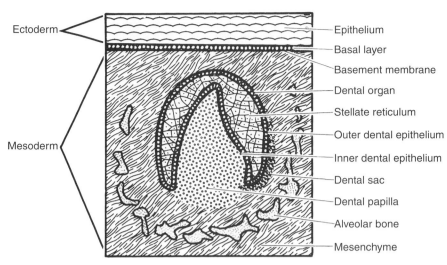

**Figure 12-19** Diagram of the morphodifferentiation stage of the life cycle of the tooth in an approximately 18-week-old fetus.

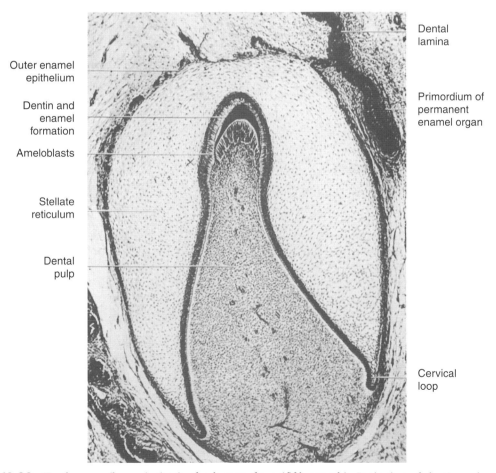

**Figure 12-20** Tooth germ (lower incisor) of a human fetus (fifth month). Beginning of dentin and enamel formation. The stellate reticulum at the tip of the crown reduced in thickness. "X" designates inset (see Fig. 12-21). (From Diamond M, Applebaum E: *J Dent Res* 21:403, 1942.)

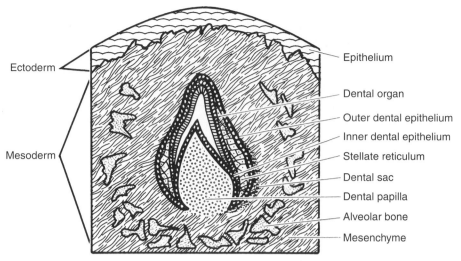

Ectoderm

Mesoderm

Epithelium

Dental organ

Outer dental epithelium

Inner dental epithelium

Stellate reticulum

Dental sac

Dental papilla

Alveolar bone

Mesenchyme

**Figure 12-23**   Diagrammatic representation of the apposition stage of the life cycle of the tooth.

This accounts for the layered appearance of enamel and dentin.[3] The organized special tissues now deposit incremental layers of enamel and dentin matrix. The matrices layered by ameloblasts and odontoblasts begin from a growth center along the dentinoenamel and dentinocemental junctions (Figs. 12-24 and 12-25).

*Calcification*

Calcification occurs with an influx of mineral salts within the previously developed tissue matrix (Fig. 12-26). The chemical structure of enamel consists of approximately 96% inorganic material and approximately 4% organic material and water. The inorganic portion is composed

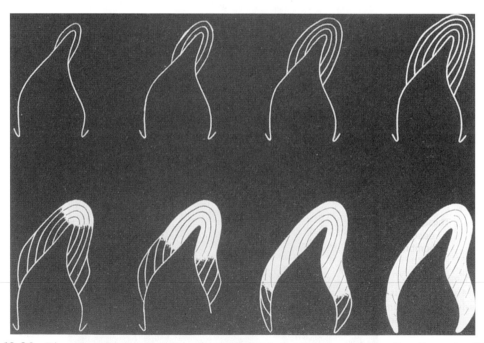

**Figure 12-24**   Diagrammatic representation of enamel matrix formation and maturation. Formation follows an incremental pattern; maturation begins at the tip of the crown and proceeds cervically in cross-relation to the incremental pattern. (From Bhasker SN, editor: *Orban's Oral Histology and Embryology,* 11th ed. St. Louis, Mosby, 1990.)

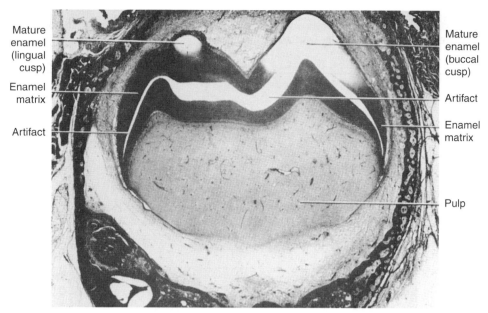

Figure 12-25   Buccolingual section through a deciduous molar. Maturation of the enamel has started in the lingual cusp; it has fairly well progressed in the buccal cusp. Note the gradual transition between the enamel matrix and the fully matured enamel. (From Bhasker SN, editor: *Orban's Oral Histology and Embryology,* 11th ed. St. Louis, Mosby, 1990.)

primarily of calcium and phosphorus, with a small portion of many other compounds and elements, such as carbon dioxide, magnesium, and sodium, to mention a few (Table 12-4).

Calcification begins with the precipitation of enamel in the cusp tips and incisal edges of the teeth and continues with the production of more layers on these small points of origin. Therefore, the older or more mature enamel is found at the cusp tips or incisal edges, and the new enamel is at the cervical region (see Figs. 12-24 and 12-25).

The calcification of enamel and dentin is a very sensitive process that takes place over a long period. Therefore, calcification irregularities noted in any fully developed tooth can often be equated with a specific systemic disturbance.[1] In the cross-section of the clinical crown of a

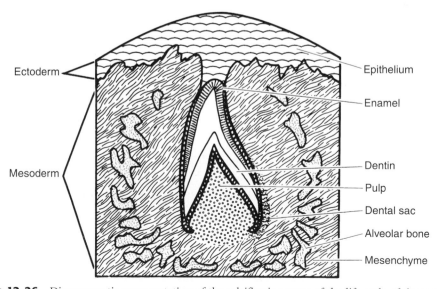

Figure 12-26   Diagrammatic representation of the calcification stage of the life cycle of the tooth.

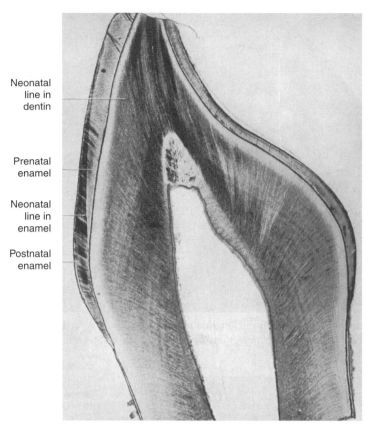

Neonatal
line in
dentin

Prenatal
enamel

Neonatal
line in
enamel

Postnatal
enamel

**Figure 12-29** Neonatal line in the enamel. Longitudinal ground section of a primary cuspid. (From Schour I: *JADA* 23:1947-1950, 1936. Copyright by the American Dental Association. Reprinted by permission.)

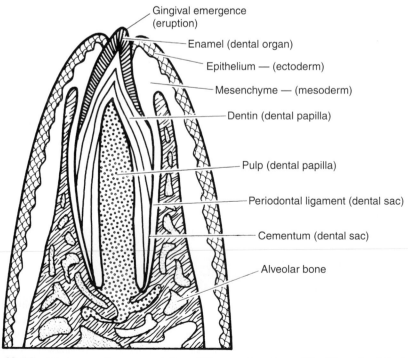

Gingival emergence
(eruption)

Enamel (dental organ)

Epithelium — (ectoderm)

Mesenchyme — (mesoderm)

Dentin (dental papilla)

Pulp (dental papilla)

Periodontal ligament (dental sac)

Cementum (dental sac)

Alveolar bone

**Figure 12-30** Diagrammatic representation of the eruption stage of the life cycle of the tooth.

stellate reticulum is now called Hertwig's epithelial root sheath, which is responsible for the size and shape of the root and eruption of the tooth (Fig. 12-31).[3]

Eruption can be categorized into three different phases: (1) preeruptive phase, (2) eruptive phase (prefunctional), and (3) eruptive phase (functional). The preeruptive phase is that period during which the tooth root begins its formation and begins to move toward the surface of the oral cavity from its bony vault. The prefunctional eruptive phase consists of that period of development of the tooth root through gingival emergence. Most eruption tables report the time that the tooth can be first seen in the mouth (Figs. 12-32 and 12-33). The tooth root is usually approximately one half to two thirds of its final length at the time of gingival emergence.

After the tooth has erupted into the oral cavity and meets its antagonist (opposing tooth in the opposite arch), it is considered to be in the functional eruptive phase. Teeth remain a dynamic unit in that some type of movement, no matter how slight, is always taking place. Teeth continue to move and erupt as necessary as the body continues to change throughout life.[3]

There has been considerable speculation about the causes of tooth eruption. Some examples of causes of tooth eruption often cited are (1) root formation, (2) proliferation of Hertwig's epithelial root sheath, (3) proliferation of the connective tissue of the dental papilla, (4) simultaneous growth of the jaw, (5) pressures from muscular action, and (6) apposition and resorption of bone. Because of this myriad of processes happening at the time of eruption, it is difficult to single out

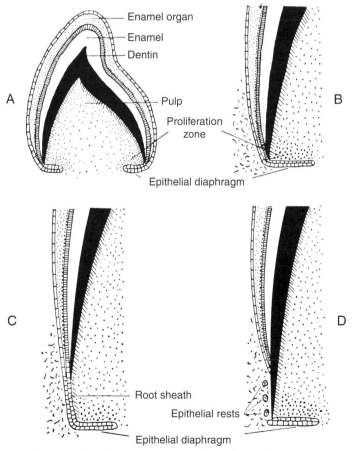

**Figure 12-31**  Three stages in root development. **A,** Section through a tooth germ showing the epithelial diaphragm and proliferation zone of the pulp. **B,** Higher magnification view of the cervical region of **A. C,** Imaginary stage showing the elongation of Hertwig's epithelial sheath between diaphragm and future cementoenamel junction. Differentiation of odontoblasts in the elongated pulp. **D,** In the cervical part of the root, dentin has been formed. The root sheath is broken up into epithelial rests and is separated from the dentinal surface by connective tissue. Differentiation of cementoblasts. (From Bhasker SN, editor: *Orban's Oral Histology and Embryology,* 11th ed. St. Louis, Mosby, 1990.)

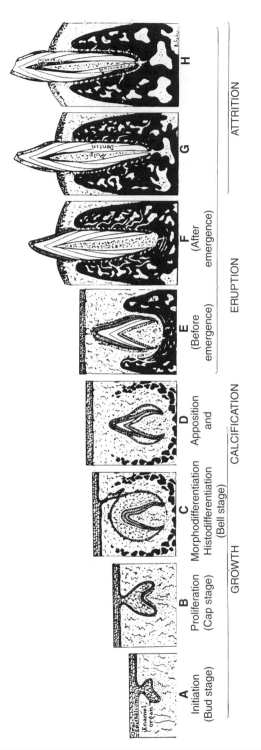

**Figure 12-35** Diagrammatic representation of the life cycle of the tooth. (Reproduced by permission from Sharawy M, Bhussry BR: Development and growth of teeth. In: Bhaskar SN, editor: *Orban's Oral Histology and Embryology*, 11th ed. St. Louis, Mosby, 1990. Modified from Schour I, Massler M: *JADA* 27:1785, 1940. Copyright by the American Dental Association. Reprinted by permission.)

molars.[1] With the exception of the third molars, all permanent teeth demonstrate hard tissue formation by 3 years of age (see Table 12-5).[2]

See Box 12-1 for a glossary of terms from this section.

## REFERENCES

1. Brauer JC, Demeritt WW, Higley LB et al: *Dentistry for Children.* New York, McGraw-Hill, 1959.
2. Finn SB: *Clinical Pedodontics.* Philadelphia, Saunders, 1973.
3. Orban BJ: *Oral Histology and Embryology.* St. Louis, Mosby, 1957.
4. Schour I, Massler M: Studies in tooth development: the growth pattern of human teeth. Part II. *JADA* 27:1918-1931, 1940.

## COGNITIVE CHANGES

*Jimmy R. Pinkham*

Even relatively recently, the human infant has been regarded because of his or her helplessness as a cognitively incompetent creature. Many psychologists now recognize that there is cognitive ability in the newborn. In fact, there is evidence that newborns can experience sensations of pain, touch, and changes in bodily position. Also, it is now known that infants can from the first day of life smell, see, and hear. Cognitive competence explains how and why an infant explores a nursing mother's fingers and studies her face.

In 1984, Mussen and coworkers noted that there are four major areas of cognitive development during the first year of a child's life.[2] The first is the area of perception. Even very young infants have the ability to perceive movement, facial relationships, and color (see Table 12-1).

The second prominent cognitive area is the recognition of information. It is now known that infants can recognize certain stimuli such as a face when viewed from various and different observational angles. In such a case, it is contended that children have developed mental schemes or representations of things encountered in their consciousness and that these schemes contain some but not all of the crucial elements of the object or event. This allows them to recognize the similarity of new objects compared with old ones because of their ability to generalize on these crucial elements.

## TABLE 12-5

### Chronology of the Human Dentition

| Tooth | Hard Tissue Formation Begins | Amount of Enamel Formed at Birth | Enamel Completed | Eruption | Root Completed |
|---|---|---|---|---|---|
| **Primary Dentition** | | | | | |
| *Maxillary* | | | | | |
| Central incisor | 4 mo in utero | Five sixths | $1\frac{1}{2}$ mo | $7\frac{1}{2}$ mo | $1\frac{1}{2}$ yr |
| Lateral incisor | $4\frac{1}{2}$ mo in utero | Two thirds | $2\frac{1}{2}$ mo | 9 mo | 2 yr |
| Cuspid | 5 mo in utero | One third | 9 mo | 18 mo | $3\frac{1}{4}$ yr |
| First molar | 5 mo in utero | Cusps united | 6 mo | 14 mo | $2\frac{1}{2}$ yr |
| Second molar | 6 mo in utero | Cusp tips still isolated | 11 mo | 24 mo | 3 yr |
| | | | | | |
| *Mandibular* | | | | | |
| Central incisor | $4\frac{1}{2}$ mo in utero | Three fifths | $2\frac{1}{2}$ mo | 6 mo | $1\frac{1}{2}$ yr |
| Lateral incisor | $4\frac{1}{2}$ mo in utero | Three fifths | 3 mo | 7 mo | $1\frac{1}{2}$ yr |
| Cuspid | 5 mo in utero | One third | 9 mo | 16 mo | $3\frac{1}{4}$ yr |
| First molar | 5 mo in utero | Cusps united | $5\frac{1}{2}$ mo | 12 mo | $2\frac{1}{4}$ yr |
| Second molar | 6 mo in utero | Cusp tips still isolated | 10 mo | 20 mo | 3 yr |
| | | | | | |
| **Permanent Dentition** | | | | | |
| *Maxillary* | | | | | |
| Central incisor | 3-4 mo | — | 4-5 yr | 7-8 yr | 10 yr |
| Lateral incisor | 10-12 mo | — | 4-5 yr | 8-9 yr | 11 yr |
| Cuspid | 4-5 mo | — | 6-7 yr | 11-12 yr | 13-15 yr |
| First bicuspid | $1\frac{1}{2}$-$1\frac{3}{4}$ yr | — | 5-6 yr | 10-11 yr | 12-13 yr |
| Second bicuspid | 2-$2\frac{1}{4}$ yr | — | 6-7 yr | 10-12 yr | 12-14 yr |
| First molar | at birth | Sometimes a trace | $2\frac{1}{2}$-3 yr | 6-7 yr | 9-10 yr |
| Second molar | $2\frac{1}{2}$-3 yr | — | 7-8 yr | 12-13 yr | 14-16 yr |
| *Mandibular* | | | | | |
| Central incisor | 3-4 mo | — | 4-5 yr | 6-7 yr | 9 yr |
| Lateral incisor | 3-4 mo | — | 4-5 yr | 7-8 yr | 10 yr |
| Cuspid | 4-5 mo | — | 6-7 yr | 9-10 yr | 12-14 yr |
| First bicuspid | $1\frac{3}{4}$-2 yr | — | 5-6 yr | 10-12 yr | 12-13 yr |
| Second bicuspid | $2\frac{1}{4}$-$2\frac{1}{2}$ yr | — | 6-7 yr | 11-12 yr | 13-14 yr |
| First molar | at birth | Sometimes a trace | $2\frac{1}{2}$-3 yr | 6-7 yr | 9-10 yr |
| Second molar | $2\frac{1}{2}$-3 yr | — | 7-8 yr | 11-13 yr | 14-15 yr |

After Logan and Kronfeld: JADA *20*, 1933 (slightly modified by McCall and Schour). Copyright by the American Dental Association.

## BOX 12-1
### Glossary—cont'd

**Initiation:** A stage of the life cycle of the tooth identified as the first point of its development.

**Mesenchyme:** The embryonic connective tissue; that part of the mesoderm whence are formed the connective tissues of the body as well as the blood vessels and lymphatic vessels.

**Mesoderm:** The middle of three layers of the primitive embryo.

**Morphodifferentiation:** A stage of the life cycle of the tooth identified as that period producing form or shape.

**Odontoblast:** One of the cylindrical connective tissue cells that form the outer surface of the dental pulp adjacent to the dentin. They are connected by protoplasmic processes. Each odontoblast has a long, thread-like process, the dental fibril (or fiber of Tomes), which extends through the dentinal tubule to the dentoenamel junction.

**Odontoclast:** One of the cells that help to absorb the roots of the primary teeth. They occur between the primary teeth and the erupting permanent teeth.

**Periodontal ligament:** *Periodontal*—situated or occurring around a tooth; pertaining to the periodontal membrane that attaches the tooth to alveolar bone.

**Periodontal membrane:** The connective tissue occupying the space between the root of a tooth and the alveolar bone and furnishing a firm connection between the root of the tooth and the bone.

**Proliferation:** The reproduction or multiplication of similar forms; a stage in the life cycle of the tooth bud just after the initiation stage.

**Sharpey's fibers:** Cementum is the covering of the tooth root surface. There is also a cementoid tissue covering the cementum, and it is lined with cementoblasts to maintain a dynamic state. There are connective tissue fibers passing through these cementoblasts from the periodontal ligament into the cementum. The embedded portion of the fiber in the cementum is the Sharpey's fiber.

**Stellate reticulum:** *Stellate*—shaped like a star or stars; *reticulum*—a network, especially a protoplasmic network in cells; *stellate reticulum*—the reticular connective tissue–like epithelium forming the enamel pulp of the developing tooth.

**Tooth bud:** The initial identification of the developing tooth by the expansion of certain cells in the basal layer of the oral epithelium (ectoderm only).

**Tooth germ:** The rudiment of a tooth, consisting of a dental sac and including the dental papilla and dental organ (enamel organ).

---

Piaget,[3] much of the intellectual development of the child from birth to the age of 2 years results from the actions of the child with objects in the environment. Although Piagetian theory is not without some controversy regarding its accuracy, it is extremely useful to researchers, clinicians, parents, and other observers of infants because Piaget based his conclusions on observations of his own children's behavior. The behaviors he saw are common to all children.

In 1954, Piaget described the first 2 years of life as a period of sensorimotor development, which he divided into six discrete stages.[3] Piaget contended that during this time the child must develop knowledge in the following three areas:

1. *Object permanence:* Objects continue to exist even when they are not perceivable by the child.
2. *Causality:* Objects have uses, and events have causes. Piaget used the term *circular reaction* (primary, secondary, and tertiary) to describe the changes that occur in this area. A primary circular reaction describes recreating an already known satisfying action, such as thumb sucking. A secondary circular reaction is the recreating of an accidentally discovered cause and effect. Tertiary circular reactions involve experimentation, and, as one might guess, such behaviors often exasperate the child's parents.
3. *Symbolic play:* One object can represent another.

The language development of the infant is, at first, very slow. The mean expressive vocabulary of an 18-month-old is 10 words. At this time, the receptive vocabulary of the child is considerably higher than the expressive vocabulary. Toward the end of the second year, the expressive vocabulary of children develops extraordinarily quickly. In 1983, Levine and colleagues noted that at 3 years of age the mean vocabulary of a child is 1000 words.[1]

Table 12-1 coordinates the six stages of the sensorimotor stage of development with cognition, play, and language development.

## REFERENCES

1. Levine MD, Carey WB, Crocker AC et al: *Developmental Behavioral Pediatrics.* Philadelphia, Saunders, 1983.
2. Mussen PH, Conger JJ, Kagan J et al: *Child Development and Personality,* 6th ed. New York, Harper and Row, 1984.
3. Piaget J: *The Construction of Reality in the Child.* New York, Basic Books, 1954.

## EMOTIONAL CHANGES

*Jimmy R. Pinkham*

There are many human emotions, such as shame, guilt, anger, joy, fear, and sadness. Emotions can be discerned by observing behavioral reactions (crying), measuring physiologic responses (faster heart rate), or ascertaining a person's thoughts and reactions ("I'm depressed").

In assessing the emotional state of young children, the latter two methods of discernment are of little or no value. As a general rule, in the first year of a child's life adults assign whatever emotion they believe that the child should feel in a particular situation. Thus, a wide range of interpretation exists. When an 18-month-old child spills milk, one parent may interpret the child's crying as frustration over his or her awkwardness, another as guilt for the mistake, and another as fear of or sadness about having nothing else to drink.

It is also evident that in older children and adults, the true description of an emotion is very much influenced by how a person reacts to, analyzes, and studies his or her own feelings. Thus, for the same stimulus one person may laugh and another may cry. In very young children, ascertaining such subtleties as these is not possible. The excited babbling of a 3-month-old, which parents label as joy, may more appropriately be called simply excitement.

There appears to be an awakening of emotional states within the child between 4 months and 10 months of age. In 1984, Mussen and colleagues noted that infants were capable of displaying fearful behavior as well as anger or frustration.[4] As a child approaches his or her first birthday, sadness on separation from a parent, joy on reunion, and jealousy of peers or siblings become reliable findings.

Infant and childhood fears are interesting to clinicians who treat children and must be taken into account when formulating a strategy for dealing with the child. Uncertainty and certainty are a pair of elements that emerge early in infancy and can lead to fear or lack of fear. For instance, if the first time the jack in a jack-in-the-box jumps up it startles the child, the child may avoid the toy until later, when he recognizes at what part of the tune the jack will jump out. Avoiding startling situations is important in helping children react in new environmental situations.

Fear of strangers is almost a universal finding after 7 to 12 months of age, although its intensity varies from child to child. Another very common fear in this age group is fear of separation from the parents. This fear starts around 6 months of age, peaks between 13 and 18 months of life, and then declines. The basis for the onset of this fear is probably the result of developing a remembrance of the parent even when the parent is not present, that is, object permanence. Because of this mental process, separation becomes distressful. In 1974, Goin-DeCarie suggested that infants with a dysfunctional relationship with their mothers develop permanency much later than those whose mothers have been consistent and affectionate.[2]

The onsets and peaks of separation anxiety appear to be the same in children from a variety of cultures, although the rate of diminishment of the fear varies greatly.[3] It should be noted that the problem of separation anxiety is fairly well controlled by most children by 36 to 40 months of age and by many children by 32 to 36 months of age. In 1967, Ainsworth concluded that children who have strong relationships with their primary caregivers could utilize that relationship as a place from which to venture into wider social circles by exploration.[1] Conversely, children with poorly developed relationships with their caregivers are not able to undertake such exploration because they lack a sense of security.

## REFERENCES

1. Ainsworth MDS: Infancy in Uganda: *Infant Care and the Growth of Attachment.* Baltimore, Johns Hopkins Press, 1967.

## Microbiology of Dental Caries

The presence of microorganisms in dental plaque has been known since van Leeuwenhoek observed them under his microscope in 1683. In 1924 a British physician, J. K. Clark, isolated strain of *Streptococcus* from a carious lesion in a child. He named it *Streptococcus mutans*. In the 1960s, Keyes and others demonstrated with laboratory animals that dental caries is a transmissible, infectious disease.[12,17] The seven species of *Streptococcus* associated with dental caries in laboratory animals and in man are collectively known as the "mutans streptococci." All are members of the *S. viridans* group. The two species responsible for the initiation of dental caries in man are *S. mutans* and *S. sobrinus*. Mutans streptococci have been correlated with caries in numerous cross-sectional epidemiologic studies. They are currently presumed to have the major role in the initiation of the lesion, even though they are not the first to colonize the tooth surface.[19] Mutans streptococci are considered to be essential but not solely sufficient for the production of dental caries. *Lactobacillus acidophilus* and *L. casei* also have been associated with dental caries. These species are minimally involved in lesion initiation but are believed to have a role in the caries progression. Increasing attention in recent cariology research is being given to the relative cariogenic potential of various combinations of plaque bacteria, including some strains of *Actinomyces*.[24]

Cariogenic bacteria possess three properties that enable them to function in the disease process. They are *adherent* to teeth, they produce acid (are *acidogenic*), and they can live and function within the acid environment (are *aciduric*).

### Transmission of Mutans Streptococci

Mutans streptococci have evolved along with humans to fill their ecological niche in the human oral cavity. They have generally been beneficial parasites, competing with perhaps more harmful species for the environment and protection provided by the oral cavity. However, when human diets began to include sucrose and other refined carbohydrates, mutans streptococci began to exert harmful effects in the form of acid production and the initiation of dental caries.

"Classic" studies on the transmission of mutans streptococci suggested that mutans streptococci have only a weak ability to colonize the oral cavity, and that they require a hard, non-desquamating surface, such as that provided by teeth, for colonization.[2,8] Because their ecological niche is on the tooth surface, mutans streptococci were not found in the mouths of infants until the later stages of primary tooth eruption. Subsequently it was shown that mouth-to-mouth transmission of mutans streptococci takes place between mothers and their children.[3] Successful implantation into the infant is also related in part to the size of the inoculum,[3] the frequency of small-dose inoculations,[20] and a minimal size for an infective dose.[27,29] Infants appear to acquire a genotype of *S. mutans* that is identical to the mother's, although mothers harbor a more heterogeneous population of *S. mutans* than do their infants at the time of acquisition.[7] This "vertical transmission" appears to involve primarily the mother, since the strains obtained by the infant show higher fidelity with those of the mother (more than 90%) compared to the father. Transmission may occur in two ways. *Direct transmission* involves the comingling of the parent's and child's saliva, as during kissing. *Indirect transmission* involves the placement of objects (spoon, pacifier, infant's fingers) into the parent's mouth, then into the infant's mouth. It has also been believed that a "window of infectivity" opens for some period of time during the development of the primary dentition. Caufield et al. detected mutans streptococci in 25% of their sample of infants by age 19 months and in 75% by 33 months.[8] The precise width of the window for individual infants may vary and was not determined in their study.

Transmission of mutans streptococci can be delayed, perhaps even prevented, by instituting intensive preventive programs designed to reduce the numbers of mutans streptococci in mothers as their infants begin to erupt teeth.[18,23] Reductions in the likelihood of transmission and the degree of transmission have been demonstrated when mothers were treated with fluoride, chlorhexidine, or xylitol-containing chewing gum.

Horizontal transmission of mutans streptococci is now thought to occur. Mattos-Graner et al.[21] isolated mutans streptococci from nursery school children aged 12 to 30 months and reported that many children were colonized with mutans streptococci strains of identical genotypes. Van Loveren and coworkers[30] demonstrated a likelihood for horizontal transmission when a child becomes colonized with mutans streptococci after age 5 years. A third study has suggested horizontal transmission among 13- to 24-month-old children in day nursery settings.[26]

Recent studies also suggest that *S. mutans* may be transmitted at an earlier age, prior to the eruption of teeth. Tanner and colleagues,[25] using DNA probe technology, reported the presence of mutans streptococci in 55% of plaque samples and 70% of tongue scrapings from a sample of 57 children ages 6 to 18 months. Wan et al.[32] evaluated 60 preterm and 128 full-term infants, all age 3 months. The authors were able to cultivate *S. mutans* from 34% of the full-term infants and 20% of the preterm infants (30% overall prevalence). There was a significant relationship between the presence of *S. mutans* and developmental (Bohn's) nodules. In a subsequent study, Wan et al.[33] detected *S. mutans* in 50% of preterm and 60% of full-term infants age 6 months. Factors associated with colonization included increased frequency of sugar intake, breast-feeding, and habits that allowed the transfer of saliva from mother to child. Noncolonization was associated with multiple courses of antibiotics. In a follow-up study of the same infants, Wan et al.[34] demonstrated that the prevalence of *S. mutans* colonization increased with age, so that by 24 months of age, 84% of the infants harbored the bacteria. Factors associated with colonization in this study were sweetened fluids taken to bed, frequent sugar exposure, snacking, sharing foods with adults, and maternal *S. mutans* levels of greater than $10^5$ colony-forming units/ml of saliva. Noncolonization was associated with tooth-brushing and multiple courses of antibiotics. The mean age of *S. mutans* colonization in dentate infants was 15.7 months. Overall, the data from Wan et al.[34] established the presence of *S. mutans* from birth to 24 months of age. These studies raise doubts about the tenet that a hard, non-shedding surface is required for mutans streptococci colonization. The furrows of the tongue appear to be an important ecological niche for the early colonization of these species.

*Formation of Plaque*

The initial bacterial colonization of teeth probably begins with organisms other than mutans streptococci, which do not have great ability to adhere to teeth.[28] The mechanisms of initial colonization include (1) adherence of bacteria to pellicle or the enamel surface; (2) adhesion between bacteria of the same or different species; and (3) subsequent growth of bacteria from small enamel defects and from cells initially attached to tooth structure.[13] Plaque development continues with the formation of extracellular polymer chains via the breakdown of sucrose into its two main components, glucose and fructose (Fig. 12-40). The polymers are synthesized from each of these components. Chains of glucose and fructose, termed glucans and fructans, respectively, are sticky, gelatinous substances that further enhance the bacteria's ability to adhere to the tooth and to each other. Glucans and fructans also affect the rate at which saliva can enter the plaque to buffer the acid and reverse the demineralization process.

Intracellular metabolism of carbohydrates leads to the production of acids, chiefly lactic, that can depress plaque pH from a resting level of about 6 to a value of 4 within minutes of contact with a fermentable carbohydrate. Fructans, which are more soluble than glucans, may also serve as a reservoir of easily catabolized polysaccharide for the bacteria to utilize when other substrates are not available. Without further carbohydrate challenge, the plaque pH requires about 20 minutes to return to its resting value.

## Histopathology of Smooth Surface Lesions

The earliest clinical sign of the caries process on smooth enamel surfaces is the white-spot lesion, an area of white, chalky, opaque enamel typically seen under a layer of plaque at the gingival margin

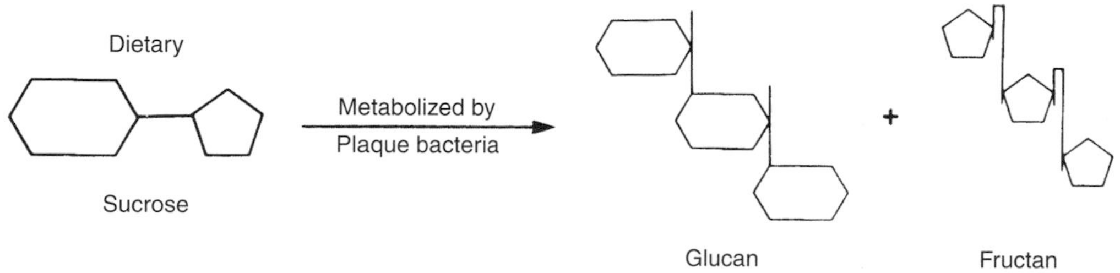

**Figure 12-40** Breakdown of dietary sucrose into glucan and fructan.

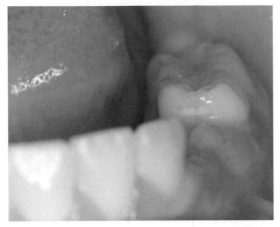

**Figure 12-41** White spot lesion on mesial surface of primary mandibular second molar, below contact area. Created by long-standing plaque, it is now visible after exfoliation of primary first molar.

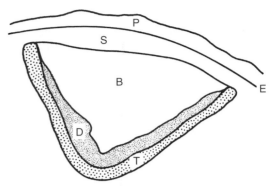

**Figure 12-42** Diagram of an early enamel lesion (white spot), illustrating plaque *(P)*, enamel surface and pellicle *(E)*, intact surface layer *(S)*, body of the lesion *(B)*, dark zone *(D)*, and translucent zone *(T)*.

of tooth surfaces. It can also be seen on the proximal tooth surfaces that become exposed after exfoliation of an adjacent primary tooth (Fig. 12-41). The white-spot lesion is an indication that the underlying enamel has decalcified. In cross-section the lesion is conical, with its apex toward the dentin. During the early stages of development, the lesion may not be visible on a bitewing radiograph.

The enamel lesion has been divided by Silverstone and coworkers[22] into histologic zones that correspond to the changes produced in the enamel (Fig. 12-42). The surface zone is the relatively unaffected superficial enamel that acts as a diffusion gradient, allowing minerals (fluoride, calcium, phosphate, and other ions) to pass in and out of the enamel. Only 5% to 10% of the mineral content is lost from the surface layer. Below this zone is the body of the lesion, the principal area of demineralization, representing about 60% mineral loss. In developed lesions, this area roughly corresponds to the radiographic image as seen on bitewing films. The third zone, called the dark zone because of its appearance under polarized light microscopy, represents an area of mineral loss intermediate to the two preceding zones. The advancing front of the lesion, the translucent zone, has sustained a mineral loss similar to that of the surface zone (5% to 10%). Unless steps are taken to arrest and reverse this process, the lesion will continue to advance toward the dentin. As it approaches the dentinoenamel junction, the lesion spreads laterally, and the previously intact surface layer breaks down, creating clinically detectable cavitation.

The histopathologic mechanism of pit and fissure caries is somewhat different from that of smooth surface lesions; consequently, approaches to the prevention of the two types of caries are different. The use of fluoride in its various forms, improved oral hygiene, and dietary control are primarily effective in combating smooth surface lesions. Pit and fissure sealants and preventive resin restoration techniques are used to control pit and fissure lesions. The histopathologic processes and prevention of pit and fissure lesions are discussed in Chapter 32.

*Demineralization-Remineralization*
One of the most important concepts that have evolved in cariology in the past several decades is the demineralization and remineralization of enamel. The caries process is no longer thought of as linear, beginning with acid demineralization of enamel and ending in a clinically detectable lesion. Rather, the process appears to be a dynamic one, involving both the loss of enamel mineral content and its replacement, with surface enamel functioning as a diffusion matrix. Enamel is composed of mineralized crystals surrounded by a water-protein-lipid matrix that occupies 10% to 15% of the total volume. This matrix provides relatively large channels through which acids, minerals, fluoride, and other ions may pass in both directions.

Under normal oral conditions, equilibrium is established between mineral loss and mineral gain. The balance can be disturbed, however, by environmental factors in the oral cavity, such as plaque fluid pH and the presence or absence of fluoride. Acid production by plaque creates an environment with a lowered pH at the enamel surface, leading to dissolution of subsurface enamel crystals. Calcium, phosphorus, and other minerals diffuse out through the enamel surface in the process known as demineralization.

The presence of fluoride in the oral environment, even in very low concentration, can affect the equilibrium of this process in the opposite manner, leading to remineralization. This fluoride may come from the saliva, the plaque fluid, or from the demineralized enamel itself. During remineralization, fluoride facilitates the diffusion of calcium and phosphorus back into the lesion where partially dissolved hydroxyapatite crystals are rebuilt into fluoridated hydroxyapatite. This latter structure is now more resistant to acid dissolution than were the original crystals.[11] True "repair" of the original early lesion takes place.

Thus, development of dental caries must be viewed as a dynamic process taking place on all plaque-covered surfaces. As long as the surface layer remains intact, remineralization of the lesions is possible and a restoration may be avoided. The clinician must recognize the importance of the surface layer of the white-spot lesion and avoid the temptation to penetrate it with the explorer. Doing so will create an irreversible lesion that must be restored. The lesion in its early stages may not be detectable on a radiograph. However, many small lesions that are radiographically limited to enamel can be managed non-invasively with fluoride. This is predominantly true in permanent teeth, which have a much thicker enamel layer than primary teeth. The clinician must also bear in mind that carious lesions are larger clinically than they appear on radiographs. Clinically cavitated lesions may also undergo remineralization, such as is the case with some chronic carious lesions, but restorations obviously cannot be avoided in these situations.

## Diet

The dietary components primarily responsible for the development of dental caries are refined (or fermentable) carbohydrates, including various sugars. Refined carbohydrates can be broken down in the oral cavity by salivary amylase into simple sugars that can be metabolized by mutans streptococci and other acidogenic bacteria. Cariogenic bacteria metabolize these fermentable carbohydrates and produce organic acids, principally lactic acid, which causes the loss of mineral content from the tooth structure (see "Histopathology of Smooth Surface Lesions" above).

Sucrose has been implicated more than any other carbohydrate in the caries process. The relationship between the sucrose content of the diet and the resultant dental caries describes a sigmoid curve that rises steeply when sucrose-rich foods are consumed frequently. The curve plateaus at high levels of sucrose intake, indicating that the sucrose content of the diet has become saturated and that increases in sucrose content beyond that level do not increase caries development to a significant extent.

Interactions between dietary carbohydrate and other caries risk factors are complex. The frequency of refined carbohydrate intake is as important, or perhaps more important, than the amount of total carbohydrate in the diet. Other food-related factors can enhance or lessen a food's cariogenicity, such as its pH, action in stimulating saliva, retainability or ease of clearance, fat content, and its susceptibility to metabolism by mutans streptococci. It is difficult, then, to rank foodstuffs on the basis of their cariogenicity.

Much of what we know about diet and caries was derived from the Vipeholm study, conducted among institutionalized adults in Sweden in 1945–1952.[14] The major findings of that study were as follows: (1) sugar consumption at meals can cause a slight increase in caries activity; (2) sugar consumption between meals creates a definite increase in caries activity; (3) sugar in sticky form produces a marked increase in caries activity; (4) caries activity differs among individuals with the same diet; and (5) caries activity declines when sugar is withdrawn from the diet.

A recent comparison of the mutans streptococci levels of children in Africa, Europe, and North America revealed that salivary counts of these microorganisms are comparable in the three populations, even though the overall levels of dental caries vary substantially.[31] Diet does not have a strong influence on the levels of mutans streptococci levels, but it does substantially determine the level of dental caries. Thus, the study concluded that differences in the caries levels among the three populations are more influenced by diet than levels of mutans streptococci.

## Saliva and Other Host Factors

Human saliva is a critical regulating factor in the caries process. It is supersaturated with calcium and phosphorus; thus it aids in the maturation process of normal enamel and promotes remineralization of demineralized enamel. It contains bicarbonate and other buffers, and so mitigates the effects of acid production by plaque bacteria. Saliva also contains proteins, immunologic components, and antibacterial compounds. It contains low levels of fluoride that become concentrated in dental plaque. The resting pH of saliva is normally around 7.0, but it may vary from about 5.5 to 8.0. Salivary flow may be reduced in children with chronic diseases, by medications, and by radiation treatment involving the head and neck. Salivary flow may be stimulated by gustatory and masticatory stimulation, preferably with sugar-free gums and candies.

Other host factors include the quality of the enamel, the depth of pits and fissures, and the individual's exposure to fluoride. Enamel hypoplasia, even at subclinical levels, increases the susceptibility of enamel to decay. There is evidence that premature/very low birth weight children are at increased risk for enamel hypoplasia.

## Early Childhood Caries

Early childhood caries (ECC) is a specific form of severe dental caries that affects infants and young children.[1] It is defined as the presence of more than one decayed (noncavitated or cavitated lesions), missing (due to decay), or filled tooth surface in any primary tooth in a child 71 months or younger.[9,16] This presentation of dental caries was formerly termed "baby bottle tooth decay" and "nursing bottle caries." Any sign of smooth surface caries in a child younger than 3 years is indicative of severe ECC. Between the ages of 3 and 5, severe ECC is defined as one or more cavitated, missing (due to caries), or filled smooth surface in primary maxillary anterior teeth or a decayed, missing, or filled surface (dmfs) score of greater than 4 (age 3), greater than 5 (age 4), or greater than 6 (age 5).[15] A feature of ECC not implicit in its definition is the typically rapid progression of the decay.

ECC is a result of the interaction of the factors involved in other types of dental caries (cariogenic bacteria, refined carbohydrates, and host factors). However, the dietary factors also include

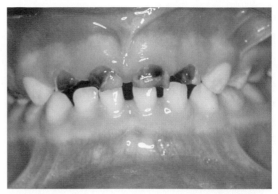

**Figure 12-43** Early childhood caries demonstrating severe dental caries in primary maxillary incisors.

frequent consumption of liquids containing fermentable carbohydrates, particularly through a nursing bottle at sleep times. Juices, sodas, infant formula. and sweetened beverages have been implicated in ECC. When taken via nursing bottle while the infant sleeps, these liquids pool around the maxillary incisors and can cause rapidly progressive, severe destruction of tooth structure (Fig. 12-43). The association between cow's milk and ECC is somewhat controversial. Many anecdotal reports have implicated milk as an etiologic factor for ECC. However, laboratory studies have shown that milk is not cariogenic and may even protect tooth surfaces because of its high calcium content.[4] Human breast milk has been implicated in ECC among children who engage in prolonged, unrestricted nursing. However, studies with humans have not indicated that human milk is cariogenic.[10] There may be other factors at work in families that engage in prolonged, unrestricted breastfeeding that promote the development of ECC.

The American Academy of Pediatric Dentistry recommends that infants not be put to sleep with a bottle and that unrestricted nocturnal breastfeeding be avoided after the eruption of the first primary tooth. Parents should encourage their infant to drink from a cup as the child approaches the first birthday; weaning from the bottle should be done at 12 to 14 months of age. Bottles or no-spill ("sippy") cups should not be used for repetitive consumption of liquids containing fermentable carbohydrates. Oral hygiene measures should be in place at the time of the eruption of the first tooth. The child's initial oral health consultation should occur within 6 months after the eruption of the first tooth but no later than 12 months of age.[1]

# REFERENCES

1. American Academy of Pediatric Dentistry: Reference manual. *Pediatr Dent* 25:24, 2003.
2. Berkowitz RC, Turner J, Green P: Primary oral infection of infants with *Streptococcus mutans. Arch Oral Biol* 25:221, 1980.
3. Berkowitz RJ, Turner J, Green P: Maternal salivary levels of *Streptococcus mutans* and primary oral infection of infants. *Arch Oral Biol* 26:147, 1981.
4. Bowen WH, Pearson SK, Rosalen PL et al: Assessing the cariogenic potential of some infant formulas, milk and sugar solutions. *JADA* 128:865, 1997.
5. Brunelle JA, Carlos JP: Changes in the prevalence of dental caries in U.S. school children, 1961–1980, *J Dent Res* 61(special issue):1346, 1982.
6. Brunelle JA, Carlos JP: Recent trends in dental caries in U.S. children and the effect of water fluoridation. *J Dent Res* 69(special issue):723-727, 1990.
7. Caufield PW, Walker TM: Genetic diversity within *Streptococcus mutans* evident from chromosomal DNA restriction fragment polymorphisms. *J Clin Microbiol* 27:274, 1989.
8. Caufield PW, Cutter GR, Dasanayake AP: Initial acquisition of mutans streptococci by infants: evidence for a discrete window of infectivity. *J Dent Res* 72:37, 1993.
9. Drury, TF, Horowitz AM, Ismail AI et al: Diagnosing and reporting early childhood caries for research purposes. *J Public Health Dent* 59:192, 1999.
10. Erickson PR, Mazhari E: Investigation of the role of human breast milk in caries development. *Pediatr Dent* 21:86, 1999.
11. Feagin F, Patel PR, Koulourides T, Pigman W: Study of the effect of calcium, phosphate, fluoride and hydrogen ion concentrations on the remineralization of partially demineralized human and bovine enamel surfaces. *Arch Oral Biol* 16:535, 1971.
12. Fitzgerald RJ: Dental caries research in gnotobiotic animals. *Caries Res* 2:139, 1968.
13. Gibbons RJ, van Houte J: On the formation of dental plaques. *J Periodontol* 44:347, 1973.
14. Gustafsson BE, Quensel C-E, Lanke LS et al: The Vipeholm dental caries study. *Acta Odontol Scand* 11:232, 1954.
15. Ismail AI, Sohn W: A systematic review of clinical diagnostic criteria of early childhood caries. *J Public Health Dent* 59;171, 1999.
16. Kaste LM, Drury TF, Horowitz AM et al: An evaluation of NHANES III estimates of early childhood caries, *J Public Health Dent* 59:198, 2000.
17. Keyes PH: The infectious and transmissible nature of experimental dental caries. *Arch Oral Biol* 1:304, 1960.
18. Kohler B, Bratthall D, Krasse B: Preventive measures in mothers influence the establishment of the bacterium *Streptococcus mutans* in their infants. *Arch Oral Biol* 28:225, 1983.
19. Loesche WJ, Rowan J, Straffon LH, Loos PJ: Association of *Streptococcus mutans* with human dental decay. *Infect Immun* 11:1252, 1975.
20. Loesche WJ: Role of *Streptococcus mutans* in human dental decay. *Microbiol Rev* 50:353, 1986.
21. Mattos-Graner RO, Li Y, Caufield PW et al: Genotypic diversity of mutans streptococci in Brazilian nursery children suggests horizontal transmission. *J Clin Microbiol* 39:2313, 2001.
22. Silverstone LM, Johnson NW, Hardie JM et al: *Dental Caries: Aetiology, Pathology, and Prevention.* London, Macmillan Press Ltd., 1981.
23. Söderling E, Isokangas P, Pienihäkkinen K et al: Influence of maternal xylitol consumption on mother-child transmission of mutans streptococci: 6-year follow-up. *Caries Res* 35:173, 2001.
24. Syed SA, Loesche WJ, Pape HL Jr, Grenier E: Predominant cultivable flora isolated from human root surface caries plaque. *Infect Immun* 11:727, 1975.
25. Tanner ACR, Milgrom PM, Kent R Jr: The microbiota of young children from tooth and tongue samples. *J Dent Res* 81:53, 2002.
26. Tedjosasongko U, Koazi K: Initial acquisition and transmission of mutans streptococci in children at day nursery. *J Dent Child* 69:284, 2002.
27. van Houte J, Burgess RC, Onose H: Oral implantation of human strains of Streptococcus mutans in rats fed sucrose or glucose diets. *Arch Oral Biol* 21:561, 1976.
28. van Houte J, Gibbons RJ, Pulkinen AJ: Adherence as an ecological determinant for streptococci in the human mouth. *Arch Oral Biol* 16:1131, 1971.
29. van Houte J, Green DB: Relationship between the concentration of bacteria in saliva and colonization of teeth in humans. *Infect Immun* 9:624, 1974.
30. van Loveren C, Buijs JF, ten Cate JM: Similarity of bacteriocin activity profiles of mutans streptococci within the family when the children acquire the strains after the age of 5. *Caries Res* 34:481, 2000.
31. van Palenstein Helderman WH, Matee MI, van der Hoeven JS et al: Cariogenicity depends more on diet than the prevailing mutans streptococci species. *J Dent Res* 75:535, 1996.
32. Wan AKL, Seow WK, Walsh LJ et al: Association of streptococcus mutans infection and oral developmental nodules in pre-dentate infants. *J Dent Res* 80:1945, 2001.
33. Wan AKL, Seow WK, Purdie DM et al: Oral colonization of Streptococcus mutans in six-month-old predentate infants. *J Dent Res* 80:2060, 2001.
34. Wan AKL, Seow WK, Purdie DM et al: A longitudinal study of Streptococcus mutans colonization in infants after tooth eruption. *J Dent Res* 82:504, 2003.

establishing a doctor-family relationship. Care is begun with nonthreatening preventive services; if an emergency occurs, parents know where to turn; if questions arise, reliable and trusted information is available; if treatment is needed, a firm foundation of trust has been built. The surgeon general's report notes quite clearly that those children who have a dentist are more likely to receive preventive services.[18] From the standpoint of a general dental practice, the one-stop, family orientation is a strong factor in success.

### Impart Optimal Fluoride Protection

Fluoride remains dentistry's best preventive tool, and optimal fluoride exposure is a tenet of early intervention. The current concern about fluorosis gives even more importance to oversight of fluoride exposure during the period when teeth are at greatest risk, in the first 3 years of life. Physician-driven fluoride supplementation has not been very effective, and with current recommendations of the Centers for Disease Control and Prevention that require caries risk to be added to the equation, dentist involvement is crucial to maximize anticaries benefit and minimize fluorosis risk.[7]

### Use Anticipatory Guidance to Arm Parents in the Therapeutic Alliance

Parental involvement has become a tenet of child health care. Because infant oral health is so heavily weighted toward risk assessment and protective factors at home, the parent becomes a cotherapist. In the first 3 years of life, there is no routine preventive message as the child develops a full primary dentition, becomes mobile, and makes his or her first forays away from the family in daycare. The dentist must empower the parent to provide prevention but even more to anticipate the oral health implications in the rapidly changing child.

## CONCEPTS OF INFANT ORAL HEALTH

### Risk Assessment

An infant presents a clean slate in terms of acquired conditions and diseases, but as the child grows and expands his or her world, risk increases. Taking a broad view of risk that goes beyond infectious disease and encompasses trauma and injury, orthodontic problems, and compliance issues helps ensure total oral health. Risk assessment is defined as identification of factors known or believed to be associated with a condition or disease for purposes of further diagnosis, prevention, or treatment. An essential part of the infant oral health visit is a specialized history addressing risk. Risk assessment is an offshoot of wellness theory in that a child may exhibit risk but not demonstrate overt disease. By eliminating the risk factors before disease occurs, the disease process can be prevented in the immediate future as well as in the long term. An example would be the infant sleeping with a bottle of sweetened liquid but with no overt dental caries. Intervention would be focused on eliminating the habit and diminishing the risk of early childhood caries. Table 13-1 depicts the Caries Assessment Tool (CAT) developed by the American Academy of Pediatric Dentistry, which can be used by different health professionals to identify risk for dental caries in children of all ages, beginning at 6 months.

### Anticipatory Guidance

The concept of anticipatory guidance is long established in pediatric care but relatively new to dentistry. Our preventive message has tended to be static and not tailored to the developmental stage of the patient. Throughout childhood and later life, environment and growth and development force change; the infant is very different from the school-aged child and lives in a broader, more complex world. Even in adulthood, the elderly patient's needs are far different from those of a middle-aged person. Anticipatory guidance is defined as proactive counseling of parents and patients about developmental changes that will occur in the interval between health supervision visits that includes information about daily caretaking specific to that upcoming interval. Anticipatory guidance is the complement to risk assessment; addressing protective factors is aimed at preventing oral health problems. An example of anticipatory guidance would be to discuss ambulation of the child at the initial dental visit and warn parents about possible tooth trauma that often occurs as the infant stands to walk. Authors have recommended that anticipatory guidance areas include oral development, diet and nutrition, fluoride adequacy, oral habits, injury

## TABLE 13-1

### Caries Assessment Tool (CAT)

| | LOW RISK | MODERATE RISK | HIGH RISK |
|---|---|---|---|
| Clinical conditions | No carious teeth in past 24 mo<br>No enamel demineralization (enamel caries white-spot lesions)<br><br>No visible plaque; no gingivitis | Carious teeth in the past 24 mo<br>One area of enamel demineralization (enamel caries white-spot lesions)<br><br>Gingivitis[a] | Carious teeth in the past 12 mo<br>More than one area of enamel demineralization (enamel caries white-spot lesions)<br>Visible plaque on anterior (front) teeth<br>Radiographic enamel caries<br>High titers of mutans streptococci<br>Wearing dental or orthodontic appliances[b]<br>Enamel hypoplasia[c] |
| Environmental characteristics | Optimal systemic and topical fluoride exposure[d]<br><br>Consumption of simple sugars or foods strongly associated with caries initiation[e] primarily at mealtimes<br>High caregiver socioeconomic status[f]<br><br>Regular use of dental care in an established dental home | Suboptimal systemic fluoride exposure with optimal topical exposure[d]<br><br>Occasional (e.g., 1–2) between-meal exposures to simple sugars or foods strongly associated with caries<br>Midlevel caregiver socioeconomic status (e.g., eligible for school lunch program or SCHIP)<br>Irregular use of dental services | Suboptimal topical fluoride exposure[d]<br><br>Frequent (e.g., 3 or more) between-meal exposures to simple sugars or foods strongly associated with caries<br>Low-level caregiver socioeconomic status (e.g., eligible for Medicaid)<br>No usual source of dental care<br>Active caries present in the mother |
| General health conditions | | | Children with special health care needs[g]<br>Conditions impairing saliva composition/flow[h] |

From American Academy of Pediatric Dentistry, Council on Clinical Affairs. Policy on use of a caries-risk assessment tool (CAT) for infants, children and adolescents. *Pediatr Dent* 25:18, 2002.

[a]Although microbial organisms responsible for gingivitis may be different from those primarily implicated in dental caries, the presence of gingivitis is an indicator of poor or infrequent oral hygiene practices and has been associated with caries progression.

[b]Orthodontic appliances include both fixed and removable appliances, space maintainers, and other devices that remain in the mouth continuously or for prolonged time intervals and that may trap food and plaque, prevent oral hygiene, compromise access of tooth surfaces to fluoride, or otherwise create an environment supporting dental caries initiation.

[c]Tooth anatomy and hypoplastic defects such as poorly formed enamel, developmental pits, and deep pits may predispose a child to develop dental caries.

[d]Optimal systemic and topical fluoride exposure is based on the American Dental Association /American Academy of Pediatrics guidelines for exposure from fluoride drinking water and/or supplementation (Ref. 4) and use of a fluoride dentifrice.

[e]Examples of sources of simple sugars include carbonated beverages, cookies, cake, candy, cereal, potato chips, French fries, corn chips, pretzels, breads, juices, and fruits. Clinicians using caries risk assessment should investigate individual exposures to sugars known to be involved in caries initiation.

## TABLE 13-1
### Caries Assessment Tool (CAT)–cont'd

[f]National surveys have demonstrated that children in low-income and moderate-income households are more likely to have dental caries and more decayed or filled primary teeth than children from more affluent households. Also, within income levels, minority children are more likely to have caries. Thus, sociodemographic status should be viewed as an initial indicator of risk that may be offset by the absence of other risk indicators.

[g]Children with special health care needs are those who have or are at increased risk for a chronic physical, developmental, behavioral, or emotional condition and who also require health and related services of a type or amount beyond that required by children generally.

[h]Alteration in salivary flow can be the result of congenital or acquired conditions, surgery, radiation, medication, or age-related changes in salivary function. Any condition, treatment, or process known or reported to alter saliva flow should be considered an indication of risk unless proven otherwise.

prevention, and oral hygiene.[15] These six areas capture the major concerns related to major oral conditions of dental caries, periodontal disease, trauma, and malocclusion.

### Health Supervision

Regular, comprehensive preventive and therapeutic dental care for every child is far superior to fragmented episodic care and therefore is a worthwhile goal. Health supervision is defined as the longitudinal partnership between dentist and family individualized to focus on health outcomes for that family and child. This is a departure from the "every 6 months" approach that is common to dental practice and that frankly has no strong basis. Some children require more frequent supervision visits and others less. The health supervision interval is the alternative to the traditional recall period, and the health outcome is the desired changes monitored at each interval. In infant oral health, the dentist assesses risk at the beginning of the interval, offers preventive advice using anticipatory guidance, and administers necessary treatment or prevention in the dental office. Outcomes are the measures that indicate success. These can be physical (reduction in gingival inflammation), cognitive (understanding of the caries process), or behavioral (elimination of the nighttime bottle habit). For example, the presence of plaque on primary teeth in infants is a strong predictor of future dental caries, so after oral hygiene instruction parents can monitor success by looking for the presence of plaque.[2] A desired outcome would be absence of plaque. Parents leave armed not only with tools (anticipatory guidance) to effect outcomes but also with measures (outcomes) they can look for

and that the dentist also uses at the end of the supervision interval to determine success.

## INFANT ORAL HEALTH AS A DIAGNOSTIC PROCESS

The best way to envision the infant oral health visit is to compare it with the traditional medical model used for diagnosis of disease. The medical model uses a stepwise approach beginning with a chief complaint, history, physical examination, differential diagnosis, and treatment plan. Infant oral health intervention assumes that the child has no disease but may be prone to disease due to risk behaviors such as nighttime bottle use or lack of fluoride. Conceptually, these risk factors will eventually lead to disease if not addressed; conversely, if the risk factors are eliminated, the child will be free of disease.

In infant oral health, the chief complaint may be absent or may be considered a generic interest in prevention. The infant oral examination is the well-baby visit for oral health. The health history is replaced with a very focused risk-based history aimed at predisposing factors for dental conditions. The patient examination looks for physical factors that predispose the child to oral disease primarily, but also for existing disease. The differential diagnosis is replaced with a risk profile that is individualized to the child. Instead of a treatment plan, the family receives anticipatory guidance with directives to eliminate risk and impart protective factors. They are given measurable outcomes to determine progress toward wellness. Both of these factors make the parents a part of the therapeutic alliance. The recall interval is designed around appropriate time frames to give parents time to address risk and for the dentist to reassess progress and ensure that disease has not manifested.

## ELEMENTS OF THE INFANT ORAL HEALTH VISIT

### Risk Assessment

The parent or guardian is the historian for the child. In Chapter 18, the general health history is discussed in depth. In this chapter, we will focus on historical elements related to oral disease risk. Box 13-1 is the history form recommended by the American Academy of Pediatric Dentistry for infant oral health. Historical risk elements can be divided into perinatal factors, diet and nutrition, fluoride adequacy, habits, injury prevention, oral

development, and hygiene/prevention. The clinician should combine the general health history responses with those focused on risk of oral disease to form an individual historical risk profile for the child.

Perinatal factors are important because of the attendant oral effects and medical treatment for premature birth. While experts have concluded that prematurity does not predispose to increased risk of dental caries,[5] some low birth weight children receive special diets, have hypoplastic dentitions,[17] and have developmental disabilities that place them at higher risk. Diet and nutrition questions focus on the frequency of sugar consumption, use of a bottle with sweetened liquids, and special diets. More than three exposures to sugar per day places the child in a higher caries risk category.[3] Fluoride adequacy refers to the adequacy of drinking water to provide optimal

---

### BOX 13-1

#### Risk Assessment Form for Infant Oral Health

**Health History**
Did birthmother have problems during pregnancy?
Was the child premature?
Was child's birth weight low?
Were there any complications at birth?
Has your infant been ill?
Is your child on any medication?
Notes _____

**Diet and Nutrition**
Is/was your child breastfed?
Does your child sleep with a bottle?
Does your child drink from a cup?
Is your child on a special diet?
Notes _____

**Fluoride Adequacy**
Do you know the fluoride level of your water?
Do you have well water?
If yes, has the water been tested?
Do you use bottled water?
Do you use a water conditioner or filtration system?
Does your child take fluoride supplements?
If yes, please list _____
Do you use a fluoridated toothpaste for your child?
Notes _____

**Oral Habits**
Does your child use a pacifier?
Does your child suck a thumb or finger(s)?
Does your child grind teeth day or night?
Notes _____

**Injury Prevention/Trauma**
Is your child walking?
Is your home childproofed?
Do you use a car seat for your child?
Has your child had an oral/facial injury?
Notes _____

**Oral Development**
Does your child have any teeth?
Child's age (in months) when first tooth erupted
_____
Has your child experienced teething problems?
Have you noticed any oral problems in your child?
Notes _____

**Oral Hygiene**
Do you clean your child's teeth/gums?
Do you use a toothbrush to clean your child's teeth?
Do you use toothpaste to clean your child's teeth?
Notes _____

From American Academy of Pediatric Dentistry: Risk assessment. In: *ABCs of Infant Oral Health.* Chicago, The Academy, 2000.

fluoride but also addresses the proper role of dentifrice in reducing the likelihood of fluorosis. The discussion of habits establishes a baseline for families and enables the dentist to counsel early on the risk and benefit of behavioral habits throughout early childhood. Historical information on injury prevention moves beyond purely dental trauma to general health issues like child-proofing and car seat use. Oral development is covered to assess presence of teeth, eruptive disorders, and teething problems. Finally, the parent is questioned about oral hygiene for the baby; such questioning should lead to a discussion of tooth cleaning implements, positioning of the child, and family routines.

## Oral Examination and Assessment of Clinical Risk Factors

The oral examination of the infant is a quick process but differs from the typical child examination in several ways:

- Use of a dental chair is unnecessary and the least preferred approach.
- The parent participates as a learner and immobilizer.
- Teaching about the oral cavity occurs during the examination process.
- The child may cry which is desirable and useful.

The preferred approach to infant examination is the knee-to-knee position (Fig. 13-1) in which parent and dental provider sit facing each other. Their knees should touch and ideally, mesh slightly, creating a flat surface on which the child can rest. The infant initially is held facing the parent and then reclined onto the lap of the dentist. The parent has the infant's legs straddling the torso and uses elbows to hold the feet in place. The parent holds the child's hands and the dentist, looking down, stabilizes the child's head. The examination can occur wherever a suitable light source can be found. The closeness of the parent and provider may concern some parents and should be explained before the procedure begins.

During the examination, which may take only seconds, the dentist also has the opportunity to demonstrate oral hygiene, point out oral structures of importance, as record findings. Most infants will cry briefly during the examination, affording a wide open mouth! Parents may need to be assured that infants who cry are normal, healthy babies and the response is expected. At the completion of the examination, the child is returned to the parent who can cuddle and console as needed.

Children this age are far more likely to see a physician regularly, so delays in cognitive, physical, emotional, and gross motor areas are usually known to parents. However, dentists should be familiar with developmental milestones for children from birth to 3 (Table 13-2) and advise families of the need for evaluation if none has been done when problems are noted or suspicion of developmental problems exists. Furthermore,

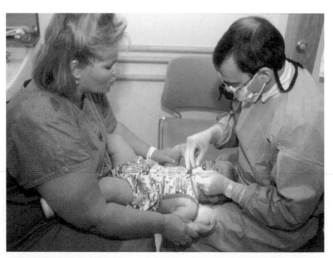

**Figure 13-1**    Knee-to-knee clinical examination position for dentist, child, and parent. Parent and dentist face each other with knees touching while parent holds child on lap with child facing parent. Parent carefully lays child in dentist's lap while holding child's hands.

## TABLE 13-2
### Selected Developmental Characteristics of the Child Aged 6 Months to 3 Years

| 6–9 MO | 12–13 MO | 24 MO+ |
| --- | --- | --- |
| **Intellectual Development** | | |
| Opens for a spoon | Copies sounds and actions | 3- to 4-word sentences |
| Imitates actions of adults | Understands simple commands | Puts toys in groups |
| Turns to locate sounds | Tries to accomplish simple acts | Name 5 body parts |
| | | |
| **Gross/Fine Motor Skills** | | |
| Rolls over | Stands with hand held | Scribbles; draws shapes |
| Becomes able to sit independently | Sits without support | Kicks/throws ball |
| Picks up objects with fingers | Feeds self raisins | Puts on/takes off clothes |
| | | |
| **Psychological Development** | | |
| Laughs and squeals with delight | Shows affection to adults | Changeable feelings |
| Screams if annoyed | Fear of strangers | Recognizes emotions |
| Dental Implications | | |
| Needs physical support | Fear of separation | Understands commands |
| Can hold bottle alone | Sippy cup use | Prone to falls/trauma |
| | | |
| **Physiologic Height (75th percentile):** | | |
| Boys = 69.7–74.0 cm | 77.7 cm | 89.9 cm |
| Girls = 67.8–72.4 cm | 76.3 cm | 88.7 cm |
| | | |
| **Weight (75th percentile):** | | |
| Boys = 8.49–9.88 kg | 10.91 kg | 13.44 kg |
| Girls = 7.83–9.24 kg | 10.23 kg | 12.74 kg |
| | | |
| **Pulse (90th percentile)** | | |
| 120/min | 120/min | 110/min |
| | | |
| **Respiration (50th percentile)** | | |
| 30/min | 28/min | 25/min |
| | | |
| **Blood Pressure** | | |
| 105/67 | 105/69 | 106/68 |

by knowing these milestones, child behaviors and abilities are easier to relate to anticipatory guidance with the parent.

The dentist would expect to see a healthy oral cavity in most infants. Table 13-3 shows several oral conditions of infants and their management. In addition, in Chapter 2, other pathologic conditions of infancy, including dental lamina cysts (Bohn's nodules and Epstein's pearls), congenital epulis, eruption cyst, and neuroectodermal tumor of infancy, are covered. These would be rare occurrences; in most infants, the dentist should look for developmental status, quality of dentition in terms of caries or hypoplasia, and presence of plaque on teeth. Table 13-4 describes some of the normal characteristics of the oral cavity, as well as of the head and neck, in children younger than 3 years.

### Risk Profiling

From the historical and clinical data obtained from the parent and child, the dentist can create a risk profile using the same six areas of anticipatory guidance. The risk profile may be simple or bring into play major factors that may be difficult to surmount, such as special diet, profound disability, or malformed teeth. Parents should be provided with explanations and an estimate of the influence of a particular factor on oral health. A

## TABLE 13-3

### Infant Oral Pathology and Unusual Clinical Findings

| CONDITION DESCRIPTION AND ILLUSTRATION | CLINICAL FINDINGS AND MANAGEMENT |
| --- | --- |
| Normal predentate infant oral cavity 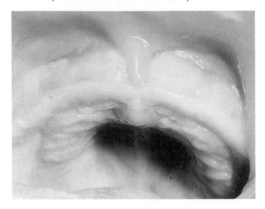 | No teeth present<br>Rugae present on palate<br>Tooth bud bulges prominent<br>Tissues pink and healthy<br>High labial frenum |
| Natal and neonatal teeth 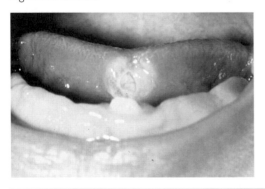 | Natal teeth present at birth and neonatal present within 30 days of birth<br>Incidence 1–2 per 6000 births<br>90% are primary; 10% supernumerary; 85% mandibular<br>Extract supernumeraries; primary teeth left if not highly mobile<br>Can be aspiration risk; nursing obstacle |
| Riga-Fede disease 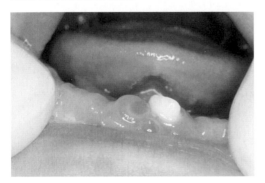 | Actually traumatic ulcer of ventral surface of tongue from tooth<br>May cause active bleeding and discomfort<br>Treatment options are observation; cessation of breastfeeding or removal/smoothing of the offending tooth |

useful visual for risk profiling is also the CAT of the American Academy of Pediatric Dentistry, which can be given to parents with risk factors for their child circled or underlined.[3] The CAT lets parents see where their child is in the risk spectrum and, perhaps more importantly, where the child needs to be.

### Anticipatory Guidance

The equivalent of a non-orthodontic treatment plan for the infant is placed in terms of anticipatory guidance. Box 13-2 is another form approved by the American Academy of Pediatric Dentistry for use in infant oral health. It is a checklist of the most typical recommendations

**TABLE 13-4**

**Elements of Head and Neck Examination of Infants**

| STRUCTURE | DIAGNOSTIC TECHNIQUE | NORMAL CHARACTERISTICS |
| --- | --- | --- |
| Head | Visualization | Disproportionately large |
| Hair | Visualization | Thin and fine |
| Scalp | Visualization/palpation | Open fontanels |
| TMJ | Palpation/manipulation | Short condyles/ flat fossae |
| Skin | Visualization | Soft, smooth |
| Neck | Palpation | Weak musculature<br>Soft airway cartilage |
| Lips | Visualization | Full, Cupid's bow |
| **Oral Cavity** | | |
| Dental arches | Visualization | Edentulous/tooth bulges |
| Frenula | Visualization | High placement on alveolus |
| Palate | Visualization | Prominent median raphe/rugae |
| Gingivae | Visualization | Pink, hydrated, flaccid around teeth |

for infants and can be added to for unique recommendations. The anticipatory guidance should be couched in temporal terms appropriate for the desired outcome. If a child is sleeping with a bottle, or if there are incipient white-spot lesions on the teeth due to plaque accumulation, then the dentist should make recommendations on how to stop the bottle habit or improve hygiene and then reevaluate at an appropriate interval. Anticipatory guidance also presumes that developmental information should cover the period until the next health supervision visit. Box 13-3 shows a list of topics that should be considered when covering anticipatory guidance.

## GROWTH AND DEVELOPMENT TREATMENT PLANNING

In rare instances, there may be an orthodontic or craniofacial component to the infant oral health visit, as would be the case with a child with a cleft lip or palate or a significant craniofacial abnormality. These patients should be referred to a team for management and followed routinely by the primary care dentist for basic oral health needs.

Parents often express interest in occlusal development and may press the dentist to discuss future orthodontic needs. Growth is difficult to predict, but the dentist ought to take the oppor-

tunity to discuss eruption, spacing, and occlusion with parents as a part of anticipatory guidance. Chapter 18 discusses early orthodontic treatment planning at an age when treatment is far more realistic in terms of child cooperation.

### Nonnutritive Sucking Habits

In addition to asking whether a child has any cavities, parents ask questions about their young child's habits, particularly thumb and pacifier habits. Such questions are common because oral habits are very prevalent in young children and negative effects of long-term habits on the dentition have been documented for more than a century. Traditionally, dentists' involvement in nonnutritive sucking habits occurred only after prolonged habits produced clear damage to the dentition and raised parental concern. The dentist was consulted in an effort to stop the nonnutritive sucking habit. This scenario still occurs with frequency, but early anticipatory guidance aimed at preventing the prolongation of oral habits is a much more constructive, effective role that dentists can have in nonnutritive sucking habits. However, before such guidance can be given the dentist must have a thorough understanding of how and why nonnutritive sucking habits develop, their effects on oral structures, and what duration of habitual behavior may cause harm.

## BOX 13-2

### Parent Information Form for Infant Oral Health

Child's Next Dental Care Visit _____

**Diet and Nutrition**
Discontinue breastfeeding/bottle
No at-will nursing
Modify breastfeeding/bottle
Only water in sleep-time bottles
Encourage use of a spill-proof cup
Cup only at age 12 months
Weaning plan _____
Decrease sugar intake
Decrease carbohydrate intake
Change diet _____

**Fluoride Adequacy**
Obtain home fluoride analysis
Contact _____
Suggested fluoride supplementation _____
Increase water intake to supplement feedings
Recommended toothpaste _____

**Oral Habits**
Thumb/finger sucking habit—Discourage by age
_____

Pacifier use—Discourage by age _____
Use pacifier that conforms to lips and cheeks
    and supports the lips
Bruxing or other habit _____

**Injury Prevention/Trauma**
Child has experienced oral injury
Childproof your home
Use infant/child care seat
Other protective device _____

**Oral Development**
Total primary teeth erupted _____
Next tooth to erupt _____
Child requires further assessment _____

**Oral Hygiene**
Use a soft toothbrush
Do not use toothpaste
Use a smear/pea-sized amount of toothpaste
Special instructions _____

From the American Academy of Pediatric Dentistry. Risk Assessment. In *ABCs of Infant Oral Health.* Chicago, 2000, AAPD.

## BOX 13-3

### Topic Areas for Anticipatory Guidance

**Oral Development**
Dental and oral milestones
Eruption of the first tooth
Development of occlusion
Teething and tooth eruption times
Anatomical landmarks

**Fluoride Adequacy**
Water evaluation and supplementation
Breastfeeding
Formula feeding
External sources of fluoride
Safety and toxicity
Dentifrice and topical agents

**Oral Hygiene**
Mouth cleaning
*Streptococcus mutans* testing
Tooth cleaning implements
Positioning and supervision

**Diet and Nutrition**
Bottle-related dental caries
Weaning
Role of carbohydrates
Role of and identification of plaque

**Habits**
Nonnutritive sucking
Pacifiers

**Injury Prevention**
Child abuse and neglect
Car safety
Child proofing
Electric cord safety
Emergency instructions

## Origins of Nonnutritive Sucking Habits

Sucking behaviors are believed to arise from psychological needs and from the physiologic need for nutrition, so that normally developed infants have an inherent, biological drive for sucking. Psychoanalytic theory and learning theory differ in their explanations of why human infants possess a sucking drive and why it persists beyond infancy[9] but are in agreement that this drive is a normal developmental characteristic. According to psychoanalytic theory, nonnutritive sucking behaviors (such as pacifier, thumb, or finger sucking) arise out of erotic pleasure derived from oral stimulation, a characteristic phase of normal human development. Persistence of substantial nonnutritive sucking habits beyond this so-called oral phase (roughly age 3 years) reflects a psychological disturbance suggestive of inability to manage stress or anxiety. Conversely, learning theory suggests that nonnutritive sucking is an adaptive response that is often rewarded and that becomes a learned habit, without psychological abnormality. Given the prevalence of nonnutritive sucking behaviors in normally developed children, the learning theory explanation is the most widely accepted, although for some children prolonged thumb or pacifier sucking beyond the preschool years may reflect a psychological disturbance.

## Prevalence of Nonnutritive Sucking Habits

Early prevalence studies of nonnutritive sucking habits generally found that 70% to 90% of children had some history. More recent studies found habits to be almost universal in infants. For example, a study in Iowa reported that well over 90% of children engaged in nonnutritive sucking at some time during the first year of life.[19] Prolonged nonnutritive sucking habits may have consequences for the orofacial structures, so prevalence of prolonged habits is more important to consider than are habits in infancy. Studies have shown that, on average, children cease habits by 24 to 36 months of age, and those who continue tend to be from better educated or higher income families.[1] Numerous studies document that thumb and finger sucking habits are more likely to persist than are pacifier habits.[19] Pacifier habits rarely persist beyond the preschool years due to peer pressure at the time of kindergarten enrollment, so it has been suggested that when a digit habit develops, a pacifier be substituted for the digit.[10]

Duration of a habit is perhaps the single most important factor to consider in assessing risk for habit-induced malocclusions, but other factors should also be considered including the amount of time a child engages in a particular habit per day and the intensity of the child's sucking. For example, a child who sucks on a pacifier for only a few minutes before falling asleep at night would be expected to be at less risk for malocclusion than a child who has a pacifier in the mouth several hours a day with frequent occasions where the sucking was intense enough to be heard.

## Effects and Mechanisms of Nonnutritive Sucking Habits on the Dentition

Numerous studies published prior to the mid-1960s found that, in general, finger sucking leads to reduced overbite as well as increased overjet and protrusion of the maxillary incisors and a narrowing of maxillary posterior arch width.[11]

Studies of the primary dentition have found sucking habits to be associated with a higher prevalence of malocclusion in the primary dentition, including class II canine and molar relationships, anterior open bite, increased overjet, decreased maxillary arch width, and increased lower arch width, resulting in increased likelihood of posterior crossbite. Habits that persist between 36 and 48 months are associated with significantly increased overjet, as well as significantly increased prevalence of anterior open bite and posterior crossbite, and this worsens with more time. Thus, for each year a habit persists beyond 24 months, the prevalence of certain malocclusions (anterior open bite, excessive overjet, posterior crossbite) more than doubles. Digit habits are more commonly associated with excessive overjet and anterior open bite, whereas pacifier habits are associated with posterior crossbites and class II canine relationship. Pacifier habits even if discontinued at age 2 represent an increased risk for malocclusion; longer duration of pacifier habits are associated with open bite and posterior crossbites; crossbites are more likely to persist after habits stop, whereas open bites and excessive overjet are associated with continued habits. Open bites tended to resolve with the cessation of pacifier habits. Comparisons between conventional pacifiers and so-called orthodontic pacifiers have suggested that there is little, if any, difference in their effects on orofacial structures.

Differing digit and pacifier effects on the oro-facial structures are likely due to different forces applied. Pacifiers, presumably because they extend further into the mouth, tend to force the tongue downward applying lateral outward pressure against the lower arch. At the same time, the sucking action activates the muscles surrounding the mouth so as to increase cheek pressure resulting in greater medial force applied to the upper arch. Pacifiers tend to widen the lower arch and narrow the upper arch resulting in posterior crossbite. Fingers or thumbs, due to the weight of the arm, tend to apply forward and slightly upward pressure on the maxillary incisor region, with accompanying backward and downward pressure on mandibular incisors, so the net effect of digit habits is greater overjet as well as a tendency toward open bite.

The risk of acute otitis media (middle ear infection) may be higher among children using pacifiers. Pacifier use has also been linked to early cessation of breastfeeding, including developing countries where lack of breastfeeding may have particularly detrimental effects on children's health. Pacifier use may be beneficial in reducing sudden infant death syndrome, a benefit that potentially far outweighs the risks associated with acute otitis media or breastfeeding cessation.[12]

### Recommendations

Traditional thinking has held that as long as habits cease by age 6 or 7 years, effects reverse so habits are of little consequence. This was based mostly on clinical observations, not longitudinal data. More recent studies have demonstrated that longer duration is associated with higher prevalence of malocclusions, and durations as short as 24 months may increase the risk of certain malocclusions. To minimize the risk of habit-induced malocclusion, such habits should be eliminated by 24 months of age. Because digit habits are likely to cause malocclusions of greater severity than those caused by pacifier habits, and because digit habits are more difficult to overcome than pacifier habits, substitution of a pacifier habit for a digit habit may be advisable. Pacifier habits have been associated with decreased risk for sudden infant death syndrome, along with increased risk for early cessation of breastfeeding and otitis media, but only in infancy. Thus given the physiologic and psychological need for sucking in the first year of life, it is not prudent to recommend elimination of habits prior to 12 months of age.

## OFFICE READINESS FOR INFANT ORAL HEALTH

Infant care represents a deviation from routine office practice in several ways. It may be done primarily by an auxiliary person rather than by the dentist. It does not routinely require the same armamentarium that would be used for a patient requiring a dental prophylaxis and tray-delivered fluoride. The site can be in the operatory but can just as well be in a well-lit, comfortable conference room or play area. Radiographs would be considered unusual in most infant visits, and patient napkin, cotton rolls, and other trappings of a typical dental examination are for the most part absent.

A dental record is still required but may be abbreviated. However, the essentials of a history, examination record, treatment plan, and progress notes remain. Patient education brochures and other instructional material should be directed to this particular age group. The dental team can be enlisted in developing the time, place, and procedure for infant oral health in the office. It offers them the chance to use their knowledge to educate, and the opportunity to work with small children is for most pediatric dental staff a joy.

Finally, in a busy office, the placement of the infant dental appointment requires some thought because it ties up personnel and, if done outside the dental operatory area, necessitates a change in staff flow patterns.

## REFERENCES

1. Adair SM, Milano M, Lorenzo I, Russell C: Effects of current and former pacifier use on the dentition of 24- to 59-month-old children. *Pediatr Dent* 17:437-444, 1995.
2. Alaluusua S, Malmivirta R: Early plaque accumulation: a sign for caries risk in young children. *Comm Dent Oral Epidemiol* 22:273-276, 1994.
3. American Academy of Pediatric Dentistry: Reference manual 2003–2004. *Pediatr Dent* 25:54, 2003.
4. American Academy of Pediatrics, Section on Pediatric Dentistry: Oral health risk assessment timing and establishment of the dental home. *Pediatrics* 111:1113-1116, 2003.
5. Burt BA, Pai S: Does low birthweight increase the risk of caries? A systematic review. *J Dent Educ* 65:1024-1027, 2001.

6. Caulfield PW: Dental caries—a transmissible and infectious disease revisited: a position paper. *Pediatr Dent* 19:491-498, 1997.
7. Fluoride Recommendations Work Group: Recommendations for using fluoride to prevent and control dental caries in the United States. *MMWR Morb Mortal Wkly Rep* 50(August):1-42, 2001.
8. Johnsen D, Gerstenmaier JH, DiSantis TA, Berkowitz RJ: Susceptibility of nursing-caries children to future decay. *Pediatr Dent* 8:168-170, 1986.
9. Johnson ED, Larson BE: Thumb-sucking: literature review. *J Dent Child* 60:385-391, 1993.
10. Larsson E: Dummy and finger sucking habits with special attention to their significance for facial growth and occlusion. 1. Incidence study. *Swed Dent J* 64:667-672, 1971.
11. Larrson E: Dummy- and finger-sucking habits with special attention to their significance for facial growth and occlusion. 4. Effect on facial growth and occlusion. *Swed Dent J* 65:605-634, 1972.
12. Mitchell EA, Taylor BJ, Ford RPK et al: Dummies and sudden infant death syndrome. *Arch Dis Child* 68:501-504, 1993.
13. Nowak AJ: Rationale for the timing of the first oral evaluation. *Pediatr Dent* 19:8-11, 1997.
14. Nowak AJ, Casamassimo PS: The dental home. A primary care oral health concept. *JADA* 133:93-98, 2000.
15. Nowak AJ, Casamassimo PS: Using anticipatory guidance to provide early dental intervention. *JADA* 126:1156-1164, 1995.
16. Seale NS, Casamassimo PS: Access to dental care for children in the United States: a survey of general practitioners. *JADA* 134(12):1630-1640, 2003.
17. Seow WK: Effects of premature birth on oral growth and development. *Aust Dent J* 42:85-90, 1997.
18. US Department of Health and Human Services: *Oral Health in America: A Report of the Surgeon General.* Bethesda, Md, National Institute of Dental and Craniofacial Research, National Institutes of Health, 2000.
19. Warren JJ, Levy SM, Nowak AJ, Tang S: Nonnutritive sucking behaviors in pre-school children: a longitudinal study. *Pediatr Dent* 22:187-190, 2000.

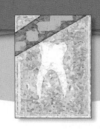

# CHAPTER 14
## Prevention of Dental Disease

*Arthur Nowak and James J. Crall*

Dental caries and periodontal diseases are reported to be among the most common bacterial diseases affecting humans. Even though substantial reductions in the levels and severity of these diseases and their sequelae have been documented in most Western nations, millions of children (and adults) continue to experience caries, periodontal disease, tooth loss, and malocclusions, much of which could be prevented if only they engaged in daily oral hygiene practices, had optimal systemic and topical fluorides, maintained sound dietary practices, and sought professional care on a regular basis. Dental diseases and their sequelae are largely preventable.

The goal of this chapter is to provide clinicians with a plan that can help infants, children, and young adults to be free from oral disease. The plan involves many participants, not only dental personnel but also children, their parents, and anyone interested in or responsible for a child's health and well-being. Planning for a lifetime of oral health should begin shortly after conception, prior to the initiation of oral disease, and should continue on a regular basis to ensure that risk factors for oral diseases are recognized early and dealt with effectively throughout pregnancy, infancy, childhood, and adolescence.

The mouth has a major role in the life of a human being. All nutrients must pass through it; it helps create the sounds and expressions through which we communicate with others; and it is a major component of our overall appearance. Therefore, a healthy mouth with a full complement of teeth and a stable, aesthetic occlusion is a goal that we should all promote and seek to achieve for the patients under our care.

## PRENATAL COUNSELING

For more than a century, the medical profession has recognized the importance of providing prenatal counseling and care to expectant mothers. With recent studies reporting an association between the presence of maternal periodontitis at 21 to 24 weeks gestation and preterm births,[42] between clinical periodontitis at delivery and preeclampsia,[16] and between *Streptococcus mutans* levels in mothers and caries experience in their offspring,[50] there has been renewed interest in the oral health of women during pregnancy.[52] The dental profession can make an important contribution in this primary preventive effort by attending to women's oral health during pregnancy and providing prenatal counseling related to infant oral health and oral development.

Prenatal counseling generally is provided in conjunction with programs conducted in community hospitals or neighborhood health centers. Programs also have been developed for office-based settings. Regardless of where the program is conducted, close collaboration among members of the various health professions and community support groups (e.g., dentists, physicians, nurses, nutritionists, social workers) is important to ensure appropriate scheduling of presentations and reinforcement of concepts.

Although many oral health counseling programs have been developed in recent years, the goals of the programs are similar (Box 14-1). Regardless of the setting, time allotted, and staff involved, the program should be individualized to the greatest extent possible and should provide parents with information about the development of oral structures and functions, dental disease processes, and recommended preventive measures. In addition, the program should provide information on the importance of the mother's

---

### BOX 14-1
#### A Model of Prenatal Counseling

**Purpose**
- To educate parents about dental development of the child
- To educate parents about dental disease and prevention
- To provide a suitable environment for the child
- To strengthen and prepare the child and dentition for life

**Methods**
- Education concerning development, prevention, and disease
- Demonstration of oral hygiene procedures
- Counseling to instill preventive attitudes and motivation
- Evaluation of learning, acceptance, and needs

**Content**
*External Component (Parents)*
- Parents' education concerning dental disease and oral hygiene
- Parents' motivation for plaque removal program
- Changes in mother's oral health
- Intake of sweets

- Pregnancy gingivitis
- Myths and misconceptions about pregnancy and dentition
- Parent's dental treatment

**Internal Component (Parents and Child)**
- Parents' education/development of child
- Effect of life-style on child
- Habits (smoking, alcohol consumption)
- Intake of sweets
- Exposure to disease (e.g., rubella, syphilis)
- Effect of drugs on child (e.g., tetracyclines)
- Nutrition
  - Calcium
  - Vitamins
  - Fluorides
  - Essential nutrients
- Child's needs after birth
- Breastfeeding versus bottle feeding
- Fluoride supplementation
- Teething
- Hygiene
- Nonnutritive sucking
- First visit

diet and health-related behaviors during pregnancy (including the effects of drugs, tobacco, and alcohol), the importance of maternal oral health care during pregnancy, and recommended scheduling of dental treatment (Box 14-2).

During prenatal counseling, teething should be mentioned because it most likely will be the first postnatal oral issue that parents confront. Although the timing and sequence of eruption of teeth are generally predictable, variations are common and a frequent source of parental anxiety. Teething is a natural phenomenon that usually occurs with little or no problems. Nevertheless, some infants exhibit signs of systemic distress, including a rise in temperature, diarrhea, dehydration, increased salivation, skin eruptions, and gastrointestinal disturbances.[14,53,70] Increased fluid consumption, a nonaspirin analgesic, and palliative care consisting of the use of

teething rings to apply cold and pressure to the affected areas generally reduce the symptoms and result in a happier infant.[47] Lancing of tissues is usually not indicated. If symptoms persist for more than 24 hours, the infant should be examined by a physician to rule out upper respiratory infection and other common diseases and conditions of infancy.

Prenatal counseling programs also should provide guidelines for the parents about the timing of the first professional dental visit. In the past, guidelines have recommended that children without symptoms of disease be scheduled for their first dental examination beginning at age 3. More recently, however, professional guidelines have incorporated the importance of earlier attention to oral health during infancy, particularly for children at elevated risk for the development of dental caries.[4,6-10] Programs designed to provide comprehensive preventive measures have stressed the importance of initiating professional visits with risk assessment within 6 months of the eruption of a child's first tooth or no later than age 12 months.[55]

*Bright Futures: Guidelines for Health Supervision of Infants, Children, and Adolescents*[36] is a comprehensive and practical resource designed to assist health professionals and families to more effectively promote the health and well-being of children and adolescents. Recommendations include an initial dental appointment at around 12 months of age to assess the infant's risk for dental disease, completion of a clinical examination, provision of anticipatory guidance information, and a follow-up appointment.[57]

## BOX 14-2

### Dental Treatment for Women During Pregnancy

**First Trimester**
Consult with woman's physician*
Emergency treatment only

**Second Trimester**
Elective and emergency treatment
Radiographs can be used with adequate
    protection

**Third Trimester**
Emergency treatment only
Avoid supine position
Radiographs can be used with adequate
    protection

**Throughout Pregnancy**
Plaque control program for parents of child
Local anesthetic is anesthetic of choice
Avoid the use of drugs if at all possible. If
    drugs are needed, use only those proved
    safe for use during pregnancy and use in
    consultation with a physician
The use of a general anesthetic for dental
    treatment during pregnancy is
    contraindicated

*The first trimester is most crucial; however, in these litigious times it would probably be wise to consult with the woman's physician during the last two trimesters, especially if there is a major problem.

## RISK ASSESSMENT

Another innovation in designing preventive programs is based on the concept of risk assessment. The risk of developing dental disease varies among children and over time for each child. Therefore, assessing each child's risk for common dental diseases and identifying specific risk factors on a regular basis allows the practitioner to more effectively individualize oral health supervision and preventive measures.

Risk assessments for dental caries based on a single risk indicator are unlikely to reliably differentiate between those at high and low risk because caries is a complex disease process. Accordingly, various multifactorial models have been developed. Most current risk assessment models are based on a synthesis of information from available literature by experts without rigorous validation in clinical settings. The American Academy of Pediatric Dentistry recently developed the Caries Assessment Tool (CAT)[7] to assist in assessing a child's caries risk based on

clinical conditions, environmental factors, and general health conditions (Table 14-1). Depending on the findings of each assessment, a child is designated as being at low, moderate, or high risk for the development of caries. Based on the risk level, the clinician can personalize and initiate a comprehensive preventive program for the child.

## TABLE 14-1
### Recommendations for Preventive Pediatric Dental Care

Because each child is unique, these recommendations are designed for the care of children who have no important health problems and are developing normally. These recommendations will need to be modified for children with special health care needs or if disease or trauma manifests variations from normal. The Academy emphasizes the importance of very early professional intervention and the continuity of care based on the individualized needs of the child.

| AGE[1] | INFANCY 6-12 MONTHS | LATE INFANCY 12-24 MONTHS | PRESCHOOL 2-6 YEARS | SCHOOL AGE 6-12 YEARS | ADOLESCENCE 12-21 YEARS |
|---|---|---|---|---|---|
| Oral hygiene counseling[2] | Parents/ guardians/ caregivers | Parents/ guardians/ caregivers | Child/parent/ caregivers | Child/parent/ caregivers | Patient |
| Injury prevention counseling[3] | • | • | • | • | • |
| Dietary counseling[4] | • | • | • | • | • |
| Counseling for nonnutritive habits[5] | • | • | • | • | • |
| Fluoride supplementation[6] | • | • | • | • | • |
| Assess oral growth and development[7] | • | • | • | • | • |
| Clinical oral examination | • | • | • | • | • |
| Prophylaxis and topical fluoride treatment[8] | | • | • | • | • |
| Radiographic assessment[9] | | | • | • | • |

Reference Manual 2003-2004. American Academy of Pediatric Dentistry. Chicago, 2003. In *Pediatr Dent* 25:63, 2003.
[1]First examination at the eruption of the first tooth and no later than 12–18 months.
[2]Initially, responsibility of parent; as child develops, jointly with parents; then when indicated only child.
[3]Initially play objects, pacifiers, car seats; then when learning to walk; and finally sports and routine playing.
[4]At every appointment discuss the role of refined carbohydrates; frequency of snacking.
[5]At first discuss the need for additional sucking; digits vs. pacifiers; then the need to wean from the habit before the eruption of the first permanent front teeth.
[6]As per AAP/ADA *Guidelines* and the water source.
[7]By clinical examination.
[8]Especially for children at high risk for caries and periodontal disease.
[9]As per AAPD Radiographic Guidelines.
[10]Appropriate discussion and counseling should be an integral part of each visit for care.

## TABLE 14-1

### Recommendations for Preventive Pediatric Dental Care–cont'd

| AGE[1] | INFANCY 6-12 MONTHS | LATE INFANCY 12-24 MONTHS | PRESCHOOL 2-6 YEARS | SCHOOL AGE 6-12 YEARS | ADOLESCENCE 12-21 YEARS |
|---|---|---|---|---|---|
| Pit and fissure sealants | | | If indicated on primary molars | First permanent molars as soon as possible after eruption | Second permanent molars as soon as possible after eruption |
| Treatment of dental disease or injury | • | • | • | • | • |
| Assessment and treatment of developing malocclusion | | | • | • | • |
| Substance abuse counseling | | | | • | • |
| Assessment and removal of 3rd molars | | | | | • |
| Referral for regular and periodic dental care | | | | | • |
| Anticipatory guidance[10] | • | • | • | • | • |

Risk status should be reassessed periodically to detect changes in the child's clinical, environmental, and general health conditions. The American Academy of Pediatrics also endorses early risk assessment and establishment of a dental home by age 1 for infants found to be at elevated risk.[4]

## ESTABLISHING A DENTAL HOME

All children should have a place where they can receive appropriate health care provided by physicians, dentists, and other allied health professionals. The dental home should include accessible facilities and comprehensive oral health services geared to the needs of children and their families. The health provider should know the child and parent and should have established a level of trust and responsibility with the family for optimal cooperation and communication. Most parents establish such an environment early with respect to medical care for their infants and toddlers because of the Recommendations for Preventive Pediatric Health Care established by the American Academy of Pediatrics.[3] To compliment the "medical home," all infants and toddlers should have a "dental home." The dental home should provide all of the services listed in Box 14-3.

Whether this dental home is located in a private practice, a community health center, or at the neighborhood hospital, it should be supervised by dentists trained in primary pediatric care. By establishing a dental home early, parents will be appropriately counseled during the early infant years and have a facility to contact immediately in case of orofacial traumatic injury. The initial infant oral examination not only initiates the preventive oral health care process but supports the concept of the dental home. The time has come for us to join with our colleagues in medicine so that all children have both a medical and a dental home for all their health needs.[11,56]

## BOX 14-3

### Services Provided by the Dental Home

1. Schedule early dental visits at approximately 12 to 18 months of age.
2. Assess the risk of the infant and toddler for future dental disease.
3. Evaluate the fluoride status of the infant and make appropriate recommendations.
4. Demonstrate to caretakers the appropriate method for cleaning teeth.
5. Discuss the advantages/disadvantages of nonnutritive sucking.
6. Be prepared to treat the infant/toddler if early childhood caries is diagnosed or to make the appropriate referral.
7. Be available 24 hours a day, 7 days a week to deal with any acute dental problems.
8. Recognize the need for specialty consultation and referrals.

## FLUORIDE ADMINISTRATION

### Rationale

Significant reductions in the prevalence of dental caries in children have been documented in the United States and other countries over the past several decades.[46] Although the exact reasons for this decline are unknown, most experts include increased availability of fluorides as one of the primary contributing factors. In spite of these advances, caries remains a relatively common yet largely preventable disease of childhood. Because of the importance of fluoride in this regard, the contemporary dental practitioner should understand the basis for using the many available forms of fluoride.

### Mechanisms of Action

Although the precise mechanisms by which fluorides prevent dental caries are not fully understood, three general mechanisms are typically acknowledged: (1) increasing the resistance of the tooth structure to demineralization; (2) enhancing the process of remineralization; and (3) reducing the cariogenic potential of dental plaque.

The effects of fluoride are usually classified as either systemic or topical. Systemic effects can be obtained through the ingestion of foods that contain natural levels of fluoride, water that contains natural fluoride or to which fluoride has been added, dietary fluoride supplements, and some forms of fluoride mouth rinses intended for swallowing (most fluoride rinses are intended for topical application only). Topical benefits are available from the previously mentioned sources as a result of their contact with the teeth as well as from fluoride toothpastes and other more concentrated forms of fluoride that are self-administered or applied professionally.

The decision to administer various forms of fluoride depends primarily on the age of the child, his or her caries history and perceived susceptibility (i.e., risk) to develop caries in the future, and whether he or she drinks fluoridated water. For the birth-to-3 category, the principal concern is that all children receive an optimal level of systemic fluoride. For children considered to be at moderate or high risk for developing caries, optimal use of topical fluoride is also a significant consideration.

### Systemic Fluorides

#### Water Fluoridation

Water fluoridation remains the cornerstone of any sound caries prevention program. It is not only the most effective means of reducing caries, but remains the most cost-effective, cost-saving, convenient, and reliable method of providing the benefits of fluoride to the general population because it does not depend on individual compliance.[19,37] Early studies documented caries reductions of 40% to 50% in the primary dentition and 50% to 65% in the permanent dentition of children drinking fluoridated water from birth.[69] More recent studies have reported that the mean dmfs ("decayed-missing-filled surfaces") of children with continuous residence in fluoridated areas was about 18% lower than that of children with no exposure. When corrected to remove children that have been exposed to topical or supplemental fluorides, the mean dmfs was 25% lower in the group exposed continuously to water fluoridation.[17]

More than 50% of the U.S. population currently has access to drinking water containing a significant level of fluoride (>0.7 ppm). Many water supplies contain significant levels of natural fluoride, especially in the midwestern and southwestern sections of the country. Numerous fluoride-deficient community water supplies also have been artificially fluoridated at a cost of less than $0.50 per person, depending on the size of the community. In the United States during 2000, approximately 162 million persons (65.8% of the population served by public water systems) received optimally fluoridated water compared with 144 million (62.1%) in 1992.[20,21]

As part of their responsibility in promoting oral health, dentists have an obligation to educate the public about the effectiveness and safety of this proven preventive measure. Involvement at the local level in support of water fluoridation can be one of the major contributions a dentist can make to enhancing the oral health of all children in his or her community.

### Dietary Fluoride Supplements

Fluoride supplements provide an alternative source of dietary fluoride for children who do not have access to optimally fluoridated water. Included in this category are children whose public or private water supplies are fluoride deficient as well as those who reside in communities with fluoridated water but do not rely on optimally fluoridated water for their primary source of fluid intake.

For example, the use of bottled and processed waters for drinking and cooking has become popular in many communities, with total U.S. consumption estimated at more than 5 billion gallons in 2000 (more than double the amount a decade earlier).[13] Consumers are turning to these water sources as alternatives to tap water, which they believe is contaminated with microorganisms, pesticides, herbicides, industrial waste, and heavy metals. The fluoride content of these bottled waters generally has been found to exhibit wide variability, usually below optimal concentrations.[32,44,58,63,65] Regulations presently do not require bottled water manufacturers to list the fluoride concentration on the label. Hence, dentists need to be aware of the bottled water products readily available in their community and be prepared to obtain fluoride analyses when necessary. Furthermore, all parents, including those who reside in fluoridated areas, should be questioned about the sources of fluid in their infant's diet and should realize that fluoride supplements are advisable for children who consume very little fluoridated water.

Fluoride supplements can be as effective as fluoridated water in preventing caries;[26,39,67] however, their effectiveness depends largely on the degree of parental compliance. Supplements are commercially available in liquid and tablet forms, both with and without vitamins. The fluoride-vitamin formulations are not inherently superior to supplements without vitamins in terms of reducing caries. However, the combination of fluoride and vitamins may improve parental compliance, thereby providing greater benefits.[40]

Liquid preparations are recommended for younger patients who may have difficulty in chewing or swallowing tablets. Liquid supplements without vitamins are dispensed in preparations that provide a dose of 0.5 mg/ml; liquid supplements with vitamins are dispensed in preparations that provide 0.25 mg/ml and 0.5 mg/ml. Fluoride supplements in tablet form for older patients are available without vitamins in doses of 0.25, 0.5, and 1.0 mg of fluoride, and fluoride-vitamin combinations are available in 0.5- and 1.0-mg doses.

In order to obtain both topical and systemic effects, fluoride supplements should be allowed to contact the teeth prior to being swallowed. With liquid preparations, this can be achieved by placing the drops directly on the child's teeth or by placing the drops in the child's food or drink, although the latter practice may reduce the bioavailability of the fluoride. Older children should be encouraged to "chew and swish" their tablets or allow the tablets to dissolve in the mouth before swallowing to prolong the contact of the fluoride with the outer surfaces of the teeth.

The dosage of fluoride that should be prescribed depends on the age of the child and the fluoride concentration of his or her drinking water. The fluoride concentration of a central community water supply can be determined by contacting the local or state department of health or the local water authority. For persons who do not obtain their drinking water from a central supply, water samples should be tested for fluoride content. This service usually is provided by state health departments, schools of dentistry, or commercial firms. Alternatively, in-office analyses of water fluoride concentrations can be performed by clinicians using a relatively inexpensive hand-held colorimeter. Although less precise than more expensive fluoride electrodes, comparisons have shown that colorimetric assays closely correlate with electrode findings and generally result in comparable supplementation recommendations.[27] When results of electrode findings and colorimetric assays differ, corresponding supplementation recommendations based on colorime-

## TABLE 14-2
### Supplemental Fluoride Dosage Schedule

| Age | CONCENTRATION OF FLUORIDE IN WATER | | |
|-----|-----------|-------------|----------|
| | <0.3 ppm F | 0.3-0.6 ppm F | >0.6 ppm F |
| Birth–6 mo | 0 | 0 | 0 |
| 6 mo–3 yr | 0.25 mg | 0 | 0 |
| 3 yr–6 yr | 0.50 mg | 0.25 mg | 0 |
| 6 yr up to at least 16 yr | 1.00 mg | 0.50 mg | 0 |

try tend to be lower, thereby minimizing the potential for adverse outcomes (e.g., fluorosis). Because of the potential for considerable variations in fluoride levels in water obtained from different wells in the same area, it is important that each individual noncentral water source be sampled to determine accurately the appropriate level of fluoride supplementation for each patient. Table 14-2 shows the daily dosage schedule for fluoride supplementation that has been recommended by the American Academy of Pediatric Dentistry, the American Dental Association, and the American Academy of Pediatrics since 1994.[12]

Until recently, fluoride supplements were generally recommended for all children whose drinking water contained suboptimal levels of fluoride. However, consistent with the growing emphasis on risk assessment and risk-based preventive practices, recent recommendations[19] call for fluoride supplements to be prescribed for children at high risk for dental caries and whose primary drinking water has a low fluoride concentration. These newer recommendations also call for dentists, physicians, and other health care providers to weigh the risk for caries without fluoride supplements, the caries prevention offered by supplements and the potential for enamel fluorosis for children younger than 6 years. Parents and caregivers should be informed of both the benefits of protection against dental caries and the possibility of enamel fluorosis.

Observations that the prevalence of fluorosis has been significantly reduced in optimally fluoridated areas suggest that additional exposure to traditional sources of ingested fluoride may not be a major etiologic factor. That conclusion is further supported by studies suggesting that fluoride ingestion from dietary sources has remained relatively constant since the 1950s.[59] Notable exceptions in the pediatric population include a lowering of fluoride concentration in most infant formulas,[43] causing a reduction in fluoride exposure, and increased availability of fluoridated beverages in nonfluoridated areas (e.g., soft drinks prepared with fluoridated water) with the potential for additional fluoride intake.[23] This latter phenomenon has been called the "halo effect," reflecting the concept of extended water fluoridation effects beyond fluoridated communities.

The fluoride in most dietary supplements is incorporated as sodium fluoride (NaF). One milligram of fluoride is equivalent to approximately 2.2 mg of sodium fluoride. When prescribing fluoride supplements, the practitioner should clearly specify the dose that is to be dispensed in terms of fluoride ion, sodium fluoride, or both. Examples of prescriptions for dietary fluoride supplements are given in Box 14-4.

Because it is common for infants and children to experience several contacts with a physician prior to their first dental visit, dentists providing

## BOX 14-4
### Sample Supplemental Fluoride Prescription

**Eight-month-old whose drinking water contains less than 0.1 ppm fluoride:**
Rx: Sodium fluoride solution 0.5 mg/ml (0.25 mg F⁻)
   Disp: 50 ml
   Sig: Dispense 0.5 ml of liquid in mouth before bedtime

**Three-year-old whose drinking water contains 0.2 ppm fluoride:**
Rx: Sodium fluoride tablets 0.25 mg fluoride/tablet (0.55 mg NaF/tablet)
   Disp: 180 tablets
   Sig: Chew one (1) tablet, swish, and swallow after brushing at bedtime. Nothing per os (NPO) for 30 minutes.

treatment for children should become aware of the prescribing practices of local physicians and be prepared to offer advice about appropriate fluoride supplementation. In addition, dentists can provide input into local prenatal care programs so that expectant parents can be made aware of the benefits and appropriate use of fluorides.

Prescribing systemic fluorides during pregnancy to benefit the developing teeth was once a common practice in the United States. However, in 1966 the U.S. Food and Drug Administration (FDA) banned the promotion of prenatal fluoride supplements in the United States.[34] Safety was not the overriding issue in this decision. Rather, the decision was based on a lack of evidence about the effectiveness of prenatal fluoride supplements in preventing caries in offspring. Data from human studies suggest that the placenta is not an effective barrier to the passage of fluoride to the fetus and that there is a direct relationship between the serum fluoride concentrations of the mother and the fetus.[30,62] A study reported that 5-year-olds whose mothers were provided 1 mg of fluoride daily during prenatal months 4 through 9 had no statistically significant differences in their caries status than the control group. In addition, the prevalence of very mild fluorosis was low. Therefore, there continues to be little support for prenatal fluoride supplementation.[51]

## Topical Fluorides

Topical fluoride use for children up to age 3 ordinarily consists of conscientious use of a moderate amount of fluoride-containing toothpaste applied by a parent or caregiver. Children whose teeth contain structural defects or who exhibit decalcified areas or other indicators that place them at moderate or high risk for developing caries, or infants who have previously experienced severe caries (i.e., early childhood caries), may receive additional topical applications in the form of professionally administered (e.g., acidulated phosphate fluoride or fluoride varnish) or parentally given concentrated preparations. Regardless of whether toothpaste or a more concentrated form of fluoride is applied, care should be taken to minimize the amount that is used and swallowed. Parents should place a pea-sized dab of toothpaste on the brush and always supervise the brushing session so that the dentifrice and saliva are expectorated.

### Fluoride Varnish

Fluoride varnish was first introduced in Europe in 1964 under the trade name Duraphat. More than 25 years of clinical studies have since demonstrated that fluoride varnish is a safe and highly effective means of preventing decay. Clinical studies have demonstrated caries reduction rates of 25% to 75% from the use of fluoride varnish.*

Fluoride varnish first became available in the United States in 1991 when Duraflor received approval from the FDA for its use as a cavity varnish. In 1997, Duraphat also became available in the United States. Although approved for use as cavity varnishes and for the management of hypersensitivity, one of the most promising uses for fluoride varnish is in the prevention of tooth decay. The therapeutic use of fluoride varnish for caries prevention in the United States is called "off-label" use. This concept is sometimes confusing to those who may misinterpret it to mean that it is either illegal or unethical to use a product for an unapproved (as opposed to disapproved) use. However, the Federal Food, Drug, and Cosmetic (FD&C) Act does not limit the manner in which dentists may use approved drugs. It is often considered accepted medical or dental practice to use drugs for purposes other than that for which the drug originally received approval.[35]

Fluoride varnish is considered by many to be ideally suited for application to the teeth of pediatric dental patients. Its ease of application makes it attractive for use with young or precooperative patients, when topical fluoride treatments are indicated. Both Duraflor and Duraphat are 5% NaF (2.26% fluoride ion) and are therefore more concentrated than most other professionally applied fluoride products. When used clinically, only a small amount is needed. Less than 0.5 ml of varnish is usually required to coat the teeth of a young child. Other potential uses for fluoride varnish include application to identified areas of high risk such as decalcified areas, deep pits and fissures that cannot be sealed, and around orthodontic appliances in patients with poor oral hygiene.

Fluoride varnish is easy to apply by disposable brush, cotton-tipped applicator, or cotton pellets. Varnish application may be preceded by professional prophylaxis but may also be accomplished

---

*References 15, 22, 25, 48, 66, 74.

after normal brushing with a toothbrush. The teeth should be dried prior to application, either with compressed air or with dry gauze. Fluoride varnish can be applied to all tooth surfaces or may be selectively applied to sites with higher risk for caries (i.e., decalcified sites or maxillary anterior teeth in children at risk for early childhood caries). It is not necessary to wait for the varnish to dry prior to releasing the patient because the varnish sets upon contact with the oral fluids. After varnish application, the teeth should not be brushed until later in the evening or the following day so that the varnish will remain in contact with the teeth as long as possible. The varnish causes the teeth to appear yellowish, but this color disappears as the varnish wears off. With children at high risk of caries, it is recommended that the fluoride varnish be applied at intervals of 3 to 6 months. More frequent application may be desired for patients at highest risk for caries.

*Concentrated Fluorides for Home Use*

Examples of concentrated agents for topical application in the home include 0.5% acidulated phosphate fluoride 1.1% NaF gel, and 0.4% stannous fluoride ($SnF_2$) gels. $SnF_2$ gels may be preferable for younger children because a 0.4% $SnF_2$ preparation is only approximately one fourth as concentrated as 0.5% acidulated phosphate fluoride, and the gel is available without a prescription. A small amount of the gel should be brushed on the child's teeth before bedtime. The child should be encouraged to expectorate following the application but should not be allowed to eat or drink for approximately 30 minutes.

## Safety and Toxicity

When used properly, fluoride in various forms can enhance the oral health status of infants and children. As is true of many other substances, however, when used improperly these same agents have the potential to produce objectionable side effects. Therefore, each member of the dental profession has a responsibility to educate patients about the appropriate storage and use of these products.

Acute toxicity can result from the accidental ingestion of excessive amounts of fluoride. The manifestations of acute fluoride toxicity are usually limited to nausea and vomiting, but on at least one occasion the death of a child was reported.[72] The amount of ingested fluoride necessary to produce acute symptoms is directly related to the weight of the individual; therefore precautions should be employed to prevent the accidental ingestion of concentrated forms of fluoride by all children, but especially by very young children and infants. The lethal dose of fluoride for a typical 3-year-old is approximately 500 mg but would be proportionately less for a younger and smaller child.

To avoid the possibility of ingestion of large amounts of fluoride, it is recommended that no more than 120 mg of supplemental fluoride be prescribed at any one time.[5] Likewise, prescriptions for concentrated topical fluoride preparations intended for home use (e.g., 0.5% fluoride gels that contain 5 mg of fluoride/ml) should be limited to 30 to 40 ml. Ingestion of moderate volumes of fluoride mouth rinses and toothpastes containing 1 mg or less of fluoride/ml would not be expected to cause severe symptoms, although nausea and vomiting could result.

Parents should be encouraged to store these and all potentially harmful substances out of the reach of small children. If a child ingests excessive amounts of fluoride, the recommended approach is to call a local poison control center for verification, induce vomiting as quickly as possible if so instructed, and give milk every 4 hours to slow absorption.[2,54]

Repeated ingestion of lesser amounts of fluoride can result in manifestations of chronic fluoride toxicity, the most common of which is dental fluorosis. Infants and young children who cannot fully control their swallowing reflex or who do not understand that they should expectorate products intended only for topical application may regularly swallow significant amounts of fluoride toothpaste. This amount of fluoride (approximately 0.3 mg at each brushing) may be significant in children who also receive fluoride from fluoridated water, fluoride supplements, or other dietary source.[24,68] In light of concern about potential increases in the prevalence of dental fluorosis, parents should be cautioned to supervise their children closely and limit the amount of fluoride toothpaste used by young children. Use of toothpaste also may be limited for infants under age 3 who are considered to be at low risk for the development of dental caries.

Another potential source of excessive fluoride ingestion is the inappropriate prescribing of fluoride supplements. Dentists and physicians may be unaware that some water supplies in their area may contain varying amounts of natural fluoride, or they may assume that the level of fluoride is relatively consistent among sources. Unless samples of drinking water are analyzed for each patient, fluoride supplements may be prescribed when they are not indicated.[50,73]

Fluoride has a critical role in the prevention of dental caries in children. Therefore, dentists who assume responsibility for the oral health of children should be knowledgeable about the safe and appropriate use of the various forms of fluoride available.

## DIET

Information is provided in this text on the dental disease process and the relationships among host, bacteria, and substrate. It is important to establish dietary habits early in the child's life that promote physical growth and development and create an environment conducive to optimal oral health.

Although considerable research to determine the potential role of various foods in promoting dental disease continues, available evidence suggests that the solubility and adhesiveness of foods are important factors. Foods that stick to the teeth and tissues for long periods and dissolve slowly are more likely to promote the production of acids that lower the pH of the oral environment. A pH below 5.5 provides an environment for bacterial growth and decalcification of enamel.[64]

Initially, the infant's diet consists primarily of milk, whether from the breast, the bottle, or both. Bovine milk has a higher calcium, phosphorus, and protein content than human milk and contains 4% lactose compared with 7% lactose in human milk.[60] The buffering capacity of human milk is very poor. Consequently, both human and bovine milk have the potential to promote development of caries and, when inappropriately provided to infants without daily oral hygiene care, milk can lead to early childhood caries. Infants should never be given a bottle containing milk or other sweetened beverages as a pacifier to be used during the day, at naptime, or at bedtime. If a naptime or bedtime bottle is customary, the infant should be held by the parent while feeding from the bottle. Upon finishing, the infant should be placed in the bed without the bottle. If there is a need for additional sucking, a pacifier is preferable to the bottle. If parents continue to insist on prolonged use of a bottle, the contents should be limited to water.

Feeding infants by breast is popular in both the United States and Europe, especially during the months immediately following birth. The overall prevalence of breastfeeding in the United States in 2001 was 69.5%. Breastfeeding was provided at 6 months of age for 32.5% of infants; however, contrary to American Academy of Pediatrics recommendations, only 17% were exclusively breastfed at 6 months.[61]

As noted earlier, because of its composition breast milk may contribute to acid production and promote enamel demineralization. However, this generally only occurs when another carbohydrate source is available for bacterial fermentation and the buffering capacity is exceeded.[31] Infants who are breastfed truly "on demand" may suckle 10 to 40 times in a 24-hour period and are at risk for the consequences of prolonged acid production. Nevertheless, many feel that the benefits of breastfeeding outweigh any harmful effects. Dentists should advise mothers who breastfeed on demand to clean their infant's teeth frequently, verify that systemic fluoride intake is optimal, and monitor dietary habits carefully.[38]

Although surveys report that most U.S. infants are fed beikost (foods other than milk or formula for infants) by 2 months of age, pediatric nutritionists recommend that the infant's total nutritional needs be supplied from human milk or formula until 5 to 6 months of age. At 5 to 6 months, iron-fortified dry cereal is recommended followed by one to two new commercially or home-prepared foods each week. Sound eating habits established during infancy assist in the continuation of sound habits later in life. Making an infant drain the last drop from the bottle or finish the last spoonful in the dish is not recommended. Forcing infants to eat when they indicate a desire to stop may contribute to overeating, frequent snacking, and obesity in later life.[33]

Usually by the time the posterior teeth erupt and the infant is sitting in the high chair for meals, the child has been introduced to a variety of foods. Parents should be advised about appropriate snack foods that not only are nutritious but are also "safe for teeth." Finger foods (e.g., soft fruits and vegetables, cereals without sugar coatings, Jell-O cubes, salt-free crackers and cheeses) are acceptable and should be introduced as the infant develops chewing patterns and swallowing reflexes to handle these new foods. Foods with a high percentage of carbohydrates should be avoided, as should foods that stick to the teeth and are slow to dissolve.

Natural fruit juices and artificially fortified fruit juices are frequently introduced to the infant. Pediatricians recommend that juices not be given to the infant in a bottle, in a covered cup, or at bedtime. Juices should not be introduced into the diet of infants before 6 months of age and should only be given by cup. Habitual and prolonged use of juices in the bottle can lead to early childhood caries.[1]

## HOME CARE

The initiation of a program to ensure an optimal environment for oral health should begin in infancy.[10] Parents should be informed that it is their responsibility to carry out this program, with information and guidance available from the dentist and staff.

Dental professionals have long provided direction to parents about their child's dental health, with the major emphasis on caries prevention. The changing patterns of dental caries in children, increasing parental concern about other oral health issues, more single-parent families, and dentistry's ability to deal with important issues other than dental caries have broadened the counseling role in dental health care delivery for children.

Anticipatory guidance is a term that describes a proactive, developmentally based counseling system that focuses on the needs of a child at a particular stage of life. The concept of a developmentally relevant, one-on-one intervention between dentist and parent offers a popular alternative to the traditional one-sided caries prevention message. Anticipatory guidance gives parents the chance to talk about their child, get age-appropriate information, and look ahead at how growth and the environment will affect their child's oral health in the next few months. It broadens dentistry's reach into related areas that have implications for children's oral health. Finally, it gives the dental professional a consistent staged format for counseling and record keeping and avoids the common routine repetition that often fails to provide effective motivation for children and parents alike.

Appendix C suggests one approach to anticipatory guidance in pediatric dentistry. Clinicians can use the chart to formulate practice-specific information for families or to track the information given to parents, or they can modify it into an instrument useful for assessing a child's dental development. In a busy practice, this organized approach allows one clinician to pick up where another has stopped without message duplication.

The preventive program includes many facets: dietary management, optimal systemic fluorides, and ongoing plaque control. All are important, but plaque removal in the infant and young child is most often neglected and misunderstood.

Studies have confirmed that the bacteria for dental disease are present at the eruption of the primary teeth.[29] The usual source of these bacteria is the mother. Studies have shown that there is a period of infectivity, maybe as early as 6 months and before teeth are present, during which bacteria are transmitted from the mother to the child.[29] This transmission coincides with the period of active tooth eruption and increases when the first and second primary molars erupt.[18] Growth of cariogenic bacteria and certain components of the infant's diet combine to promote the development of plaque and the subsequent production of acid. This environment around the teeth is conducive to demineralization of enamel and, eventually, cavitation. In addition, the gingiva is subjected to daily insult from the products of bacterial metabolism, which can lead to marginal gingivitis.

Daily removal of plaque promotes sound enamel and healthy gingiva. Early initiation of plaque removal helps to establish a lifelong habit of oral care. A disease-free mouth brings happiness and satisfaction not only to the parents and children but also to the dental team that provided the counseling and encouragement.

Once the parents have been informed about the dental disease process and have been charged with the responsibility of cleaning their child's teeth daily, counseling should be provided about a suitable location for performing the procedure, devices for plaque removal, pros and cons of dentifrice use, positioning of the infant, and techniques for effective plaque removal. Initially, oral hygiene for the infant probably should be performed wherever the parent changes the infant's diapers. A changing table is a convenient height and usually has appropriate lighting. As the infant grows, the knee-to-knee position (see Fig. 13-1) becomes preferable. Bathrooms (the usual site for oral hygiene for older children and adults) often are crowded and not designed for infant safety.

Positioning the infant for visibility and control is important. Whether the parent uses the changing table, a bed top, countertop, or the knee-to-knee position, appropriate stabilization, visibility, and control of the lips, tongue, and cheeks are important for a thorough and pleasant hygienic experience.

Once teeth have erupted, a wet, soft-bristled brush can be gently wiped over them. When several teeth have erupted, a more thorough and systematic routine should be established in which one makes sure to clean all surfaces of the teeth in both the upper and lower jaws and especially the area near the gingiva. By this time the infant will have become stronger and may even object to the activity. The parent should be advised to be persistent. With time, the tooth cleaning activity becomes an accepted part of the daily routine.

Finding an appropriate time is important. The combination of a tired infant and an exhausted parent does not produce a favorable environment for a positive experience. Developmentally, an infant is not prepared to accept or understand the activity. Games may be developed, or music and singing used; the parent must try to create a positive experience. With time, the infant may even become less tolerant, but the parent should be encouraged to be persistent.

A thorough cleaning before bedtime is recommended. Usually the infant is given a bath. Tooth cleaning can follow immediately along with any other personal hygiene. Toward the end of the second year of life, the child will be very mobile, actively involved in play and other "grown up" activities. Parents must remember to save time at the end of a busy day for oral care. Although many 24-month-olds want to clean their own teeth, parents should understand that fine motor activity remains largely undeveloped at this age. A parent should provide supervision and removal of plaque from missed areas.

Toothbrushes are available in many shapes, colors, sizes, and designs (Box 14-5). Brushes with soft, rounded, nylon bristles are recommended. The size of the head, angle of the head to the handle, and size and shape of the handle all

## BOX 14-5

### Plaque Removal Innovations for Infants and Toddlers
*M. Catherine Skotowski, RDH, MS*

There are products in the oral health care market that assist parents in cleansing the mouth of an infant or toddler that do not resemble the traditional shape of a toothbrush. Small cotton finger cloths that fit over the finger of an adult have been marketed as a pretoothbrush for infants with very few or possibly no erupted teeth present. Not only do they help remove plaque and food debris but they assist in stimulating the gingival tissues and introduce oral cleansing at a very early age. Another popular oral cleansing device for a very young child resembles a small circular rubber ring with a few tufts of bristles at one end. The easy-to-grasp shape allows a child or an adult to stimulate the gums and cleanse the oral cavity without the risk of overinsertion.

Historically, toothbrushes for infants and toddlers have been miniature replicas of adult toothbrushes, varying primarily by size and character designs added to the toothbrush to appeal to young children. In recent years, considerable research and study have been invested in exploring better designed, more functional toothbrushes for this age group, focusing on the shape and design of the toothbrush itself. Recognizing that parents should be the primary plaque removers for young children, some manufacturers have produced toothbrushes with longer handles for easier parental brushing. Some manufacturers are designing brush heads to meet the specific needs of the developing dentition. Most still feature soft bristles, but efforts have been made to alternate the lengths of the bristles to accommodate different surfaces of the teeth. Some designs feature soft rubber padding around the brush head to make it gentle to the gums. Innovations in the shape of the handle have evolved to improve the grip as well as to promote angling of the bristles at the optimal 45 degrees.

Along with the attention focused in recent years on the shape and design of toothbrushes for young children, much research and study continue on the marketability of toothbrushes based on their color and character designs. Keeping current with the latest trends in this area is imperative because most often the consumer selects the product with the most eye appeal. The fact that the toothbrush has been designed to assist with better plaque removal is an added bonus.

depend on the infant's and parent's preference. A design that works best in their hands and can get the cleaning and massaging completed is the brush to use. Mechanical or novelty brushes also are available. Although novel, adequate documentation of advantages associated with the use of these devices (e.g., greater likelihood of sustained use) is lacking.

Infants have limited ability to expectorate. Therefore, dentifrices with fluoride should be used sparingly if at all before age 2. Fluoride from the dentifrice can appreciably increase total fluoride intake. If a fluoride dentifrice is used, a very small amount should be placed on the brush and the cleaning completely performed or supervised by the parent. Because spacing usually is present between teeth in the primary dentition, flossing is not necessary until interdental contacts have been established.

## REFERENCES

1. American Academy of Pediatrics: The use and misuse of fruit juice in pediatrics. *Pediatrics* 107:1210-1213, 2000.
2. American Academy of Pediatrics: Poison treatment at home. *Pediatrics* 112:1182-1185, 2003.
3. American Academy of Pediatrics: Recommendations for preventive pediatric health care. *Pediatrics* 105:645,2000
4. American Academy of Pediatrics: Oral health risk assessment timing and establishment of the dental home. *Pediatrics* 2003;111:1113-1116.
5. American Academy of Pediatric Dentistry: Fluoride guidelines. *Pediatr Dent* 25:67-68, 2004.
6. American Academy of Pediatric Dentistry: Guideline on infant oral health care. Available at www.aapd.org/media/policies. 2003.
7. American Academy of Pediatric Dentistry: The use of a caries-risk assessment tool (CAT) for infants, children and adolescents. Available at www.aapd.org/media/policies. 2003.
8. American Academy of Pediatric Dentistry: Guideline on infant oral health care. *Pediatr Dent* 25(special issue):54, 2003.
9. American Academy of Pediatric Dentistry: Policy on the use of a caries risk assessment tool (CAT) for infants, children and adolescents. *Pediatr Dent* 25(special issue):18-20, 2003.
10. American Academy of Pediatric Dentistry: Guidelines on periodicity of examination, preventive dental services and anticipatory guidance and oral health needs of children. *Pediatr Dent* 25:61-63, 2003.
11. American Academy of Pediatric Dentistry: Policy on the dental home. *Pediatr Dent* 25:12, 2003.
12. American Dental Association: New fluoride schedule adopted. *ADA News*, May 1994.
13. American Dental Association : The facts about bottled water. *JADA* 2003;134:1287.
14. Barlow BS, Kanellis MJ, Slayton RL: Tooth eruption symptoms: a survey of parents and health professionals. *J Dent Child* 69:148-150, 2002.
15. Bawden JW: Fluoride varnish: a useful new tool for public health dentistry. *J Public Health Dent* 58:266-269, 1998.
16. Boggess KA, Lief S, Murtha AP, et al. Maternal periodontal disease is associated with an increased risk for preeclampsia. *Obstet Gynecol* 101:227-231, 2003.
17. Brunelle JA, Carlos JP: Recent trends in dental caries in U.S. children and the effect of water fluoridation. *J Dent Res* 69 (special issue):723-727, 1990.
18. Caufield PW, Hagan TW, Cutter GR, Dasanayake AP: Infants acquire *mutans* streptococci from mothers during a discrete window. *J Dent Res* 70:814, 1991.
19. Centers for Disease Control and Prevention: Recommendations for using fluoride to prevent and control dental caries in the United States. *MMWR Morb Mortal Wkly Rep* 50(RR-14):26, 2001.
20. Centers for Disease Control and Prevention: Populations receiving optimally fluoridated public drinking water–United States, 2000. *MMWR Morb Mortal Wkly Rep* 51:144-147, 2002.
21. Centers for Disease Control and Prevention. National Center for Prevention Services: *Fluoridation Census 1992 Summary.* Atlanta: US Department of Health and Human Services, Public Health Service, 1993.
22. Clark DC, Stamm JW, Robert G, Tessier C: Results of a 32-month fluoride varnish study in Sherbrooke and Lac-Megantic, Canada. *JADA* 111:949-953, 1985.
23. Clovis J, Hargreaves JA: Fluoride intake from beverage consumption. *Commun Dent Oral Epidemiol* 16:11-15, 1988.
24. Crall JJ: Biological implications and dietary supplementation. In: Pinkham JR, editor. *Pediatric Dental Care: An Update for the 90s.* Evansville, Ind, Bristol-Myers Squibb, 1991, pp 25-27.
25. De Bruyn H, Arends J: Fluoride varnishes—a review. *J Biol Buccale* 15:71-82, 1987.
26. Driscoll W: The use of fluoride tablets for the prevention of dental caries. In: Forrester D, Schultz E, editors. *International Workshop on Fluorides and Dental Caries Reductions.* Baltimore, University of Maryland, 1974, pp 25-96.
27. Edelstein BL, Cottrel D, O'Sullivan D, Tinanoff N:

Comparison of colorimeter and electrode analysis of water fluoride. *Pediatr Dent* 14:47-49, 1992.

28. Edelstein B, Tinanoff N: Screening preschool children for dental caries using a microbial test. *Pediatr Dent* 11:129-132, 1989.

29. Edwardsson S, Mejare B: *Streptococcus milleri* (Guthof) and *Streptococcus mutans* in the mouths of infants before and after tooth eruption. *Arch Oral Biol* 23:811-814, 1978.

30. Ekstrand J, Whitford GM: Fluoride metabolism. In: Ekstrand J, Fejerskow O, Siluentone LM, editors. *Fluoride in Dentistry.* Copenhagen, Munksgaard, 1988, pp 165-166.

31. Erickson P, Mazhari E: Investigation of the role of human breast milk in caries development. *Pediatr Dent* 21:86-90, 1999.

32. Flaitz CM, Hill EM, Hicks MJ: A survey of bottled water usage by pediatric dental patients: Implications for dental health. *Quintessence Int* 20:847-852, 1989.

33. Fomon S: *Nutrition of Normal Infants.* St Louis, Mosby, 1993.

34. Food and Drug Administration: Statements of general policy or interpretation, oral prenatal drugs containing fluoride for human use. *Fed Reg,* October 20, 1966.

35. Food and Drug Administration: Use of approved drugs for unlabeled indications. *FDA Drug Bull*;12:4-5, 1982.

36. Green M, Palfrey JS, editors: *Bright Futures: Guidelines for Health Supervision of Infants, Children, and Adolescents,* 2nd ed. Arlington, Va, National Center for Education in Maternal and Child Health, 2000.

37. Griffin SO, Jones K, Tomar SL: An economic evaluation of community water fluoridation. *J Public Health Dent* 61:78-86, 2001.

38. Hallonsten AL, Wendt LK, Mejere I, et al: Dental caries and prolonged breast feeding in 18 month old Swedish children. *Int J Paediatr Dent* 5:149-155, 1995.

39. Hargreaves JA: Water fluoridation and fluoride supplementation: considerations for the future. Proceedings of a Joint IADR/ORCA International Symposium on Fluorides: Mechanisms of Action and Recommendations. *J Dent Res*(special issue) 69:765-770, 1990.

40. Hennon DK, Stookey GK, Muhler JC: The clinical anticariogenic effectiveness of supplementary fluoride-vitamin preparations. Results at the end of three years. *J Dent Child* 33:3-11, 1966.

41. Holm AK, Anderson R: Enamel mineralization disturbances in 12-year-old children with known early exposure to fluorides. *Commun Dent Oral Epidemiol* 10:335-339, 1982.

42. Jeffcoat MK, Geurs NC, Reddy MS, et al: Current evidence regarding periodontal disease as a risk factor in preterm birth. *Ann Periodontal*; 6:183-188, 2001.

43. Johnson J Jr, Bawden JW: The fluoride content of infant formula available in 1985. *Pediatr Dent* 9:33-37, 1987.

44. Johnson SA, DeBiase C: Concentration levels of fluoride in bottled drinking water. *J Dent Hyg* 77:161-197, 2003.

45. Centers for Disease Control and Prevention. Recommendations for using fluoride to prevent and control dental caries in the United States. *MMWR Morb Mortal Wkly Rep* 50 (No.RR-14) 1-42, 2001.

46. Kaste LM, Selwitz RH, Oldakowski RJ, et al: Coronal caries in the primary and permanent dentition of children and adolescents 1–17 years of age: United States, 1988–1991. *J Dent Res* 75(special issue):631-641, February 1996.

47. King DL: Teething revisited. *Pediatr Dent* 16:179-182, 1994.

48. Kock G, Petersson LG. Caries preventive effect of a fluoride-containing varnish (Duraphat) after 1 year's study. *Community Dent Oral Epidemiol*; 3:262-266, 1975

49. Kohler B, Bratthall D, Krasse B: Preventive measures in mothers influence the establishment of the bacterium *Streptococcus mutans* in their infants. *Arch Oral Biol* 1983;28:225-31.

50. Kuthy RA, McTigue DJ: Fluoride prescription practices of Ohio physicians. *J Public Health Dent* 47:172-176, 1987.

51. Leverett DH, Adair SM, Vaughan BW et al: Randomized clinical trial of the effect of prenatal fluoride supplements in preventing caries. *Caries Res* 31:174-179, 1997.

52. Livingston HM, Dellinger TM, Holden R. Considerations in the management of the pregnant patient. *Spec Care Dentist* 18:183-188, 1998.

53. Macknin ML, Piedmonte M, Jacobs J, et al: Symptoms associated with infant teething. A prospective study. *Pediatrics* 105:747-752, 2000.

54. National Institutes of Health. Fluoride overdose. Available at http://www.nlm.nih.gov/medlineplus/ency/article/002650.htm#Symptoms. 2003

55. Nowak AJ: Rationale for the timing of the first oral evaluation. *Pediatr Dent* 19:8-11, 1997.

56. Nowak AJ, Casamassimo PS: The dental home: a primary care oral health concept. *JADA* 133:93-98, 2002.

57. Nowak A, Casamassimo P: Using anticipatory guidance to provide early dental intervention. *JADA* 126:1155-1163, 1995.

58. Nowak A, Nowak MV: Fluoride concentration of bottled and processed waters. *J Iowa Dent* 75:28, 1989.

59. Pendrys DG, Stamm JW: Relationship of total fluoride intake to beneficial effects and enamel

fluorosis. *J Dent Res* 69 (special issue):529-538, 1990.

60. Rugg-Gunn AJ, Roberts GJ, Wright WG: Effect of human milk on plaque pH in situ and enamel dissolution in vitro compared with bovine milk, lactose and sucrose. *Caries Res* 19:327-334, 1985.

61. Ryan AS, Wenjon Z, Costa A: Breastfeeding continues to increase into the new millennium. *Pediatrics* 110:1103-1109, 2002.

62. Shen YW, Taves DR: Fluoride concentrations in the human placenta and maternal and cord blood. *Am J Obstet Gynecol* 119:205-207, 1974.

63. Stannard J, Rovero J, Tsamtsouris A, Gavris V: Fluoride content of some bottled waters and recommendations for fluoride supplementation. *J Pedod* 14:103-107, 1990.

64. Stephan RM: Changes in the hydrogen ion concentration on tooth surfaces and in carious lesions. *JADA* 27:718-723, 1940.

65. Tate WH, Snyder R, Montgomery EH, Chan JT: Impact of source of drinking water on fluoride supplementation. *Pediatrics* 86:419-421, 1990.

66. Tewari A, Chawla HS, Utreja A: Comparative evaluation of the role of NaF, APF, and Duraphat topical fluoride applications in the prevention of dental caries—a 2½ years study. *J Indian Soc Pedod Pre Dent* 8:28-35, 1991.

67. Thylstrup A: Clinical evidence of the role of pre-eruptive fluoride in caries prevention. *J Dent Res* 69(special issue):742-750, 1990.

68. Tinanoff N: Comment on urinary excretion of fluoride following ingestion of MFP toothpastes by infants ages two to six years. *Pediatr Dent* 7:345, 1985.

69. US Department of Health, Education, and Welfare: *Evaluatory Surveys of Long-Term Fluoridation Show Improved Dental Health.* USPHS Publication No. 84-22647. Atlanta, March 1979.

70. Wake M, Hesketh K, Lucas J: Teething and tooth eruption in infants: a cohort study. *Pediatrics* 106:1374-1379, 2000.

71. Wan AH, Seow WK, Purdie DM et al: Oral colonization of *Streptococcus mutans* in six month old predental infants. *J Dent Res* 80:2060-2065, 2001.

72. Watson WA, Litovitz TL, Rodgers GC Jr, et al: 2002 Annual report of the American Association of Poison Control Centers Toxic Exposure Surveillance System. *Am J Emerg Med* 21:353-421, 2003.

73. Woolfolk NW, Faja BW, Bagramian RA: Relation of sources of systemic fluoride to prevalence of dental fluorosis. *J Public Health Dent* 49:78-82, 1989.

74. Yanover L. Fluoride varnishes as cariostatic agents: a review. *J Can Dent Assoc* 48:401-404, 1982.

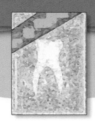

# CHAPTER 15

## Introduction to Dental Trauma: Managing Traumatic Injuries in the Primary Dentition

*Gideon Holan and Dennis J. McTigue*

An injury to the teeth of a young child can have serious and long-term consequences, leading to their discoloration, malformation, or possible loss. The emotional impact of such an injury can be far reaching. It is therefore important that the dentist treating children is:

1. Knowledgeable in the techniques for managing traumatic injuries
2. Readily available during and after office hours to provide treatment

If either of the above conditions cannot be met, the child suffering a dental injury should immediately be referred to a specialist.

The purpose of this chapter is to provide a straightforward approach to managing dental injuries in the primary dentition. Techniques for diagnosis, treatment, and follow-up care are described. Fundamental issues covered in this chapter, such as classification of injuries, history, examination, and pathologic sequelae of trauma, pertain to both the primary and permanent dentitions. Chapter 34 will focus on management of injuries to young permanent teeth and will refer to this chapter for the information just noted. The principles gleaned from both chapters should enable the dentist to manage the great majority of dental injuries encountered in children.

## ETIOLOGY AND EPIDEMIOLOGY OF TRAUMA IN THE PRIMARY DENTITION

The most frequently injured teeth in the primary dentition are the maxillary incisors. Primary molars are rarely injured, and when injury occurs it is usually due to indirect trauma (i.e., blows to the underside of the chin causing the mandible to close forcefully against the maxilla). In the primary dentition luxation injuries are more common than fractures due to the spongy nature of the bone in young children and to the lower root/crown ratio in comparison with that of permanent teeth.

By the age of 5 years about one third of boys and one fourth of girls have experienced traumatic injuries to their teeth.[6] The peak age of injuries to the primary teeth is 2 to 4 years when children are developing mobility skills. Children with protruding incisors, as in developing class II malocclusions, are two to three times more likely to suffer dental trauma than children with normal incisal overjets.

Another major cause of dental injuries in young children is automobile accidents. Unrestrained children who are seated or standing often hit the dashboard or windshield when the car is stopped suddenly. All states now have laws mandating use of child restraints in automobiles, and it is hoped that universal adoption of these laws will decrease the incidence of all trauma to children in automobile accidents.[12]

Children with chronic seizure disorders experience an increased incidence of dental trauma. Frequently, these high-risk children wear protective headgear, and the fabrication of custom mouth guards for them is indicated (see Chapter 40).

Another serious cause of dental injuries to young children is child abuse. Often overlooked by the dental profession, up to 50% of abused children suffer injuries to the head and neck. Cardinal signs of abuse are injuries in various stages of healing, tears of labial frena, repeated injuries, and injuries whose clinical presentation is not consistent with the history presented by the parent.[2] Battered children frequently lie to protect their parents or due to fear of retaliation. Dentists are required by law to report cases of suspected child abuse (see Chapter 1 for more specific details).

## CLASSIFICATION OF INJURIES TO TEETH

Tooth fractures may involve the crown, root, or both (Figs. 15-1 to 15-3; see also Figs. 34-1 to 34-3). Fractures of the crown may be limited to

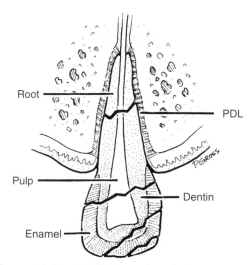

**Figure 15-1**  Classification of tooth injuries. Tooth fractures may involve enamel, dentin, or pulp and may occur in the crown or the root.

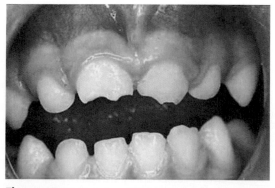

**Figure 15-2**  Fracture of enamel and dentin in both maxillary primary central incisors.

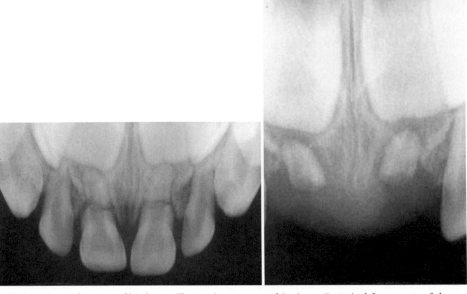

**Figure 15-3** **A,** Root fracture of both maxillary primary central incisors. **B,** Apical fragments of the root fractured maxillary primary central incisors after extraction of the coronal fragments.

the enamel, may involve the dentin, or may include the pulp. Injury to the pulp is the most complicated and demanding to manage.

As just mentioned, the most common types of injuries to primary teeth are luxation (displacement) injuries. These injuries damage supporting structures of the teeth, which include the periodontal ligament (PDL) and the alveolar bone (see Fig. 15-1). The PDL is the physiologic "hammock" that supports the tooth in its socket. Maintaining its vitality is the primary objective in the management of all luxation injuries. Several types of luxation injury occur.[6]

1. Concussion: The tooth is not mobile and is not displaced. The PDL absorbs the injury and is inflamed, which leaves the tooth tender to biting pressure and percussion.
2. Subluxation: The tooth is loosened but is not displaced from its socket.
3. Intrusion: The tooth is driven into its socket. This compresses the PDL and commonly causes a crushing fracture of the alveolar socket. See Figures 15-4 and 34-12.

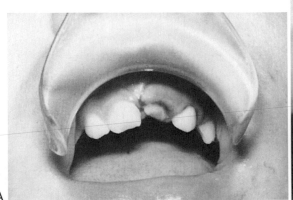

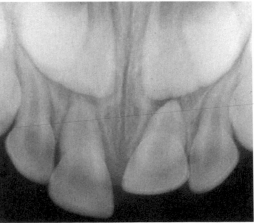

**Figure 15-4** **A,** Intruded maxillary left primary central incisor. **B,** Periapical radiograph showing the left maxillary primary central incisor after intrusion. The shortened and more opaque image of the intruded tooth, as compared with that of the right central incisor, indicates that the root has been pushed labially and away from the underlying permanent tooth.

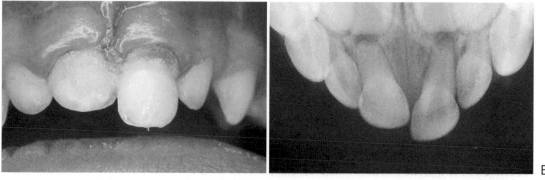

**Figure 15-5**  Extrusion of the left maxillary primary central incisor. **A,** Clinical view. **B,** Radiographic view. Notice the pulp canal obliteration in the right maxillary primary central incisor, which resulted from a previous injury.

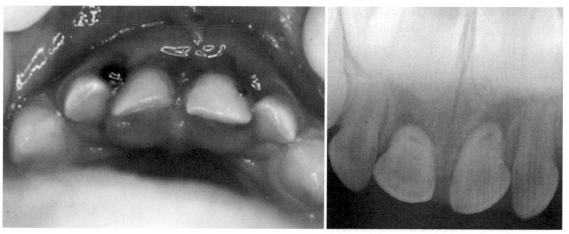

**Figure 15-6**  Lingual luxation of both maxillary primary central incisors. **A,** Clinical view. **B,** Radiographic view.

4. Extrusion: This is a central dislocation of the tooth from its socket (Figs. 15-5 and 34-13A). The PDL is usually torn in this injury.

5. Lateral luxation: The tooth is displaced in a labial, lingual, or lateral direction. The PDL is torn, and contusion or fracture of the supporting alveolar bone occurs (Figs. 15-6 and 34-13B).

6. Avulsion: The tooth is completely displaced from the alveolus. The PDL is severed, and fractures of the alveolus may occur (Figs. 15-7 and 34-14).

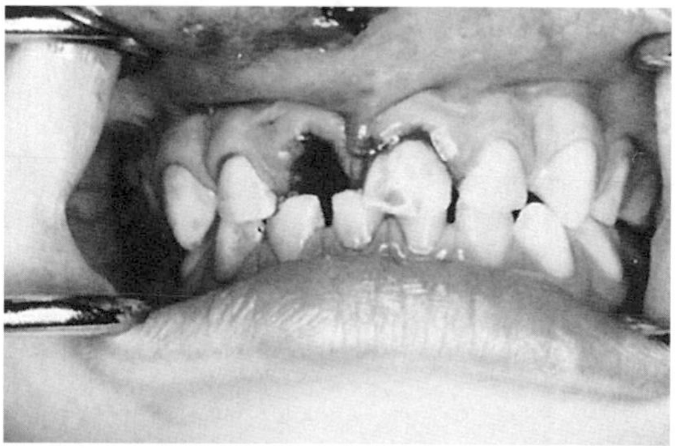

**Figure 15-7**  Avulsion of maxillary right primary central incisor.

## HISTORY

Obtaining an adequate medical and dental history is essential to proper diagnosis and treatment. The medical history should already be on record if the child suffering an injury is brought to his or

her regular dentist. Frequently, however, a parent will take an injured child to the closest dentist or to one known to treat children. Thus, with the confusion of a young injured child entering the office for possibly the first time and disrupting the day's schedule, the potential to forget to gather important historical information is great. The use of a trauma assessment form to help record data and organize the management of care is highly recommended (Fig. 15-8).

## Medical History

Routine data on the patient's general health should be obtained. Historical information particularly relevant to the dental injury includes the following:

1. Cardiac disease, which may necessitate prophylaxis against infectious endocarditis
2. Bleeding disorders
3. Allergies to medications
4. Seizure disorders
5. Medications
6. Status of tetanus prophylaxis

The issue of tetanus protection is particularly important when a child has suffered a dirty wound (an avulsion), a deep laceration, or an intrusion injury in which soil is embedded in the tissues. Wounds containing necrotic tissue, dirt, and foreign material should be cleaned and debrided as an essential part of tetanus prophylaxis. Children acquire active immunity through a series of five injections of adsorbed tetanus

---

**SCHOOL of DENTISTRY**
**DEPARTMENT of PEDIATRIC DENTISTRY**

Child's Name _____    Student _____
Age _____ Sex _____ Race _____    Faculty _____
Place of Injury _____    Chart No. _____    Date _____
Date of Injury _____
Time of Injury _____
Time Elapsed Since Injury _____

**HISTORY**
Chief Complaint _____    Previous Trauma _____
Past Medical History _____
Past Dental History _____
How Injury Occurred _____
Tetanus Protection: ☐ No    Yes ☐    Date of Last Booster _____

**EXTRAORAL ASSESSMENT**
**CNS Status**
☐ Unconsciousness    ☐ Amnesia
☐ Unequal Pupil Size    ☐ Headache
☐ Fixed Pupil    ☐ Nausea
☐ CSF from Ears    ☐ Disorientation
☐ CSF from Nose    ☐ Loss of smell
☐ Nystagmus    ☐ Seizure
☐ Vertigo
Describe _____

**Hard Tissue**
☐ Cranial Fracture    ☐ Zygoma Fracture
☐ Mandibular Fracture    ☐ Infection
☐ Maxillary Fracture
Describe _____

**Soft Tissue**
☐ Laceration    ☐ Abrasion
☐ Contusions    ☐ Infection
☐ Swelling    ☐ Embedded Maternal
Describe _____

**INTRAORAL ASSESSMENT**
**Hard Tissue**
☐ Alveolar Fracture    ☐ Palatal Fracture
Describe _____

**Soft Tissue**
☐ Lips    ☐ Frenum
☐ Buccal Mucosa    ☐ Tongue
☐ Gingiva    ☐ Palate ☐
Describe _____

**Dental Occlussion**
Molar _____    Cuspid _____
Overjet _____ mm    Overbite _____ %
Openbite _____    Crossbite _____
Classification Deviation Induced by Trauma _____
Describe _____

**RADIOGRAPHS**
☐ Periapical    ☐ Occlusal
☐ Lateral Anterior    ☐ Panorex
Other _____
Pathology _____

**Figure 15-8**    Trauma assessment form.

*Continued*

**DENTAL FINDINGS**

| Fracture | Class I | Class II | Class III | Class IV |
|---|---|---|---|---|

*Draw Injury*

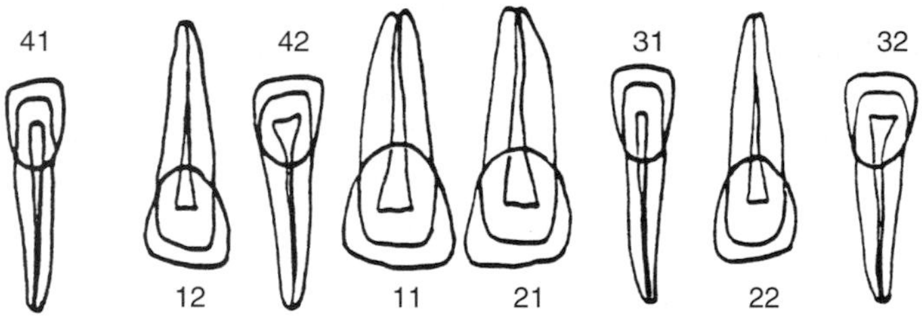

Involved Teeth _____

**Tooth Response — Pulp and PDL**

| Tooth No. | | | | |
|---|---|---|---|---|
| Exposure | | | | |
| Hemorrhage | | | | |
| Heat | | | | |
| Cold | | | | |
| Contamination | | | | |
| Percussion | | | | |
| Mobility | | | | |
| Vitalometer | | | | |

**Displacement**

☐ Intrusion       ☐ Subluxation
☐ Extrusion       ☐ Lateral Luxation
☐ Avulsion

**Color**

☐ Normal       ☐ Dark       ☐ Light

**SUMMARY AND DIAGNOSIS**

Crown _____

Pulp _____
_____

Root _____
_____

Periapical Tissue _____
_____

Alveolar Process _____
_____

Root Displacement _____
_____

Restoration _____
Fragments _____
_____

**TREATMENT**

Soft Tissues _____
Pulp _____
Restoration _____
Splinting _____
Medication _____

**Recall Follow-up**

☐ 2 weeks       ☐ 3 weeks       ☐ 6 weeks
☐ 3 months            ☐ 6 months
Other _____
_____

**Figure 15-8—cont'd**

toxoid, usually completed by the age of 4 to 6 years. These are normally administered as part of the diphtheria-tetanus-pertussis immunizations. Children should then receive a booster of tetanus toxoid at 11 to 12 years of age and every 10 years thereafter, unless the child suffers a dirty wound as just described. A booster is then indicated if the child has not received one in the last 5 years.[1] An increasing number of reports have indicated that children in the United States are not receiving their childhood immunizations appropriately. If there is any question about the adequacy of a child's tetanus protection, the child's physician should immediately be consulted.

### History of the Dental Injury

Three important questions are asked in gathering the dental history: *when, where,* and *how* did the accident occur? The time elapsed since the injury occurred is a major factor in determining the type of treatment to be provided. The dentist should also determine whether the tooth had been injured previously or whether the injury had first been treated elsewhere.

*Where* the injury occurred sheds light on its severity. Did the toddler slip and hit the coffee table in the living room, or did she fall off her parent's bicycle in the park? This information can help determine the need for tetanus prophylaxis as well as signal a need to rule out more serious injury to the child.

*How* the accident occurred obviously provides the dentist with the most information regarding severity. Serious head injuries should be ruled out by the dentist's asking if the child lost consciousness, has vomited, or is disoriented as a result of the accident. Positive findings indicate potential central nervous system injury, and medical consultation should be immediately obtained.[9] Tecklenburg and Wright note that significant head injuries can lead to symptoms many hours after the initial trauma, and they caution parents to watch for the signs noted above for 24 hours including waking the child every 2 to 3 hours through the night.[36]

As previously discussed, the possibility of child abuse can also be ruled out through a careful dental history. Any history of previous dental injuries should also be determined as their sequelae may complicate diagnosis of the current injury.

Directing attention to the specific teeth involved, the dentist should ask the child if there is spontaneous pain from any teeth. Positive findings here may indicate pulp inflammation that is due to a fractured crown or injuries to the supporting structures such as extravasation of blood into the PDL. Does the child experience a thermal change with sweet or sour foods? If so, dentin or pulp may be exposed. Are the teeth tender to touch or tender while chewing? Does the child note a change in occlusion? These findings may indicate a luxation injury or an alveolar fracture.

## CLINICAL EXAMINATION

Once the medical and dental histories are complete, the dentist is ready to begin the clinical examination. It is very tempting to focus immediately on a fractured or displaced tooth and thus miss other important injuries. A disciplined approach to a complete clinical examination should be followed in diagnosing every traumatic injury.

## Extraoral Examination

A complete examination should rule out injuries to the child's facial bones.[25] The facial skeleton should be palpated to determine discontinuities of facial bones. Extraoral wounds and bruises should be recorded. The temporomandibular joints should be palpated, and any swelling, clicking, or crepitus should be noted. Mandibular function in all excursive movements should be checked. Any stiffness or pain in the child's neck necessitates immediate referral to a physician to rule out cervical spine injury.

## Intraoral Examination

All soft tissues should be examined and any injuries recorded. The presence of foreign matter in lacerations of the lips and cheeks, such as tooth fragments or soil, should be identified. Removal at the initial appointment will eliminate chronic infection and disfiguring fibrosis.

Each tooth in the mouth should be examined for fracture, pulp exposure, and dislocation. In some crown fractures, only a very thin layer of dentin remains over the pulp, so that the pulp's outline can be seen as a pink tinge on the dentin. The dentist should be very careful not to perforate this dentin with an instrument.

Displacement of teeth should be recorded, as well as horizontal and vertical tooth mobility. Increased mobility of an injured primary tooth is an indication of damage to the PDL unless the tooth is near natural exfoliation. Reaction to palpation and percussion of teeth is recorded. Percussion sensitivity is a good indicator of PDL inflammation.

Pulpal vitality testing is not routinely performed in the primary dentition. This is because primary teeth do not respond to such tests reliably and because the test requires a relaxed and cooperative patient who can report reactions objectively. Many young children lack the ability to report their reactions to pulpal testing objectively.

## Radiographic Examination

### Indications for Radiographs
Radiographs are an important part of the diagnosis and management of dental injuries. They allow the clinician to detect root fractures, extent of root development, size of pulp chambers, peri-

apical radiolucencies, resorption, degree of tooth displacement, position of unerupted teeth, jaw fractures, and the presence of tooth fragments and other foreign bodies in soft tissues. Although some radiographs will show negative findings at the initial appointment, they are nonetheless important as baseline documentation. Subsequent radiographic evidence can thus be compared with the initial films.

*Radiographic Techniques*

There is no "standard series" of radiographs for dental injuries. All films taken should clearly show the apical areas of traumatized teeth. In cases in which root fractures are suspected, a second or third radiograph should be made from slightly different angles both vertically and horizontally to verify the location and extent of the fracture.

To determine the presence of foreign bodies such as tooth fragments in the lips or tongue, one fourth of the normal exposure time is utilized. The film is placed beneath the tissue to be examined, and the radiograph is exposed (Fig. 15-9).

*Timing of Follow-up Radiographs*

As noted previously, many pathologic changes are not immediately apparent in radiographs. After approximately 3 weeks, periapical radiolucencies that are due to pulpal necrosis can usually be detected. In addition, inflammatory root resorption may be evident at this time. After approximately 6 to 7 weeks, replacement resorption, or ankylosis, can be seen. Thus, there is adequate rationale to obtain postoperative radiographs at 1 month and 2 months following the injury. In the absence of any clinical signs or symptoms, such as development of a fistula, mobility, discoloration, or pain, additional films are not indicated until 6 months after the injury. If changes are to appear radiographically, they usually do so by this time.

## EMERGENCY CARE

### Injuries to the Hard Dental Tissues

*Cracks and Fractures of the Enamel and Dentin without Pulp Exposure*

Enamel cracks and small fractures are common findings in primary teeth (see Fig. 15-2). It is believed that even fractures exposing dentin in primary teeth have no deleterious effect on the pulp and need not be covered. In the case of larger fractures, treatment is often indicated to restore aesthetics. Various methods have been suggested to restore the fractured crown, including use of strip crowns, preformed esthetic crowns, and open-faced steel crowns (see Chapter 21).

If it is decided to avoid crown restoration, possibly due to the child's age and/or behavior, sharp edges at the fracture line can be smoothened with abrasive disks to prevent irritation to the tongue and lips. The exposed dentin should be carefully examined to ensure that there is no exposure of the pulp. If tooth fracture is associated with a wounded lip, then a radiograph of the lip should be obtained to rule out the presence of tooth fragments trapped in the soft tissue (see Fig. 15-9). Late complications, such as coronal discoloration (see below), usually are attributed not to the fractured crown but to overlooked minor displacement of the tooth and obstruction of blood supply to the pulp.

*Fractures of the Enamel and Dentin with Pulp Exposure*

Deep fracture of the crown may be associated with exposure of the pulp, usually at the pulp horn. If the pulp horn is exposed at its incisal edge

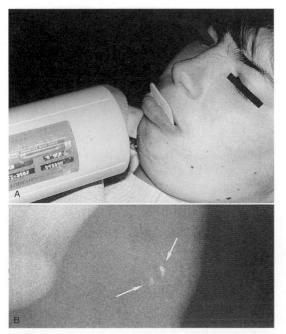

**Figure 15-9**  **A,** Positioning film to detect presence of tooth fragments in the lip. **B,** Radiograph demonstrating tooth fragments in lip (arrows).

it may not bleed and therefore may go unnoticed. A red point of blood can be seen if the pulp is exposed at a deeper level.

Several treatment options are available for crown fracture with pulp exposure in primary teeth, including pulpotomy, root canal treatment, and extraction. The vitality of the tissue and the time elapsed since the injury dictate the treatment of choice. If the pulp tissue is vital, a cervical pulpotomy can be performed (see Chapter 22). Ram and Holan suggested that a partial pulpotomy technique is indicated to preserve pulp vitality in a young primary tooth with a wide-open apex and thin root dentin walls.[30]

Pulp exposure is sometimes overlooked or neglected and no treatment rendered. The unavoidable outcome is a necrotic and infected pulp with consequent swelling or fistula. If massive external inflammatory root resorption is detected or if the follicle of the underlying permanent tooth bud is involved in the inflammatory process, the tooth must be extracted as soon as possible. Leaving such teeth untreated increases the risk of damage to the permanent incisor. If there is no evidence of inflammatory external root resorption, some clinicians attempt to save these teeth with complete pulpectomies. The principle of this treatment is complete removal of the necrotic pulp, filling the pulp canal with a resorbable paste, and providing aesthetic restoration of the crown. (For further details, see Chapter 22.)

Permanent incisors succeeding infected and root-treated primary incisors show mild enamel defects that could be attributed to both the inflammatory process and overinstrumentation during the endodontic procedure.[19]

### Crown-Root Fractures

Fractures involving both the crown and the root of primary teeth are rare. The teeth in this type of injury are split into two or more fragments, with one main fragment remaining firm and the other fragment becoming loose due to injury to its periodontal fibers (Fig. 15-10). The two fragments should be separated to determine if the pulp has been exposed. The loose fragment should be removed allowing inspection of the main fragment's exposed dentin. Pulpotomy is the suggested treatment for such exposures with subsequent aesthetic reconstruction of the crown. If the fracture goes deep into the alveolus, creating a periodontal pocket in the space previously occupied by the loose fragment, both fragments should be extracted.

### Root Fractures

Root fractures are also rare in primary teeth. Both fragments may remain close to each other, with the tooth presenting slight mobility and sensitivity to percussion (see Fig. 15-3). If the coronal fragment is pushed away from the apical part of the root, it frequently assumes a lingual inclination that may interfere with the occlusion unless the child has an open bite. In this case, the coronal fragment should be extracted. Attempts to remove the apical fragment should be avoided as such action may harm the developing permanent successor. These apical fragments usually resorb as part of the physiologic process of tooth replacement. If no disturbance to the child's occlusion exists, the tooth may be left untreated and the parents provided with instruction for thorough oral hygiene and soft diet for a limited time

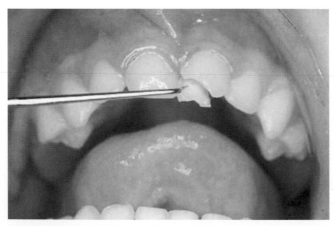

**Figure 15-10** Clinical view of a left maxillary primary central incisor with crown-root fracture. The palatal fragment is mobile and attached by gingival fibers only.

(see "Information and Instructions for Parents" below). The PDL attached to the mobile coronal fragment may recover with decrease in tooth mobility and sensitivity to percussion. Unlike permanent teeth there is no intention to cause repair of the fracture with calcified tissue in root-fractured primary teeth; thus immobilization of the tooth is unnecessary. Splinting the tooth is recommended only to alleviate sensitivity during routine function.

## Injuries to the Chin

An injury to the chin may produce a sudden forceful closure of the mandibular teeth with their maxillary opponents. As a result, a wide range of injuries may affect molar teeth.[18] These include minor enamel fractures, fractures with dentin exposure that may imitate a carious lesion on the radiograph, crown root fractures with or without pulp exposure, and injuries to the PDL (see Fig. 34-8). In addition, fracture of the mandible may occur mainly in the symphysis, mental, and subcondylar areas[23] (Fig. 15-11). These injuries have also been correlated with cervical spine fractures.[7]

The exposed dentin in fractured posterior teeth increases the risk of pulp irritation and may become carious. It can, therefore, be covered by a composite resin if the area of exposure is small. If the fracture is large or extends below the gum line, a stainless steel crown is preferable. When the pulp is exposed and the crown restorable, pulpotomy and a stainless steel crown is the treatment of choice. Otherwise, the tooth must be extracted and space maintenance considered.

## Injuries to the Supporting Tissues

### Concussion and Subluxation

Teeth suffering concussion injuries are sensitive to percussion without any additional sign. Subluxated teeth also present increased mobility and widening of the periodontal space. If the teeth are examined shortly after the injury, signs of bleeding from the gingival crevice can be seen (Fig. 15-12). Concussion and subluxation are mild injuries that often go unnoticed. Parents, if questioned, may recall the injury when a late complication develops, such as tooth discoloration (see "Coronal Discoloration"). Usually no treatment is required except thorough oral hygiene to avoid contamination of the damaged PDL (see "Information and Instructions for Parents").

### Intrusion

Intrusion is one of the most complicated injuries to the primary incisors. Clinically, the tooth may disappear completely into the surrounding tissues or the incisal part may remain visible with its clinical crown shorter than an adjacent nontraumatized tooth. Following intrusion the PDL is compressed, and the root surface is tightly pressed against the alveolar bone, resulting in reduced mobility. Percussion on an intruded tooth produces a metallic sound and does not provoke pain. Bleeding from the gingival sulcus is visible shortly after the injury. A swollen upper lip due to edema and/or hemorrhage can often be seen.

The root of the primary incisor is normally in close proximity with the labial surface of the permanent tooth. If the root of the primary tooth

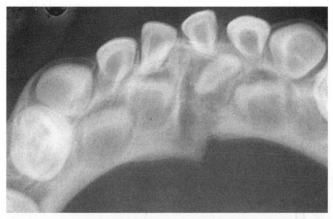

**Figure 15-11**  Fracture of the mandible in a baby as a result of trauma to the chin.

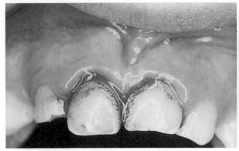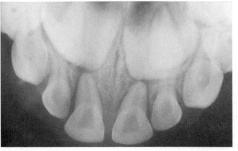

A                                                                                              B

**Figure 15-12    A,** Clinical view of subluxation of the left maxillary primary central incisor and slight extrusion of the adjacent central incisor. **B,** Radiograph of both teeth showing widening of the periodontal ligament.

is pushed against the crown of the permanent incisor, it may severely damage the developing tooth bud. Immediate removal of the primary tooth may relieve the pressure and minimize the damage.[4] It is, therefore, extremely important to determine as soon as possible after the injury if the root of the primary tooth is in contact with the permanent tooth or has been pushed in a labial direction and away from the labial surface of the permanent successor. Fortunately, the root apex of maxillary primary incisors has a labial curvature leading the root away from the permanent tooth in more than 80% of cases.[20]

Several clinical and radiographic signs support the diagnosis of labial alignment of the root:

- Palatal inclination of the crown
- Hemorrhage and hard swelling palpated in the vestibule due to fracture of the labial bone plate by the root of the primary tooth
- A shortened and more opaque image of an intruded incisor as compared to an adjacent nondisplaced tooth (see Fig. 15-4)
- Proper alignment of the permanent successor as seen on a periapical radiograph

Absence of such signs should alert the operator to suspect palatal displacement of the primary tooth root with subsequent displacement of the permanent tooth.

Some authors suggest the use of lateral extra-oral radiographs, although a recent study showed that this technique's contributions to the assessment of the relation between the root of the intruded tooth and the labial surface of the permanent tooth are most beneficial in children younger than 20 months.[22]

Intruded incisors that do not risk the permanent teeth can be left to spontaneously reerupt. Reeruption begins within 2 to 3 weeks but can be delayed for more than 6 months. In many cases the teeth do not erupt back to their original position but into a rotated alignment (see Fig. 15-21). The distance between the incisal edge of a partially intruded tooth and an imaginary line connecting the incisal edge of two adjacent unaffected teeth should be measured. Repeated measurements at recall visits allow estimation of the rate of reeruption. It should be emphasized that increase of the clinical crown (the distance between the incisal edge and the gingival margins) is not an indication of reeruption. Decrease in size of edematous gums may erroneously be viewed as reeruption.

### Extrusion
An extruded tooth is clinically elongated in comparison with adjacent unaffected teeth. The tooth presents increased mobility and sensitivity to percussion. Bleeding from the gingival sulcus can be seen shortly after the injury. A periapical radiograph of an extruded tooth will show widening of the PDL especially around the apex (see Fig. 15-5). The more the tooth moves out of the alveolar socket, the higher are the chances of disruption of the blood supply and development of pulp necrosis. Extrusions resemble lingual luxation in many features; thus the approach to both types of injuries should be similar (see below).

### Lingual Luxation
In the case of lingual luxations, the crown moves in a palatal direction while the apex is pushed labially. It is sometimes difficult to distinguish between lingual luxation and intrusion. The palatal inclination of the crown may interfere with the occlusion unless the child has an open bite. The tooth presents increased mobility and sensitivity to percussion. Signs of bleeding may be evident around the tooth (see Fig. 15-6, *A*). The

upper lip is often swollen with signs of hemorrhage due to fracture of the labial bone plate by the tooth apex. A periapical radiograph will show a radiolucent gap between the apex and the alveolar bone (see Fig. 15-6, *B*). The luxated tooth presents a shortened and more opaque image as compared to an adjacent unaffected tooth.

Many clinicians recommend extraction of severely luxated primary teeth owing to the potential damage to the succeeding permanent incisor.

Some parents insist that everything be done to save anterior primary teeth, and if the child is seen shortly after the injury and before the formation of a coagulum, the tooth can be repositioned. The tooth must then be splinted for 7 to 14 days, and root canal treatment is indicated as rupture of the blood supply to the pulp is expected in cases of severe luxation.[19] The cost/benefit of retaining these teeth and the potential for injury to the succeeding permanent teeth must be explained to the parents.

In the case of open bite without occlusal interference, the functional forces of the tongue may push the crown into a labial position. Extraction of the luxated tooth is indicated after the formation of a blood clot in the alveolus several hours after the injury and in the case of severe fracture of the labial bone plate.

Parents should be provided with strict instructions for good oral hygiene to avoid migration of microorganisms between the root and the gums with subsequent infection of the PDL (see "Information and Instructions for Parents").

### Avulsion

Avulsion of a primary incisor is a common outcome of dental trauma in young children (see Fig. 15-7). The high crown/root ratio of primary incisors and the resilience of the bone are contributing factors. In about 75% of cases involving avulsion of a primary incisor, the developing permanent successor is damaged.[32] Most articles, textbooks, and guidelines recommend that avulsed primary incisors should not be replanted owing to damage that may be inflicted to the permanent tooth during insertion of the root back to its socket.[5] Case reports suggest shortening of the root by 2 to 3 mm before replantation to avoid such damage.[10] If a child arrives at the dental office with a tooth that has been avulsed and replanted by his parents, the parents should be apprised of the risks and costs versus benefits of

keeping that tooth. A splint and root canal treatment with a resorbable paste will be required to attempt to save the tooth until its natural exfoliation and to prevent inflammatory resorption of the root.

Avulsed primary teeth should be accounted for to rule out potential aspiration. If the tooth cannot be found, the child should be referred for further evaluation by a pediatrician.[21]

## Information and Instructions for Parents

### Emergency Telephone Call

Diagnosis of traumatic injuries to primary teeth should never be based solely on information provided by parents over the telephone. Occasionally, however, parents call stating that their child injured a primary tooth and asking how urgent it is to bring the child to the dental office. The dentist's main concerns are risk of damage to the permanent teeth in case of intrusion and risk of aspiration in case of avulsion. So if the injury sounds like a serious luxation, the child should be seen as soon as possible. The management of other conditions can be postponed until the next day without risking the prognosis.

### Information and Instructions Provided at the Emergency Visit

Parents should be informed about possible complications of the injury, prognosis of the injury, and the likelihood of damage to the permanent successors. Instructions for parents are aimed at preventing late complications (e.g., infection of the PDL and pulp necrosis) following injuries to the primary teeth and detecting such complications as soon as possible. Early detection allows appropriate treatment that may prevent further damage to the injured primary tooth or to its permanent successor.

In cases of luxation injuries, parents should be given strict instructions for their child's oral hygiene. Thorough cleaning and plaque removal all around the injured teeth are imperative. Application of an antiseptic medicament, such as 0.2% chlorhexidine gluconate or 3% hydrogen peroxide, to the injured gingivae can improve the chance for healing. As preschool children may swallow the solution while rinsing it is advised to use cotton-tipped applicators soaked with the solution and gently applied to the gingival crevice of the injured teeth. This should be repeated several times a day, especially after meals, for 7 days at which time the gingival fibers are expected to heal.

The child should be placed on a soft diet for several days to avoid intense forces on the tooth and to allow its stabilization. Antibiotics are necessary only in cases of severe tooth luxation and heavy damage to the oral soft tissues.

The timing of follow-up examinations is based on the type of injury sustained. Pathologic sequelae such as pulpal necrosis and inflammatory root resorption can frequently be detected radiographically in 1 month. Parents should be instructed to bring the child in earlier if they suspect any deterioration in the condition of the injured teeth, such as redness, swelling, or the appearance of a fistula in the gums above the injured tooth and, in case of discoloration, increased mobility or sensitivity of the tooth.

## PATHOLOGIC SEQUELAE OF TRAUMA TO THE TEETH

Complications following traumatic injuries to primary teeth may appear shortly after the injury (e.g., infection of the PDL or dark discoloration of the crown) or after several months (e.g., yellow discoloration of the crown and external root resorption). It is currently not possible to accurately identify the histopathologic condition of a dental pulp based on clinical symptoms. The following terms describe a spectrum of clinical signs and symptoms that accompany inflammation and degeneration of the pulp and/or PDL.

### Reversible Pulpitis

The pulp's initial response to trauma is pulpitis. Capillaries in the tooth become congested, a condition that can be clinically apparent upon transillumination of the crown with a bright light. Teeth with reversible pulpitis may be tender to percussion if the PDL is inflamed (e.g., following a luxation injury). Pulpitis may be totally reversible if the condition causing it is addressed, or it may progress to an irreversible state with necrosis of the pulp.

### Infection of the Periodontal Ligament

Infection of the PDL becomes possible when detachment of the gingival fibers from the tooth in a luxation injury allows invasion of micro-

organisms from the oral cavity along the root to infect the PDL. Loss of alveolar bone support can be seen on a periapical radiograph (Fig. 15-13). This diminishes the healing potential of the supporting tissues. Subsequently, increased tooth mobility accompanied by exudation of pus from the gingival crevice will require extraction of the injured tooth. Parents should be informed about the risk of infection and provided with appropriate instructions to minimize such risk.

### Irreversible Pulpitis

Irreversible pulpitis may be acute or chronic, and it may be partial or total. Acute, irreversible pulpitis following a dental injury can be painful if the exudate accompanying the pulpal inflammation cannot vent. Most frequently in children, however, inflammatory exudates are quickly vented and the pulpitis progresses to a chronic, painless condition.

### Pulp Necrosis and Infection

Two main mechanisms can explain how the pulp of injured primary teeth becomes necrotic: (1) infection of the pulp in cases of untreated crown fracture with pulp exposure and (2) interrupted blood supply to the pulp through the apex in cases of luxation injury leading to ischemia. Not all luxation injuries result in a necrotic pulp.

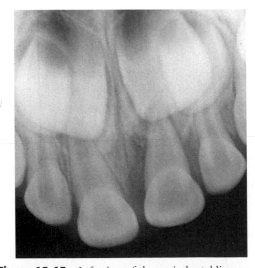

**Figure 15-13** Infection of the periodontal ligament. This radiograph shows the left maxillary primary central incisor following injury to the supporting tissues. Infection of the attachment apparatus resulted in loss of alveolar bone at the medial aspect of the root.

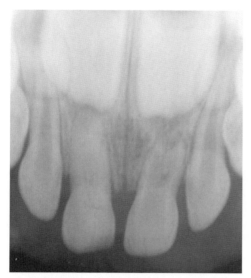

**Figure 15-14** Periapical radiograph of the premaxilla of a 42-month-old child. Both maxillary primary central incisors were injured at 18 months. The left incisor presents arrest of dentin apposition due to pulp necrosis. The pulp of the fractured right incisor reacted by pulp canal obliteration. Notice the two radiopaque stripes in the root canal.

Surprisingly, intruded primary teeth, unlike permanent teeth, maintain the vitality of their pulp.[20] While untreated teeth with exposed pulps are expected to develop swelling or fistula, injured teeth with avascular necrosis may remain asymptomatic both clinically and radiographically.[16] Loss of pulp vitality due to a traumatic injury at an early stage of root development results in the arrest of dentin apposition and cessation of root development (Fig. 15-14).

Periapical radiolucencies indicative of a granuloma or cyst are frequently evident radiographically in necrotic anterior teeth (Fig. 15-15, *A*). In addition, a parulis is often clinically evident at the level of the involved tooth's root apex (Fig. 15-15, *B*). Controversy exists regarding the most appropriate treatment of primary anterior teeth with necrotic pulps. Some clinicians treat them with a pulpectomy technique similar to that used in permanent teeth. A resorbable paste is packed into the thoroughly cleansed canal (see Chapter 22). Other clinicians choose to extract these teeth because of the potential for damage to the developing permanent tooth buds. It is generally agreed that pulpectomy is contraindicated in primary teeth with gross loss of root structure, advanced internal or external resorption, or periapical infection involving the crypt of the succedaneous tooth.

## Coronal Discoloration

As a result of trauma, the capillaries in the pulp occasionally hemorrhage, leaving blood pigments deposited in the dentinal tubules. In mild cases, the blood is resorbed and very little discoloration occurs, or that which is present becomes lighter in several weeks. In more severe cases, the discoloration persists for the life of the tooth (Fig. 15-16).

From a diagnostic standpoint, discoloration of primary teeth does not necessarily mean that the tooth is nonvital, particularly when the discoloration occurs 1 or 2 days after the injury. Dark discoloration that persists for weeks or months

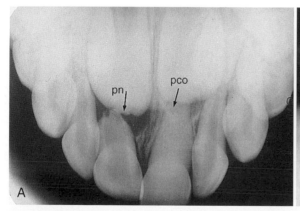
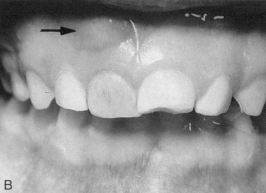

**Figure 15-15** **A,** Pulp canal obliteration *(pco)* in the patient's left primary central incisor and pulp necrosis (pn) in the right primary central incisor. **B,** In the same patient, a parulis is present at the apical level of the necrotic right central incisor *(arrow)*.

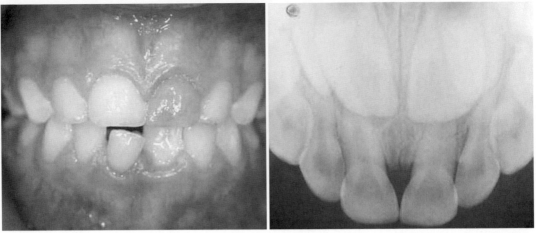

**Figure 15-16    A,** Left maxillary primary central incisor 1 year after color change due to trauma. This clinical view shows no pathologic signs except dark discoloration. **B,** Periapical radiograph showing no pathology associated with the injury.

after the injury is more indicative of a necrotic pulp.[16] Nevertheless, in the primary dentition of a healthy child, color change alone does not indicate pulp therapy or extraction of the tooth. Additional signs and symptoms of infection, such as mobility, radiographic radiolucency, swelling, fistula, or pain, must be evident before further treatment is indicated.

Crown discoloration is the external expression of changes in the pulp-dentin complex that become visible through the almost transparent enamel. Crown discoloration of primary incisors is a common posttraumatic finding and is often the only evidence of trauma to the tooth. Discoloration of a primary tooth can be noticed earlier and seen better if viewed from the palatal aspect by transillumination than by direct observation of its labial aspect. The variety of colors is traditionally divided into three main groups: pink-red, yellow, and dark (gray-brown-black).

*Pink discoloration* that is observed shortly after the injury may represent intrapulpal hemorrhage. Rupture of blood vessels in the pulp as a result of the injury allows extravasation of red blood cells into the surrounding pulpal tissue, resulting in a reddish hue of the crown that becomes visible shortly after the injury.

A reddish hue noticed long after the injury is usually due to internal resorption in the pulp chamber. In both cases follow-up is the only treatment option. While the hemorrhage eventually dissolves and disappears, the resorption process continues and results in early loss of the crown. The apical part of the root can be left untouched awaiting its spontaneous resorption. It can be removed, if necessary, but care must be taken not to damage the permanent successor.

*Yellow discoloration* of primary incisors can be seen when the dentin is thick and the pulp chamber narrower than usual. This condition is termed pulp canal obliteration (PCO). It has been shown that PCO can be seen on radiographs without the corresponding yellow discoloration of the crown.[8] Although PCO is a pathologic process, it has no known deleterious effects and therefore does not necessitate any treatment except follow-up. (See further discussion below.)

*Dark discoloration* of primary teeth is the most controversial posttraumatic complication in terms of the significance of the change in tooth color. The term "dark" refers to a variety of shades, including black, gray, brown, and intermediate hues.

When the pulp becomes necrotic or when pulpal hemorrhage occurs, red blood cells undergo lysis and release hemoglobin. Hemoglobin and hemoglobin derivatives, such as hematin molecules that contain iron ions, invade the dentin tubules and stain the tooth dark.[29,27] If the pulp remains vital and eliminates the pigments, the dark discoloration may fade with subsequent restoration of the original color.[14] If the pulp loses its vitality and cannot eliminate the iron-containing molecules, the tooth may remain discolored.

If dark-discolored primary incisors present additional signs such as swelling, fistula, or a periapical radiolucent defect, the diagnosis of pulp necrosis is easy. The controversy exists when the dark coronal discoloration is the only evidence of trauma to the tooth (see Fig. 15-16, *A*). Sonis found that 72% of these teeth exfoliated normally without any evidence of radiographic or clinical pathology.[34] Furthermore, asymptomatic primary incisors with persistent dark discoloration of the crown following trauma contain a necrotic or partially necrotic pulp.[16] It is not yet clear why some teeth gain different hues of dark discoloration. An attempt to investigate the variations in the dark colors failed to show a correlation between the various shades and the condition of the pulp.[35] Importantly, in the primary dentition of a healthy child, color change alone does not indicate a need for pulp therapy or extraction of the tooth.

## Inflammatory Resorption

Inflammatory resorption can occur either on the external root surface or internally in the pulp chamber or canal (see Fig. 34-10). It occurs subsequent to luxation injuries and is related to a necrotic pulp and an inflamed PDL.[37] It can progress very rapidly, destroying a tooth within months. Clinicians who choose to treat a patient with this condition when it occurs in the primary dentition use resorbable zinc oxide paste as an endodontic filling material.

### Internal Resorption

The predentin, an unmineralized layer of organic material, covers the inner aspect of the dentin and protects it against access of osteoclasts. When the pulp becomes inflamed, as in cases of traumatic injury, the odontoblastic layer may lose its integrity exposing the dentin to odontoclastic activity, which is then seen on radiographs as radiolucent expansion of the pulp space. Eventually this process reaches the outer surface of the root causing root perforation. If the coronal dentin is completely resorbed the red color of the resorbing tissue becomes visible through the enamel.

### External Resorption

The cementoblast layer and the precementum serve as a shield protecting the root from involvement in the perpetual remodeling process of the surrounding bone. In nontraumatized primary teeth, external root resorption is part of the physiologic process of replacing the primary dentition with permanent teeth. In primary incisors sustaining traumatic injuries, external root resorption may appear as an accelerated unfavorable pathologic reaction. A variety of patterns of pathologic external root resorption can be seen in primary incisors following traumatic injury.

*External inflammatory root resorption,* as in permanent teeth, is a rapid process characterized clinically by increased mobility of the tooth, sensitivity to percussion, a dull sound produced by percussion, and often a fistula or swelling in the gums above the tooth. Radiographically the PDL space is widened and the root surface is irregular (Fig. 15-17). This condition may develop within a few weeks of the injury. Removal of the necrotic, and probably infected, pulp may stop the resorption process; however, due to the unfavorable preexisting conditions the benefit of root canal filling aimed to save the tooth is questionable. Traumatized primary incisors with external inflammatory root resorption should, therefore, be extracted. It has been shown that root canal

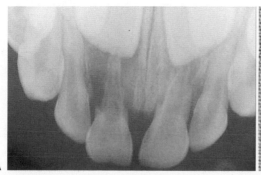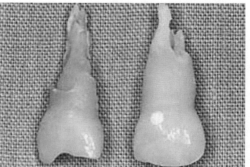

**Figure 15-17**  **A,** Periapical radiograph of the maxillary primary central incisors showing external inflammatory root resorption as a result of traumatic injury several months earlier. **B,** The affected teeth after extraction. Notice the irregularity of the resorbed root surface.

A     B     C

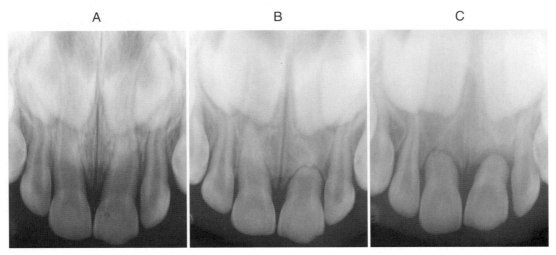

**Figure 15-18** Periapical radiograph of maxillary primary central incisors with external surface root resorption. **A,** Shortly after the injury. **B,** Twelve months after the injury. **C,** Twenty-seven months after the injury.

treatment in traumatized and infected primary incisors is highly correlated with enamel defects in the permanent teeth.[15]

*External surface root resorption* is characterized by gradual elimination of the root dentin with preservation of the PDL. The resorption process affects the apex of the root only, which becomes rounded, and progresses until natural exfoliation or traumatic avulsion occurs (Fig. 15-18). As the resorption progresses, bone replaces the space previously occupied by the root and separates the primary tooth and its permanent successor. Sometimes an intermediate stage exists in which osteoclasts attack the root along its apical half, leaving the coronal half unaffected.[28] The apical half is finally completely resorbed leaving a short-ened root with a rounded apex. The clinical appear-ance imitates that of natural but early exfoliation.

Root resorption associated with expansion of the permanent tooth follicle can be seen mainly, but not exclusively, in traumatized incisors with dark coronal discoloration (Fig. 15-19, *A*). The follicle of the permanent tooth expands gradually and often does not become visible until close to the normal shedding age, even if the teeth were injured at an early age. Expansion of the follicle of the permanent tooth is rarely expressed clinically, and dark coronal discoloration is the only reason to suspect it. Occasionally, the hard expansion of the labial bone above the injured primary incisors can be observed or better palpated (Fig. 15-19, *B*). Usually, the primary tooth sheds normally fol-lowed by normal eruption of the permanent teeth.

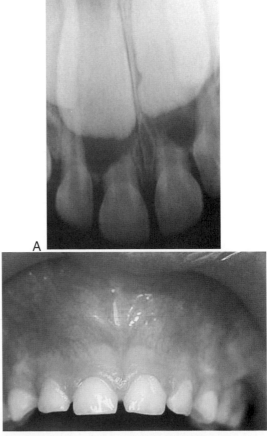

**Figure 15-19** **A,** External root resorption associated with expansion of the follicle of the developing permanent tooth. **B,** Clinical view that shows no pathologic signs except a hard expansion of the bone in the vestibule above the tooth.

Occasionally, a dilated follicle becomes infected or the permanent tooth is deflected from its normal alignment (Fig. 15-20). Immediate extraction of the primary incisors is mandatory in these cases.

## Replacement Resorption

Replacement resorption, also known as ankylosis, results after irreversible injury to the PDL. Alveolar bone directly contacts and becomes fused with the root surface.[37] As the alveolar bone undergoes normal physiologic osteoclastic and osteoblastic activity, the root is resorbed (replaced with bone; see Fig. 34-11). Ankylosed primary teeth should be extracted if they cause a delay in or ectopic eruption of a developing permanent tooth.

## Pulp Canal Obliteration

Pulp canal obliteration is the result of intensified activity of the odontoblasts that results in accelerated dentin apposition. Gradually, the pulp space narrows to a state in which it cannot be seen on a radiograph (see Figs. 15-5, B, 15-14, and 15-15, A). PCO is a common finding in primary incisors following traumatic injuries. As yet, however, the exact mode by which the impact to the tooth affects the odontoblasts is still obscure. Though scientifically defined as a pathologic process, clinically it is not regarded as having deleterious effects. Ninety percent of primary teeth that have undergone PCO resorb normally,[24] and therefore treatment in the primary dentition is usually not indicated.

## Complications Following Intrusion

Approximately two thirds of intruded primary incisors reerupt and survive without any complications more than 3 years after the injury.[20] In most cases, however, the teeth do not return to their original position but reerupt into a rotated alignment (Fig. 15-21). If the child still uses a pacifier it may occupy the space of the crown of the intruded tooth and prevent its reeruption back to the occlusal level. Intruded primary teeth may fail to reerupt if the root has been pushed out of the alveolar bone into the surrounding soft tissues (Fig. 15-22). These teeth should be extracted. Another reason for failure of intruded incisors to reerupt is damage to the PDL during the injury that results in ankylosis. It is not yet clear whether intervention is needed to remove the ankylosed tooth or if the root can be resorbed spontaneously with subsequent exfoliation of the tooth.

Periodontal breakdown due to infection is the main reason for loss of primary incisors following intrusion.[20] This can be avoided by maintaining optimal oral hygiene (see "Information and Instructions for Parents"). Surprisingly, pulp necrosis following intrusion of primary incisors is not a common finding[20] and, unlike the recommendations for intruded permanent teeth, removal of the pulp is not recommended. Even if the apex of an intruded primary incisor avoids contact

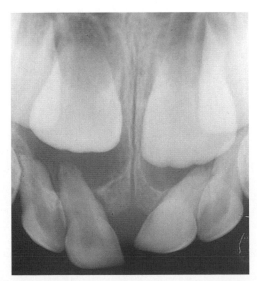

**Figure 15-20** Radiograph showing an infected expansion of the follicle of the permanent incisors with deflection of the right maxillary permanent central incisor from its normal alignment.

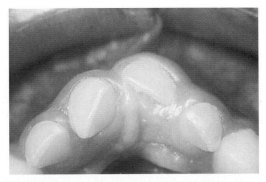

**Figure 15-21** Clinical view of the maxillary primary incisors. Both central incisors were completely intruded and reerupted several weeks after the injury but into a rotated alignment. The teeth are clinically asymptomatic.

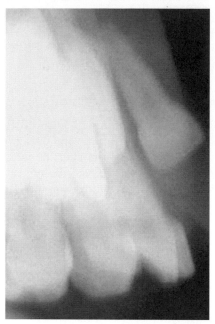

**Figure 15-22**  Lateral extraoral radiograph showing an intruded maxillary primary central incisor that has been pushed out of the labial alveolar bone plate.

with its permanent successor the permanent tooth may have still been damaged. It could have been affected during the movement of the primary tooth from its original position to its final alignment. This explains the discrepancy found between the low percentage (10% to 20%) of primary incisors pushed toward the developing permanent teeth[20] and the high percentage (69%) of affected permanent teeth following intrusion of their primary predecessors.[3]

## Complications Following Avulsion

Several outcomes of early loss of primary incisors have been described in the dental literature. Loss of space can be expected if the injury occurred prior to eruption of the primary canines[26] and in children with a crowded dentition.[13] If primary incisors are lost before the child masters articulation, speech development may be affected.[33] However, pronunciation becomes normal after eruption of the permanent teeth.[11] The impact to the primary incisor pushes the tooth into the surrounding tissues before the tooth is completely detached from the PDL. This results in damage to the permanent successors in 38% to 85% of cases.[38,31] The younger the child when injured, the higher is the prevalence of damage to the perma-

nent teeth.[32] Delayed and ectopic eruption of permanent incisors in cases of avulsion of their primary predecessors have been described and were attributed to lack of guidance, development of a scar tissue, and deflection of the developing permanent tooth bud by the injured primary incisor.[6]

## INJURIES TO DEVELOPING PERMANENT TEETH

The most damaging sequelae of injuries to primary teeth are their effects on the unerupted developing permanent teeth. Anatomically, the permanent anterior teeth develop in close proximity to the apices of primary incisors (see Fig. 15-22). Thus, a periapical pathologic process that is due to necrotic pulps, intrusion injuries, or overinstrumentation of primary root canals can irreversibly damage the permanent teeth. If the injury occurs during the development of the permanent tooth crown, enamel hypoplasia or hypocalcification may occur (Fig. 15-23). These injuries can also alter the path of the developing permanent tooth crown, causing root dilaceration or ectopic eruption. For these reasons, the clinician should plan management of injuries to primary teeth with the ultimate objective of preventing or minimizing damage to the succeeding permanent teeth. Enamel calcification of permanent central incisor crowns is usually completed by age 4 years, so the risk of injury to them is greater in children younger than that.

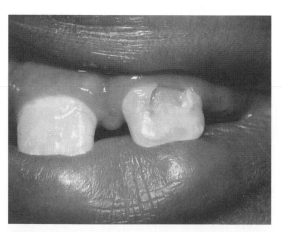

**Figure 15-23**  Hypoplasia of the patient's maxillary left permanent central incisor as a result of intrusion of a primary incisor.

# REFERENCES

1. American Academy of Pediatrics: Tetanus. In: Pickering L, editor. *2003 Red Book: Report of the Committee on Infectious Diseases,* 26th ed. Elk Grove Village, Ill, The Academy, 2003, pp 614-616.

2. American Academy of Pediatrics, American Academy of Pediatric Dentistry: Oral and dental aspects of child abuse and neglect. *Pediatrics* 104:348, 1999.

3. Andreasen JO, Ravn JJ: The effect of traumatic injuries to primary teeth on their permanent successors. II. A clinical and radiographic follow-up study of 213 teeth. *Scand J Dent Res* 79:284, 1971.

4. Andreasen JO: The influence of traumatic intrusion of primary teeth on their permanent successors. A radiographic and histologic study in monkeys. *Int J Oral Surg* 5:207, 1976.

5. Andreasen JO, Andreasen FM: Injuries to the primary dentition. In: Andreasen JO, Andreasen FM, editors: *Essentials of Traumatic Injuries to the Teeth.* Copenhagen, Munksgaard, 1990.

6. Andreasen JO, Andreasen FM: *Textbook and Color Atlas of Traumatic Injuries to the Teeth,* 3rd ed. Copenhagen, Munksgaard, 1994.

7. Bertolami CN, Kaban LB: Chin trauma: a clue to associated mandibular and cervical spine injury. *Oral Surg* 53:122, 1982

8. Borum MK, Andreasen JO: Sequelae of trauma to primary maxillary incisors.1. Complications in the primary dentition. *Endod Dent Traumatol* 14:31, 1998.

9. Davis MJ, Vogel BA: Neurological assessment of the child with head trauma. *J Dent Child* 62:93, 1995.

10. Filippi A, Pohl Y, Kirschner H: Replantation of avulsed primary anterior teeth: treatment and limitations. *ASDC J Dent Child* 64:272, 1997

11. Gable TO, Kummer AW, Lee L et al: Premature loss of the maxillary primary incisors: effect on speech production. *J Dent Child* 62:173, 1995.

12. Governors Highway Safety Association: Available at http://www.naghsr.org/html/state_info/childsafety_laws.html April 12, 2004.

13. Hargreaves JA, Craig JW: Total displacement of a tooth. In: Hargreaves JA, Craig JW, editors: *The Management of Traumatised Anterior Teeth in Children.* Edinburgh, E&S Livingstone, 1970.

14. Heithersay GS, Hirsch RS: Tooth discoloration and resolution following a luxation injury: significance of blood pigment in dentin to laser Doppler flowmetry readings. *Quintessent Int* 24:669, 1997.

15. Holan G, Topf J, Fuks AB: Effect of root canal infection and treatment of traumatized primary incisors on their permanent successors. *Endod Dent Traumatol* 8:12, 1992.

16. Holan G, Fuks AB: The diagnostic value of coronal dark-gray discoloration in primary teeth following traumatic injuries. *Pediatr Dent* 18:224, 1996.

17. Holan G: Periodontal breakdown and pathologic root resorption of primary molars following traumatic injuries to the chin: a case report. *Pediatr Dent* 19:425, 1997.

18. Holan G: Traumatic injuries to the chin: a survey in a paediatric private practice. *Int J Paediatr Dent* 8:143, 1998.

19. Holan G: Conservative treatment of severely luxated maxillary primary central incisors: a case report. *Pediatr Dent* 21:459, 1999.

20. Holan G, Ram D: Sequela and prognosis of intruded primary incisors. a retrospective study. *Pediatr Dent* 21:242, 1999.

21. Holan G, Ram D: Aspiration of an avulsed primary incisor. A case report. *Int J Paediatr Dent* 10:150, 2000.

22. Holan G, Ram D, Fuks AB: The diagnostic value of lateral extraoral radiograph in cases of intrusion of maxillary primary incisors. *Pediatr Dent* 24:38, 2002.

23. Hurt TL, Fisher B, Peterson BM, Lynch F: Mandibular fractures in association with chin trauma in pediatric patients. *Pediatr Emerg Care* 4:121, 1988.

24. Jacobsen I, Sagnes G: Traumatized primary anterior teeth: prognosis related to calcific reactions in the pulp cavity. *Acta Odontol Scand* 36:199, 1978

25. Kaban LB: Diagnosis and treatment of fractures of the facial bones in children, 1943–1993. *J Oral Maxillofac Surg* 51:722, 1993

26. Levine N: Injury to the primary dentition. *Dent Clin North Am* 26:461, 1982.

27. Marin PD, Bartold PM, Heithersay GS: Tooth discoloration by blood: an in vitro histochemical study. *Endod Dent Traumatol* 13:132, 1997.

28. Mortelitti GM, Needleman HL: Risk factors associated with atypical root resorption of the maxillary primary central incisors. *Pediatr Dent* 13:273, 1991.

29. Pindborg JJ: *Pathology of the Dental Hard Tissues.* Copenhagen, Munksgaard, 1970.

30. Ram D, Holan G: Partial pulpotomy in a traumatized primary incisor with pulp exposure: case report. *Pediatr Dent* 16:46, 1994.

31. Ravn JJ: Sequelae of acute mechanical traumata in the primary dentition. *J Dent Child* 35:281, 1968.

32. Ravn JJ: Developmental disturbances in permanent teeth after exarticulation of their primary predecessors. *Scand J Dent Res* 83:131, 1975.

33. Riekman GA, El Badrawy HE: Effect of premature loss of primary maxillary incisors of speech. *Pediatr Dent* 7:19, 1985.

34. Sonis S: Longitudinal study of discolored primary teeth and effect on succedaneous teeth. *J Pedod* 11:247, 1987.

35. Soxman JA, Nazif MM, Bouquot J: Pulpal pathology in relation to discoloration of primary anterior teeth. *J Dent Child* 51:282, 1984.

36. Tecklenburg F, Wright M: Minor head trauma in the pediatric patient. *Pediatr Emerg Care* 7:40, 1991.

37. Tronstad L: Root resorption: etiology, terminology and clinical manifestations. *Endod Dent Traumatol* 4:241, 1988.

38. von Arx T: Developmental disturbances of permanent teeth following trauma to the primary dentition. *Aust Dent J* 38:1, 1993.

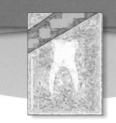

# CHAPTER 16
## Congenital Genetic Disorders and Syndromes
*Rebecca L. Slayton*

Our understanding of genetics and the genetic basis of disease has increased dramatically over the last 20 years. During this time, scientists have ascertained the sequence of the entire human genome (more than 3 billion nucleotides of DNA) and have discovered new ways that diseases and disease susceptibility are inherited.

As health care professionals, we have gained information from the Human Genome Project that provides us with many opportunities as well as challenges. This information has given us the ability to understand diseases at a molecular level. In addition, diseases that were once thought to be influenced primarily by environmental factors are now known to have genetic factors that modulate their severity. Access to the sequence of the entire human genome will facilitate the identification of additional disease genes and allow us to understand the complex interactions that occur between genes and regulatory proteins. The ability to identify single-nucleotide changes (referred to as polymorphisms) will help us understand individual risk factors for disease and how to tailor prevention and treatment strategies at an individual rather than a global level. The complete sequencing of microbial genomes will help us understand what makes some strains of bacteria more virulent than others and will aid in the development of more effective therapeutic interventions.

There are also challenges involved in the management and use of information generated by the Human Genome Project. It will be important to anticipate how this information might be used in ways that are unethical or detrimental to individuals or groups of people. Information about genetics and genetic research is reported on an almost daily basis in newspapers, magazines, and on the radio and television. This often means that a patient may hear of a new discovery before it is published in a scientific journal. Health professionals must be prepared to answer patients' questions and know how and where to refer them for additional information or counseling. Practicing dental clinicians provide the front line as diagnosticians and for referral of patients and families for genetic testing and counseling for many oral health conditions. This requires a basic understanding of the genetics of human disease, knowledge of the types of genetic testing that are available, and sensitivity to the family's concerns.

Practicing dentists are confronted daily with conditions that have either primarily or significant genetic contribution in their etiology. Common conditions such as congenitally missing teeth now are known, in many cases, to be caused by specific genetic mutations. Many syndromes involve craniofacial structures and have associated dental anomalies. Frequently, other major malformations are present in addition to the craniofacial anomalies. Advances in the Human Genome Project have led to the discovery of the genetic basis of many of these disorders that have craniofacial and dental anomalies as part of the spectrum of the disease. Understanding the disease at this level permits the practitioner to provide more precise diagnosis of the disease, more appropriate treatment, and more accurate prognosis of the outcomes of care.

Dental practitioners are aware of the environmental and behavioral risk factors that contribute to poor oral health. We routinely counsel our patients and their parents about the risks involved with cigarette smoking, smokeless tobacco, alcohol, poor oral hygiene, sweetened beverages, a diet high in carbohydrates, and traumatic injuries to the head and mouth. We know that the two most common dental diseases—dental caries and periodontal disease—are complex with both environmental and genetic components. As we continue to gain information about the genetic makeup of individuals, there will be additional genetic susceptibility or resistance factors identified that will influence the severity of oral diseases. Once these factors are identified, there will be tests that can be performed well before the occurrence of disease. This will permit practitioners to educate patients about the importance of their behaviors

and to tailor their preventive strategies more specifically for each patient. There will be some tests that dentists can perform in their offices, whereas others will require the use of an outside laboratory. The application of appropriate tests and ultimately the interpretation of the test results and the management of the oral disease will be the responsibility of the dentist. Therefore practicing dentists must understand the basis of the test, how it is performed, and how the results are interpreted. Understanding the basis for many of the genetic tests available today requires an understanding of basic genetic concepts as well as the current technologies that are available for testing.

## BASIC GENETIC CONCEPTS

A person's genome is made up of the DNA in all 46 chromosomes in the nucleus of each cell of the body. Each cell has 23 pairs of chromosomes. One chromosome of each pair was inherited from each parent. Two of the chromosomes are called sex chromosomes (X and Y) whereas the remaining chromosomes (numbered 1 through 22) are called autosomes. Males have one X and one Y chromosome; females have two X chromosomes. In each cell of a female, one of the X chromosomes is randomly inactivated. This is an important determinant of the severity of X-linked genetic disorders, as will be discussed later. The tool used to look at all of the chromosomes in a cell and to determine the sex of a fetus from amniotic fluid is called a karyotype (Fig. 16-1). This technique also identifies major chromosomal anomalies such as triploidy (an extra chromosome), translocations of one part of a chromosome to another, or large chromosomal deletions.

Each chromosome is made up of double-stranded DNA helix composed of a series of four nucleotides and a sugar-phosphate base. Each of the four nucleotides (adenine, thymine, cytosine, and guanine) is paired with a specific complementary nucleotide to form the double helix. Adenine always pairs with thymine, and cytosine always pairs with guanine. The ability of a single strand of DNA to bind to a complementary strand of DNA or RNA forms the basis of many of the diagnostic tests performed today.

Genes are sequences of DNA that are transcribed into messenger RNA and then translated into proteins. Each chromosome contains thou-

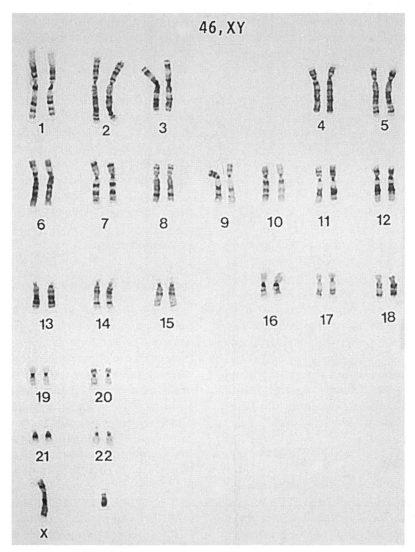

**Figure 16-1**    Karyotype of a normal male.

sands of genes. The entire human genome is estimated to have between 35,000 and 50,000 genes. The exquisite control of gene expression is essential for the proper growth, development, and functioning of an organism.

Although each cell contains the same DNA and therefore the same genes, only a small percentage of those genes are active or expressed depending on the time of development and the type of cell. Cells in the epidermis need different proteins than cells in the developing tooth or in the kidney, and each cell type has a complex regulatory process to ensure that the right genes are expressed and translated into the necessary proteins at the proper time.

## MOLECULAR BASIS OF DISEASE

Traditionally, genetic diseases have been thought of in terms of mendelian inheritance patterns. This means that a mutation present in a gene transmitted to a child from one or both parents results in the child's either having the disease or being a carrier of the disease. As we have learned more about genetics, additional mechanisms of inheritance have been identified that make it more challenging to predict both the occurrence and the severity of disease. It is not uncommon for a genetic disease to be the result of a new mutation. In this case, there would be no history of the disorder on either side of the family. Other types of nonmendelian inheritance patterns include imprinting, DNA triplet repeat expansion, mitochondrial DNA defects, and complex disorders in which multiple genes may be involved and in which sequence changes increase or decrease a person's susceptibility to disease.

# INHERITANCE PATTERNS

## Autosomal Dominant

In autosomal dominant inheritance, the transmission is vertical from parent to child. An affected parent has a 50% chance of passing along the defective gene to either sex child. It may occur in the family initially as a new mutation or may have been present in the family for multiple generations. Dentinogenesis imperfecta is an example of an autosomal dominant disorder. The gene for type I dentinogenesis imperfecta has been identified (dentin sialophosphoprotein) and is located on chromosome 4. Other autosomal dominant disorders include achondroplasia (short-limbed dwarfism), some forms of amelogenesis imperfecta, and Marfan syndrome.

## Autosomal Recessive

An autosomal recessive disorder is only manifest when an individual has two copies of the mutant gene. Most frequently, each parent has one copy of the defective gene and is a carrier, and there is a 25% chance that both mutant genes will be passed on to their offspring. It is equally likely that males and females will be affected. Fifty percent of the time the offspring will get one copy of the mutant gene from one parent and will be a carrier, and 25% of the time the offspring will get two normal copies of the gene. Although autosomal recessive disorders are relatively uncommon, the carrier status in certain populations can be significant. For example, 1 in 25 people of northern European descent are carriers of cystic fibrosis.[5]

## X-Linked

Mutations in genes located on the X chromosome result in X-linked genetic disorders. Since females have two X chromosomes and one is randomly inactivated in each cell, they are carriers and do not normally manifest the disorder. Males, on the other hand, only have one X chromosome, which

is inherited from their mother. A son has a 50% chance of inheriting the defective gene from his mother and manifesting the disease. A daughter also has a 50% chance of inheriting the defective gene from her mother but will then be a carrier. X-linked disorders often appear to skip a generation because an affected male will only pass the affected X chromosome to a daughter and she will serve as a carrier to the next generation. Disorders with X-linked inheritance include hemophilia, X-linked hypohydrotic ectodermal dysplasia, fragile X syndrome, and X-linked amelogenesis imperfecta. Occasionally, as a result of nonrandom X inactivation, females may have mild symptoms of an X-linked disorder.

## Chromosomal Anomalies

In the previous examples, defects in one or both copies of a gene were responsible for the occurrence of a genetic disorder. Some disorders result from defects in chromosomes that result in extra copies of one or more genes, entire deletions of one or more genes, or translocation of one part of a chromosome with another. Generally, chromosomal anomalies result in multiple physical defects as well as mental and developmental delay. Down syndrome is the result of a trisomy (three copies) of all or part of chromosome 21. The duplicated part of the chromosome leads to an extra copy of all the genes on that part of the chromosome. The dosage of gene products in each cell is highly regulated. Extra copies of genes lead to excess gene products that interfere with the necessary balance in the cell. Frequently extra or missing chromosomal material results in miscarriages and/or multiple birth defects.

## Multifactorial Inheritance

Most common diseases of adulthood (such as diabetes, hypertension, and manic depression) as well as most congenital malformations (cleft lip/palate and neural tube defects) are the result of multiple genes and gene-environment interactions, rather than a single gene defect. This is also true for the most common dental diseases (periodontal disease and dental caries). Multifactorial traits are thought to result from the interaction between multiple genes with multiple environmental factors. The most convincing evidence for this type of inheritance is twin studies. If a trait is multifactorial, with a significant genetic component, monozygotic (identical) twins will both have the disease significantly more frequently than dizygotic (fraternal) twins. This has been demonstrated for dental caries among twins raised apart in multiple studies and provides strong evidence that there is a genetic component to dental caries susceptibility.[1,3]

## Nontraditional Inheritance

Other types of inheritance patterns that do not fit the traditional mendelian patterns and that have been identified fairly recently are *imprinting* and *triplet repeat expansion*. Imprinted genes are turned off by methylation of the gene. This process controls the level of expression of a particular gene in the offspring. Depending on whether the imprinted gene is inherited from the mother or father determines if the child has a particular disease. In some cases, if the imprinted gene is inherited from the father, the child has one disease, but if the same imprinted gene is inherited from the mother, he or she has a different disease.

*DNA triplet repeat expansion* is a phenomenon where strings of repeated nucleotides increase in number. For example, within a particular gene, there may be 200 copies of the trinucleotide repeat "TAG." Smaller numbers of repeats are often referred to as a premutation but when expanded in an offspring may cause the gene to be inactivated (often due to methylation). Diseases caused by this type of defect include Huntington chorea and fragile X syndrome.

## DENTIST AS DYSMORPHOLOGIST

The word *dysmorphic* describes faulty development of the shape or form of an organism. Facial features in a child are frequently referred to as dysmorphic when they vary from what is considered normal. Features such as the spacing between the eyes, the position and shape of the ears, and the relative proportions of the maxilla and mandible either are within the range of normal or vary enough to be considered dysmorphic. Many genetic syndromes result in dysmorphic facial features that frequently help to diagnose the syndrome. For example, children with Down syndrome have inner epicanthal folds, up-slanting palpebral fissures, and maxillary hypoplasia. This causes unrelated children with Down syndrome to have a similar appearance to each other.

There are four basic mechanisms that result in structural defects during development. The first is malformation, the second is deformation due to mechanical forces, the third is disruption where there is a breakdown of tissues that were previously normal, and the fourth is dysplasia. Dysplasia is caused by a failure of normal organization of cells into tissues.[8] It is not uncommon for humans to have at least one "minor" malformation. This includes things such as hair whorls, inner epicanthal folds, aberrant positioning of oral frenula, or preauricular pits. Although the occurrence of single anomalies such as these are relatively common and often present as a familial trait, there are a number of studies that have demonstrated that a child who has three minor anomalies has a much greater chance of having a major anomaly such as a defect in brain or heart development.[14-16] This illustrates why it is important for health care professionals to be careful observers of their patients and to be familiar with the facial features that are considered to be normal or aberrant.

In general, the children seen in a dental practice fit into one of three categories. They may be normally developed in every way; they may have been diagnosed with a developmental anomaly of some type (either physical or mental); or they may have a developmental anomaly that has not been diagnosed. Pediatric dentists and general dentists are in the unique position of seeing their patients on a regular basis, even when the patient does not perceive a dental problem. This is in contrast to the typical physician who may only see patients when they are ill. This frequent interaction between dentists and their patients gives the dentist the opportunity to observe a child's growth and development and to note changes that are not within the range of normal. As health care professionals, it is incumbent on all dentists to recognize disease in their patients and to make the appropriate referral for definitive diagnosis and treatment.

Dentists are trained to observe and examine the mouth, face, and other craniofacial structures. Coincidentally, many inherited diseases in humans involve malformations of the craniofacial region. Accurate diagnosis of developmental anomalies and their related disorders relies on the ability of the clinician to recognize and differentiate between normal and dysmorphic physical characteristics. According to the text *Smith's Recognizable Patterns of Human Malformation,* 12 of the 26 categories of malformations used for diagnostic purposes involve features of the head or neck.[8] Several are limited to oral structures such as hypodontia, microdontia, micrognathia, and cleft lip/palate. In addition, having an understanding of the full spectrum of malformations associated with certain syndromes is essential for the safe and effective treatment of patients with these disorders.

Because dentists concentrate their diagnostic expertise on the face and mouth, they may be more likely to observe anomalies that are suggestive of major developmental malformations. Dentists who can recognize potential genetic disorders can also provide a valuable service to their patients by offering appropriate referral to a medical geneticist or a genetic counselor.

## Ocular Anomalies

Minor anomalies that affect the eyes and ocular region include widely spaced eyes (hypertelorism) (Fig. 16-2), inner epicanthal folds (Fig. 16-3) slanting of the palpebral fissures (upward or downward) (Figs. 16-4 and 16-5), a single eyebrow (synophrys), blue sclera and coloboma of the iris (cat-eye) (Fig. 16-6).

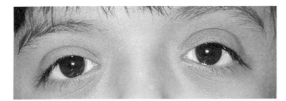

**Figure 16-2**    Hypertelorism.

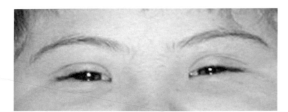

**Figure 16-3**    Inner epicanthal fold.

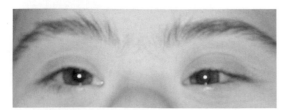

**Figure 16-4**    Up-slanting palpebral fissures.

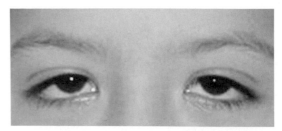

**Figure 16-5**    Down-slanting palpebral fissures.

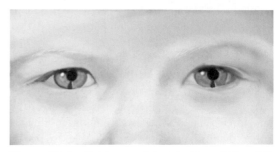

**Figure 16-6**    Coloboma of the iris. (From Kaban LB, Troulis MJ: *Pediatric Oral and Maxillofacial Surgery.* St Louis, Saunders, 2004.)

## Auricular Anomalies

There are a number of minor anomalies that affect the outer ear (auricle) and the preauricular region. These include preauricular tags or pits (Fig. 16-7), low-set and malformed ears (Fig. 16-8), protruding ears, and slanted ears.

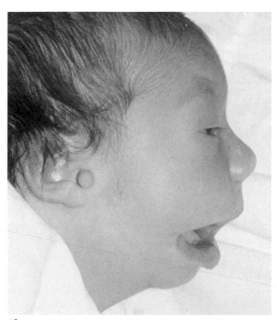

**Figure 16-7**    Ear tag. (From CameronA, Widmer R: *Handbook of Pediatric Dentistry.* London, Mosby International Limited, 1997.)

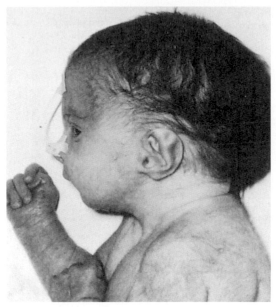

**Figure 16-8** Low set and malformed ears. (From Nussbaum RL, McInnes RR, and Willard HF: *Thompson & Thompson Genetics in Medicine*, 6E, Philadelphia, Saunders, 2001.)

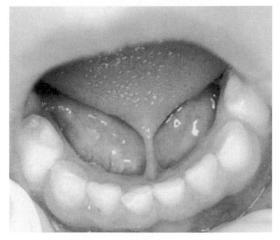

**Figure 16-10**  Ankyloglossia.

## Anomalies of the Mouth and Oral Region

Cleft lip alone or combined with a cleft palate, although not a minor anomaly, can occur independently from other malformations and is then considered nonsyndromic. Other anomalies in this region include lower lip pits (Fig. 16-9), bifid uvula, macroglossia, and prominent or full lips. Attached frenula as is seen with ankyloglossia (Fig. 16-10) is also a fairly common anomaly in the oral region.

## Dental Anomalies

Anomalies of tooth development are relatively common and may occur as an isolated finding or in association with other minor and major anomalies. Hypodontia is the developmental absence of one or more primary or permanent teeth. Although there are a number of syndromes in which hypodontia is a feature, the occurrence of one or more missing teeth (other than third molars) is estimated to be 6%. Anomalies of teeth follow patterns that reflect the time in development when the malformation occurs. For example, disruptions in tooth initiation result in hypodontia or supernumerary teeth, whereas disruptions during morphodifferentiation lead to anomalies of size and shape such as macrodontia (Fig. 16-11), microdontia (Fig. 16-12), taurodontism (Fig. 16-13) and dens invaginatus (Fig. 16-14). Disruptions that occur during histodifferentiation, apposition, and mineralization result in dentinogenesis imperfecta (Fig. 16-15), amelogenesis imperfecta (Fig. 16-16), dentin dysplasia, and enamel hypoplasia (Fig. 16-17).

Aside from managing the oral health of patients, a dentist's first responsibility is to recognize disease, whether it is in the mouth or in another part of the body. The second responsibility is to know what to do when anomalies are identified in a patient. We are fortunate to be in an era where there is a wealth of information at our fingertips. With access to a computer and the Internet, both health care practitioners and the lay public can find information about a specific disorder in minutes. There are a number of extremely valuable and reliable resources on the

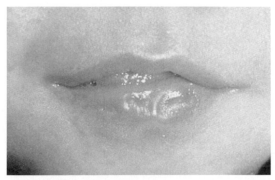

**Figure 16-9**  Lower lip pits. (From Cameron A, Widmer R: *Handbook of Pediatric Dentistry*. London, Mosby International Limited, 1997.)

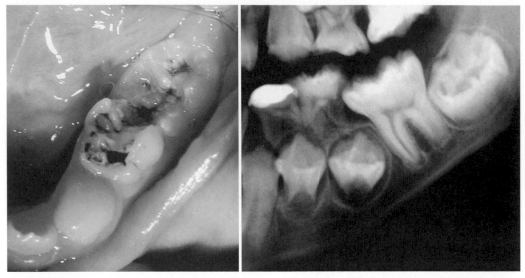

**Figure 16-11**    (**A**) Clinical and (**B**) radiographic images of primary molars with macrodontia.

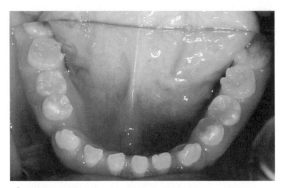

**Figure 16-12**    Permanent teeth with microdontia.

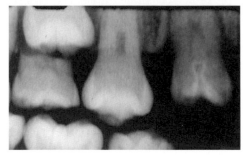

**Figure 16-14**    Radiographic image of permanent canine with dens invaginatus.

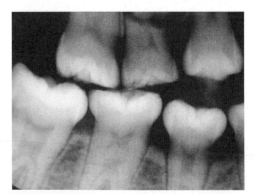

**Figure 16-13**    Permanent molars with taurodontism.

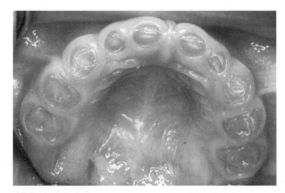

**Figure 16-15**    Dentinogenesis imperfecta in the primary dentition.

Internet including databases of published research articles, databases for inherited or rare diseases, and websites dedicated to information about specific syndromes (Box 16-1). For those without access to the Internet, there are a variety of valuable and frequently updated textbooks that provide information about syndromes that have craniofacial anomalies.[6,8]

Why is it important for dentists to pay attention to potential developmental problems with their child patients, and what should dentists do if a developmental anomaly or syndrome is

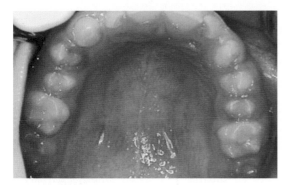

**Figure 16-16** Amelogenesis imperfecta in the permanent dentition.

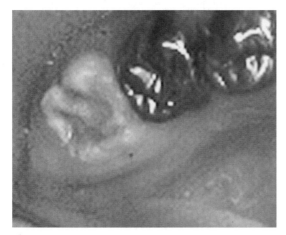

**Figure 16-17** Enamel hypoplasia of a permanent first molar.

suspected? First, the dentist is responsible for the patient's overall health, not just the health of the mouth or teeth. Patients rely on health care providers to diagnose problems and inform them of those problems so they can get appropriate and timely treatment. Second, there are many syndromes with features that influence how a dentist provides care for patients. For example, many children with Noonan syndrome have a congenital heart defect that necessitates the use of prophylactic antibiotics prior to dental treatment. Patients with Down syndrome frequently have congenital cardiac anomalies and, in addition, are at higher risk for periodontal disease as adults. Both of these characteristics require that a dentist modify the way he or she provides treatment to such patients.

When an anomaly is suspected but not diagnosed, the dentist should know how to gather the appropriate background information from the parent and, if necessary, refer the patient to a medical geneticist for further evaluation. Most teaching hospitals have a department of medical genetics that a child could be referred to for evaluation. In some areas, there are also outreach clinics where medical geneticists and genetic counselors travel to smaller towns to evaluate patients. Availability of genetic counselors in a particular area can be determined from the website of the National Society of Genetic Counselors (http://www.nsgc.org/resourcelink.asp). The database can be searched by entering a zip code and the number of miles a patient is able or willing to travel for care. As with any referral, it is important to send a letter to the physician or genetic counselor explaining why you are sending the patient for evaluation.

When discussing potential developmental anomalies with parents, it is important to be very sensitive to their concerns and to avoid causing undue alarm. Depending on the circumstances, it may be best to observe the child at multiple appointments (assuming there are treatment needs) and to get to know the family better before broaching the subject. On the other hand, when there are clear or obvious concerns and a timely diagnosis is indicated, an immediate referral should be made. One disorder that a dentist is likely to be the first to diagnose is ectodermal dysplasia. Frequently, parents become concerned when their 2- or 3-year-old child does not have any visible teeth or has conically shaped teeth. This should be recognizable to a dentist who sees children as being a developmental anomaly that should be further investigated. At this age, children frequently also have sparse hair, but the combination of hypodontia, sparse hair, and dry skin should cause a dentist to refer this child to determine if he or she has a form of ectodermal dysplasia. Similarly, if a child who is 10 or 12 years old has not lost any primary teeth, a dentist should investigate further to determine the reason the teeth have not exfoliated. In children with cleidocranial dysplasia, multiple supernumerary teeth are present that block the eruption of the permanent teeth but there is also a genetic defect that keeps teeth from erupting even after the supernumerary teeth are removed.

Because the genetic defects that cause many dominantly inherited syndromes can occur as new mutations, frequently the child is the first person in the family to experience the disorder. It is always important to ask about family history of disease, but absence of disease in the family does not preclude the occurrence of disease in the offspring.

When the child has already been diagnosed with a particular disorder, frequently the disorder is rare enough that a dentist may not have heard of it. In this case, it is important to gather as much information about the characteristics of the disorder prior to treating the child. Again, one of the most useful resources for this is the Internet. The database known as Online Mendelian Inheritance in Man (OMIM; http://www3.ncbi.nlm.nih.gov/entrez/query.fcgi?db=OMIM&cmd=Limits) is maintained and updated regularly by Johns Hopkins University. The database can be searched by entering the name of the syndrome or by entering clinical characteristics of the syndrome, such as hypodontia and sparse hair. After searching for a particular term, the database will give a list of disorders that include that term within the text of the description of the disorder. In addition, there are references that are linked to the National Library of Medicine's database of published literature, PubMed (see Box 16-1), so that abstracts for articles about the disorder can be easily accessed or downloaded. This is a free database that is available to anyone with an Internet connection. Information about syndromes is also available via the National Organization for Rare Disorders (NORD). Basic information about the syndrome is available at no charge, but to get detailed information it is necessary to purchase a subscription to the site.

## SYNDROMES WITH CRANIOFACIAL ANOMALIES

It is not possible in a single chapter to discuss every syndrome that includes malformations involving the face or mouth. The following section focuses on a subset of these disorders that are either more commonly seen in the dental office or have such dramatic dental and oral manifestations that all dentists should be aware of them. It is recommended that every dental office has access to information about genetic disorders via both the Internet and one or more textbooks.

### Down Syndrome

Inheritance pattern. Chromosomal; sporadic
  Gene(s). Trisomy 21
  General manifestations. Mental deficiency; hypotonia; cardiac anomaly in about 40%; dry skin
  Craniofacial/dental manifestations. Brachycephaly; inner epicanthal folds; up-slanting palpebral fissures; small ears; microdontia; decreased risk for dental caries; increased risk for periodontal disease[8]
  Dental treatment considerations. When treating children with Down syndrome (Fig. 16-18), the primary concerns are to determine the need for subacute bacterial endocarditis prophylaxis and the child's ability to cooperate. If a child has had surgery to repair a congenital heart defect, he or she may or may not need subacute bacterial endocarditis prophylaxis depending on when the surgery was performed and on the presence of any

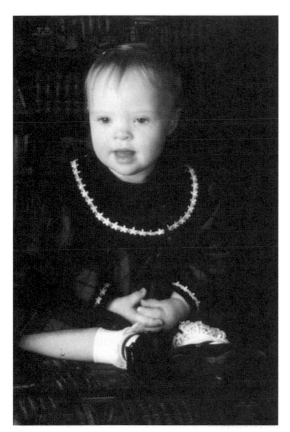

**Figure 16-18** Typical facies of a child with Down syndrome including flat nasal bridge, epicanthal folds, and up-slanting palpebral fissures.

residual defect. This should be confirmed with the parent or with the child's cardiologist. The behavior of children with Down syndrome varies from one child to another just as it does for normally developed children. It is not fair to assume in advance that a child will be uncooperative for dental treatment. On the other hand, some children and young adults with Down syndrome are extremely stubborn and very difficult to examine in the traditional dental setting. When behavior is an issue, it may be necessary to use oral sedation, general anesthesia, and/or referral to a specialist in order to provide quality care for the patient. It is important to note that patients with Down syndrome are much more susceptible to periodontal disease. The dentist should make this clear to the parent and should stress early development of good oral hygiene habits including thorough, supervised daily tooth brushing with a fluoridated toothpaste, flossing, and, when necessary, the use of an antibacterial mouth rinse such as 0.12% chlorhexidine.

## Ectodermal Dysplasia/Hypodontia

Inheritance pattern. X-linked recessive, autosomal dominant, autosomal recessive

Gene(s): Ectodermal dysplasia 1 *(ED1)*[9]; ectodysplasin 1 *(EDAR)*[17]; muscle segment homeobox homolog 1 *(MSX1)*[23]; paired box gene 9 *(PAX9)*.[21]

General manifestations. Sparse hair; dry skin; absence of sweat glands; normal mental status[8]

Craniofacial/dental manifestations. Full lips; small nose; hypodontia; conical or malformed teeth; deficient alveolar ridge

Dental treatment considerations. There are more than 150 forms of the ectodermal dysplasia syndromes that affect one or more of the tissues derived from the ectoderm (Figs. 16-19 and 16-20). Although the most well-known condition is the X-linked anhidrotic form, there are also autosomal dominant and autosomal recessive forms with symptoms that range from mild with hypodontia only to severe with many structures affected along with a cleft lip and palate (ectrodactyly–ectodermal dysplasia–clefting syn-

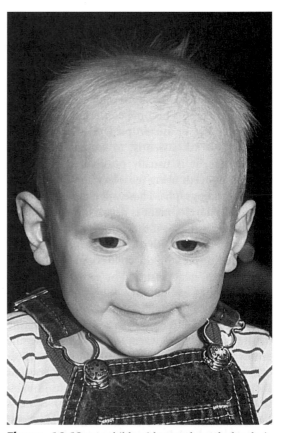

**Figure 16-19** A child with ectodermal dysplasia showing sparse hair.

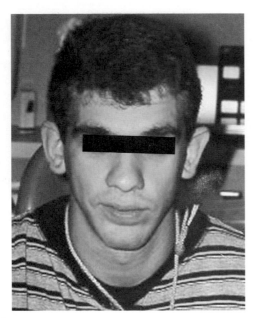

**Figure 16-23** A young man with fragile X syndrome.

## Dentinogenesis Imperfecta

Inheritance pattern. Autosomal dominant or sporadic

Gene(s). Dentin sialophosphoprotein (DSPP)[24]

General manifestations. Normal intelligence; good general health unless in combination with osteogenesis imperfecta

Craniofacial/dental manifestations. Both primary and permanent teeth are affected; teeth are blue-gray or brown; susceptible to extreme wear; pulpal obliteration and dental abscesses

Dental treatment considerations: The severity of this disorder varies considerably from one child to another both within families and between families (see Fig. 16-15). In addition, the appearance of the primary dentition does not reliably predict the appearance of the permanent dentition. In the primary dentition, stainless steel crowns are frequently used to prevent excessive wear of the molars. This should be initiated once wear is apparent on the molars. For some children this may occur as early as 2 years of age whereas for others it may occur later. Abscessed primary teeth require pulp therapy but may need to be extracted if significant pulpal obliteration has occurred. When aesthetics becomes a concern for the child or family, this can be addressed in the primary dentition using aesthetic anterior crowns or partial overdentures. In the permanent dentition, tray bleaching has been used to lighten the

shade of the teeth, and then composite or porcelain veneers may be used on the anterior teeth. As adults, most individuals require full-coverage crowns and frequently root canal therapy. Every effort should be made to maintain the teeth as long as possible to maximize the options the individual has as an adult. Consulting with other dental specialists to assist in planning for future treatment is recommended. If parents report a history of fractures, the child should be referred for a medical evaluation to rule out osteogenesis imperfecta.

## Amelogenesis Imperfecta

Inheritance pattern. Autosomal dominant, autosomal recessive, X-linked, sporadic

Gene(s). Amelogenin (AMG)[13]; enamelin (ENAM)[20]

General manifestations. Normal intelligence; good general health

Craniofacial/dental manifestations. Enamel defects that affect both dentitions; appearance is yellow-brown to orange depending on subtype; teeth are sensitive, susceptible to wear, and may also have taurodontism in molars

Dental treatment considerations. There are 3 major categories of amelogenesis imperfecta and 14 subtypes. More in-depth discussion of the subtypes can be found in Chapter 3 of this textbook. Dental treatment considerations require that the clinician understand the characteristics of the different subtypes prior to developing a treatment plan. In general, treatment concerns fit into a few general categories. Most subtypes are susceptible to wear and require full crown coverage to minimize this. In the primary dentition, this is usually accomplished by placing stainless steel crowns on all the primary molars. A combination of veneers and full-coverage cast crowns may be used in the permanent dentition. Frequently, transitional restorations must be made during the adolescent years until the permanent teeth are fully erupted. Other concerns with this group of disorders include tooth sensitivity, aesthetics, susceptibility to dental caries, and malocclusion. It is not unusual for there to be delayed or partial eruption of permanent premolars and molars that require gingival surgery to expose the crown and orthodontic forces to move them into place prior to restoration. Because of the many complicated issues involved in treating patients with amelogenesis imperfecta, it is recommended that such patients be treated by a team of dental specialists who have had experience with this disorder. When that is not an option due to geographic or other constraints, every effort should be made to consult colleagues who have had experience with this disorder prior to treatment (see Fig. 16-16).

## Treacher Collins Syndrome

Inheritance pattern. Autosomal dominant or sporadic

Gene(s). Treacher Collins-Franceschetti syndrome 1 *(TCOF1)*[22]

General manifestations. Normal intelligence; conductive deafness; occasional congenital heart defect

Craniofacial/dental manifestations. Down-slanting palpebral fissures; malar hypoplasia; lower lid coloboma; mandibular hypoplasia; malformation of external ear; cleft palate

Dental treatment considerations: The severe micrognathia in some patients with Treacher Collins syndrome contributes to dental crowding and may make intubation difficult if treatment under general anesthesia is required (Fig. 16-24). Frequently, orthognathic surgery is required during childhood or adolescence. Dental practitioners should consult with the child's physician to confirm the absence of other medical conditions such as congenital heart defects that might dictate modifications in how dental treatment is delivered.

## Van der Woude Syndrome

Inheritance pattern. Autosomal dominant or sporadic

Gene(s). Interferon regulatory factor 6 *(IRF6)*[11]

General manifestations. Normal intelligence; good general health

Craniofacial/dental manifestations. Lower lip pits; cleft lip/palate; cleft uvula; hypodontia

Dental treatment considerations: Cleft lip and/or palate may occur as a solitary finding or as part of a syndrome (Fig. 16-25). Children with Van der Woude syndrome may have lower lip pits alone or in combination with cleft lip and/or cleft palate. Because the symptoms are limited and because affected individuals have normal intelligence, this disorder could be confused with non-syndromic cleft lip/palate. It is important that children with cleft lip/palate or with lip pits only be seen and evaluated by a craniofacial anomalies team to determine the cause and heritability of their disorder. In addition, this type of team approach is important for providing coordinated, timely treatment of children with cleft lip/palate. Most hospitals have cleft lip/palate or craniofacial teams that include specialists from the following disciplines: plastic and/or oral surgery, pediatric dentistry, orthodontics, speech pathology, prosthodontics, social work, and medical genetics.

## Osteogenesis Imperfecta

Inheritance pattern. Autosomal dominant or sporadic

Gene(s). Type I collagen *(COL1A1, COL1A2)*[2]

General manifestations. Moderate to severe bone fragility; short stature; normal intelligence; hearing impairment in adulthood; hyperextensible joints; deformity of limbs

Craniofacial/dental manifestations. Triangular facies; blue sclera; occasional dentinogenesis imperfecta; delayed eruption of teeth

Dental treatment considerations. Osteogenesis imperfecta is a heterogeneous disorder resulting

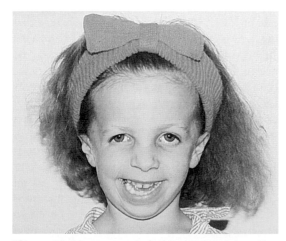

**Figure 16-24**  Facies of a child with Treacher Collins syndrome.

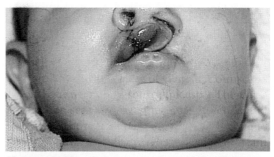

**Figure 16-25**  Cleft lip/palate in a child with Van der Woude syndrome

from both quantitative and qualitative defects in type I collagen. There are four distinct subtypes of osteogenesis imperfecta with symptoms that range from mild to severely deforming to lethal. Osteogenesis imperfecta type I is the mildest form and may go undiagnosed until the child's first fracture. In some cases, parents of children with an undiagnosed mild form of osteogenesis imperfecta have been accused of child abuse when an unreported previous fracture is detected radiographically. It is important for a physician to rule out osteogenesis imperfecta when questions of previous fractures are being evaluated. Osteogenesis imperfecta type II is lethal at birth or shortly thereafter, and dental professionals are not likely to have exposure to children with this form of the disease. The most severe, deforming variety of osteogenesis imperfecta is type III. These children have extreme bone fragility and by childhood may have had as many as 30 fractures. They are frequently not ambulatory and have a history of surgeries that includes placement of rods in their legs and spine. Dental treatment of patients with osteogenesis imperfecta should be done with great care and with guidance from the parent to determine what the child can tolerate. Active or passive immobilization of patients with osteogenesis imperfecta is not recommended for obvious reasons. If behavior at a young age makes treatment in the traditional dental setting unfeasible, other options such as sedation or general anesthesia should be considered. Osteogenesis imperfecta type IV is intermediate in severity between type III and type I. These children have moderate short stature, bone fragility, and significant bone deformity. Sclera is normal and often dentinogenesis is present in children with osteogenesis imperfecta type IV. When a child with dentinogenesis imperfecta presents in a dental office, especially when there is no history of this disorder in the family, the dentist should raise the possibility that the child also has osteogenesis imperfecta. A referral to a medical geneticist for evaluation is appropriate if there is any doubt about the diagnosis.

## Hypophosphatasia

Inheritance pattern. Autosomal dominant, autosomal recessive, or sporadic

Gene(s). Alkaline phosphatase *(ALPL)*[7]

General manifestations. Normal or short stature; bone fragility; bowed lower extremities

Craniofacial/dental manifestations. Premature loss of teeth due to lack of cementum; craniosynostosis

Dental treatment considerations. There are four forms of hypophosphatasia that range from mild to lethal. The milder form that presents in childhood after 6 months of age results in premature loss of primary teeth and craniosynostosis. All types demonstrate decreased levels of serum alkaline phosphatase. Although this is a relatively rare disorder, dentists should be aware of its existence so that an appropriate referral can be made. Frequently, the first sign of this disorder is the premature loss of a mandibular primary incisor without a history of trauma. The exfoliated tooth typically has no root resorption, and histologic analysis will show a lack of cementum. In the mild form of this disorder, the dental manifestations may be the only symptoms.

## GENETIC TESTING

The majority of genetic tests available today are used to diagnose specific inherited disorders such as cystic fibrosis, Huntington disease, or fragile X syndrome. These tests are performed and interpreted by medical geneticists or genetic counselors for the most part. Genetic tests for inherited disorders involve screening for specific mutations or chromosomal disruptions. A second category of genetic tests screens for genetic risk factors for various disorders that have a genetic component. This includes disorders such as familial breast cancer and Alzheimer disease. Testing positive for one of these risk factors does not guarantee that one will get the disease, but it does indicate that an individual is at increased risk of developing the disease. This information allows one to make changes in their life to decrease other risk factors for that disease. Identification of genetic risk factors for dental caries and for periodontal disease is the goal of a number of dental researchers. It is conceivable that in the near future in-office tests will be available to determine the caries risk or periodontal disease risk of an individual patient based on a series of genetic tests. Using the results of these tests, the dentist will be able to develop a targeted prevention plan to minimize the severity of disease for that individual.

## Decision Tree to Assess Inherited Disorders

Most dentists recognize the importance of investigating suspected inherited disorders in their patients. However, it may not be something that a dentist is faced with very often, and it is difficult for many private practitioners to know where to start and how to get the necessary information. Access to the Internet has made this task both easier and more complicated at the same time. The purpose of this section is to demonstrate how a dentist with access to the Internet can get information about a genetic disorder and then find the appropriate referral source for the patient. This process will vary somewhat depending on the nature of the disorder, the location of the dental practice, and the dental practitioner's level of experience with the Internet. It is meant to be one example of how a dentist can assist a family in getting the necessary information or treatment needed.

Case 1: David and Matthew are 12-year-old twin boys in good general health. Their mother has brought them to the dentist because she is concerned about the appearance of their teeth and wants to know what options are available to treat them. The clinical and radiographic evaluation of the face and mouth of both boys reveals complete permanent dentition with no dental caries, generalized microdontia, taurodontism of permanent first and second molars, and dens invaginatus of all four permanent canines. The mother is aware that the teeth are unusual and reports that other family members have similar dental findings. One method for investigating this disorder is described below and shown graphically in a decision tree.

1. Do other members of the family have this? Yes

Are both males and females affected? No; only males are affected.

2. Has this disorder been described in the literature?

To determine this, search the Online Mendelian Inheritance in Man (OMIM) database by entering the following URL and the search terms that describe the disorder: *http://www3.ncbi.nlm.nih. gov/Omim/searchomim.html*

**Search terms:** microdontia, taurodontism, dens invaginatus

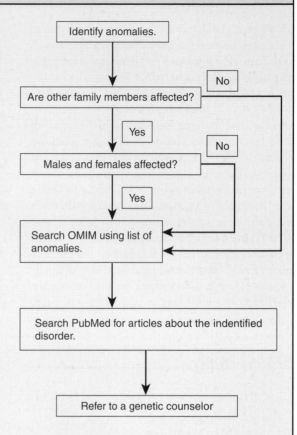

**Results:** One entry with a paper written by Casamassimo et al. in 1978. To look for additional references, search PubMed using the author name (Casamassimo) and one or more of the previous search terms.

**Results:** Two references are found, the above-mentioned article as well as a second article by Ettinger, Casamassimo, and Nowak that discusses management of a similar case.

3. Should patient be referred to medical genetics for evaluation?

If yes, find a genetic counselor in your area by entering the URL: *http://www.nsgc.org/*

If no, discuss findings of papers with mother and make plans for necessary treatment.

## ETHICAL, LEGAL, AND SOCIAL IMPLICATIONS OF THE HUMAN GENOME PROJECT

In the past, patients have not been denied dental insurance because of preexisting dental disease, and it is very unusual for a patient to have a thorough dental examination in order to qualify for dental benefits. The result is that dentists may not be aware of the potential for discrimination to which some patients are susceptible because of their health history. Genetic testing that identifies a person's risk for disease before they have any manifestations of the disease introduces a new level of information about an individual's health and insurability that has not been available in the past. Information about risk for disease may interfere with an individual's ability to get a job or to obtain health, life, or disability insurance. In many cases, the ethical, legal, and social implications of the information learned from the Human Genome Project are still being evaluated.

## REFERENCES

1. Boraas JC, Messer LB, Till MJ: A genetic contribution to dental caries, occlusion and morphology as demonstrated by twins reared apart. *J Dent Res* 67:1150-1155, 1988.
2. Byers PH, Wallis GA, Willing MC: Osteogenesis imperfecta: translation of mutation to phenotype. *J Med Genet* 28:433-442, 1991.
3. Conry JP, Messer LB, Boraas JC et al: Dental caries and treatment characteristics in human twins reared apart. *Arch Oral Biol* 38:937-943, 1993.
4. Crawford DC, Acuna JM, Sherman SL: FMR1 and the fragile X syndrome: human genome epidemiology review. *Genet Med* 3:359-371, 2001.
5. Gelehrter T, Collins FS: *Principles of Medical Genetics.* Baltimore, Williams & Wilkins, 1990.
6. Gorlin RJ, Cohen MM, Hennekam RCM: *Syndromes of the Head and Neck.* New York, Oxford University Press, 2001.
7. Henthorn PS, Raducha M, Fedde KN et al: Different missense mutations at the tissue-non-specific alkaline phosphatase gene locus in autosomal recessively inherited forms of mild and severe hypophosphatasia. *Proc Natl Acad Sci U S A* 89:9924-8, 1992.
8. Jones K: *Smith's Recognizable Patterns of Human Malformation.* Philadelphia, Saunders, 1997.
9. Kere J, Srivastava AK, Montonen O et al: X-linked anhidrotic (hypohidrotic) ectodermal dysplasia is caused by mutation in a novel transmembrane protein. *Nat Genet* 13:409-416, 1996.
10. Kim K, Ruprecht A, Jeon K et al: Personal computer-based three-dimensional computed tomographic images of the teeth for evaluating supernumerary or ectopically impacted teeth, *Angle Orthod* 73:614-621, 2003.
11. Kondo S, Schutte BC, Richardson RJ et al: Mutations in IRF6 cause Van der Woude and popliteal pterygium syndromes. *Nat Genet* 32:285-289, 2002.
12. Kremer EJ, Pritchard M, Lynch M et al: Mapping of DNA instability at the fragile X to a trinucleotide repeat sequence p(CCG)n. *Science* 252:1711-1714, 1991.
13. Lagerstrom M, Dahl N, Nakahori Y et al: A deletion in the amelogenin gene (AMG) causes X-linked amelogenesis imperfecta (AIH1). *Genomics* 10:971-975, 1991.
14. Leppig KA, Werler MM, Cann CI et al: Predictive value of minor anomalies. Association with major malformations. *J Pediatr* 110:531-537, 1987.
15. Marden P, Smith D, McDonald MJ: Congenital anomalies in the newborn infant, including minor variations. *J Pediatr* 64:357-371, 1964.
16. Mehes K, Mestyan J, Knoch V et al: Minor malformations in the neonate. *Helv Pediatr Acta* 28:477-483, 1973.
17. Monreal AW, Ferguson BM, Headon DJ et al: Mutations in the human homologue of mouse dl cause autosomal recessive and dominant hypohidrotic ectodermal dysplasia. *Nat Genet* 22:366-369, 1999.
18. Mundlos S, Otto F, Mundlos C et al: Mutations involving the transcription factor CBFA1 cause cleidocranial dysplasia. *Cell* 89:773-779, 1997.
19. Osborne LR, Martindale D, Scherer SW et al: Identification of genes from a 500-kb region at 7q11.23 that is commonly deleted in Williams syndrome patients. *Genomics* 36:328-336, 1996.
20. Rajpar MH, Harley K, Laing C et al: Mutation of the gene encoding the enamel-specific protein, enamelin, causes autosomal-dominant amelogenesis imperfecta. *Hum Mol Genet* 10:1673-1677, 2001.
21. Stockton DW, Das P, Goldenberg M et al: Mutation of PAX9 is associated with oligodontia. *Nat Genet* 24:18-19, 2000.
22. The Treacher Collins Syndrome Collaborative Group: Positional cloning of a gene involved in the pathogenesis of Treacher Collins syndrome. *Nat Genet* 12:130-136, 1996.
23. Vastardis H, Karimbux N, Guthua SW et al: A human MSX1 homeodomain missense mutation causes selective tooth agenesis. *Nat Genet* 13:417-421, 1996.
24. Zhang X, Zhao J, Li C et al: DSPP mutation in dentinogenesis imperfecta Shields type II. *Nat Genet* 27:151-152, 2001.

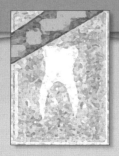

# PART 3

# THE PRIMARY DENTITION YEARS: THREE TO SIX YEARS

The 3- to 6-year-old age group is a group in which the dental needs have changed dramatically in the past several years. The good news is that the caries-free child now exists who, because of fluoride, home care, proper nutrition, and sealants, has no decay at all or, at most, only very modest decay. The bad news is that there are still children who for a variety of reasons need restorative care and sometimes extensive restorative care, including stainless steel crowns and pulp therapy. There are also children who have had extractions and damaging interproximal decay who need space maintenance and, in some instances, space regaining.

The oral habits acquired by children in the first 3 years, which often were of no concern to the parent or clinician, become of concern now. Sometimes the possible detrimental effects of these habits are easily discernible even by the untrained eye. Patient management is included along with hospital dentistry in this section because the majority of patient management problems that a dentist will encounter will probably occur in this age group. At the same time, this age group, with its skills at talking to people and relating to them, is one that many clinicians find delightful. Dentists who enjoy dentistry for children certainly enjoy working with this age group.

## TABLE 17-1

### Cephalometric Angles: A Comparison Between Preschoolers (4–5 years) and Adults

|  | VANN (N = 32)* | ADULT[†] |
| --- | --- | --- |
| SNA | 82.9 | 82.0 |
| SNB | 78.1 | 80.0 |
| SNPg | 77.4 | 83.0 |
| ANB | 4.9 | 2.0 |
| FNA | 89.1 | 88.0 |
| FNB | 84.4 | 87.0 |
| FNPg | 85.5 | 88.0 |
| IMPA | 85.2 | 92.0 |
| FMIA | 65.9 | 65.0 |
| UI-SN | 92.4 | 104.0 |
| UI-F | 97.6 | 110.0 |
| 1-1 | 148.4 | 130.0 |
| M | 67.5 | 69.0 |
| Y axis | 58.5 | 59.0 |
| OCC-SN | 18.8 | 14.5 |
| SN-MP | 35.3 | 32.0 |
| FMA | 29.2 | 25.0 |

From Vann WF et al: *J Dent Child* 45:45-52, 1978.
*All children in this study were between their fourth and fifth birthdays.
[†]Generally accepted adult norms borrowed from Downs, Steiner, and Tweed.

children (4.9 degrees) than in adults (2.0 degrees).

The soft tissue prominence of the nose and to some extent the mandible continue to increase consistently with some reduction in overall facial convexity (Fig. 17-2).[1] It is hard to judge the underlying skeletal configuration from the soft tissue in this age group. Vertically, there is a lowering of the palatal vault with sutural growth and apposition on the oral side of the palate and resorption on the nasal side. There is an even greater lowering of the lowest point of the chin, but the mandibular plane (lower border of the mandible) stays parallel to its original orientation. This occurs because condylar growth exceeds the vertical maxillary growth, which prevents opening of the mandibular plane angle. It is clearly wrong to think of these as nongrowing years for the face.

There is obviously considerable growth in the transverse direction during this time period as well (Fig. 17-3).[1] Remember that this growth comes to an end earlier than that in other dimensions, so attention to problems in this dimension is important. Transverse maxillary growth during this time period is largely the result of midpalatal sutural changes, whereas the growth of the body and angles of the mandible are the result of apposition and resorption (Fig. 17-4).

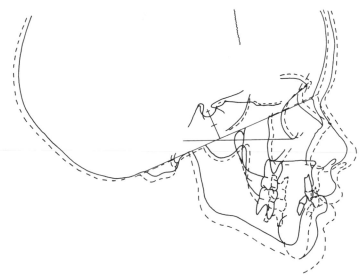

**Figure 17-2**  This anterior cranial base superimposition of the Bolton standard for 3- and 6-year-olds demonstrates the magnitude of anteroposterior and vertical skeletal growth during this period as well as the soft tissue change. (Redrawn from Broadbent BH Sr, Broadbent BH Jr, Golden WH: *Bolton Standards of Developmental Growth.* St Louis, Mosby, 1975.)

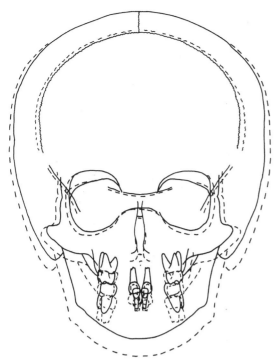

**Figure 17-3** This anterior cranial base superimposition of the Bolton standard for 3- and 6-year-olds demonstrates the magnitude of transverse and vertical skeletal growth during this period. (Redrawn from Broadbent BH Sr, Broadbent BH Jr, Golden WH: *Bolton Standards of Developmental Growth.* St Louis, Mosby, 1975.)

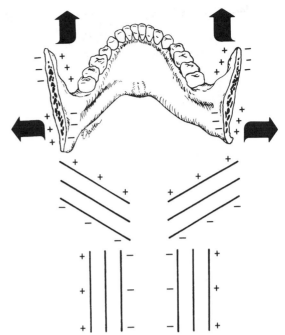

**Figure 17-4** Cross-section through the rami and coronoid processes, illustrating how these areas of the mandible can be visualized as following the V principle. (From Ranly DM: *A Synopsis of Craniofacial Growth.* New York, Appleton-Century-Crofts, 1980. Adapted from Enlow DH, Harris DB: A study of the postnatal growth of the human mandible. *Am J Orthod* 50:25, 1964.)

Posterior maxillary and mandibular growth (sutural growth in the maxilla and endochondral growth in the mandible) helps to accommodate the emerging permanent first molars. There is some appositional growth at the dentoalveolar ridges as the permanent anterior teeth erupt.

Consistent with eruption of the new permanent teeth is the continued eruption of the primary teeth (Fig. 17-5). Often the magnitude of this vertical change is unappreciated. It is also obvious that the permanent anterior teeth will occupy a more anterior and protrusive position in the face.

## REFERENCES

1. Broadbent BH Sr, Broadbent BH Jr, Golden WH: *Bolton Standards of Developmental Growth.* St Louis, Mosby, 1975.
2. Ranly DM: *A Synopsis of Craniofacial Growth.* New York, Appleton-Century-Crofts, 1980.
3. Vann WF, Gilley GJ, Nelson RM: A cephalometric analysis for the child in the primary dentition. *J Dent Child* 45:1, 1978.

## Dental Changes

*Clemons A. Full*

Table 12-5 in Chapter 12 presents a chronology of human dentition. This table demonstrates that the entire primary dentition has completed root development by 3 years of age. This is a relatively stable period clinically for the primary dentition, which was very active before its eruption was completed by 24 to 36 months and before root formation was completed by age 3 years. However, this is a significant period of time for the development of the clinical crowns of the permanent dentition and their subsequent eruptions. There will also be some root resorption of the primary incisors for most children during the last 6 months of this period.

ages of 3 and 6 and is paralleled by an equally dramatic socialization process. During these years, a child's sense of sexual identity emerges, and a certain degree of masculine or feminine qualities is adopted by the child. A sense of identity and a concept of self-esteem also emerge during these years.

One dramatic difference between the child from birth to age 3 and the child from age 3 to age 6 is the development of self-control. Preschool children can be taught methods of self-control, such as distracting themselves when they become impatient or when they are receiving a local anesthetic from a dentist. They can be taught to monitor their own behavior. During the preschool years, the conscience of the child develops, and he or she becomes capable of feeling guilty or anxious if and when he or she violates a moral norm.

An understanding of aggression is important for parents of preschool children and for other adults who deal with preschool children. Aggression is often caused by a child's inability to exert self-control. There are two kinds of aggression. One is called instrumental aggression and is designed for achieving a goal such as taking a piece of candy from a sibling. The other is hostile aggression, and this type is intended to cause hurt or pain to another person. During the preschool years the frequency of instrumental aggression should decline. Children who remain hostilely aggressive during the preschool years are children who come from families in which parents and other children are also overtly aggressive. A parenting philosophy that is inconsistent and unclear in the enforcement of rules has also been linked with aggressive behavior in children.[1]

In summary, at the sixth birthday a child is certainly not emotionally mature but is emotionally complex. He or she is capable of feeling friendship and hostility, acting out aggression, and experiencing guilt and anxiety. This is a child who is susceptible to praise and can suffer hurt feelings. Much of the literature available in bookstores for children in this age group covers "how people feel about things." Obviously, these children can relate to the emotions of other people.

## REFERENCE

1. Mussen PH, Conger JJ, Kagan J et al: *Child Development and Personality,* 6th ed. New York, Harper and Row, 1984.

## SOCIAL CHANGES

*Jimmy R. Pinkham*

Ages 3 to 6 are a time of enormous social growth in the child. Two-year-olds, for example, cannot for the most part play with a peer. Their play is at best separate but parallel. For example, a pair of 2-year-olds may play in the same sandbox, but there is no relationship between the project of one and the project of the other. By age 3 a child can understand taking turns, and by age 4 cooperative play is possible. By age 6, a child is capable of simple team games.

Between ages 3 and 6, children need to gain an understanding of their own personal identification and how they are to relate to other people, including nurturing parents, siblings, peers, and authority figures. During these years, a value system develops, self-discipline is imposed on basic urges, and a consciousness that enables the child to feel guilt emerges. The social transformations of preschoolers ensure that their lives will never be the same.

Many theories seek to explain the reasons for the dramatic psychosocial transitions that take place in this age group. The medical-psychoanalytical theory asserts that sexual fantasies and the guilt associated with these fantasies, which at first take the form of an unusual feeling for the parent of the opposite sex (Oedipus or Electra complex), are the underlying reasons for personality changes. As a child seeks a way to resolve these problems, he or she is forced into identification with the parent of the same sex and into the adoption of a system of morality, complete with its code of values. This code of moral values has been labeled the *superego.* Behaviorists ascribe the assumption of sex-appropriate roles and social values to the effects of reinforcement, both positive and negative, during this period. Social learning theories explain the changes during this period as the product of the influences of parenting and parental behavior. Some theorists believe that as the child becomes conscious of the reasons behind systems of things, she or he is better able to recognize and be allegiant to the reasoning that underlies social order and values.

Regardless of the theoretical position one may subscribe to, it cannot be denied that the role of parents is extremely powerful in the preschooler's life. In 1983, Shonkoff pointed out that anyone observing the play of preschoolers will note that the fantasies they enact are rich in relation to sexual and adult values.[1] He further noted that many parents have often been embarrassed by their children's acting out realistic domestic situations that have occurred in the home.

There continues to be considerable debate in the literature about where stereotypical sex roles merge and how much they are controlled biologically or culturally. There are data that suggest that boys are inherently more aggressive than girls. Conversely, preferences for activities such as active sports and playing with dolls are certainly influenced by reinforcement. It can also be argued that a medium such as television may in a given situation provide information that stereotypes a child's behavior and that media in general may have more influence than the parents in some situations.

## REFERENCE

1. Shonkoff JP: Patterns of variation over time: preschool. In: Levine MD, Carey WB, Crocker AC et al, editors. *Developmental-Behavioral Pediatrics.* Philadelphia, Saunders, 1983, pp 97-107.

## EPIDEMIOLOGY AND MECHANISMS OF DENTAL DISEASE

*Steven M. Adair*

Development of a full complement of healthy primary teeth is important for proper oral function and general health. Aside from the specific early childhood caries patterns discussed in Chapter 12 primary teeth are benefiting from the general reduction in dental caries that has taken place in many industrialized nations during the past 30 years. Still, dental caries is the single most common disease among children, with a prevalence five times that of asthma.[13] Dental caries in children is found in disproportionately higher numbers among children in lower income groups.[21] It has been estimated that about 80% of dental decay occurs in 20% of children, and those are largely children of poverty.[10] This chapter will discuss the epidemiology of caries in the primary dentition and etiologic factors in the caries process at this age.

## EPIDEMIOLOGY OF DENTAL CARIES IN THE PRIMARY DENTITION

Data regarding the prevalence of caries in the primary dentition have not been systematically collected on populations as large as those surveyed in permanent dentition studies. There is, however, a body of literature on U.S. children spanning several decades from which trends can be ascertained. Table 17-2 illustrates a selected number of these reports. Direct comparisons cannot be drawn because of the various ways (dmfs, deft, etc.) in which the data are reported, the variety of populations studied, fluoridation status of the communities, and a host of other variables that are not consistent across studies. Inspection of Table 17-2 reveals that caries in the primary dentition remains a problem, at least for certain segments of the population. Three surveys of 3- to 6-year-old children enrolled in Head Start programs found mean caries experiences ranging from 2.37 to almost 10 decayed, extracted, and filled primary tooth surfaces (defs) or 4.8 to 11.07 decayed, missing, and filled primary tooth surfaces (dmfs).[9,11,18]

Some rough comparisons are possible. Hennon et al.[7] found a mean defs of 6.16 in fluoride-deficient areas of Indiana in 1969 among 36- to 39-month-olds. Johnsen et al.[9] reported a mean defs of 4.7 among 3½- to 5-year-old subjects in fluoride-deficient areas of Ohio almost 20 years later. Two studies conducted in Philadelphia demonstrate the effects of fluoridation in that city. The subjects in the first study[22] were born when Philadelphia was a fluoride-deficient community, although the city had become fluoridated by the time of the survey. The second survey 12 years later[3] demonstrated lower mean defs rates among the 3- to 5-year-old children.

Recent surveys, while demonstrating a trend for caries reductions in the primary dentition, indicate that by age 3 perhaps 25% to 65% of children will have been affected by dental caries. Edelstein and Tinanoff[6] found that 30.5% of 200 children younger than 6 had caries detectable by visual or radiographic findings. Speechley and Johnston's data[16] indicate that the general decline in dental caries may be reversing in the primary dentition, at least in some parts of the world.

Table 17-3 demonstrates differences in primary dentition caries in U.S. children aged 2 to 5 years. Between the early 1970s and the period

## TABLE 17-2
### Selected Surveys of Caries in the Primary Dentition of U.S. Children

| Study | Subject Age | DEFS | DEFT | DMFS | DMFT | DFS | DFT | Percent Caries Free | Remarks |
|---|---|---|---|---|---|---|---|---|---|
| Savara and Suher, 1954[15] | 1 yr | | 0.67 | | | | | 78 | Portland, OR |
| | 2 | | 0.83 | | | | | 77 | Fluoridation |
| | 3 | | 2.72 | | | | | 38 | status not |
| | 4 | | 4.05 | | | | | 39 | given |
| | 5 | | 4.76 | | | | | 22 | |
| | 6 | | 5.13 | | | | | 17 | |
| Wisan et al., 1957[22] | 2 yr | 0.6 | | | | | | | Philadelphia |
| | 3 | 2.2 | | | | | | | FD when |
| | 4 | 3.6 | | | | | | | subjects |
| | 5 | 3.5 | | | | | | | were born |
| Bronstein, 1969[3] | 3 yr | 0.47 | 0.38 | | | | | 85 | Philadelphia |
| | 4 | 1.57 | 1.13 | | | | | 71 | OF |
| | 5 | 2.27 | 1.60 | | | | | 58 | |
| Hennon et al., 1969[7] | 18–23 mo | 1.75 | | | | | | | FD areas, |
| | 36–39 mo | 6.16 | | | | | | | Indiana |
| Weddell and Klein, 1981[20] | 24–35 mo | 1.15 | | | | | | | OF |
| Johnsen et al., 1986[9] | 3½–5 | | | | | | | | Ohio: |
| | | 3.3 | 2.3 | | | | | | Urban OF |
| | | 4.7 | 2.8 | | | | | | Urban FD |
| | | 3.3 | 2.0 | | | | | | Rural OF |
| | | 4.7 | 2.8 | | | | | | Rural FD |
| Trubman et al., 1989[18] | 3 yr | 2.37 | 1.34 | | | | | | Mississippi |
| | 4 | 4.91 | 2.58 | | | | | | Head Start |
| | 5 | 7.33 | 3.53 | | | | | | Program |
| | 6 | 9.99 | 4.32 | | | | | | |
| Louie et al., 1990[12] | 3½–5½ | | | | 4.8 | 2.97 | 36 | | California: OF |
| | | | | | 7.44 | 4.03 | 30 | | FD |
| | | | | | 11.74 | 5.13 | | | Hawaii |
| | | | | | 11.07 | 5.4 | | | Micronesia |

*FD*, Fluoride-deficient community water supply; *OF*, optimally fluoridated community water supply.

1988–1994, the number of untreated carious primary tooth surfaces declined by about 30% overall. However, percent decline for children living at or below poverty level was not as great as that for children living above the poverty line.[4] Other data from the 1988–1994 period indicate that the percentages of children with at least one decayed or filled primary tooth were higher among lower socioeconomic groups (Table 17-4).[20]

## LOCATION OF DENTAL CARIES IN THE PRIMARY DENTITION

The distribution of caries among occlusal, facial-lingual, and proximal surfaces as illustrated in Table 17-2 clearly demonstrates the differential effect of fluoride on the various surfaces of primary teeth. In optimally fluoridated communities, caries reduction on proximal and facial-lingual

## TABLE 17-3

**Number of Untreated Carious Primary Teeth and Surfaces Among 2- to 10-Year-Old Children, NHANES I (1971–1974) and NHANES III (1988–1994)[4]**

| SUBJECT CHARACTERISTICS | TEETH | | PERCENT DIFFERENCE | P VALUE | SURFACES | | PERCENT DIFFERENCE | P VALUE |
|---|---|---|---|---|---|---|---|---|
| | NHANES I | NHANES III | | | NHANES I | NHANES III | | |
| All | 0.96 | 0.67 | -30% | <.01 | 1.58 | 1.26 | -20% | .13 |
| At or below poverty | 1.25 | 1.12 | -10% | .53 | 2.17 | 2.19 | +1 | .97 |
| Above poverty | 0.88 | 0.47 | -47% | <.01 | 1.42 | 0.86 | -39% | <.01 |

*NHANES*, National Health and Nutrition Examination Study.

## TABLE 17-4

### Percentage of Children Ages 2–5 Years with Decayed and Filled Primary Teeth by Income Level[21]

| INCOME LEVEL (% OF FPL) | PERCENTAGE WITH AT LEAST ONE DECAYED PRIMARY TOOTH (SE) | PERCENTAGE WITH AT LEAST ONE FILLED PRIMARY TOOTH (SE) |
|---|---|---|
| 0–100 | 29.7 (2.7) | 9.3 (1.6) |
| 101–200 | 24.4 (2.3) | 9.3 (1.6) |
| 201–300 | 12.2 (1.6) | 7.8 (1.5) |
| >301 | 6.0 (1.2) | 6.5 (1.3) |
| Total sample | 18.7 (1.2) | 8.7 (0.9) |

FPL, Federal poverty level; SE, standard error of the percentage.

surfaces leads to 41% of the caries occurring on the occlusal surfaces. In fluoride-deficient communities, a somewhat more uniform distribution is seen, with a higher proportion of proximal lesions and proportionately fewer occlusal lesions.[12] The prevalence of proximal lesions is higher than that reported for permanent teeth by a factor of 3 to 4.

Within the primary dentition, individual tooth susceptibility is determined to a large extent by tooth and dental arch morphology. Primary first molars in both arches are less susceptible to occlusal caries because of the relative lack of deep pits and fissures on that tooth as compared with primary second molars. The broad contact area between primary first and second molars contributes to a high proportion of proximal caries occurring at those surfaces. The distal surface of the primary second molar has no approximating tooth until the permanent first molar erupts. Thus, it is relatively unaffected by caries until age 6 or 7, after which it becomes more susceptible. The caries susceptibility of the distal surface of the primary canine and the mesial surface of the primary first molar is similar, and both are less affected than the first molar–second molar contact area. The canine–first molar contact area is less broad. In the mandibular arch this contact area serves as the primate space and thus is often free cleansing.

## ETIOLOGIC FACTORS

The etiologic factors discussed in Chapter 12 apply to primary as well as permanent teeth. However, studies have indicated that differences may exist between younger and older children for some of the factors. Saliva, one of the host factors, differs among preschool children in its levels of lysozyme activity and IgA concentration.[5,19] Salivary flow rate is lower among younger children, and lower among girls than boys.[2] The concentrations of certain salivary solutes, notably amylase and phosphate, increase during the first year, whereas others (potassium, sodium, protein) decrease during the same time. The net effect of these changes is unclear at this time.

The increased use of antibiotics, especially in young children, has been suggested as another possible cause of the decline in caries in the primary dentition. Administration of antibiotics during the eruption of teeth may delay colonization by mutans streptococci and allow the establishment of other bacteria in the occlusal pits and fissures.[11] Early establishment of mutans streptococci in the mouths of infants may lead to a greater caries experience by age 4.[1]

An increased frequency of sugar consumption in early childhood has been linked to caries levels, as might be expected. Primary dmft scores greater than 3 have been correlated with intakes of more than 95 g/day, whereas scores below 3 are associated with daily sugar consumption of less than 50 g.[17] Pacifiers dipped in honey and other sweeteners have been shown to be detrimental to the dentition. Rampant caries is not uncommon among 3- and 4-year-olds who practice this habit.[8] Another contributing factor for children who are continuously on medication is the high sugar content of some formulations.[14]

Many other factors contribute to the risk of caries in children. Such predisposing factors include oral hygiene, socioeconomic status, and nutrition, but the major interactions occur between a susceptible host, dietary sucrose, and the presence of cariogenic microflora.

# REFERENCES

1. Alaluusua S, Renkonen O-L: *Streptococcus mutans* establishment and dental caries experience in children from 2 to 4 years old. *Scand J Dent Res* 14:453, 1983.

2. Andersson R, Arvidsson E, Crossner C-G et al: The flow rate, pH and buffer effect of mixed saliva in children. *J Int Assoc Dent Child* 5:5, 1974.

3. Bronstein E: A survey of caries-experience among the preschool children of Philadelphia. *J Public Health Dent* 29:24, 1969.

4. Brown LJ, Wall TP: Trends in untreated caries in primary teeth of children 2 to 10 years old. *JADA* 131:93, 2000.

5. Camling E, Kohler B: Infection with the bacterium *Streptococcus mutans* and salivary IgA antibodies in the mothers and their children. *Arch Oral Biol* 32:817, 1987.

6. Edelstein B, Tinanoff N: Screening preschool children for dental caries using a microbial test. *Pediatr Dent* 11:129, 1989.

7. Hennon DK, Stookey GK, Muhler JC: Prevalence and distribution of dental caries in preschool children. *JADA* 79:1405, 1969.

8. Holt RD, Joels D, Bulman J et al: A third study of caries in preschool aged children in Camden. *Br Dent J* 165:87, 1988.

9. Johnsen DC, Bhat M, Kim MT et al: Caries levels and patterns in head start children in fluoridated and non-fluoridated, urban and non-urban sites in Ohio, USA. *Community Dent Oral Epidemiol* 14:206, 1986.

10. Kaste LM, Selwitz RH, Oldakowski JA et al: Coronal caries in the primary and permanent dentition of children and adolescents 1–17 years of age: United States, 1988–1991. *J Dent Res* 75(special issue):631, 1996.

11. Loesche WJ: Decline in *Streptococcus mutans*-associated caries secondary to medical usage of antibiotics. In: Hamada S et al, editors. *Molecular Microbiology and Immunology of* Streptococcus mutans. Amsterdam, Elsevier, 1986.

12. Louie R, Brunelle JA, Maggiore ED et al: Caries prevalence in Head Start children, 1986–87. *J Public Health Dent* 50:299, 1990.

13. National Center for Chronic Disease Prevention and Health Promotion (n.d.). *Preventing Dental Caries.* Retrieved May 1, 2004 from http://www.cdc.gov/nccdphp/pe_factsheets/pe_oh.htm.

14. Roberts IJ, Roberts GJ: Relation between medicines sweetened with sucrose and dental disease. *Br Med J* 2:14, 1979.

15. Savara BS, Suher T: Incidence of dental caries in children 1 to 6 years of age. J Dent Res 33:808, 1954.

16. Speechley M, Johnston DW: Some evidence from Ontario, Canada, of a reversal in the dental caries decline. *Caries Res* 30:423, 1996.

17. Sreebny LM: Sugar availability, sugar consumption and dental caries. *Community Dent Oral Epidemiol* 10:1, 1982.

18. Trubman A, Silberman SL, Meydrech EF: Dental caries assessment of Mississippi Head Start children. *J Public Health Dent* 49:167, 1989.

19. Tweetman S, Lindner A, Modeer T: Lysozyme and salivary immunoglobulin A in caries free and caries susceptible pre-school children. *Swed Dent J* 5:9, 1981.

20. Weddell JA, Klein AI: Socioeconomic correlation of oral disease in six- to thirty-six-month children. *Pediatr Dent* 3:306, 1981.

21. Vargas CM, Crall JJ, Schneider DA: Sociodemographic distribution of pediatric dental caries. *JADA* 129:1229, 1998.

22. Wisan JM, Lavell M, Colwell FH: Dental survey of Philadelphia preschool children by income, age and treatment status. *JADA* 55:1, 1957.

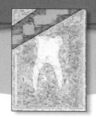

# CHAPTER 18

## Examination, Diagnosis, and Treatment Planning

*Paul S. Casamassimo, John R. Christensen, and Henry W. Fields, Jr.*

## DIAGNOSIS FOR NONORTHODONTIC PROBLEMS

The examination of the 3-year-old child often represents a youngster's first dental experience, although earlier examinations are advocated by most pediatric dentists and the American Academy of Pediatric Dentistry for diagnostic, preventive, and treatment purposes. For a child who has not had a dental examination previously, the new environment, new people, and manipulation of tissues can be difficult or overwhelming.

An initial examination of a child this age can also be stressful for the dentist, who is faced with a potential behavior problem, no clinical baseline, and the challenge of providing both immediate and long-term planning and treatment.

The initial examination is a first experience for both dentist and patient and provides an opportunity to establish a course of dental health for years to come. Of particular interest in the examination of the 3- to 6-year-old are the following factors:

1. Limited existing health history
2. No clinical baseline data
3. Behavioral unknowns
4. A primary dentition occlusion with limited predictive value
5. Preventive needs that must be assessed

All of the above must be addressed during evaluation of a child this age, especially if this is the child's initial dental visit.

## PATIENT RECORDS

The nature of health care record keeping in dentistry has evolved from a historical or financial repository to a vital working document. The bare essentials for a pediatric dental record are a health history, examination record, treatment plan, and series of visit notes. Parental or guardian consent should be obtained and recorded at the initial visit. Adjunctive records such as study casts and preventive and dietary forms or analyses also should be kept with the record, if indicated. The history form should permit updating and summary.

The possibilities for a dental examination record for children are endless.

Many practitioners opt for a standard form or use the one they employed in dental school. No clear-cut guidelines exist for choice of a pediatric dental tooth chart, but there are some basic requirements from a medicolegal standpoint and from the standpoint of providing a developmental history. The examination record should do the following:

1. Adequately record both developmental status and existing pathosis of teeth and supporting structures as well as head and neck
2. Record facial and occlusal status
4. Record oral hygiene, periodontal, and intraoral soft tissue status
5. Indicate findings from radiographic and other diagnostic tests

The tooth chart need not be anatomically correct, and in many cases a diagram of teeth is of more value. It is critical that the charting system address both primary and permanent teeth so that each record entry provides an up-to-date developmental profile. In addition to a notation of the presence or absence of a tooth, as is done with adults, the mobility of primary teeth and clinically evident eruption of teeth are noted in the pediatric dental chart. Current child safety concerns strongly suggest making an initial chart of the dentition, including restorations and abnormalities. For many children this age, the absence of restorations or caries makes this an academic exercise.

Periodontal probing of all teeth is not routine, but the dental chart should provide an area for noting deep pocketing or loss of attachment in some manner. The nature of this notation requires simply adequate baseline data to accomplish treatment and follow-up.

Many practitioners develop individual approaches to prevention that can be efficiently addressed on the examination record. A serial chart of oral hygiene performance or gingival scores can be helpful. Other helpful items on the examination record are vital signs, medical alerts, behavior notes, and unusual findings. Reasons for deferring radiographic examination should be noted in the record. These data provide quick reference for the dentist at chairside.

Recent changes in patient privacy procedures, procedure coding, expected assessments, and dental disease risk assessment suggest that today's dental examination record (history and physical) should incorporate other measurement scales. These might include any or all of the following:

1. A caries risk assessment based on the Caries Assessment Tool of the American Academy of Pediatric Dentistry (see Chapter 13), or some other instrument that accounts for clinical and historical risk factors. This can be a list of factors or simply a choice of high, medium, or low risk.
2. An initial pain or behavior assessment that provides the dentist with a sense of the child's cooperation or state of oral health upon initial examination. Some clinicians use a set of diagrammatic "faces" ranging from happy to sad. Others use a version of the Frankl behavior scale, which is a four-point selection ranging from definitely positive to definitely negative.

The treatment plan should indicate the sequence of care and permit notation of the date of completion of individual procedures. Each visit's progress note indicates what was done and any notable occurrences. The advent of the computerized record has made use of dental coding a must. Treatment plans generated in the office ought to include current dental codes to facilitate communication both within and outside the office.

## THE HISTORY

The parent or guardian is the historian for the child. The dentist needs to address both real and perceived problems. Parents may provide erroneous and unverified information simply because the information has not been tested by the health system. Two such examples are reported heart murmurs and allergies. Parents may have been informed of a murmur but are unaware of its seriousness. Parents also may confuse nausea with a true allergic reaction. The dentist may be required to address these concerns directly with a physician to obtain accurate information. In other situations, a long-established or past problem may have been forgotten or dismissed as unimportant.

A general health history form can be used to determine a child's health background if attention is given to specific elements that relate to children. The dentist should be well versed in conditions that relate specifically to children. Table 18-1 provides a list of health items that are particularly common in the 3- to 6-year-old group. The American Dental Association offers a contemporary history form specifically designed for children that covers most childhood health issues.

A short and noncontributory history was unusual in this age group in the past, but with the improvement in infant health practices and home care, immunization, and early intervention, many routine problems and illnesses have been reduced. On the other hand, a growing number of infants survive who would have perished previously. Although some develop normally, a substantial number are physically or mentally compromised and require alternative and more complex health care approaches. It is not uncommon in this age group to have parents note normal development or simply indicate a vague delay in speech or motor skill. This may be the result of the failure to fully diagnose a disability or because the parent is reluctant to accept that the child may have a problem.

The dentist's review of a checklist with annotations can be used to complete an accurate medical history. Significant findings should be explained in the record. Any health history should be finalized by a summary of the status of the child, especially in the areas of drug allergies, surgical procedures and related problems, cardiac abnormalities, and developmental status. Many pediatric dental records are designed so that this summary appears on the examination form to preclude paging through the record for important information. This also serves to confirm that the dentist has reviewed the history and made a decision about its impact on treatment.

The dental history should be comprehensive. Many parents have not thought to characterize their child's dental history other than the eruption of the first tooth. The dental history should cover, at a minimum, past problems and care, fluoride experience, current hygiene habits, and an eruption-developmental profile. Table 18-1 addresses the essential elements of the dental history. The most contemporary approach to the dental history uses a developmental model that permits the parent to address age-specific issues. For example, the health history may ask about bottle use, weaning, access to sweets, and other dietary issues to cover a range of ages on one form. The checklist approach to the health history permits a "not applicable" choice when a child has outgrown a set of questions. This developmental approach provides an age-specific set of findings that can be converted to preventive instruction in the anticipatory guidance counseling by dental staff.

## THE EXAMINATION

The examination encompasses six major sections: behavioral assessment; general appraisal; and head and neck, facial, intraoral, and radiographic examinations.

### Behavioral Assessment

A complete behavioral assessment is discussed in Chapter 23. The general appraisal and chairside examination provide two opportunities to observe behavior and initially assess potential cooperation.

### General Appraisal

The general appraisal addresses the child's physical and behavioral status. The classic areas of this appraisal include gait, stature, and presence of gross signs and symptoms of disease. The normal 3- to 6-year-old is ambulatory, well coordinated in basic tasks, engaging, and physically healthy in appearance. Table 18-2 lists physical and behavioral milestones for the 3- to 6-year-old child. The dentist should incorporate these markers mentally into a profile for evaluation of the child's status. The general appraisal of the child is best accomplished in the waiting room or similar nonthreatening environment. This appraisal

## TABLE 18-1

### Selected Health History Considerations with Common Findings in the 3- to 6-Year-Old Group

| AREA OF CONCERN | COMMON FINDINGS |
| --- | --- |
| **General Health** | |
| Allergies | Probably related to food and other environmental allergens; may have allergy to medications such as antibiotics; rash is common manifestation; false allergies often reported |
| Asthma | May be reported; triggering factors usually known; medications also well known; impact of dental intervention usually not known |
| Bleeding | Parent may suggest excessive bruising without real problem |
| Blood transfusion | May have been performed at birth |
| Childhood infections | Immunizations will have occurred, or there is a clear history of having had a specific illness such as measles or chickenpox |
| Development | Poor parental knowledge for normal children; for those with developmental delays, a good history of diagnostic procedures and status |
| Heart | Functional murmur may exist, or parent may have been told of a murmur |
| Hypertension | Usually unknown, unless child has chronic problem |
| Illnesses | Probable history of upper respiratory infections |
| Jaundice | Possible at birth |
| Medications | Probably has taken acetaminophen (Tylenol) as necessary; may have received amoxicillin or other antibiotic |
| Surgical procedures | Possible tonsillectomy or adenoidectomy; possible ear tubes; circumcision seldom noted as procedure |
| Seizures | Possibly febrile; may be on seizure medication for only one seizure |
| **Dental Health** | |
| Bottle use | Probably considered not to contribute to decay |
| Developmental/eruption | Knowledge may be limited to eruption dates of first teeth, unless consistently very early or late |
| Fluoride | May know water status; possible vitamin with fluoride supplementation |
| Habits (thumb sucking) | Will be well known to parent if present |
| Home care | Usually confined to tooth brushing; may be largely left to child |
| Previous care | Possibly none; no dentist or care rendered |
| Reaction to care (behavior) | Possibly none; likely poor or tentative |
| Trauma to teeth and chin | Possible, but usually left untreated unless serious; commonly upper teeth and chin |

This table suggests usual or common responses to questions put to parents of this age group for the average child, but it does not suggest a norm or most frequent response for all children.

should be followed by clarification of any abnormal findings and discussion of potential behavior problems with the parent.

The role of vital signs in the general appraisal is twofold. The first purpose is to identify abnormalities, and the second is to satisfy the medicolegal role of providing baseline health data for emergency situations. Vital signs may be distorted if the child is upset or anxious. Taking vital signs of blood pressure, pulse, and respiration may be put off until the child has become accustomed to the environment, but these data must be obtained before any drugs are administered. Weight should be obtained and recorded in a conspicuous location on the chart so that the information is available in an emergency. Height should also be recorded and, together with weight, should serve as an index of physical development.

## TABLE 18-2

### Selected Developmental Characteristics of the 3- to 6-Year-Old Child

| 3-YEAR-OLD | 4-YEAR-OLD | 5-YEAR-OLD |
|---|---|---|
| **Intellectual Development** | | |
| Gives first and last name | Recognizes colors | Names four colors |
| Counts three objects | Counts four objects | Counts 10 objects |
| States own age and sex | Tells a story | Asks about the meaning of words |
| **Gross/Fine Motor Skills** | | |
| Puts on shoes | Dresses without supervision | Dresses and undresses |
| Pedals tricycle | Balances on one foot | Hops on one foot |
| Copies a circle | Copies cross and square | Draws a triangle |

**Psychological**
The 3- to 6-year-old is in the *phallic* stage of development. During this period, the child undergoes *oedipal* conflicts, which may lead to opposite-sex parental preference. The child may exhibit some aggression with siblings. By age 6, the child may be ready to surrender some dependency toward parents.

| | | |
|---|---|---|
| **Dental Implications** | | |
| Needs maternal presence, especially during stress | May be difficult and aggressive | Should leave parent for treatment |
| Fear of separation | Responds to verbal direction | Proud of possessions |
| Visual fear | Auditory fear | Bodily harm fear |
| **Physiological Height (75th percentile)** | | |
| Boys = 97.5 cm | Boys = 106 cm | Boys = 113 cm |
| Girls = 97 cm | Girls = 104.5 cm | Girls = 111.5 cm |
| (Growth rate for this period is approximately 6-8 cm/yr) | | |
| **Weight (75th percentile)** | | |
| Boys = 15.5 cm | Boys = 18 cm | Boys = 20 cm |
| Girls = 15.5 cm | Girls = 17.5 cm | Girls = 19.5 cm |
| (Growth rate for this period is approximately 2 kg/yr) | | |
| **Pulse (90th percentile)** | | |
| 105/min | 100/min | 100/min |
| **Respiration (90th percentile)** | | |
| 30/min | 28/min | 26/min |
| **Blood Pressure** | | |
| 100/60 | 100/60 | 100/60 |

## Head and Neck Examination

Examining a 3-year-old requires attention to both clinical findings and the patient's behavior in the dental setting. Stated differently, the product (dental findings) cannot be separated from the process (patient's behavior) of the examination. The examination provides a moderately threat-ening environment for development of behavioral interactions between dentist and child.

Table 18-3 outlines the elements and expectations for a thorough head and neck examination. The process begins with an orientation about what is to occur. What will take place at each step in the examination should be described by the dentist. The tell-show-do technique, which

## TABLE 18-3

### Elements of Head and Neck Examination

| STRUCTURE | DIAGNOSTIC TECHNIQUE | NORMAL CHARACTERISTICS | SELECTED ABNORMAL FINDINGS/POSSIBLE CAUSES |
|---|---|---|---|
| **Head** | | | |
| Hair | Visualization | Quality<br>Thickness<br>Color | Dryness/malnutrition, ectodermal dysplasia<br>Baldness/child abuse, self-abuse, chemotherapy<br>Infestation/neglect |
| Scalp | Visualization | Skin color<br>Dryness<br>Ulceration | Scaling/dermatitis<br>Sores/abuse, infection, neglect |
| Ears | Visualization<br>Palpation<br>Assessment of hearing | Intact and normally formed external ear and auditory canal<br>Gross normal hearing | Malformed ears and canals/genetic malformation syndrome (e.g., Treacher Collins)<br>Conductive and neurologic hearing loss/trauma, developmental disability |
| Eyes | Visualization<br>Assessment of vision | Position and orientation in fact<br>Movement of eyes<br>Vision<br>Reaction to light | Variation in separation and orientation/genetic malformation syndromes<br>Cranial nerve damage/trauma, developmental disability |
| Nose | Visualization | Normal size, shape, function, and location | Malposition/genetic malformation syndrome (e.g., median facial cleft)<br>Misshapen/ectodermal dysplasia, congenital syphilis, achondroplasia<br>Discharge/upper respiratory tract infection (URI), asthma, allergy<br>Poor smell, cranial nerve damage |
| Lip | Visualization<br>Assessment of function | Speech, closure<br>Integrity<br>Absence of lesions | Poor closure/lip incompetence<br>Clefting/genetic clefting syndrome<br>Asymmetry/Bell's palsy or cranial nerve damage<br>Ulceration/herpes infection |
| Temporomandibular joint | Visualization<br>Palpation<br>Auscultation | Symmetry in function<br>Smooth movement<br>Absence of pain<br>Range of motion (maximum) | Deviation/trauma<br>Crepitus, pain/temporomandibular joint disorder<br>Limitation/arthritis, trauma |
| Skin | Visualization | Color<br>Tone<br>Moisture<br>Absence of lesions | Edema/cellulitis, renal disorder<br>Redness/allergic response<br>Dryness/dehydration, ectodermal dysplasia<br>Ulceration/infectious disease, abuse |
| Chin | Visualization | Absence of scar | Scar indicates previous mandibular trauma |

*Continued*

## TABLE 18-3

### Elements of Head and Neck Examination—cont'd

| STRUCTURE | DIAGNOSTIC TECHNIQUE | NORMAL CHARACTERISTICS | SELECTED ABNORMAL FINDINGS/POSSIBLE CAUSES |
|---|---|---|---|
| **Neck** | | | |
| Lymph nodes | Palpation | Normal size, mobility | Increased size/infection, neoplasia<br>Fixation/neoplasia |
| Thyroid | Palpation | Normal size | Increased size/goiter, tumor |
| **Oral Cavity** | | | |
| Palates | Visualization<br>Palpation<br>Assessment of function | Integrity<br>Absence of lesion<br>Normal function | Cleft/genetic syndrome<br>Ulceration/herpes, mononucleosis, or other infection, abuse<br>Petechiae/sexual abuse<br>Deviation/cranial nerve damage |
| Pharynx | Visualization | Normal color | Normal size of tonsils<br>Redness/URI, tonsillitis |
| Tongue | Visualization<br>Palpation<br>Assessment of function | Normal color<br>Range of motion<br>Absence of lesions | Redness/glossitis<br>Ulceration/herpes, aphthous, or other infection, trauma<br>Deviation/cranial nerve damage<br>Limited movement/cerebral palsy |
| Floor of mouth | Visualization<br>Palpation | Salivary function<br>Absence of swelling<br>Absence of lesions | Swelling/mucocele, sialolith<br>Ulceration/aphthous ulceration or other infection, abuse |
| Buccal mucosa | Visualization<br>Palpation | Absence of lesions<br>Absence of swelling<br>Salivary function | Ulceration/cheek bite, abuse<br>Swelling/salivary gland<br>Infection, mumps |
| Teeth | Visualization<br>Palpation<br>Percussion | Normal development<br>Morphologic appearance<br>Occlusion<br>Color<br>Integrity<br>Mobility<br>Hygiene | Absence/delayed eruption/congenital absence, genetic syndromes<br>Extra teeth/supernumerary, cleidocranial dysplasia<br>Abnormal morphologic appearance/microdontia, macrodontia, fusion<br>Abnormal color/amelogenesis or dentinogenesis imperfecta, staining, pulpal necrosis, caries<br>Fracture/trauma, abuse, caries<br>Mobility/periapical infection, trauma, bone loss conditions, exfoliation<br>Malposition/malocclusion, trauma<br>Pain/periapical involvement |

involves explanation, demonstration, and finally completion of a step, is usually the way the diagnostic process is handled. Positive or negative responses from the child should be encouraged. Children also should be warned and supported prior to the dentist's making positional changes or beginning intraoral manipulation.

Parental presence is always a matter of controversy. Initial parental involvement may be encouraged to allow a transition to be made from a dentist-parent to a more direct dentist-child relationship. This supported transition is important for children younger than 3 years of age but is less threatening for children near school age. Each child reacts differently to having a parent in the operatory, and the dentist must assess the benefit of that presence on the developing relationship he or she has with that child. It is within the parent's purview to request to be present during the examination and treatment, but it is within the practitioner's purview to choose not to treat the child under those circumstances. Growing numbers of practitioners allow parents in the treatment setting, and most data indicate that parents are neutral factors.

The examination must involve evaluation of the head and neck. Palpation to identify enlarged and fixed lymph nodes or other swellings is critical. Many children of this age have swollen nodes, but the nodes are usually movable and confined to the lower face and jaws and are indicative of minor infection. Swollen nodes in the neck and clavicular region are more rare and may indicate more serious ailments.

Critical to a thorough examination of the head and neck is evaluation of form and function. The cranial nerves, speech, and mandibular function should be evaluated. However, a complete cranial nerve examination need not be performed because careful observation of sensory and motor function and the child's responses can indicate nerve status to a significant degree. Normal conversation can be used to identify gross speech pathosis. While palpating the craniofacial structures, the dentist should talk with the child and observe his or her responses. Asking the child to open and demonstrate maximal opening and maximal intercuspation allows the child to perform simple tasks. Mandibular movements should be observed for deviation and restriction of range of movement. The child should also be asked to move the mandible from side to side and to protrude it. Restriction of these movements may identify functional and morphologic problems that are developmental or the result of trauma.

Verbal responses also serve as behavioral signals of the child's adaptation. A child's cooperation, nonverbal communication, and physiologic responses often suggest stable, improving, or deteriorating behavior. Because the examination setting is only moderately threatening, it provides a good opportunity to develop cooperation.

The manual examination should address any physical variations as well as the strength and mobility of structures. The visual aspect of the process should address color changes, asymmetry, and marked physiologic responses such as sweating or trembling.

## Facial Examination

A systematic facial examination is one portion of a complete orthodontic evaluation that describes skeletal and dental relationships in three spatial planes: anteroposterior, vertical, and transverse. The steps include a description of the overall facial pattern, the positions of the maxilla and mandible, and the vertical facial relationships. Next, the position of the lips is determined. Finally, facial symmetry is assessed, and the maxillary dental midline is located relative to the facial midline.

### Overall Facial Pattern

First, the facial profile is evaluated in the anteroposterior plane. An assumption is made that the soft tissue profile reflects the underlying skeletal relationship. To begin the examination, the child should be seated in an upright position, looking at a distant point. Three points on the face are identified: the bridge of the nose, the base of the upper lip, and the chin.

Line segments connecting these points form an angle that describes the profile as convex, straight, or concave (Fig. 18-1). A well-balanced profile in this age group is slightly convex. A well-balanced profile in the anteroposterior dimension has an underlying skeletal relationship that is labeled class I (see Fig. 18-1, A). This terminology is used because most class I skeletal relationships also have Angle class I or end-to-end permanent first molar dental relationships and flush terminal plane or mesial step second primary molar relationships. Furthermore, the canine relationships usually will be class I, and there will be overjet

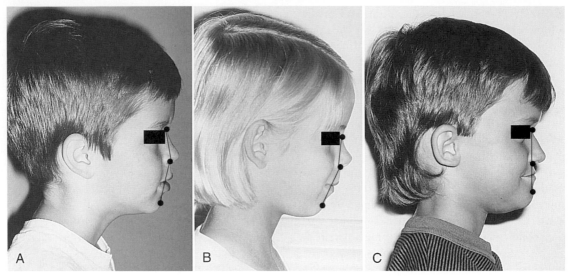

**Figure 18-1** **A,** Class I skeletal relationship is characterized by a well-balanced profile in the anteroposterior dimension. These relationships can be judged by mentally connecting the points of the bridge of the nose, the base of the upper lip (maxilla), and the soft tissue chin (mandible). This line should be slightly convex. **B,** A Class II skeletal relationship is characterized by a truly convex profile. **C,** A Class III skeletal relationship is characterized by a straight or concave profile.

of 2 to 5 mm. The Angle dental classification is described in a later section.

An assessment of the overall profile gives a general feeling for the skeletal relationships, but this evaluation does not diagnose the reason for the relationships. Some children in this age group have extremely convex profiles (see Fig. 18-1, *B*). This is consistent with a class II skeletal relationship, and these patients usually have class II permanent first molar relationships and distal step second primary molar relationships, class II canine relationships, and increased overjet. Other children have straight or concave profiles (see Fig. 18-1, *C*). These are usually found with class III permanent first molar relationships and mesial step second primary molar relationships, class III canine relationships, and negative overjet.

### Positions of the Maxilla and Mandible

If the profile is excessively convex or concave, the clinician can try to determine which skeletal component is contributing to the problem. This is a necessary step if orthodontic treatment is being considered. When one knows the problem, one can direct appropriate treatment. It is extremely rare, however, to treat an anteroposterior problem in the primary dentition.

Specifically, in this diagnostic step, the antero-posterior position of the maxilla and mandible

are determined. A vertical reference line is extended from the bridge of the nose (the anterior aspect of the cranial base), and the position of other soft tissue points is noted relative to the reference line (Fig. 18-2). If the maxilla is properly oriented relative to other skeletal structures, the base of the upper lip will be on or near the vertical line. The soft tissue chin will be slightly behind the reference line if the mandible is of proper size and in the correct position. If the maxilla is positioned significantly in front of the vertical reference line, the patient is said to exhibit maxillary protrusion. If the maxilla is substantially behind the line, the patient exhibits maxillary retrusion. The position of the mandible is described in the same way.

So, if the overall skeletal pattern is significantly convex (class II), the reason is a maxilla positioned in front of the line (maxillary protrusion), a mandible positioned behind the line (mandibular retrusion), or both. Class II skeletal relationships are sometimes caused by one jaw alone but are often the result of some combination of maxillary protrusion and mandibular retrusion.

Conversely, if the facial pattern is straight or extremely concave (class III), the reason is a maxilla positioned behind the line (maxillary retrusion), a mandible positioned in front of the line (mandibular protrusion), or both. Again,

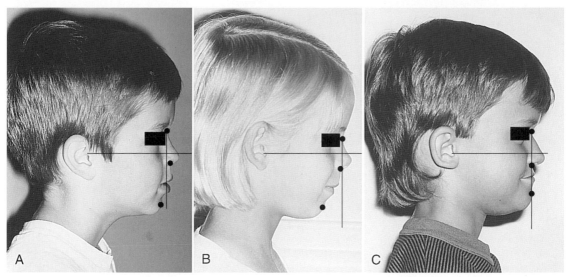

**Figure 18-2** The contributions to the skeletal malocclusion can be estimated extraorally by determining the positions of the maxilla and mandible. A perpendicular reference line is established beginning at the soft tissue bridge of the nose. The positions of the maxilla and mandible are related to this line. If the base of the upper lip and nose are anterior to this line, the maxilla is protrusive. If these points are posterior to this line, the maxilla is retrusive. Similarly, the soft tissue chin is determined to be anterior (protrusive) or posterior (retrusive) to this line. **A,** This patient has normal relationships for one younger than 6 years. **B,** This patient has a significantly convex facial profile (class II), which is contributed to by a near-normal maxilla that is near the line and a clearly retrusive mandible that is posterior to the line. **C,** This patient has a normal maxilla and a protrusive mandible.

both jaws usually contribute to the skeletal dysplasia.

Some caution must be exercised because soft tissue profile relationships do not always accurately reflect the underlying skeletal relationships. Research has shown that the 3- to 6-year age group is especially difficult to classify accurately from a profile analysis.[4] In addition, vertical facial relationships influence the anteroposterior relationships. This interaction between the horizontal and vertical planes of space and its effect on the profile is discussed later.

*Vertical Facial Relationships*
The third portion of the facial examination is an evaluation of the vertical relationships. Proportionality is judged by dividing the face into thirds. The upper third extends from approximately the hair line to the bridge of the nose, the middle third from the bridge of the nose to the base of the upper lip, and the lower third from the base of the upper lip to the bottom of the chin (Fig. 18-3). These thirds are approximately equal, or the lower third is slightly larger in well-proportioned faces.

Vertical problems tend to be manifest below the palate in the lower third of the face.[3] The short-faced person tends to have a lower facial

third that is smaller than the other thirds (see Fig. 18-3, *C*). The long-faced patient has a lower facial third that is larger than the other thirds (see Fig. 18-3, *B*).

*Lip Position*
Next we advocate an evaluation of the anteroposterior lip position to give an estimation of the anteroposterior incisor position. Incisor position is grossly reflected in lip contour and posture. Lip posture is assessed by drawing an imaginary line from the tip of the nose to the most anterior point on the soft tissue chin. The lips normally lie slightly behind this line; however, in the 3- to 6-year-old child, the lower lip is generally 1 mm anterior to the line (Fig. 18-4). Two facts must be kept in mind. First, lip protrusion is characteristic of different ethnic groups, and lips that are considered protrusive in one group may not be considered protrusive in another. For example, African-Americans and Asians tend to have more lip protrusion than do people of northern European descent. Second, the lips are evaluated in the context of the nose and chin. A large nose and chin can accommodate more protrusive lips, whereas a small nose and chin require less protrusive lips to be proportional.

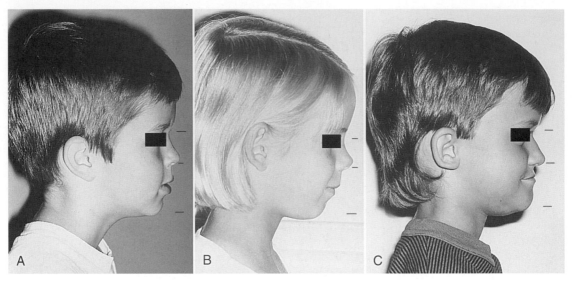

**Figure 18-3**    Vertical facial proportions can be evaluated by dividing the face into thirds and then comparing the middle third to the lower third. **A,** In a well-proportioned face, the facial thirds are equal or the lower third is slightly larger. **B,** A child with long lower facial third. **C,** A child with short vertical facial dimensions has a proportionately smaller lower facial third.

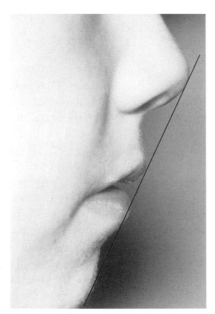

**Figure 18-4**    The anteroposterior position of the lips is determined by drawing a line from the tip of the nose to the most anterior point on the soft tissue chin. The upper lip normally should lie slightly behind the line, whereas the lower lip should lie slightly in front of this line in the 3- to 6-year-old child.

### Facial Symmetry

Transverse facial dimensions are examined to rule out true facial asymmetry. Facial symmetry is best evaluated with the patient reclined in the dental chair and the dentist seated in the 12 o'clock position. Hair is pulled away from the face, and a piece of dental floss can be stretched down the middle of the upper face to aid in judging lower face symmetry. The mandible should be either at rest or in centric relation position. Maximal intercuspation or centric occlusion positions can be affected by dental interferences during closing.

All faces show a minor degree of asymmetry, but marked asymmetry is not normal (Fig. 18-5).

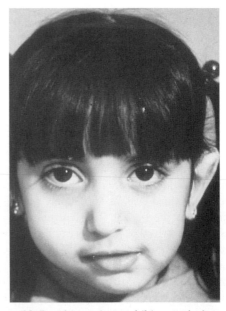

**Figure 18-5**    This patient exhibits marked asymmetry that is the result of a congenital fusion of the left condyle and coronoid process to the temporal bone.

Deviations or asymmetric positioning of the eyes, ears, or nose may be symptoms of cranial synostosis, an undiagnosed syndrome, or severe trauma. A child with these findings should be referred to appropriate professionals for a complete evaluation.

Asymmetry usually manifests in the lower facial third whereas upper facial asymmetry is extremely rare. In this age group, a deviation of the midpoint of the mandible to one side or another may be due to true asymmetry, but it is most often indicative of a posterior crossbite and mandibular shift due to a dental interference. Posterior crossbites and mandibular shifts are two findings that are discussed later in the chapter.

The maxillary dental midline should be compared with the upper facial midline. This helps determine where the midline of the mandibular teeth is relative to the face when it is compared with the upper dental midline.

## Intraoral Examination

The armamentarium for the intraoral examination includes mirror, explorer, gauze, and periodontal probe. Additional materials are disclosing solution, dental floss, toothbrush, and scaler.

The intraoral examination begins with an excursion around the oral cavity, noting its general architecture and function. The fingers should be used to identify soft tissue abnormalities of the cheeks, lips, tongue, palate, and floor of the mouth before instruments are placed in the mouth. Children in this age group often permit oral inspection with "just fingers," and the dentist can use this technique as a springboard to obtain cooperation for the use of mirror and explorer. The mirror should be the first instrument introduced. This is usually readily accepted by the child owing to its familiarity and nonthreatening shape.

Young children are sometimes uncooperative. If they are, a decision must be made early about how to manage the behavior. Parental assistance can be used to obtain an examination of the oral cavity. Use of physical restraint by the dentist without parental consent is risky and is not advisable. Parents are more likely to accept restraint in conjunction with an emergency examination than with a routine examination.

An important portion of the intraoral examination is directed to the teeth. Each of the 20 primary teeth should be explored and scrutinized visually. Selective periodontal probing may be performed, but the yield is likely to be minimal because of the infrequency of irreversible attachment loss in the primary dentition.

### Occlusal Evaluation

Another portion of the intraoral examination is the systematic analysis of the occlusion in three spatial planes. In addition, each dental arch is analyzed individually to describe arch form and symmetry, spacing and crowding, and the presence or absence of teeth. Arch analysis is best performed on diagnostic study models; however, diagnostic casts are usually not indicated in this age group unless there is some need to further study the intraoral findings or if tooth movement is contemplated.

### Alignment

Dental arches can be categorized as either U shaped or V shaped. The mandibular arch is normally U shaped, whereas the maxillary arch can be either shape. The dental arch should be symmetrical in the anteroposterior and transverse dimensions. Individual teeth are compared with their antimeres to determine if there is anteroposterior or transverse symmetry.

The ideal arch in the primary dentition has spacing between the teeth. Two types of spaces are identified. The first type, primate space, is located mesial to the maxillary canine and distal to the mandibular canine. Developmental space is the space present between the remaining teeth (Fig. 18-6). Anterior spacing is desirable in the primary dentition because the permanent incisors are larger than their primary precursors. Although the presence of primate and developmental spacing does not ensure that the permanent dentition will erupt without crowding, these spaces usually alleviate some crowding during the transition from the primary to the mixed dentition. Crowding or overlapped teeth in the primary dentition may occur, although it is rare. True crowding in the primary dentition is usually not regarded as encouraging (Fig. 18-7). Crowding of isolated teeth, however, is sometimes due to space loss or indicative of a sucking habit. Lower anterior teeth can be tipped lingually into a crowded position as a result of constant pressure from a sucking habit.

Although it seems elementary, the clinician should carefully count the number of teeth in the mouth. Children in this age group should have all their primary teeth present. Those with delayed

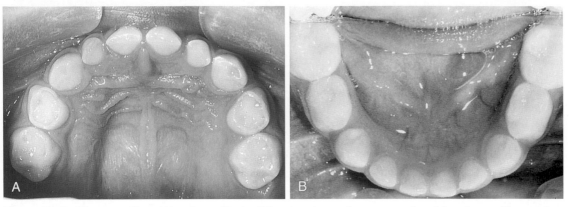

**Figure 18-6**    These maxillary (**A**) and mandibular (**B**) arches show primate spaces (mesial to the maxillary canines and distal to the mandibular canines) and developmental spacing (space between the remaining teeth).

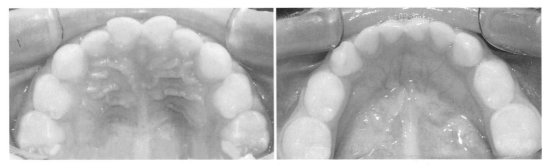

**Figure 18-7**    These maxillary (**A**) and mandibular (**B**) arches show a lack of primate and developmental spaces.

dental eruption may have either a very slow but normal sequence of eruption or some isolated eruption problem. To distinguish the two, the eruption sequence of the child is compared with the normal sequence of eruption, and the eruption pattern on the right side is compared with that on the left. If the sequence seems to be appropriate, dental development is probably slow. If, however, the patient's eruption pattern deviates from the normal sequence and there are differences between the contralateral sides of the mouth, further investigation is warranted to determine whether teeth are missing or are impeded from erupting. The maxillary lateral incisor is the most common missing tooth in the primary dentition.[9]

Counting the teeth also reveals the presence of supernumerary or extra teeth. Approximately 0.3% of children have supernumerary teeth in the primary dentition. The prevalence of fused and geminated teeth is approximately 0.1% to 0.5%.[9] One can usually distinguish fusion of two primary teeth from gemination without the aid of

radiographs by counting the number of teeth. If two teeth are fused, there should be 9 teeth in the arch, one of which is very large, rather than 10 teeth. If gemination has occurred, there should be 10 teeth in the arch and one will be very large. A radiograph may be necessary to confirm the preliminary diagnosis of fusion or gemination. Fused primary teeth show two distinct and independent pulp chambers and canals with union of the dentin. Geminated primary teeth show two crowns and two pulp chambers connected to a single root and pulp canal (Fig. 18-8).

### Anteroposterior Dimension

After the maxillary and mandibular arches have been examined for symmetry, spacing, and number of teeth, the relationship of the two arches to each other is examined. In the anteroposterior dimension, primary molar and canine relationships are determined and compared with the skeletal classification. In the primary dentition, molars are called flush terminal plane, mesial step, or distal step (Fig. 18-9). Primary canines are clas-

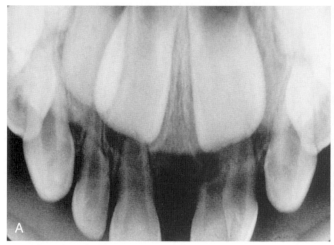
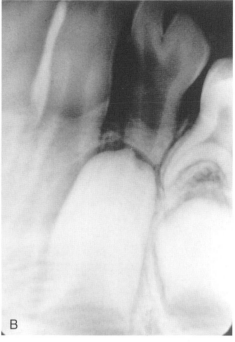

**Figure 18-8**   Supporting radiographs such as these are often necessary to distinguish fusion from gemination. **A,** These fused primary teeth are joined only at the dentin and have independent pulp chambers and canals. **B,** This geminated primary tooth has a large crown and a common pulp canal. (Photos courtesy of Dr. W. F. Vann.)

sified as class I, class II, class III, or end-to-end. These dental classifications generally reflect the skeletal classification.

Primary molar relationships, as described by the distal surfaces of the primary second molar, are worthy of attention not only because they describe the relationship of the primary mandibular teeth to the primary maxillary teeth but also because these surfaces guide the permanent molars into occlusion and determine the permanent molar relationships. Documenting primary molar relationships also allows one to follow the effects of growth or treatment.

Overjet, the horizontal overlap of the maxillary and mandibular incisors, is measured in millimeters (Fig. 18-10). It may be more helpful to describe overjet as ideal, excessive, or deficient rather than as a millimetric measure.

*Transverse Relationship*

The transverse relationship of the arches is examined for midline discrepancies and posterior crossbites. The midline of each arch is compared with the other and with the midsagittal plane. Remember that the upper midline was evaluated to the facial midline during the facial evaluation.

A large midline discrepancy is unusual in the early primary dentition, and clinicians should be suspicious of a mandibular shift. The presence of a mandibular shift is often indicative of a posterior crossbite with a centric relation to centric occlusion shift.

If a posterior crossbite is encountered, the clinician should try to determine the cause. The majority of posterior crossbites are due to constriction of the maxillary arch. This is one situation in which diagnostic casts are helpful to aid in or confirm the diagnosis. After the arch at fault is identified, an attempt is made to determine whether the crossbite is bilateral or unilateral. If models are available, they can be measured to determine whether teeth are equidistant from the midpalatal raphe. If models are not available, the determination must be made clinically. The first step is to guide the mandible into centric relation. If teeth are in crossbite on both sides of the arch when the mandible is in centric relation, the child has a bilateral crossbite. If the teeth are in crossbite on only one side of the arch when the mandible is in centric relation, the crossbite is unilateral (Fig. 18-11). It is important to check that the mandible is in centric relation because a

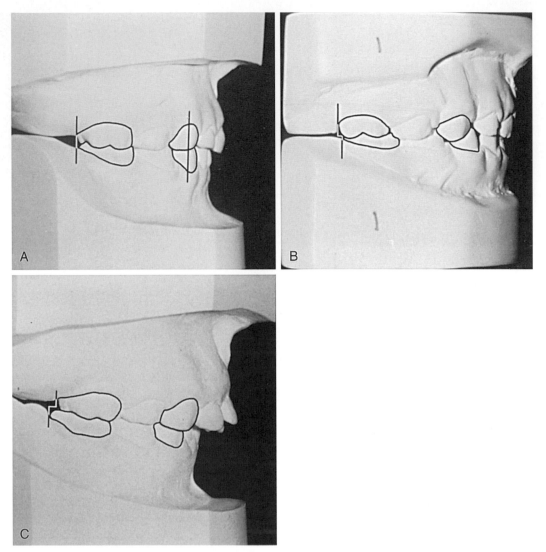

**Figure 18-9   A,** In the primary dentition, an occlusion is classified according to the relationship of the mandibular second molars and canines to the maxillary second molars and canines. In this example, the distal surface of the mandibular second molar is flush with the distal surface of the maxillary second molar. This primary molar relationship is called flush terminal plane. The long axis of the mandibular canine is coincident with the long axis of the maxillary canine. This is described as an end-to-end canine relationship. **B,** In this example, the distal surface of the mandibular molar is mesial to the distal surface of the maxillary molar. This primary molar relationship is termed mesial step. The maxillary canine is positioned in the embrasure between the mandibular canine and the first molar. This is described as a class I canine relationship. **C,** In this example, the distal surface of the mandibular molar is distal to the distal surface of the maxillary molar. This primary molar relationship is called distal step. The maxillary canine is positioned in the embrasure between the mandibular canine and the lateral incisor. This is described as a class II canine relationship.

bilateral crossbite appears to be unilateral if the mandible shifts laterally into maximal intercuspation (Fig. 18-12). The child shifts the jaw because the teeth do not fit well together, and the bite is uncomfortable because of dental interferences. A true unilateral crossbite that is due to a unilateral maxillary constriction in the primary dentition is rare but can occur.

*Vertical Dimension*

Overbite, the vertical overlap of the primary incisors, is measured and recorded in millimeters or as a percentage of the total height of the mandibular incisor crown (see Fig. 18-10) and is approximately 2 mm in the primary dentition. Deep bite is the complete or nearly complete overlap of the primary incisors. Anterior open

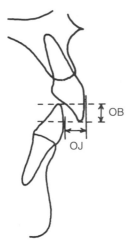

**Figure 18-10**  Overjet (OJ) is the horizontal overlap of the maxillary and mandibular central incisors and is measured from the most anterior point on the facial surfaces of these teeth. Overbite (OB) is the vertical overlap of the incisors and is measured from the incisal edge of one incisor to the other. Overbite can be recorded in millimeters or as a percentage of overlap of the total length of the mandibular incisor.

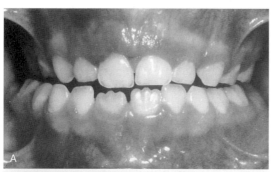

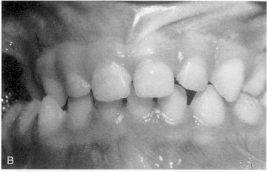

**Figure 18-11**  It is important to determine the patient's centric relation to identify the etiology of the problem and the treatment needs. **A,** This patient has a bilateral posterior crossbite when the teeth are positioned in centric relation. **B,** This patient has a unilateral posterior crossbite when the teeth are positioned in centric relation. These two patients will be approached differently for treatment.

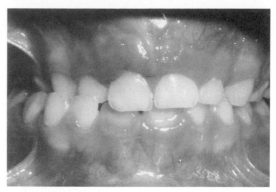

**Figure 18-12**  The same patient pictured in Figure 18-11A, with the teeth in centric occlusion. This emphasizes the importance of determining centric relation occlusion because it is the basis for most treatment decisions. Although this looks remarkably similar to the occlusion in 18-11B, the differences disclosed by the centric relation occlusion will result in different treatment.

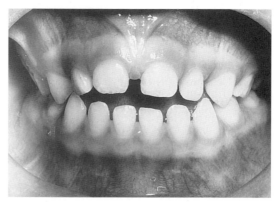

**Figure 18-13**  This patient exhibits an anterior open bite (the absence of vertical overlap). Anterior open bite, especially an asymmetric anterior open bite, is most commonly caused by a sucking habit in this age group.

bite, the absence of vertical overlap, is usually indicative of a sucking habit in this age group (Fig. 18-13). If the patient and parent deny the existence of a sucking habit, further investigation into the cause of open bite is needed. Skeletal malocclusion, ankylosed anterior teeth, condylar fracture or the sequela of trauma, and degenerative diseases such as juvenile rheumatoid arthritis may account for the open bite and should be investigated.

Ankylosis, the fusion of tooth to bone, is common in the primary dentition (Fig. 18-14). Although an ankylosed tooth cannot erupt further, the unaffected adjacent teeth will continue to erupt. This creates the illusion that the ankylosed

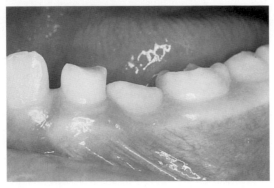

**Figure 18-14**  Ankylosis, the fusion of tooth to bone, is common in the primary dentition. This patient has an ankylosed primary mandibular first molar that is below the plane of occlusion.

tooth is submerged in the bone. The prevalence of ankylosed teeth is between 7% and 14% in the primary dentition.[2,5] In addition, 50% of patients with an ankylosed tooth have more than one ankylosis. The following is a list of the most commonly ankylosed teeth in the primary dentition:[2]

1. Mandibular primary first molar
2. Mandibular primary second molar
3. Maxillary primary first molar
4. Maxillary primary second molar

A number of eruption and exfoliation problems have been blamed on ankylosed teeth. However, longitudinal studies indicate that ankylosed primary teeth exfoliate normally and allow normal eruption of succedaneous teeth.[5,6] An ankylosed tooth discovered during this developmental stage should not be removed routinely unless a large marginal ridge discrepancy develops between it and the unaffected adjacent teeth. If a marginal ridge discrepancy develops, the adjacent teeth may tip into the space occupied by the ankylosed tooth and cause space loss.

## SUPPLEMENTAL ORTHODONTIC DIAGNOSTIC TECHNIQUES

If diagnostic casts are necessary, an appropriate impression tray must be chosen. Properly fitted trays seat comfortably in the mouth and extend far enough posteriorly to cover the most distal tooth and either the maxillary tuberosity or the mandibular retromolar pad. The trays should be of a nonperforated variety that hold the impres-

sion material and express the excess material into the vestibule. Expression of the excess material into the vestibule is desirable because it displaces the soft tissues, which allows the dentoalveolar morphology to be clearly viewed on the cast. The trays also can be lined with wax, which aids in tissue displacement and makes seating the tray into position more comfortable.

After the appropriate tray has been selected, the alginate is mixed and placed in one tray. For either arch, the tray should be rotated laterally into the mouth and firmly seated, first posteriorly against the palate or the retromolar pad. This technique limits the posterior flow of alginate and forces excess alginate anteriorly and laterally. The tray is then rotated and seated over the anterior teeth. Finally, the tray is held in place until the alginate has set. After the upper and lower impressions are obtained, a wax bite is made by placing a softened piece of baseplate wax between the teeth and having the patient close in centric occlusion. The wax is cooled with air and serves to orient the casts properly during trimming.

Impressions should be wrapped in moist paper towels and stored in sealed plastic bags or poured soon in white plaster because the alginate will dehydrate and distort if exposed for more than a few minutes. The plaster is thoroughly mixed usually using a vacuum spatulator to reduce bubbles and then vibrated into the impression and flowed from one tooth to another to prevent air entrapment, which results in holes in the models. Separate plaster bases are poured, and the impressions are inverted on the bases when the plaster is partially set. After the plaster has set, the trays are carefully separated from the casts to prevent breaking of the teeth.

The maxillary cast is trimmed so that the top of the base is parallel to the occlusal plane. The back of the upper cast is trimmed perpendicular to its top and the midpalatal raphe. The maxillary and mandibular casts are occluded, and the back of the mandibular base is trimmed parallel to the top of the maxillary cast. Finally, the sides of the casts are trimmed symmetrically, which allows the clinician to judge arch symmetry (Fig. 18-15). For a discussion of digital casts, see Chapter 30.

### Radiographic Evaluation

The dentist requires radiographs to make a thorough diagnosis or problem list in the 3- to 6-year-old child. Children in this age range may find it

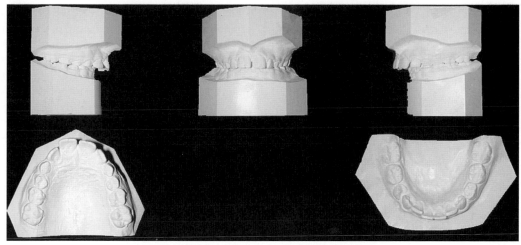

**Figure 18-15** Well-trimmed diagnostic casts can aid in the evaluation of intra- and interarch occlusal problems and serve as documentation of a patient's pretreatment status when evaluating treatment of growth changes.

difficult to cooperate with the radiographic procedures, in which case the radiographic examination should be deferred until behavior improves or can be managed. Introduction of the child to intraoral radiography can be managed as discussed in Box 18-1.

For the primary dentition, no radiographs are indicated when all proximal surfaces can be visu-

alized and examined clinically. When the proximal surfaces cannot be visualized and clinically examined, bitewing radiographs are indicated to determine the presence of interproximal caries (Fig. 18-16). Other projections are indicated in the following circumstances: history of pain, swelling, trauma, mobility of teeth, unexplained bleeding, disrupted eruption pattern, or deep

---

### BOX 18-1

#### Introducing a Child to Intraoral Radiography

1. Use a tell-show-do introduction with a camera analogy. It helps to do a dry run, showing an unexposed packet of film and an exposed radiograph to explain the process. By positioning the film and the x-ray machine, the dentist can also determine whether a child will cooperate for an exposure, preventing unproductive irradiation.

2. Match film size to comfort. Many children have difficulty with the film impinging on the lingual soft tissue of the mandible. In some cases, bending the anterior corners helps, but this may lower the diagnostic quality of the radiograph. Another technique is to place the film vertically to minimize anteroposterior size.

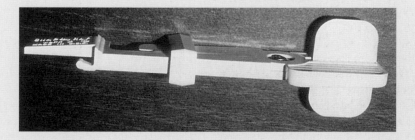

3. Obtain the least difficult radiograph first to acquaint the child with the procedures. Anterior occlusal films are usually easiest.

4. Be certain that all settings are made on the

machine and that the apparatus is positioned before positioning the film. Some children can hold a film for only a short period because of the gag reflex, discomfort, or a short attention span.

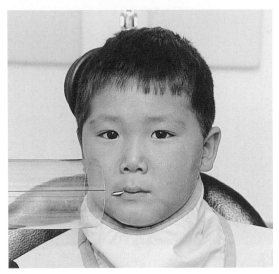

**Figure 18-16**  The proper technique for obtaining a posterior bitewing radiograph (no. 0 film) is critical because it is used frequently. The tube head should have a vertical angulation of +10 degrees and a horizontal angulation such that the face of the cone is parallel to the film packet with the beam directed to the open embrasures. The film packet should be placed lingual to the teeth with the child biting on the tab. The film should be placed anteriorly to obtain a view of the distal surfaces of the canines. Asking the child to smile so as to show the teeth often helps to orient the beam and prevents overlap.

carious lesions.[8] These views include the maxillary (Fig. 18-17, *A*) and mandibular (Fig. 18-17, *B*) periapical views and the maxillary (Fig. 18-17, *C*) and mandibular (Fig. 18-17, *D*) occlusal views.

An occlusal-sized film can be used to obtain a lateral jaw radiograph in children of this age if needed to identify pathosis and if a panoramic film is not obtainable. The lateral jaw film can be made by having the child hold the film or lie on his or her side, as shown in Figure 18-18.

Pediatric (0 size) films should be used most often, with the exception of the occlusal films, which are no. 2 size. The Snap-a-Ray (Rinn Corporation, Elgin, Ill.) device has been used for film positioning in this age group with great success because of its small size and light weight. Other positioning instruments can be used, but some thought should be given to the size and weight of the instrument that must be placed intraorally. The patient should be adequately protected from unnecessary radiation. A lead apron and collar are necessary to provide thyroid and gonadal protection. A 16-inch or longer cone

further reduces skin exposure. Ideally, rectangular collimation should be used, but movement by children of this age may result in less than ideal radiographs with an extremely truncated beam. Prior to exposure of the radiographs, the ability of the child to cooperate must be assessed to prevent unnecessary radiation exposure. When parents assist, they must be adequately shielded, pregnancy must be ruled out, and the parent must demonstrate the ability to stabilize the film and patient before exposure.[10] Dental personnel should refrain from holding films because of the risks of repeated exposure.

A concerned parent may ask about frequency of films. The American Academy of Pediatric Dentistry[1] advises the use of radiographic exposure at a rate necessary to maximize detection of abnormalities yet minimize exposure to ionizing radiation. Table 18-4 lists selection criteria for pediatric radiographs in the 3- to 6-year-old child. All radiographs should be made only after a clinical examination and history have been completed.

## TREATMENT PLANNING FOR NONORTHODONTIC PROBLEMS

The process of diagnosis of disease is a complicated one based on clinical, historical, and supportive data. A problem list may be preferable to a series of diagnoses because the list represents a presumption that treatment will be provided. A synthesis of all data is required. The practical portions of the diagnostic process consider the following:

1. Existence of an abnormal state
2. Determination of cause
3. Alternatives or options to correct the problem
4. Anticipated benefits, immediate and long term
5. Problems or requirements for accomplishing treatment

A primary consideration is denoting an abnormal state, such as caries or a nonvital pulp. A problem list helps to separate those abnormalities that are in need of management from those that are simply identified. For example, a carious primary molar in a 6-year-old is a problem; a loose carious mandibular incisor may not be if it is

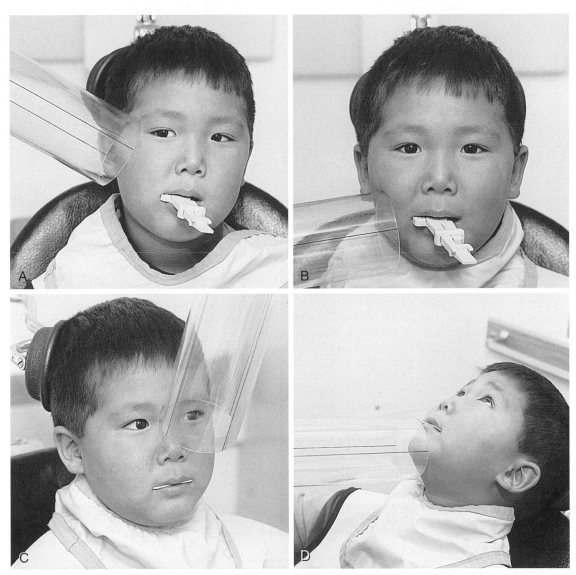

**Figure 18-17**   The following techniques are commonly used to obtain supplementary views. **A,** Maxillary periapical view (no. 0 film). Vertical angulation: Beam at right angle to film; starting angle of +30 degrees. Horizontal angulation: Face of cone parallel to facial surface of teeth. Film placement: With film in jaw of holder, holder is placed between the maxillary and mandibular teeth with dimpled surface of film against the lingual surfaces of teeth. Child bites on larger sides of jaws. **B,** Mandibular periapical view (no. 0 film). Vertical angulation: Beam at right angle to film; starting angle of ~5 degrees. Horizontal angulation: Face of cone parallel to facial surface of teeth. Film placement: With film in jaws of holder, holder is placed between the maxillary and mandibular teeth with dimpled surface of film against the lingual surfaces of teeth. Child bites on larger sides of jaws. **C,** Maxillary occlusal view (no. 2 film). Vertical angulation: +60 degrees, with beam directed downward. Horizontal angulation: Beam directed along midsagittal plane. Film placement: Film packet is placed between maxillary and mandibular teeth so that it is parallel to floor. Film is oriented so that the long dimension extends to the right and left. The child bites gently on the film while seated upright. **D,** Mandibular occlusal view (no. 2 film). Vertical angulation: ~15 degrees, with beam directed upward. Horizontal angulation: Beam directed along midsagittal plane. Film placement: Film packet is placed between the maxillary and mandibular teeth, and child is instructed to bite gently on the film. Patient is reclining so that the chin is extended. Bisecting angle technique is used.

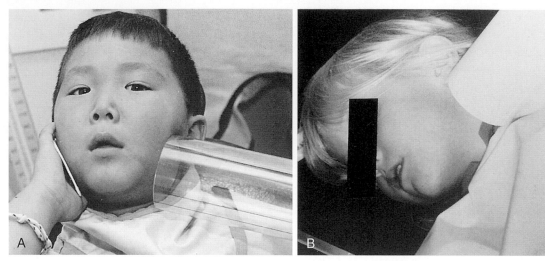

**Figure 18-18**    Lateral jaw techniques. **A,** Child is seated upright with head tilted approximately 20 degrees. Film packet is held or taped across area to be exposed. Beam is directed from side opposite film through the tissues at about −10 degrees. The central beam is directed perpendicular to the film and is aimed at the center of the film. **B,** This technique can be used for an active child or a patient with cerebral palsy. The dental chair is reclined, and the patient lies on one side with the head tilted. Pillows can be used to stabilize the body and head. The film is placed between the child and the chair, and the beam angulation is adjusted accordingly.

about to exfoliate. Identification of the cause of the abnormality is critical to determine short- and long-term treatment. A manageable cause most often results in both short- and long-term success. Caries is a largely environmental condition that can be managed with great likelihood of success in both the short and long term. On the other hand, dentinogenesis imperfecta is genetic and has a guarded and limited prognosis.

For most patients, no single treatment plan is ideal. A variety of alternatives must be considered and based on the child's health, cooperation,

---

### TABLE 18-4
#### Selection Criteria and Guidelines for Pediatric Radiographs in the 3- to 6-Year-Old Child

| PROJECTION | CRITERIA | FREQUENCY |
|---|---|---|
| Posterior bitewing | Proximal surfaces of posterior teeth cannot be examined clinically<br>Child is cooperative | At initial examination if contacts closed<br>Semi-annually if interproximal surfaces have been restored, until child achieves low-risk status* or is caries-free; also semi-annually if child is at high risk*<br>Annually to 24-month interval if child is caries-free at initial bitewing examination |
| Posterior periapical | Suspected pathosis<br>Confirmed pathosis<br>Child is cooperative | As needed to diagnose and monitor treatment or patient condition |
| Anterior occlusal | Suspected pathosis<br>Confirmed pathosis<br>Child is cooperative | Same as above |

Excerpted from The Selection of Patients for X-Ray Examinations: Dental Radiographic Examinations. VSDHHS, PHS, FDA (HHS Publication FDA 88-8273), US Government Printing Office, Washington, DC, 1988.
*High risk for dental caries may be associated with (1) poor oral hygiene, (2) fluoride deficiency, (3) prolonged or inappropriate nursing, (4) high-carbohydrate diet, (5) poor family dental health, (6) developmental enamel defects, (7) developmental disability or acute medical problem, or (8) genetic abnormality.

# Patients with Special Health Care Needs
*Paul S. Casamassimo*

Care of special-needs patients is a responsibility shared by general dentists and pediatric dental specialists. By definition, pediatric dentistry is the specialty charged with care of the special child. As is the case with dentistry for all children, however, the general dentist cares for the vast majority of persons with disabilities and chronic illnesses. In addition, children with disabilities grow and need to transition into the adult care community.

A basic skill set for the dentist who wants to commit to care of special patients includes the following:

1. Knowledge of the medical elements of conditions in order to understand the biological processes and therapies that may affect oral health delivery, such as congenital heart disease
2. Knowledge of oral health implications of conditions, such as precocious periodontal disease in Down syndrome or gingival overgrowth in transplantation patients
3. Essential management skills to communicate with, stabilize, and manage patients in the care setting
4. Awareness of the social, therapeutic, and cultural milieu of those with special health care needs

A functional or problem-oriented view of dental care for the special patient offers a way for dentists to organize education, staff training, and integration of these patients into a practice. The functional view establishes a number of problem areas or obstacles to care that must be addressed before the special patient can be treated successfully. These problem areas are not unique to patients with special health care needs but occur more often and in constellations with persons with disabilities and chronic illnesses. For example, many patients, whether disabled or not, experience fear or difficulty in connection with paying for care. Many patients bring with them chronic or short-term medical problems that are acquired during their life with a practice. The disabled patient may cluster a number of problem areas, some of which may be severe, and challenge the practice's ability to keep that patient in the practice family. On the other hand, in today's world, with aging baby boom and burgeoning elderly populations, with the Americans with Disabilities Act, and with continuing advances in medical care, the black-and-white concept of disabled versus nondisabled is blurring. Every dentist can count those fragile elderly persons, children with learning disabilities or asthma, and adults with acquired

heart disease on multiple medications in their practice family.

The specific terminology of problem areas or obstacles may vary by author, but the following summary should suffice to explain the basic concepts and give the motivated clinician a start in developing a practice philosophy and method.

1. *Accessibility*: The person with a disability experiences physical, mental, and system-wide obstacles to access. The most overt would be an architectural barrier. More subtle are attitudes of staff, community transportation limits, and office decoration that blocks access, confuses the poorly sighted, or inhibits wheelchairs, walkers, or canes. An office "accessibility audit," perhaps conducted by a person who is disabled, can point out overt and hidden obstacles.

2. *Psychosocial*: The person with special care needs may develop in an environment of chronic care, painful procedures, and emphasis on aspects of health other than dentistry. Families may be preoccupied with a disability, ignoring oral health. The clinician may be faced with a high-anxiety, low-dental-IQ patient and family.

3. *Financial*: Cost of dental care is an issue for many patients. Persons with special health care needs may not have incomes yet be beset with competing medical costs. Such individuals may qualify for public assistance, yet these programs often reimburse at rates that discourage dentist participation. The practice committed to care of special-needs patients will learn about public and private programs, work with families, and develop realistic treatment plans.

4. *Communication*: The dentist-patient chairside relationship demands a functional communication cycle of both parties involving input, processing, and output. The patient with special needs may have compromised senses (input), have intellectual limitations (processing), or have speech difficulties (output). Less obvious may be the compromises the dentist contributes such as equipment noise (input), preoccupation with a dental procedure (processing), and use of dental terminology (output). Effective chairside communication may require the sophistication of a signing interpreter or the simplicity of a pad and pencil.

5. *Medical*: Special health needs often translate to chronic illness and polypharmacy. Dentists are faced with pathologic processes and therapeutic procedures that present risks for the patient and complicate treatment. Congenital heart disease, drug interactions, and susceptibility to infection are

## Patients with Special Health Care Needs—cont'd

just a few of the overlying concerns the special-needs population brings to dental practice.

6. *Mobility and stability*: Dental offices are designed for fully functional human beings, but many individuals who would describe themselves as such have difficulty in positioning, reclining for long periods, or even fitting in the contours of the chair. Some patients with special needs require stabilization, support, and assistance entering or leaving the dental chair.

7. *Preventive*: Basic oral hygiene home care may have to be supplemented with fluoride rinses, antimicrobials, saliva substitutes, and other adjunctives. Special-needs patients may need special instruction for self-care, and the dentist's problem-solving skills are called into play. Again, the continuum of "special need" includes the child with cerebral palsy as well as the healthy adult on saliva-reducing medication.

8. *Treatment planning*: The ideal treatment plan is the one that is right for that patient. The special-needs patient may need and want treatment that balances cost, longevity, difficulty of achievement, aesthetics, and function. These principles are common to all patients, but with special-needs patients the combination often challenges conventional thinking.

9. *Continuity of care*: A crisis often brings the special-needs patient to the dentist, and the myriad of problems such an individual experiences can force him or her into oral neglect. The culture of special-needs care brings together a variety of professionals concerned with the health of these patients, and dentistry must sit at this table. Similarly, dentists must expand outside the cottage-care concept and utilize the physical therapist, psychologist, medical subspecialist, and other nondental professionals in achieving dental treatment goals.

Dentistry as a health science must be available for all patients no matter how extreme their special needs. In the development of the specialist in pediatric dentistry it is implied that an essential feature of that educational growth be directed to understanding and giving care to special-needs children. Generalists find this domain of dentistry to be challenging and one that requires additional knowledge and skills above and beyond their dental education.

Although the work is challenging, the gratifying emotional rewards of taking care of patients with special needs are difficult to describe. The dentistry rendered is also received by the caretakers of these patients with vast appreciation for the dentist and the dental staff.

---

parental finances, and the anticipated benefits to be derived from the treatment. These issues are shared by dentist and parent. For example, extraction of decayed primary teeth may be preferred to restoration if pulpal therapy is likely to be unsuccessful. Another example is the choice of a stainless steel crown rather than a three-surface amalgam restoration in a decay-prone person because fewer surfaces will be left exposed to recurrent decay.

A frank assessment of the cooperation and involvement in the child's treatment by the family must be considered. Dental treatment is necessarily a cooperative effort, with success resting on both personal and professional maintenance. The behavioral plan is critical to the success of the treatment plan in general. For the 3- to 6-year-old child, the methods of behavior management to be used must be included in the treatment plan. The sequencing of behavior management, obtainment of consent for medications, and reasonable alter-

natives to recommended procedures should be covered in discussion of the behavioral plan with the parents. Some dentists prefer to explain and obtain consent for all behavior procedures they might be liable to use at the initial case presentation.

Generally, acute infection and pain are managed first. Hopelessly involved teeth should be extracted, although this is a rude introduction to dental care for the young child. If numerous large lesions are present, they may be excavated and interim restorations placed. Use of glass ionomer cement offers some additional preventive benefit with its fluoride release. This "first aid" approach reduces the chance of decay progression with resultant pain and reduces the difficulty in cleaning while reducing the deleterious oral flora. If deep lesions and chronically pulpally involved teeth are not painful, they can be incorporated in a treatment plan that proceeds by quadrant or sextant.

## Early Caries Detection
*James S. Wefel*

Traditional caries detection is based on the Radike technique, which includes visual, tactile, and radiographic analyses. The explorer, for example, is used to determine the extent of the obvious visual lesions. It can also be used quite aggressively to identify defects and incipiences. With an increase in our understanding of the caries process, such as the knowledge that subsurface lesions may remineralize, a less aggressive approach in probing is now advocated. The consensus is that one could compromise the relatively intact surface and spread bacteria from one tooth or site to another with aggressive probing. This is an example of the profession trying to move from the surgical to the medical model in the management of dental caries. It has also led to a desire to manage the disease process with a preservative or preventive dentistry approach; therefore the need for risk assessment and early caries detection becomes obvious. This has led to a reevaluation of our current visual, tactile, and radiographic approach as well as investigations into the use of newer diagnostic aids. The explosion of research in this area of diagnostic aids has resulted in studies of the validity and reliability of these techniques to measure tissue changes occurring prior to the traditional detection of "holes in teeth." This is critical for early intervention and a reduction in the need for restorative procedures.

These caries detection techniques include:

1. Electrical conductivity measurements (ECM)
2. Laser fluorescence using the Diagnodent unit (KaVo-IR)
3. Ultrasound measurements (UM)
4. Quantitative light fluorescence (QLF)
5. Optical coherence tomography (OCT)
6. Fiberoptic transillumination (FOTI)
7. Digital imaging fiberoptic transillumination (DIFOTI)
8. Direct digital radiography (DDR)

These techniques are currently being refined, tested for reliability in vitro and in vivo, and tested for validity against a gold standard. The data are not all in as to which techniques may be applicable in the near future and which have been able to be adapted for practical clinical use. Currently available in the marketplace are an ECM unit, DIFOTI, QLF, and KaVo-IR (Diagnodent) devices. Potential problems remain such as restricted access to various surfaces, plaque presence as a confounder, initial versus significant demineralization, wet versus dried surfaces, and so forth. Thus the applicability to measure all surfaces is limited as is the capability to detect minor tissue changes as well as severe tissue changes with one methodologic approach. The need to redefine "caries" as measurable "tissue change" and not the traditional "cavitated lesion" is necessary to make the most of a preventive or preservative dentistry model. Each investigator may have a different view as to the level or the time at which caries should be detected. The epidemiologist needs a method to monitor disease at an earlier point than cavitation, whereas the clinician may desire an adjunct in diagnosing active disease necessitating restoration. The ideal technique will allow the clinician to detect the earliest change in the tissue, to follow lesion progression through the white-spot lesion stage, to aid in the decision for restorative treatment, and to detect secondary caries around the restoration. Current techniques are striving to these ends.

### REFERENCES

1. Stookey GK, editor: *Early Detection of Caries. Proceedings of First Annual Indiana Conference.* Held in May 1996. Cincinnati, Ohio, Sidney Printing Work, 1997.
2. Stookey GK, editor: *Early Detection of Dental Caries II. Proceedings of Fourth Indiana Conference.* Held in May 1999. Cincinnati, Ohio, SpringDot, 2000.

All factors being equal, restorative care often is easiest in the maxillary posterior areas. The infiltration injections are easiest for the patients to tolerate. One can then move to the mandibular posterior sextants. Seldom are the mandibular anterior teeth involved unless rampant decay is present.

Finally, the maxillary anterior teeth can be approached. This is a good final selection because the injections are uncomfortable, and some families will not pursue necessary care if the maxillary anterior teeth are restored first and aesthetics are good.

When restorative care is complete and the patient and parent demonstrate that they can maintain good oral health, orthodontic care, whether active or space maintenance, can be considered. It is best if space maintenance can be implemented in the first 6 months after necessary extractions because space loss is most common during this period.

# REFERENCES

1. American Academy of Pediatric Dentistry: *Oral Health Policies: Dental Radiographs in Children.* Chicago, The Academy, 1985.
2. Brearly IL, McKibben DH: Ankylosis of primary molar teeth: parts I and II. *J Dent Child* 40:54-63, 1973.
3. Fields HW, Proffit WR, Nixon WL et al: Facial pattern differences in long-faced children and adults. *Am J Orthod* 85:217-223, 1984.
4. Fields HW, Vann WF: Prediction of dental and skeletal relationships from facial profiles in pre-school children. *Pediatr Dent* 1:7-15, 1979.
5. Kurol J, Koch G: The effect of extraction on infraoccluded deciduous molars: a longitudinal study. *Am J Orthod* 87:46-55, 1985.
6. Messer LB, Cline JT: Ankylosed primary molars: results and treatment recommendations from an eight-year longitudinal study. *Pediatr Dent* 2:37-47, 1980.
7. Pfefferle JC, Machen JB, Fields HW, Posnick WR: Child behavior in the dental setting relative to parental presence. *Pediatr Dent* 4:311-316, 1982.
8. University of Texas Dental School at San Antonio: *Pediatric Dentistry Radiography: Early Eruptive Stage (5 Years and Under).* San Antonio, The University, 1987.
9. Valachovic RW, Lurie AG: Risk-benefit considerations in pedodontic radiology. *Pediatr Dent* 2:128-146, 1980.
10. White SC: Radiation exposure in pediatric dentistry: current standards in pedodontic radiology with suggestions for alternatives. *Pediatr Dent* 3:441-447, 1982.

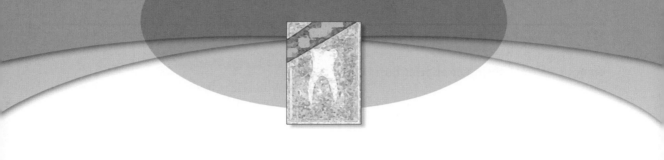

# CHAPTER 19
## Prevention of Dental Disease

*Arthur Nowak and James J. Crall*

With the complete eruption of all primary teeth, the preschool child enters a relatively short period of dental stability in preparation for the loss of the first primary tooth and the lengthy process of eruption of the permanent teeth. Historically, many preschoolers' first dental examination has occurred during this period; however there is growing recognition that a dental home should be established much earlier for all children, and especially for high-risk children. Instructions are provided for appropriate oral hygiene techniques and topical fluoride use. Adjustments in optimal systemic fluoride supplementation should be considered if the child is not living in a fluoridated community and is at high risk.

Dietary management may now become a problem. This is the period of development of strong preferences for and aversions to specific foods. The effect of commercials from television, radio, and the press begins to take its toll. Children are frequently sent to a childcare facility for a quasi-educational experience, a baby-sitting service, or a true preschool developmental experience. Meals may be prepared by surrogate parents, lunches may be packed by parents to be consumed later, snacks may be provided by peers or care providers, and control of the quality and quantity of the diet is sometimes greatly sacrificed.

With the end of the day in sight and the "I want to watch just one more TV program" routine common, the daily supervised oral hygiene routine may be sacrificed for the quick 30-second unsupervised brushing. It is amazing how quickly parents assume that 4-year-old children can be responsible for their own oral hygiene when they cannot even comb their hair or print their name clearly.

## FLUORIDE ADMINISTRATION

### Dietary Fluoride Supplementation

Steps to ensure an optimal dietary intake of fluoride should continue to be a primary concern with children 3 to 6 years of age. For children who do not have access to fluoridated drinking water, this means continuing to provide adequate fluoride supplementation. By age 3 most children are able to chew and swallow tablets; therefore, prescriptions for supplemental fluoride should be changed accordingly to reflect this change in developmental status. The recommended supplemental fluoride dosage schedule also requires an increase in the amount of fluoride prescribed after a child reaches 3 years of age. The recommended daily dosage of supplemental fluoride for children aged 3 to 6 is 0.5 mg for those whose drinking water contains less than 0.3 ppm of fluoride and 0.25 mg for those whose water contains between 0.3 and 0.6 ppm. Children whose drinking water contains more than 0.6 ppm of fluoride do not require any supplementation. Although the potential for producing dental fluorosis on permanent anterior teeth will have diminished in this age group owing to substantial crown formation, the practice of analyzing samples of each child's drinking water prior to prescribing supplemental fluoride should continue. Analysis can be requested from the local public health department, family dentist, or commercial laboratories.

Because parental compliance continues to play a key role in determining the effectiveness of these supplements, efforts to reinforce parental motivation should be made. One method of assessing parental compliance is to monitor the need to rewrite supplemental fluoride prescriptions at recall visits. The dosage of fluoride prescribed should be noted in each patient's record whenever a prescription is written. Parents who indicate no need for an additional prescription when the patient's record suggests that the previously prescribed supplement should have been consumed should be questioned about the number of tablets remaining. A large existing supply suggests poor compliance during the period prior to the recall visit.

### Topical Fluoride Therapy

Topical fluorides have an increasingly important role in the 3- to 6-year-old group. The child's ability to use fluoride dentifrices increases throughout this period, although restraint in the amount of toothpaste used at each brushing should continue. Professional topical applications are often initiated during this interval. One mode of topical application that is generally not recommended for the younger members of this age group is the use of fluoride mouth rinses because most preschoolers are unable to avoid swallowing some of these solutions.

### Professional Applications of Fluoride

Topical application of highly concentrated forms of fluoride has been provided in clinical settings for 50 years. The most commonly used agents have included 8% to 10% solutions of stannous fluoride as well as 2% sodium fluoride and 1.23% acidulated phosphate fluoride (APF), the latter two compounds being available in solution, gel, and foam formulations. Numerous studies conducted prior to 1980 reported caries reductions averaging approximately 30% following use of these agents.[4,17] However, several studies, including a large-scale national demonstration program,[3] have reported a more limited effect from semiannual applications of these agents (i.e., caries reductions of roughly 25%), especially in fluoridated areas.[5] Fluoride varnish has become a popular topical agent for preschool children and children with special health care needs, and has been recommended for conditions in which decalcified enamel secondary to poor plaque removal or poor feeding practices is present.[21,25]

### Indications for Professional Topical Fluoride Applications

The questions of when and for whom topical application of fluoride should be provided in the dental office are the source of some controversy. One school of thought invokes the argument that professional fluoride application is a primary preventive measure and should be provided to all children to minimize the potential for development of new carious lesions. Part of the historical basis for this approach relates to the lack heretofore of validated methods to predict whether an individual patient is likely to develop caries.

Advocates of this philosophy tend to focus only on the potential benefits that might be achieved from topical fluoride application while ignoring the costs associated with providing the service.

Others feel that the decision to provide topical fluoride therapy should be based on the factors that have been shown to be associated with the risk of developing caries in groups or in individuals (e.g., access to fluoridated drinking water, use of other forms of topical fluoride, degree of spacing between teeth). Their approach is to consider the likelihood that each patient develops disease according to these factors and then to recommend professional topical fluoride therapy for those considered to be at significant risk for developing caries. Proponents of this philosophy tend to consider the costs associated with providing the service as well as the potential benefits.

The validity of the second approach obviously depends on the degree of accuracy with which one is able to predict which persons are more likely to experience caries. Several approaches aimed at differentiating high-risk from low-risk patients have recently been developed but as yet have not been rigorously evaluated.[1,7] As methods of caries prediction are refined over time, the argument for individualizing preventive treatments is likely to become increasingly compelling.

## Cost-Benefit Considerations

In a private practice setting the patient's willingness or ability to pay for different forms of treatment usually is an important factor in determining what types of services are provided. In the case of public programs or private third-party payors, the decision to provide reimbursement for various services may be based on a more formal analysis of the relationship between the costs and benefits associated with those services. The ratio of costs to benefits has historically been higher for topical fluoride applications provided in dental offices than for other types of preventive services or for the same services provided in other settings. Consequently, professional topical fluoride treatments have not been recommended as a public health measure because of their unfavorable cost-benefit ratio. Documented changes in caries levels and patterns of decay in children in the United States have pushed these ratios even higher. Specifically, four large-scale studies[3,10,14,15] have reported that a substantial proportion of

school-aged children in the United States are caries free and that a relatively small percentage of children account for a large percentage of all tooth decay.[24] Also, in addition to the overall decline in the level of caries, there has been a decrease in the proportion of smooth-surface caries and a corresponding increase in the proportion of pit and fissure caries. The combination of these factors seems to be associated with a reduction in the effectiveness of concentrated topical fluoride therapy in terms of the actual number of surfaces saved from becoming carious during a given period.[3]

Changes of this nature have led some interested parties to call for a reexamination of the manner in which various preventive measures are provided. In an era when increased attention is being focused on measures for controlling all types of health care costs, some have proposed that consideration be given to making preventive dental services more cost effective. One means of improving the cost-benefit ratio of topical fluoride therapy would be to provide this therapy in settings other than dental offices (e.g., at school or in the home) by self-application techniques. Another previously mentioned method that could also apply to preventive services provided in dental offices would be to identify patients who are more likely to develop caries and target preventive services to those individuals.

A factor that has been repeatedly demonstrated to be associated with a reduction in both the risk of developing caries and the relative effectiveness of topical fluoride therapy is the availability of drinking water containing fluoride. Studies have shown that topical fluorides are considerably more effective in reducing the incidence of decay in nonfluoridated areas compared with fluoridated areas.[5] Therefore, the cost of preventing a carious lesion in a fluoridated area by means of professional topical fluoride therapy is significantly greater than the cost of preventing a lesion in a nonfluoridated area. From a cost-benefit perspective, this suggests that in fluoridated areas topical fluoride treatments should be reserved for patients who have a history of moderate to high caries development or who belong to proven high-risk categories.[5] Those who do not seem to be particularly prone to developing caries, especially smooth-surface decay, would probably benefit more from other forms of prevention such as occlusal sealants.

The question of which preventive services should be provided for a particular child in the dental office remains an individual issue for dentists and their patients (or parents in the case of children). Accordingly, the final decision about professional preventive services must be made by the child's parents based on informed consideration of costs and expected benefits. However, the influence of third-party coverage for different types of services can significantly affect this decision and ultimately the care received by the child.

## Prophylaxis Prior to Topical Fluoride Treatment

Another issue related to the effectiveness of professional topical fluoride therapy, which also has implications for lowering the cost-benefit ratio, concerns the need for the prophylaxis that has traditionally been provided prior to fluoride application. Research in both laboratory and clinical settings has shown that the ability of a variety of topical fluoride agents to penetrate dental plaque and deposit fluoride in the enamel is not significantly reduced by the presence of an organic layer on the tooth surface.[9,11,22] This concept has been tested further in a 3-year clinical study that demonstrated that the effectiveness of a professionally administered APF gel treatment in preventing caries was not influenced by prior prophylaxis.[18]

It has been pointed out that elimination of the prophylaxis could significantly reduce the labor cost of delivering topical fluoride treatments.[5] The practical implications of these findings in terms of a dental office are (1) that the decision to provide thorough prophylaxis, less rigorous cleaning (i.e., toothbrushing prior to fluoride treatment), or no cleaning prior to fluoride treatment can be made individually, depending on the condition of the patient, and (2) that several children could be treated simultaneously, thereby reducing the time and cost of the procedure.[17]

Some persons insist that prophylaxis is an excellent way to introduce children to the sensations associated with the use of a handpiece in the mouth. Others point out that cleaning the teeth prior to an examination makes for a more thorough assessment. While both appear to be valid considerations, the practitioner should realize that elimination of this step does not appear to adversely affect the caries protection provided by topical fluoride therapy in most cases.

## Methods of Application

The most popular professional topical fluoride agents in use today are APF and sodium fluoride. APF was developed as a solution containing 1.23% fluoride at pH 3.2.[5] For decades fluoride varnish has been used in Europe and Scandinavia for topical application. Recent studies show that fluoride varnish is as effective as a gel in preventing approximal lesions.[21] Less time is required to place the varnish, and therefore the treatment may be more cost effective than the use of gel.

Applications of APF or sodium fluoride should be provided to at-risk patients semiannually in disposable polystyrene trays via a gel or foam as a vehicle. The recommended application time for both APF and sodium fluoride is 4 minutes. Manufacturers of foam products suggest a 1-minute application, although clinical data on the effectiveness of this approach generally are lacking.[5] Most studies report the use of 4-minute applications of topical fluoride gel or foam. Enamel uptake is similar with both types at 4 minutes, but when foam is used, about one fifth the amount is used. This reduces fluoride retention by the patient and potential postapplication side effects.[26]

Advantages of the foam or gel tray systems include (1) generally good patient acceptance, (2) a relatively long shelf-life of the agents, (3) control over the areas to which fluoride is applied, and (4) minimization of personnel time because the application process usually involves treating both arches simultaneously. Occasionally a child is not able to tolerate the use of two trays at once; in these instances, each arch may have to be treated separately.

The usual procedure involves (1) selecting an appropriately sized tray; (2) dispensing a small amount of gel (approximately 1.5 ml per tray) or foam into each tray; (3) drying the teeth in the maxillary and mandibular arches with gauze or a stream of air prior to placing the trays; (4) inserting the trays and checking for proper coverage; (5) inserting a saliva ejector; and (6) asking the child to bite down and close his or her lips around the saliva ejector. A saliva ejector should always be used during topical fluoride applications with trays to minimize the swallowing of these highly concentrated agents. Following the topical application, the saliva ejector should be used for at least 30 seconds to remove any excess fluoride remaining.

## Considerations for Special Patients

As in any age group, some children require special consideration with respect to their need for fluoride therapy or the manner in which this therapy must be provided (Box 19-1). Specifically, alternative approaches should be available for children with developmental disabilities or medical conditions that either place them at higher risk for caries or limit their ability to obtain fluoride in the usual manner.

For example, patients with cerebral palsy may find it difficult to tolerate the trays used for topical fluoride applications. Topical fluorides may have to be applied with a brush or cotton swab in these persons. Fluoride varnishes can be applied quickly to dried interproximal or other at-risk tooth surfaces. Children who are being treated with irradiation or chemotherapy often experience ulcerative degeneration of the soft tissues, causing them to be extremely sensitive to preparations having a low pH (i.e., APF) or to certain flavoring agents. A diluted, neutral, non-irritating formulation should be provided for these patients. Children with chronic renal failure may experience elevated serum fluoride levels for prolonged periods following ingestion of concentrated fluoride preparations owing to their kidney impairment. Because they also have been noted to have a lower incidence of caries than matched controls, systemic or professional topical fluorides are not recommended for these patients.[6] These are just a few of the many types of patients who require modification of the usual preventive practices.

---

### BOX 19-1

### Adaptive Oral Hygiene for the Child with Special Needs
*Gayle J. Gilbaugh*

Good oral health is an important aspect of every child's well-being and general health. For the child with special needs it is both a health and a social issue. Lack of regular home care can lead to dental disease causing a painful and unsightly mouth. This can interfere with daily functions such as eating, sleeping, and making friends. A child with special needs does not need this additional burden. A healthy smile boosts the child's morale, enhances self-esteem, and is a part of total well-being.

Unfortunately, daily oral hygiene can be a challenge for children with special health care needs and their caregivers. Some children with disabilities may be capable of cleaning their own teeth whereas others may find it physically and mentally difficult or impossible. In these cases, a caregiver needs to provide some assistance. The child should be encouraged to brush by himself first with the caregiver providing follow-up care.

Daily oral hygiene should be built into the schedule and require a minimum of frustration for the child and caregiver. The basic tooth cleaning concepts are the same as for any child and should be accomplished daily. For the child with special health care needs, achieving the goals may require some adaptations and a little ingenuity.

Historically there have not been many commercial oral care products that were tailored for people with special health care needs. However, nowadays a wide variety of cleaning devices, products, and adaptations are available. It is important for the dental professional to keep abreast of such products in order to make appropriate recommendations.

The chart below lists potential oral hygiene challenges and techniques or devices that may be of assistance. All adaptations should be individualized according to the needs of a particular child.

| POTENTIAL OBSTACLE | TECHNIQUE/DEVICE |
| --- | --- |
| Access to the child | Avoid small confined bathrooms<br>Use a room with plenty of space for maneuvering<br>Good light source |
| Difficulty expectorating | Use a minimal amount (smear) of toothpaste<br>A bulb syringe or portable power suction can be used for expectoration<br>Antimicrobial agents and fluoride can be applied with a toothbrush, cotton swap, or toothette if indicated |

*Continued*

## DIETARY MANAGEMENT

A number of factors begin to emerge during the preschool period that can have a profound effect on the growth and development of children as well as on their dental health. Following the large gains in growth during the first 3 years of life, the preschool child's rate of growth slows markedly. Therefore, caloric requirements should be reduced accordingly, but a balanced diet need not be sacrificed. Because it is becoming common for both parents to be employed when a child reaches the age of 3 years, the management and control of the child's diet that was maintained during the first 3 years of life may become threatened. When preschoolers are sent off to a baby sitter, grandparents, or daycare center, children are introduced to new environments, food selections, and management styles. It is no wonder that they become confused, begin to question routine dietary practices, and even stop eating foods that were once favorites.

By this time the effect of television begins to be felt. The preschooler may be exposed to 2 to 8 (or more) hours of television on any day. Advertisements during this period are numerous, and unfortunately most are for food items, all of which the preschooler seems to want when he or she accompanies the parents to the market for the weekly shopping.

Fortunately, during this period children are still willing to try new foods. Parents need to experiment not only with new foods but also with the preparation of these foods. In addition, the presentation of foods is most important. Appropriate amounts of a variety of colorful foods go a long way to increasing children's consumption at mealtime.

Although preschoolers seem to be always busy, they have an increasing amount of "idle" time because of their decreasing willingness to take a morning or afternoon nap. With more time available, reinforcement from the comments heard on television, and the encouragement of peers, snacking increases during this period. Appropriate snacking is encouraged. It is only when snacks are restricted to foods heavy with salt, fats, or refined carbohydrates of a consistency that adheres to the teeth and oral tissues or dissolves slowly that there will be a problem. Parents, teachers, and caretakers must be educated or told by parents or guardians about the kinds of snacks that are best for their children. On special occasions, such as birthday parties, Halloween, or Valentine's Day, a special treat of sweets can be suggested. At all other times snacks should be selected from a list of foods that have been shown to be "friendly to teeth."

Fortunately, preschoolers are highly impressionable and can be greatly influenced by experiences within the family. Therefore, meal times are important "classrooms" in which they learn and observe the feeding practices of older siblings and their parents. A friendly, congenial atmosphere at mealtime without threats ("You'd better eat all your food or you'll get no dessert") or badgering from siblings goes a long way toward establishing positive dietary practices.

It is because of these factors that the dentist may find it difficult to encourage parents to modify dietary practices when they are implicated in dental disease. Although many approaches are available to the dental team, no one approach is successful all the time. The approach used must be individualized to the personality of the practice, the willingness of the family to learn, and the specific dental problems encountered. Although many studies on the effect of diet and dietary practices on dental disease have been and continue to be conducted, there continues to be considerable reluctance as well as controversy about the approach to be used by the dental team.

Although historically sucrose has been implicated as the major carbohydrate necessary for acid production, we now know that other simple carbohydrates can produce acid (e.g., corn sweeteners, commonly used in processed and convenience foods, and fructose and glucose, which occur naturally in honey, fruits, and vegetables). Therefore, it is no longer simply a matter of recommending that the patient reduce his or her sucrose intake. Over the years, sucrose has been appreciably replaced in the food industry with fructose and other sweeteners. The critical factor that remains is the potential for this food to produce acid that lowers the pH in and around the tooth in the presence of plaque. Many foods have been tested and found to lower pH to 5.5 or lower (Box 19-2).[20]

Other critical factors are the tendency of a food to adhere to the teeth, the rate at which a food dissolves, the potential for a food to stimulate saliva production, and the potential for a food to buffer the production of acid. It has been

## BOX 19-2

### Foods that Cause the pH of Interproximal Plaque to Fall Below 5.5

Apples, dried
Apples, fresh
Apple drink
Apricots, dried
Bananas
Beans, baked
Beans, green canned
White bread
Whole wheat bread
Caramels
Cooked carrots
Cereals, presweetened and regular
Chocolate milk
Cola
Crackers, soda
Cream cheese
Doughnuts
Gelatin-flavored dessert
Grapes
Milk, whole
Milk, 2%
Oatmeal
Oranges
Orange juice
Pasta
Peanut butter
Potato, boiled
Potato chips
Raisins
Rice
Sponge cake, cream-filled
Tomato, fresh
Wheat flakes

suggested[19] that a food with a low cariogenic potential would have the following attributes:

1. A relatively high protein content
2. A moderate fat content to facilitate oral clearance
3. A minimal concentration of fermentable carbohydrates
4. A strong buffering capacity
5. A high mineral content, especially of calcium and phosphorus
6. A pH greater than 6.0
7. The ability to stimulate saliva flow

Although foods have been identified with these characteristics, it remains difficult to assist parents

in the selection of a diet and dietary practices that are best for the individual family.

## DIETARY COUNSELING

Although the dental profession recognizes the role of good nutrition and appropriate dietary practices in achieving and maintaining good oral health, the execution of the process has been difficult to promote. Fortunately, parents now appear to be more aware of these issues, they are willing to listen, and many are even ready to make some changes. The Dietary Guidelines for Americans (available at www.usda.gov) provides information for families' nutritional requirements, promoting health, supporting active lives, and reducing major risk factors.23 When used in conjunction with the Food Guide Pyramid, parents have practical information on making choices from the food groups and the number of servings from each group each day (available at www.nal.usda.gov). How can the dentist and his or her staff help them?

In families with a preschool child and no dental disease, the approach would be quite different from that recommended for families with a preschool child with dental disease. For all children, the dentist should ask the parents the following questions during the initial interview to develop a baseline for further dietary assessment:

1. At what age was the child weaned from the breast or bottle?
2. If the child was still on the breast or bottle after 1 year of age, what was the frequency and duration of use?
3. When were solids introduced?
4. Were baby foods commercially prepared or homemade?
5. How many meals are served presently? Does the family eat together?
6. Who selects the menu and prepares the food?
7. Are snacks provided? Are they given at home, in nursery school, or by a baby sitter? As a parent do you choose the snacks? If not, do you know what they are?
8. Is the child a good eater? Does he or she eat a balanced diet? If not, what are the problem areas?

2. Barnhart WE, Hilles HL, Leonard GJ, Michaels SE: Dentifrice usage and ingestion among four age groups. *J Dent Res* 53:1317, 1974.

3. Bell RM, Klein SO, Bohannan HM, et al: Analysis of DFMS increments. In *Treatment Effects in the National Preventive Dentistry Demonstration Program,* Santa Monica, Rand Corporation, 1984, pp 19-41.

4. Brudevold F, Naujoks R: Caries-preventive fluoride treatment of the individual. *Caries Res* 12(suppl 1):52-64, 1978.

5. Centers for Disease Control and Prevention: Recommendations for using fluoride to prevent and control dental caries in the United States. *MMWR Morb Mortal Wkly Rep* 50 (RR-14):26, 2001.

6. Crall JJ, Nowak AJ: Clinical uses of fluoride for the special patient. In: Wei SHY, editor. *Clinical Uses of Fluorides.* Philadelphia, Lea & Febiger, 1985, pp 193-201.

7. Featherstone JD, Adair SM, Anderson MH et al: Caries management by risk assessment: consensus statement. *J Calif Dent Assoc* 31:257-269, 2003.

8. Isman B, Newton R, Bujold C, Baer MT: A planning guide for dental professionals serving children with special health care needs. University of Southern California Affiliated Program, Children's Hospital, Los Angeles, 2000.

9. Joyston-Bechal S, Duckworth R, Braden M: The effect of artificially produced pellicle and plaque on the uptake of $^{18}$F by human enamel in vitro. *Arch Oral Biol* 21:73-78, 1976.

10. Kaste L, Selwitz R, Oldakowski RJ, et al: Coronal caries in the primary and permanent dentition of children and adolescents 1–17 years of age: United States 1988– 1991. *J Dent Res* (special issue) 75:631-641, 1996.

11. Klimek J, Hellwig E, Ahrens G: Fluoride taken up by plaque, by the underlying enamel and by clean enamel from three compounds in vitro. *Caries Res* 16:156-161, 1982.

12. Levy SL, McGrady JA, Bhwride P et al: Factors affecting dentifrice use and ingestion among a sample of US pre-schoolers. *Pediatr Dent* 22:389-394, 2000.

13. Levy SM, Zarei MZ: Evaluation of fluoride exposure in children. *J Dent Child* 58:467-473, 1991.

14. National Institute of Dental Research: Summary of findings. In: *The Prevalence of Dental Caries in United States Children, 1979–1980.* NIH Publication No. 82-2245, December 1981, pp 5-8.

15. National Institute of Dental Research: *Oral Health of United States Children: The National Survey of Dental Caries in U.S. School Children: 1986–1987.* NIH Publication No. 89-2247, 1989, pp 6-8.

16. Nowak AJ, Skotowski MC, Cugini M, Warren PR: A practice based study of a children's power toothbrush: efficacy and acceptance. *Compendium* 23:25-32, 2002.

17. Ripa LW: Professionally (operator) applied topical fluoride therapy: a critique. *Clin Prev Dent* 4:3-10, 1982.

18. Ripa LW, Leske GS, Sposato A, Varma A: Effect of prior toothcleaning on bi-annual professional acidulated phosphate fluoride topical fluoride gel-tray treatments: results after three years. *Caries Res* 18:457-464, 1984.

19. Schachtele CF: Changing perspectives on the role of diet in dental caries information. *Nutr News* 45:13-15, 1982.

20. Schachtele CF, Jensen ME: Can foods be ranked according to their cariogenic potential? In: Guggenheim B, editor. *Cariology Today.* Basel, Karger, 1984, pp 136-146.

21. Seppa L, Leppönen T, Hausen H: Fluoride varnish versus acidulated phosphate fluoride gel: a 3 year clinical trial. *Caries Res* 28:327-330, 1995.

22. Tinanoff N, Wei SHY, Parkins FM: Effect of a pumice prophylaxis on fluoride uptake in tooth enamel. *JADA* 88:385-389, 1974.

23. US Department of Agriculture and US Department of Health and Human Services: *Nutrition and Your Health: Dietary Guidelines for Americans,* 4th ed. Hyattsville, Md, Department of Agriculture, 1995.

24. Vargas CM, Crall JJ, Schneider DA: Sociodemographic distribution of pediatric dental caries: NHANS III, 1988-1994. *J Am Dent Assoc* 129: 1229-1234, 1998.

25. Weinstein P, Domoto P, Koday M, Leroux B: Results of a promising open trial to prevent baby bottle tooth decay: a fluoride varnish study. *J Dent Child* 61:338-341, 1994.

26. Whitford G, Adair S, Hanes CM, et al: Enamel uptake and patient exposure to fluoride: comparison of APF gel and foam. *Pediatr Dent* 17:199-203, 1995.

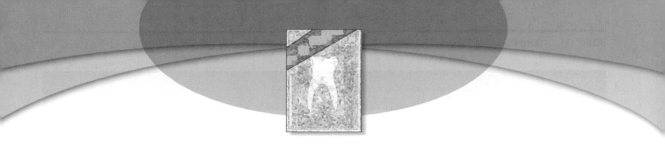

# CHAPTER 20
## Dental Materials

*Kevin James Donly and Adriana Segura*

Restorative materials used in pediatric restorative dentistry are commonly the same as those used in restorative dentistry in general. This chapter is intended to identify commonly used materials in pediatric dentistry and provide information that applies specifically to their use. Many materials are available, and in many cases, clinical considerations will dictate the choice of the appropriate material. Table 20-1 identifies the most commonly used materials in pediatric restorative dentistry and the relevant clinical considerations. Chapters 21, 32, and 39 will discuss the specific clinical uses of dental restorative materials.

## BASES AND LINERS

The use of bases and liners is important in pediatric dentistry. Bases and liners are available to reduce marginal microleakage from the restoration and to prevent sensitivity to the underlying tooth structure. Traditionally, preparations of calcium hydroxide, zinc oxide–eugenol, and zinc phosphate were the materials of choice. Presently, glass ionomer cement is also a common base.

### Calcium Hydroxide

Calcium hydroxide cements are supplied in a visible light–cured system and a two-paste system. A catalyst paste containing calcium hydroxide, zinc oxide, and zinc stearate in ethylene toluene sulfonamide reacts with a base paste containing calcium tungstate, calcium phosphate, and zinc chemical setting and increases the working time. When using zinc phosphate cement as a base, additional zinc oxide powder is placed in the mixture to provide a thick consistency, increasing the strength and decreasing the hardening time of the cement.

## Glass Ionomer Cement

Glass ionomer cement has become a commonly used basing agent. It has the ability to create a physicochemical bond to tooth structure and to release fluoride. Glass ionomer cement consists of calcium aluminosilicate glass particles mixed with polyacrylic acid. The initial reaction stage involves the ionization of polyacrylic acid, which leads to a change in the polymer chains from a coiled to linear form. The hydrogen ions produced by ionization attack the calcium aluminosilicate glass, which also contains fluoride, and causes the release of metal and fluoride ions. The majority of the metal cations ($Ca^{2+}$, $Al^{3+}$), divalent or trivalent, respectively, are bound by the ionized polymer to form cross-linked salt bridges. Calcium and aluminum ions bind to polyacrylic acid at the carboxyl groups, and a gel phase is precipitated to form a matrix of the hardening cement. Calcium carboxylates are formed first as a firm gel due to the rapid binding of calcium to the polyacrylic acid chains. This initial set has the property of being carvable, but at this stage the ionomer is very susceptible to water absorption. Likewise, the free aluminum ions are susceptible to diffusion from moisture contamination and thus are lost from the cement because they are unable to cross-link with the polyacrylic acid chains. Isolation of prepared teeth with a rubber dam is recommended. Aluminum salt bridges are then formed with the polyacrylic acid matrix, and the cement hardens. The trivalent aluminum ions ensure a much stronger cross-linking than is possible with the calcium divalent bonds alone. The slower reaction of aluminum ions is attributed to the more stringent steric requirements imposed by a trivalent ion on polyanion chain configuration.

Glass ionomer can bond to dentin by free hydrophilic carboxyl groups in the cement, promoting surface wetting to form hydrogen bonds at the tooth interface. At the same time, an ionic exchange occurs at the interface, with calcium ions being displaced by phosphate ions. Some manufacturers recommend removing the smear layer, created during cavity preparation, with polyacrylic acid. This tooth "conditioning" provides an uncontaminated tooth surface for bonding.

Tartaric acid is added to the glass ionomer cement to accelerate the rate of hardening without decreasing the working time. Itaconic acid may be placed in glass ionomer mixtures to increase the reactivity of the polyacrylic acid to the glass, and polymaleic acid may be added to modify the reaction.

Studies have shown that glass ionomer bases and liners exhibit less marginal microleakage than zinc oxide–eugenol, zinc phosphate, and calcium hydroxide,[30,40] thereby preventing bacterial penetration. Fluoride is released from glass ionomer cement by dissolution and diffusion. Glass ionomer bases and liners have demonstrated the inhibition of secondary caries formation.[15,28,32,35] The fluoride released is taken up by both the enamel and dentin adjacent to the material.[13,24,25,58] This fluoride aids in creating an inhibition zone that is not susceptible to demineralization, when compared with areas adjacent to non–fluoride-releasing materials.[19,29]

Glass ionomer cements are supplied in anhydrous and hydrous forms. Due to the viscosity of the hydrous form, mixing the cement may be difficult. The anhydrous form has a longer shelf life because the polyacrylic acid is dehydrated and placed in the powder. It is critical that glass ionomer be mixed according to the manufacturer's instructions. If the cement is too thick (the thickness of zinc phosphate cement), it will not provide sufficient water to complete the reaction, and dentin sensitivity may be encountered; the necessary water will be obtained from the dentin, causing sensitivity due to hydraulic pressures created within the dentin.

Resin-modified glass ionomer cement preparations are available and can be light cured.[42] Photoinitiated polymers have been placed in the glass ionomer cement formulation to provide light polymerization. Although these resin-modified glass ionomer cements can be light cured, the material sets as a true cement, with an acid-base reaction taking place; therefore, the material will chemically set without light curing.

Glass ionomer cement has a coefficient of thermal expansion similar to that of tooth structure, can protect an underlying base and dentin, and has the advantages of bonding to resin-based composite and releasing fluoride to inhibit secondary decay.

## Glass Ionomers as Dental Adhesives
*Joel H. Berg*

Glass ionomers used as adhesives have been "underpromoted." Because of the timing of their introduction coinciding with the launch of the third-generation resin adhesives, any awareness about their potential effectiveness as dentin adhesives has been significantly superimposed by the massive weakness promulgated regarding resin adhesives. In addition, this high level of awareness concerning resin adhesives has resulted in a multitude of sometimes superfluous studies investigating and comparing resin-based dentin adhesives in lieu of any possible studies that otherwise may have been performed examining glass ionomers as dentin adhesives. In the meantime, at least one manufacturer has introduced a (resin-modified) glass ionomer dentin adhesive. Several studies have noted the excellent bond strength as well as the chemical nature of the bond between glass ionomer adhesives and the underlying dentin.[1] Although some have suggested using glass ionomers as adhesives only for the dentin (while covering the enamel with a "pure" resin) because of marginal discoloration and accompanying aesthetic concerns, many excellent studies have clearly demonstrated the potential advantages of glass ionomer adhesives.[1] Their shrinkage is minimal, while their attachment to dentin is by covalent bonding as opposed to an entirely physical connection created via etching the surface.

### REFERENCES

1. Berg JH: Glass ionomer cement. *Pediatr Dent* 24:430-438, 2002.

## CAVITY VARNISHES

Cavity varnishes are resins that are insoluble in oral fluids. Varnish is to be used with amalgam restorations; it inhibits surface bonding of resin-based composite systems, dentin-bonding systems, and glass ionomer systems as well as prevents the fluoride released from glass ionomer from gaining access to the restoration and tooth interface. The purpose of cavity varnishes is to reduce microleakage at restoration margins and inhibit penetration of corrosion products from amalgam into dentin, thereby preventing tooth discoloration adjacent to restorations. The varnishes do not prevent thermal sensitivity.

## DENTIN-BONDING AGENTS

Dentin-bonding agents have been incorporated into the restorative dentistry armamentarium. Previously, dentin- or enamel-bonding agents fell into two groups. The first was halophosphorous esters of 2,2-bis[4-(2-hydroxy-3-methacryloyl-oxypropyloxy)phenyl] propane (BIS-GMA). The second group was categorized as polyurethanes. The polyurethanes are halophosphorous esters of hydroxyethyl methacrylate (HEMA). Both of these dentin-bonding agents relied on a phosphate-calcium bond for retention.

Removing the smear layer was found to increase the effectiveness of the dentin-bonding agents. The newer bonding agents include conditioning or primer components that remove or alter the smear layer over the dentin. This results in the creation of a mechanical bond by the infiltration of monomers into a zone of demineralized dentin, where the monomers polymerize and interlock with the dentin matrix.[22] A majority of the contemporary dentin-bonding agents

### Dentin-Bonding Resins
*Franklin Garcia-Godoy*

Dentin-bonding resins have become an integral part of restorative dentistry.[1] Research indicates that both permanent and primary dentin can be effectively bonded with adhesives.[2] Strict adherence to application instructions is recommended to enhance bonding because every product has unique directions for each system.

### REFERENCES

1. Garcia-Godoy F, Donly KJ: Dentin/enamel adhesives in pediatric dentistry. *Pediatr Dent* 24:462-464, 2002.
2. Swift EJ Jr: Dentin/enamel adhesives: review of the literature. *Pediatr Dent* 24:456-461, 2002.

are similar to those previously discussed or composed of 4-methacryloxyethyl trimellitic anhydride.

Self-etching primers have been developed to offer the convenience of etching and priming simultaneously. Although some preliminary research demonstrates excellent bonds to dentin and enamel, caution is advised. The products must be used as instructed by the manufacturer, particularly focusing on agitation of the product during placement and the recommended length of application time.[27, 62]

## RESTORATIVE MATERIALS

### Amalgam

Traditionally, amalgam was the material of choice for class I and class II restorations. Today amalgam continues to be an effective restorative material.[26,45] A 3-year study of the clinical performance of 260 amalgam restorations (86.4% class II) demonstrated 254 to be successful.[46] It is important to understand the clinical makeup and setting reaction of amalgam to correlate restoration successes and failures with the fundamental properties of the material.

#### Amalgamation

Dental amalgam consists of an alloy mix of silver, copper, tin, and, in some cases, zinc particles combined with mercury. The alloy particles have either a spherical or comminuted (lathe-cut) configuration. The unreacted alloy particles are termed the silver-tin (gamma) phase. These particles are combined with mercury, the mercury actually acting as a wetting agent of the alloy particles to initiate the setting reaction termed amalgamation. The particle surfaces react with mercury to form a cementing matrix, consisting of the gamma 1 and gamma 2 phases. The gamma-1 phase employs the binding of silver and mercury ($Ag_2$-$Hg_3$). The gamma 2 phase involves the binding of tin and mercury ($Sn_7$-$Hg$). The gamma 2 phase is responsible for early fracture and failure of the comminuted particle amalgam restorations. Tin cannot be eliminated from the alloy because of its importance in the setting reaction and control of dimensional change of amalgam. To avoid the detrimental gamma 2 phase, copper was introduced into the amalgamation reaction. The copper replaced the tin-

mercury phase with a copper-tin phase ($Cu_5$-$Sn_5$). The copper-tin matrix decreases the corrosion of tin, preventing secondary weakening with subsequent fracture of the restoration.

The amount of mercury needed to complete the amalgamation reaction is contingent on the alloy composition and particle configuration but usually falls between 42% and 54% of the amalgam mix. When mercury exceeds 55%, there is a detrimental reduction in amalgam strength. Spherical alloy particles, with the addition of copper, require less mercury than comminuted particles to complete the amalgamation process. It is important to point out that once amalgamation occurs, unreacted mercury is not available; the mercury is alloyed with silver, tin, or copper. Although it has been brought to the attention of the public that mercury is present in the amalgam restoration, the results of controlled clinical research indicate that mercury from amalgams has no toxic effects.[1] Zinc is present in some alloy mixes to act as a scavenger for oxygen, which inhibits the formation of copper, silver, or tin oxides that weaken the amalgam restoration. Using preencapsulated amalgam or strictly following the manufacturer's recommendations for dispensing, trituration, and manipulation is a critical factor in achieving successful restoration.

#### Properties

Hardening amalgam may expand or contract depending on the type and manipulation of the material. The American Dental Association[8] requires that there may be no more than 20 $\mu$m/cm of expansion or contraction after 24 hours.

The compressive strength required by the Council on Dental Materials and Devices[8] for amalgam is 11,600 psi (88 $MN/m^2$) after 1 hour. Tensile strength is substantially lower; therefore, cavity preparation design becomes critical. The preparation should have a design that allows the amalgam to be condensed as a "bulk" of material, avoiding shallow depths and a thin isthmus where fracture may occur. Comminuted and spherical low-copper amalgam demonstrates decreased marginal fracture resistance. This is partially due to the increased creep of these amalgams. Creep is the dimensional change that occurs when amalgam sustains a load during mastication, a result of the viscoelastic property of amalgam. The American Dental Association requires that an amalgam have a maximum of 5% creep to be certified.

Corrosion, a chemical or electrochemical deterioration of amalgam, occurs at the surface or subsurface. Deterioration may be due to pitting or scratching secondary to poor condensation, carving, or finishing of amalgam, which allows food or saliva components to attack the chemical matrix. Dissimilar metals in contact can also cause corrosion, a galvanic action that encourages the materials to go into solution. Pitting occurs, and food entrapment within the pits subsequently causes further corrosion. The gamma 2 phase (tin-mercury) is most susceptible to corrosion; therefore, the spherical high-copper amalgams are the least susceptible. Although extensive corrosion can lead to restoration failure, minimal corrosion in conjunction with creep allows open restoration margins to be packed full enough with corrosion byproducts to significantly close these margins.

*Condensation*

Amalgam should be placed and condensed immediately after trituration, according to the manufacturer's recommendations. Placement of amalgam in small increments is appropriate. Condensation allows force to be applied for material adaptation with a minimum of excess mercury. Use of small condensers with firm pressure on small increments of amalgam minimizes voids within the final restoration. A delay in condensation should be avoided; the effective removal of excess mercury becomes more difficult owing to the initial hardening that occurs before initiating condensation. This in turn decreases restoration strength and increases the creep in the material. Moisture contamination should also be controlled because excess moisture causes delayed expansion, particularly in zinc-containing alloys. The use of a rubber dam can prevent moisture contamination and isolate the working field effectively.

*Finishing and Polishing*

Finishing and polishing of the amalgam surface is highly recommended. Small scratches and pits can be removed with finishing burs, and abrasive stones and rubber points impregnated with abrasives. The final polish can be accomplished with a tin oxide compound. Care should be taken to use water when polishing to avoid the vaporization of mercury from the amalgam. Most amalgam restorations should not be polished for 24 hours, although the spherical high-copper amalgam can be polished almost immediately because its strength is obtained rapidly.

## Resin-Based Composite

Resin-based composite has become one of the most widely used contemporary restorative materials during the past 20 years. Currently, resin composite is used for sealants and for class I, II, III, IV, and V restorations in primary and permanent teeth.[7,14] Resin-based composite restorations have been accepted primarily because of their excellent aesthetic qualities. Other advantages include relatively low thermal conductivity, preservation of tooth structure in cavity preparation, and advances in the stability of compositional properties of the material.

Conventional resin-based composites were viscous fluid involatile monomers (BIS-GMA) that have filler particles incorporated into the resin. Bowen[6] formulated the BIS-GMA resin by synthesizing a dimethacrylate monomer, the product of the reaction between bisphenol A and glycidyl methacrylate. Many contemporary composite restorative materials contain dimethacrylate monomers (BIS-GMA) as the major component of the matrix phase. A relatively low-viscosity monomer (triethylene glycol dimethacrylate [TEGDMA]), which helps produce the desired handling qualities of the material, is an important component of the matrix phase. Figure 20-1 schematically illustrates the chemical structure of BIS-GMA, and Figure 20-2 illustrates the chemical structure of TEGDMA.

Incorporated into the monomer matrix are filler particles. A small number of available products contain urethane dimethacrylates rather than the BIS-GMA matrix. Initially, fused quartz and various glasses were incorporated into the BIS-GMA monomer as filler particles, providing a reinforced resin composite. The fillers were coated with a vinyl silane coupling agent, the silane chemically bonding with the polymer matrix.[50] These particles were usually irregularly shaped to provide mechanical retention in the resin.

Composites available today contain quartz, colloidal silica, borosilicate glasses, and glasses containing barium, strontium, and zinc. Excluding quartz and colloidal silica, these filler particles give the material radiopacity, which is clinically advantageous during radiographic examination. Contemporary posterior resin-based composites contain a high percentage by volume of filler particles. This composition provides wear resistance and more stability. Thermal expansion and polymerization contraction are both reduced by increasing the volume percentage of filler parti-

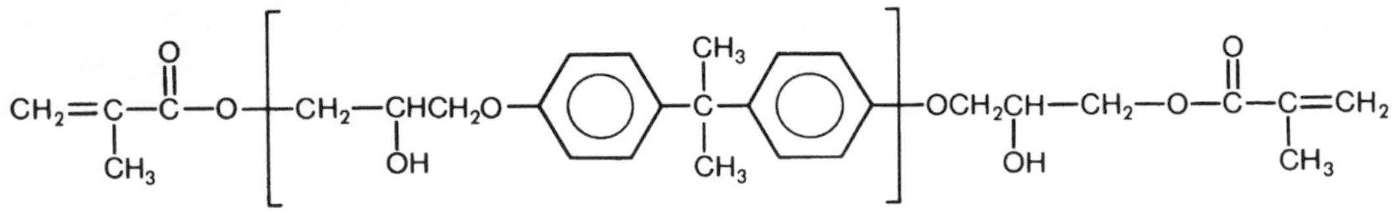

**Figure 20-1** Chemical composition of 2,2-bis[4-(2-hydroxy-3-methacryloyloxypropyloxy)phenyl] propane (BIS-GMA).

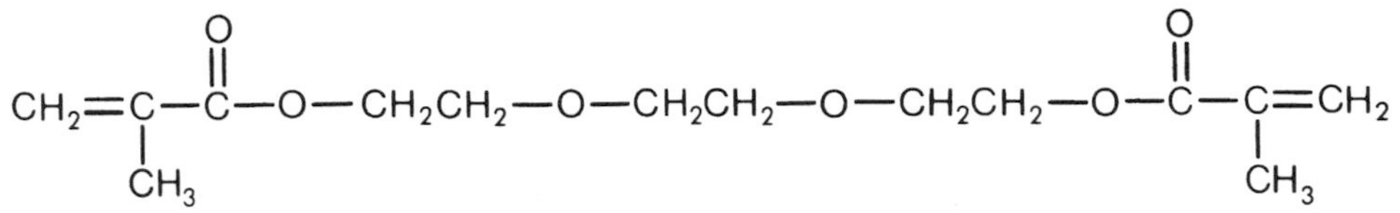

**Figure 20-2** Chemical composition of triethylene glycol dimethacrylate (TEGDMA).

cles. The increased filler content, needed for wear resistance, requires a decrease in matrix resin polymer, therefore allowing for a reduction in the amount of shrinkage that occurs upon polymerization. As the concentration of filler particles increases, the modulus of elasticity increases and tends to minimize shrinkage.[55]

Resin-based composites absorb water, yet hygroscopic expansion is very infrequently sufficient to compensate for polymerization shrinkage.[2,5] Therefore, the incremental placement and polymerization of composite resin are critical during restorative care.[16,21,37,56]

### Chemically Polymerized Resin-Based Composite
The traditional chemically activated resin-based composites form cross-links during copolymerization of methyl methacrylate and ethylene glycol dimethacrylate. The dimethacrylate monomers polymerize, by means of free radical–initiated polymerization, to form the organic matrix of a three-dimensional network. This highly viscous monomer can undergo free radical addition polymerization to provide a rigid cross-linked polymer. Usually the benzoyl peroxide present in one paste acts as the initiator, whereas a tertiary amine (dihydroxyethyl-p-toluidine) acts as the catalyst in the other paste.[9]

### Visible-Light-Polymerized Resin-Based Composite
Today most resin-based composites are visible-light-activated materials. This allows for more control in the placement of the composite into a cavity preparation; the application can easily be done in increments. The visible-light-activated composites usually contain a diketone initiator

(camphor quinone) and an amine catalyst (dimethylaminoethyl methacrylate). The diketone absorbs light at approximately 470-nm wavelength to form an excited state, which, together with the amine, results in ion radicals to initiate free radical polymerization.[54,59]

In attempts to reduce polymerization shrinkage, longer resin molecules than BIS-GMA have been placed in resin-based composite. An example would be EMA-6, which can be found in Z250 (3M ESPE Dental Products, St Paul, MN).[64]

Problems that may be associated with light-activated resin-based composites include polymerization toward the light source, sensitivity of composite to ambient light, and variability in the depth of polymerization due to the intensity of light penetration. Polymerization toward the light source may cause the composite resin to pull away from the preparation. Sensitivity of resin-based composite to ambient light may cause initial polymerization before placement of the material into the preparation. Variability in the depth of light penetration, differences in light intensity, light source active diameter, and time of light exposure can result in variations of polymerization. The benefits of light-activated resin composites include ease of manipulation, control of polymerization, and lack of need for mixing. Since mixing is not required with light-activated composites, there is less chance of air being incorporated into the material and therefore fewer voids.

### Resin-Based Composite Wear
Early resin-based composites, used for posterior restorations, exhibited excessive occlusal wear. Studies have shown that when conventional composites are placed in high stress concentration

areas, excessive wear occurs.[20,39,44,51] Further investigation pursued factors that might influence the rate of wear, such as the size and hardness of the filler particles, the amount of porosity within the material, and the method of polymerization.[38] It was found that the ceramic filler particles nearly always remained intact. There was no evidence of wear on the particles; they were found to be hard enough to cause wear of the unfilled resin during mastication until the resin matrix was gradually worn from the particles. Once a critical portion of the filler particle was exposed, it was easily dislodged. Although there seemed to be a correlation between the size of the filler particle and its hardness (larger particles possessing a more critical hardness), substantially larger particles were found to accelerate the wear. Therefore, the hardness of particles is not necessarily the most significant factor affecting wear; particles that have adequate hardness, are distributed within minimal unfilled resin, and have the least abrasion potential during mastication are ideal.[3,34]

Porosity has been shown to be a major factor in the wear rate of posterior resin-based composites.[38,49] All resin restorations contain a certain degree of porosity. These porosity defects, the occurrence of voids, can be minimized by careful insertion and polishing of the material. The use of light-cured composites avoids the mixing process, which creates fewer voids and increases abrasion resistance. Problems of wear appear to be improved with newer composites. Composite resins are vacuum packed to decrease porosity. It is important to note that mixing shades for aesthetics may cause an increase in porosity. This problem is created due to the incorporation of air during the mixing process. Current posterior resin-based composites show minimal wear. This has been achieved by incorporating a variety of particle sizes into the polymer matrix. The increased filler content results in a decrease of matrix resin polymer. The mechanism of wear is hypothesized to be due to the loss of the resin matrix. Increasing wear resistance is believed to be possible because the filler particles are situated in close proximity, thereby leaving little unfilled resin exposed.

### Marginal Adaptation

The use of resin-based composites for restoring posterior teeth has historically presented the problem of marginal leakage at the resin-tooth interface.[12,51] This marginal leakage caused teeth with posterior resin-based composite restorations to be more prone to secondary caries than teeth with amalgam restorations. Failure of the composite to bond to the cavity preparation walls and voids in the restorative material have been identified as the cause of inadequate marginal adaptation. This problem has been reduced by (1) using contemporary posterior resin-based composites, which contain a high volume of filler that decreases polymerization shrinkage, (2) using an enamel bevel, (3) using newer dentin-bonding agents and glass ionomer cements, and (4) acid etching the enamel.

### Formulations

**Enamel-Bonding Agents.** The use of phosphoric acid (35% to 50%) results in an acid-etched surface on enamel that creates an effective mechanical bond with the BIS-GMA enamel-bonding agent. Enamel-bonding agents are placed over the acid-etched enamel prior to composite placement. The bonding agents are merely unfilled dimethacrylates and are used because they can easily penetrate the etched enamel surface due to the low viscosity. The resin matrix of the composite resin will then chemically bond to the bonding agent.

**Sealants.** The use of pit and fissure sealants has been effective in preventing occlusal caries for more than two decades.[52,57] Sealants are composed of a BIS-GMA resin structure used in resin-based composites. The BIS-GMA monomer is diluted with low-weight dimethacrylate monomer to make the sealant material a fluid that can easily penetrate the pits and fissure of occlusal surfaces. Sealants are available in two component systems that self-polymerize when mixed and light-polymerized systems.

Although the use of sealants is an excellent preventive technique, there remained at first the concern that caries could occur at sealant margins or where the sealant had partially broken away. The concept of adding fluoride-releasing resins was examined for caries inhibition and found to be effective in vitro.[33,36]

**Microfilled Resin–Based Composite.** Microfilled resin–based composite has silane-treated colloidal silica filler particles in a BIS-GMA resin. Traditional microfilled composites contained approximately 50% (by volume) filler particles. Because of the high percentage of resin matrix, the particle configuration, and the small particle size (less than 1 μm in diameter), this resin composite is easily polishable and reaches a high luster. Microfilled composites are recommended for restorations that are highly visible yet encounter minimal stress during mastication. The low percentage of filler results in a decrease in strength and an increase in wear. To compensate for polymerization shrinkage, some of the BIS-GMA resin in the composite is prepolymerized by the manufacturer.

More highly filled (greater than 70% by volume) microfilled resin–based composites are available and can be effectively utilized in areas where greater wear and stress is anticipated.

**Macrofilled Resin–Based Composite.** Macrofilled resin–based composite has silane-treated filler particles (approximately 80% by volume) in a BIS-GMA resin. The particle sizes are much larger than those found in microfilled systems. Although these particles are larger than those found in the microfilled composites, they are smaller than the conventional resin-based composite particles. The high filler particle percentage increases wear resistance. Because most of these resin composites are used for posterior restorations, the material is usually radiopaque from the filler type.

**Hybrid Resin–Based Composite.** Hybrid resin–based composites have a combination of small and large particles, representing the size of the particles found in microfilled and macrofilled resin–based composites, respectively. The high percentage of filler particles provides strength and wear resistance, yet the smaller filler particles allow for particles to arrange in close proximity to each other, which can provide minimal polymerization shrinkage and improved polishability compared with macrofilled composite. These resin-based composites are considered for restorations that may have stress-bearing areas during mastication but must have a well-polished surface.

**Nanofilled Resin–Based Composite.** Since the introduction of resin-based composites, filler particle size has become smaller. More recently, nanofilled composites have been introduced, which contain very small filler particles. These resins can offer the strength of a highly filled resin, as well as polishability due to the small particles.

### Glass Ionomer

#### Anterior Restorations

Preparations of glass ionomer are available in various shades that can be used for anterior restorations.[4,11] The use of glass ionomer for ante-rior restorations is limited to class III and class V preparations. The low fracture resistance and mechanical bonding strength to enamel make its use impractical for class IV restorations. Retention of glass ionomer restorations in class V restorations, when the gingival margin is not in enamel, may demonstrate advantages. The fluoride release from glass ionomer restorations has been shown to inhibit development of secondary caries.[17,23,60,63]

#### Posterior Restorations

The major disadvantage of glass ionomer cement as a posterior restorative material is its susceptibility to fracture and wear. Metal particles have been added to glass ionomer cement to increase the strength and wear resistance for posterior restorations. Fracture resistance remains a concern, and critical decisions should be made when using the material for posterior restorations. Investigation has demonstrated the clinical success of resin-modified glass ionomer cement as a posterior restorative material in the primary dentition.[10,17,43] Again, the fluoride release and bonding capabilities are advantages of the glass ionomer cement.

### Compomers

Compomers have become available and are recommended for use as a pediatric dental restorative material.[31,41,48,53] Compomers are actually a cross between resin-based composite and glass ionomer cement.

The compomers are expected to bring the favorable properties of resin-based composite, such as wear resistance, color stability, and polishability, to the material. An acid-base reaction takes place within the compomer material but is not the primary setting reaction; therefore, visible light polymerization is necessary to complete the setting reaction. Compomers are utilized in conjunction with methacrylate primers that bond to enamel, dentin, and compomer restorative material; therefore, manufacturers consider the etching of tooth structure prior to restoration placement optional.

## CEMENTS

Cements are frequently used in pediatric dentistry. Their primary use is for the cementation of stainless steel crowns and orthodontic bands.

**TABLE 20-2**

**Comparison of Dental Cements**

| Cement | Composition | Working Time | Setting Time | Compressive Strength | Bond Strength to Dentin | Release of Fluoride | Pulpal Response | Removal of Excess |
|--------|-------------|--------------|--------------|----------------------|-------------------------|---------------------|-----------------|-------------------|
| Ideal | — | Medium | Short-medium | Very high | High | Yes | None | Easy |
| Zinc phosphate | Zinc oxide<br>Phosphoric acid | Medium | Medium | Medium | None | No | Low-medium | Easy |
| Polycarboxylate | Zinc oxide<br>Polycarboxylic acid | Short | Short | Low-medium | Low-medium | No | None | Medium-difficult |
| Glass ionomer | Silicate glass containing Ca, Al, F<br>Polycarboxylic acid | Short-medium | Short | High | Medium | Yes | Low | Moderate |
| Zinc silicophosphate | Zinc oxide and silicate<br>Phosphoric acid | Medium | Medium | High | None | Yes | Medium | Easy |
| Zinc oxide and eugenol | Zinc oxide<br>Eugenol | Long | Medium | Low-medium | None | No | None | Easy |
| Reinforced zinc oxide and eugenol | Zinc oxide reinforced with EBA or alumina or polymer<br>Eugenol | Long | Medium-long | Low-medium | None | No | None | Easy |

Adapted from Farah JW, Powers JM: *Dental Advisor* 2(1):3, 1985.

Zinc phosphate, polycarboxylate, zinc oxide–eugenol, and glass ionomer are the cements most commonly used. These cements were previously discussed in the section on bases and liners. When used as luting cements, adjustments may be made in the mix of the cement to provide properties needed for cementation. For example, less powder is placed in zinc phosphate cement when it is being used as a luting cement than when it is being used as a base or liner. The particles in glass ionomer cement are usually larger in size than those found in glass ionomer bases. There is less particle surface area available for reaction in the cement, and therefore the cement sets slower than the base and allows more working time. The importance of the accuracy in liquid-powder ratio of glass ionomer cement has been discussed. Encapsulated, premeasured cement is available and may be considered for clinical use.

The various cements most commonly utilized in pediatric dentistry and their clinical considerations are noted in Table 20-1 and Table 20-2.

# REFERENCES

1. American Dental Association Divisions of Communication and Scientific Affairs and Department of State Government Affairs: When your patients ask about mercury in amalgam. *JADA* 120:395-398, 1990.
2. Asmussen E: Composite restorative resins. Composition versus wall to wall polymerization contraction. *Acta Odontol Scand* 33:337-344, 1975.
3. Bayne SC, Taylor DF, Sturdevant JR et al: Protection theory for composite wear based on 5-year clinical results. *J Dent Res* 67:120(Abstract no. 60), 1988.
4. Berg, JH: Glass ionomer cements. *Pediatr Dent* 24:430-438, 2002.
5. Bowen RL, Rapson JE, Dickson G: Hardening shrinkage and hygroscopic expansion of composite resins. *J Dent Res* 61:654-658, 1982.
6. Bowen RL: Dental filling material comprising vinyl-silane treated fused silica and a binder consisting of the reaction product of bisphenol and glycidyl methacrylate. U.S. Patent 3,066,112, 1962.
7. Burgess JO, Walker R, Davidson BS: Posterior resin-based composite: review of the literature. *Pediatr Dent* 24:465-479, 2002.
8. Council on Dental Materials and Devices: Revised American Dental Association Specification No. 1 for Alloy for Dental Amalgam. *JADA* 95:614-617, 1977.
9. Craig RG: Chemistry, composition and properties of composite resins. Symposium on Composite Resins in Dentistry. *Dent Clin North Am* 25:219-239, 1981.
10. Croll TP, Bar Zion Y, Segura A, Donly KJ: Clinical performance of resin-modified glass ionomer cement restorations in primary teeth: a retrospective evaluation. *JADA* 132:1110-1116, 2001.
11. Croll, TP, Nicholson JW: Glass ionomer cements in pediatric dentistry: review of the literature. *Pediatr Dent* 24:423-429, 2002.
12. Derkson GD, Richardson AS, Waldman RJ: Clinical evaluation of composite resin and amalgam posterior restorations: two year results. *J Can Dent Assoc* 4:277-279, 1983.
13. Diaz-Arnold AM, Holmes DC, Wistrom DW, et al: Short-term fluoride release/uptake of glass ionomer restoratives. *Dent Mater* 11:96-101, 1995.
14. Donly KJ, Garcia-Godoy F: The use of resin-based composite in children. *Pediatr Dent* 24:480-488, 2002.
15. Donly KJ, Ingram C: An in vitro caries inhibition of photopolymerized glass ionomer liners. *J Dent Child* 64:128-130, 1997.
16. Donly KJ, Jensen ME: Posterior composite polymerization shrinkage in primary teeth: an in vitro comparison of three techniques. *Pediatr Dent* 8:209-212, 1986.
17. Donly KJ, Segura A, Kanellis M, Erickson RC: Clinical performance and caries inhibition of resin-modified glass ionomer cement and amalgam restorations. *JADA* 130:1459-1466, 1999.
18. Donly KJ, Wild TW, Jensen ME: Posterior composite Class II restorations: in vitro comparison of preparation designs and restoration techniques. *Dent Mater* 6:88-93, 1990.
19. Donly KJ: Enamel and dentin demineralization inhibition of fluoride-releasing materials. *Am J Dent* 7:275-278, 1994.
20. Eames WB: Clinical comparison of composite, amalgam, and silicate restorative materials. *JADA* 89:1111-1117, 1974.
21. Eick DJ, Welch FH: Polymerization shrinkage of composite resins and its possible influence on postoperative sensitivity. *Quintessence Int* 77:103-111, 1986.
22. Erickson RL: Mechanism and clinical implications of bond formation for two dentin bonding agents. *Am J Dent* 2:117-123, 1989.
23. Ewoldsen H, Herwig L: Decay-inhibiting restorative materials: past and present. *Compend Cont Educ Dent* 19:981-992, 1998.
24. Forsten L: Fluoride release and uptake by glass ionomers and related materials and its clinical effect. *Biomaterials* 19:503-508, 1998.
25. Forsten L: Resin-modified glass ionomer cements: fluoride release and uptake. *Acta Odontol Scand* 53:222-225, 1995.
26. Fuks A: The use of amalgam in pediatric dentistry. *Pediatr Dent* 24:448-455, 2002.
27. Garcia-Godoy F, Donly KJ. Dentin/enamel adhesives in pediatric dentistry. *Pediatr Dent* 24:462-464, 2002.

28. Garcia-Godoy F, Jensen ME: Artificial recurrent caries in glass ionomer–lined amalgam restorations. *Am J Dent* 3:89-93, 1990.

29. Griffin F, Donly KJ, Erickson RC: Caries inhibition of three fluoride-releasing liners. *Am J Dent* 5:293-295, 1992.

30. Heys RJ, Fitzgerald M: Microleakage of three cement bases. *J Dent Res* 70:55-58, 1991.

31. Hickel R: Glass ionomer, cements, hybrid-ionomers and compomers. Long term clinical evaluation. *Trans Acad Dent Mater* 9:105-112, 1996.

32. Hicks MJ, Flaitz CM, Silverstone LM: Secondary caries formation in vitro around glass ionomer restoration. *Quintessence Int* 17:527-532, 1986.

33. Hicks MJ, Flaitz CM: Caries-like lesion formation around fluoride-releasing sealant and glass ionomer. *Am J Dent* 5:329-334, 1992.

34. Jaarda MJ, Wang RF, Lang BR: A regression analysis of filler particle content to predict composite wear. *J Prosthet Dent* 77:57-67, 1997.

35. Jensen ME, Wefel JS, Hammesfahr PD: Fluoride-releasing liners: in vitro recurrent caries. *Gen Dent* 39:12-17, 1991.

36. Jensen ME, Wefel JS, Triolo PT, Hammesfahr PD: Effect of a fluoride-releasing fissure sealant on artificial enamel caries. *Am J Dent* 3:75-78, 1990.

37. Jorgensen KD, Asmussen E, Shimokobe H: Enamel damage caused by contracting restorative resins. *Scand J Dent Res* 83:120-122, 1975.

38. Leinfelder KF, Roberson TM: Clinical evaluation of posterior composite resins. *Gen Dent* 31:276-280, 1983.

39. Leinfelder KF, Sluder TB, Santos JF, Wall JT: Five year clinical evaluation of anterior and posterior restorations of composite resin. *Oper Dent* 5(2):57-65, 1980.

40. Manders CA, Garcia-Godoy F, Barnwell GM: Effect of a Copal varnish, ZOE or glass ionomer cement bases on microleakage of amalgam restorations. *Am J Dent* 3:63-66, 1990.

41. Marks LA, Weerheijm KL, van Amerongen WE et al: Dyract versus Tytin class II restorations in primary molars: 36 months evaluation. *Caries Res* 33:387-392, 1999.

42. Mitra SB: Property comparisons of a light-cure and a self-cure glass ionomer liner. *J Dent Res* 68A (Abstract no. 740):274, 1989.

43. Mjör IA, Dahl JE, Moorhead JE: Placement and replacement of restorations in primary teeth. *Acta Odontol Scand* 60:25-28, 2002.

44. Osborne JW, Gale EN, Ferguson GW: One-year and two-year clinical evaluation of composite resin vs. amalgam. *J Prosthet Dent* 30:795-800, 1973.

45. Osborne JW, Summitt JB, Roberts HW: The use of dental amalgam in pediatric dentistry: review of the literature. *Pediatr Dent* 24:439-447, 2002.

46. Osborne JW: Three-year clinical performance of eight amalgam alloys. *Am J Dent* 3:157-159, 1990.

47. Pereira JC, Manfio AP, Franco EB, Lopes ES: Clinical evaluation of Dycal under amalgam restorations. *Am J Dent* 3:67-70, 1990.

48. Peters MCRB, Roeters FJM: Clinical performance of a new compomer restorative in pediatric dentistry. *J Dent Res* 73A(Abstract no. 34):106, 1994.

49. Phillips RW, Lutz F: Status reports on posterior composites. Council on Dental Materials, Instruments and Equipment. *JADA* 107:74-76, 1983.

50. Phillips RW, Swartz ML, Norman RD: *Materials for the Practicing Dentist.* St Louis, Mosby, 1969, pp 182-191.

51. Phillips RW: Observations on a composite resin for class II restorations: two year report. *J Prosthet Dent* 28:164-169, 1972.

52. Ripa LW: Sealants revisited: an update of the effectiveness of pit-and-fissure sealants. *Caries Res* 27(suppl 1):77-82, 1993.

53. Roeters JJ, Frankenmolen F, Burgersdijk RC, Peters TC: Clinical evaluation of Dyract in primary molars: 3 year results. *Am J Dent* 11:143-148, 1998.

54. Ruyter IE: Monomer systems and polymerization. In: Vanherle C, Smith DC, editors. *Posterior Composite Resin Dental Restorative Materials.* Utrecht, Peter Szulc, 1985, pp 109-135.

55. Ruyter IE: Polymerization and conversion in composite resins. In: Taylor DF, editor. *Proceedings of the International Symposium on Posterior Composite Resins* (held in Chapel Hill, NC, October 1982), University of North Carolina, Chapel Hill, NC, 1984, pp 255-286.

56. Segura A, Donly KJ: Posterior composite polymerization shrinkage recovery following hygroscopic expansion. *J Oral Rehabil* 20:495-499, 1993.

57. Simonsen RJ: Retention and effectiveness of dental sealants after fifteen years. *JADA* 122:34-42, 1991.

58. Skartveit L, Tveit AB, Totdal B et al: In vivo fluoride uptake in enamel and dentin from fluoride-containing materials. *J Dent Child* 58:97-100, 1990.

59. Smith DC: Posterior composite dental restorative material: materials development. In: Vanherle G, Smith DC, editors. *Posterior Composite Resin Dental Restorative Materials.* Utrecht, Peter Szulc, 1985, pp 47-60.

60. Souto M, Donly KJ: Caries inhibition of glass ionomers. *Am J Dent* 7:122-124, 1994.

61. Straffon LH, Corpron RL, Bruner FW, Daprai F: Twenty-four-month clinical trial of visible-light-activated cavity liner in young permanent teeth. *J Dent Child* 58:124-128, 1991.

62. Swift EJ: Dentin/enamel adhesives: review of the literature. *Pediatr Dent* 24:456-461, 2002.

63. ten Cate JM, van Duinen RN: Hyper-mineralization of dentinal lesions adjacent to glass-ionomer cement restorations. *J Dent Res* 74:1266-1271, 1995.

64. Z250, Material Data Sheet, 3M ESPE, St Paul, Minn.

## Pediatric Dentistry Restorative Materials Adhesion Made the Difference
*Theodore P. Croll*

Remarkable advances in dental restorative materials in the 1980s and 1990s are irrevocably changing pediatric restorative dentistry.[9] The children of the 21st century will probably learn about "silver fillings" from history books, the Internet, and their parents' stories.

The ideal direct-application dental restorative material would have the following properties and characteristics:

- Is biocompatible with the dental pulp and nontoxic in the mouth
- Adhesively bonds to dentin and enamel, and the bonded interface is impervious to oral fluids
- Has fracture strengths, wear resistance, and compressive strength at least equivalent to that of enamel, and its physical properties should not diminish in the oral environment over time
- Should be dimensionally stable during application and throughout the hardening reaction and have a coefficient of thermal expansion compatible with that of surrounding tooth structure
- Should be virtually insoluble in the mouth
- Should strengthen residual tooth structure by its adhesive properties
- Should be tooth colored
- Has easy handling characteristics, ideal working time, and hardens significantly on command
- Can be placed quickly, easily, and comfortably
- Would be of reasonable cost for the dentist and patient (parent)

It is apparent that the ideal restorative material for children's teeth has not yet been developed. However, today's dentists have more options than ever before when considering how to restore carious, malformed, or traumatically injured primary and permanent teeth. With the "ideal" in mind, the chief types of dental restorative materials for children in the 21st century are as follows:

1. Silver amalgam
2. Traditional glass-ionomer cements (self-hardening)
3. Glass ionomer silver-cermet cement
4. Stainless steel crowns (primary molars and canine teeth)
5. Stainless steel crowns with prefabricated resin veneer facings (incisors)
6. Resin composites
7. Resin-modified glass-ionomer cements
8. Polyacid modified resin composites

The use of *silver amalgams, traditional glass ionomer cements,* and *glass ionomer silver cement* (Ketac-Silver [3M ESPE]) is declining in the United States. Silver amalgams served dentists treating children very well in the 19th and 20th centuries, but now adhesive tooth-colored materials are proving so durable and reliable that silver amalgam is becoming a less desirable alternative. The traditional glass ionomer restorative cements, including the cermet cement, harden initially in about 4 to 5 minutes. The light-hardened resin-modified glass ionomers have a hard initial set after 40 seconds of light curing. In addition, fracture strengths and wear resistance are improved in the resin-modified materials, so if a polymerizing light is available there are no advantages to use of the self-hardening materials.

*Stainless steel crowns* for primary canines[4] and molars[8] and permanent molars[3,5] are strong, durable, and can remain in place for 5 to 10 years or more with no additional treatment. They can also be repaired if worn through. Modern steel crown forms are precontoured and have excellent anatomic form, so dentists have a much easier time adapting these crowns to properly prepared teeth. The new self-hardening resin-modified glass ionomer luting cements, with their improved physical properties, will undoubtedly make stainless steel crown recementation a rare occurrence.

A most welcome addition to pediatric dentistry restorative material inventories has been the *preveneered stainless steel crown for primary anterior teeth.*[6] Certain dental laboratories supply anterior stainless steel crowns with resin veneer facings covering the labial, incisal, mesial, and distal aspects. When severely diseased primary incisors or canines are prepared correctly, such preveneered crowns can be cemented into place, imperceptibly restoring the child's smile. Full crown restorations for primary incisors have always been a difficult challenge for dentists treating children, and now a new, and perhaps best, option is available. Two carious primary central incisors are shown with crown restorations in place.

## Pediatric Dentistry Restorative Materials
## Adhesion Made the Difference—cont'd

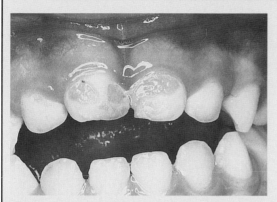

**Figure 1**   A 28-month-old child with severe nursing-related caries of the central incisors.

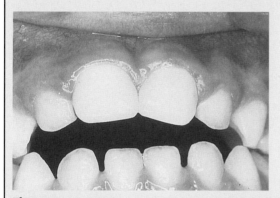

**Figure 2**   Stainless steel crowns with prefabricated resin veneer facings, 12 months after placement.

*Resin composites* are the best direct-application *enamel replacement* currently available to dentists. Via the acid-etch method, they adhesively bond to enamel and dentin and have excellent physical strength. They also can imperceptibly restore cosmetically prominent anterior teeth and have the great advantage of curing on command with light activation. The chief disadvantages of the resin composites are the need for perfect handling, material shrinkage during the polymerization reaction, and eventual marginal leakage due to forces that can open the resin–tooth structure interface. Improvements in techniques and materials and continuing developments of improved dentin and enamel bonding agents are making resin composite more attractive to clinicians. Starting in the late 1970s,[10-12] resin composites completely revolutionized management of enamel pits and fissures

in permanent teeth to the point that silver amalgam should now be considered an inferior alternative as a first restorative material for a class I lesion (personal communication, Dr. R.J. Simonsen).

*Polyacid-modified resin composite materials* (often called *compomers*) are resin composites made with a fluoride-containing glass filler and polyacid components, similar to acids used in glass ionomer materials.1 These materials do not undergo a significant acid/base hardening reaction and therefore must be light cured. They cannot be classified as glass ionomer systems. Dentists treating children have been using the polyacid-modified resins for primary teeth primarily because of ease of use. At this time durability and reliability of such restorative materials look promising. Examples of this class of materials include Dyract [Caulk], Compoglass (Vivadent), Hytac (ESPE), and F2000 (3M ESPE).

In 1992, *resin-modified glass ionomer restorative cements* were first marketed. The three chief products were Fuji II LC (GC), Vitremer Tri-Cure (3M), and Photac-Fil (ESPE). These cements have the favorable properties of the glass ionomer class of materials as well as a resin component that provides initial light-cure hardening in only 40 seconds. Furthermore, the resin component gives these materials improved wear resistance and fracture strengths. The resin-modified glass ionomer restorative cements are causing a veritable renaissance in pediatric restorative dentistry,[2,7,9] and improvements in the materials, or improved related materials, are inevitable. This class of materials is perhaps the most ideal *dentin replacement* ever produced.

### Summary

Even though prevention of dental caries has improved the oral health of many children, the caries problem, especially in those receiving no fluoride protection, will continue to challenge dentists well into the 21st century. Malformed and traumatically injured teeth will also continue to command much of the clinical dentist's time. Treatment planning for our youngest patients has become much more complex. Dentists need to be perpetual students, continuing to discover the advantages and disadvantages of each class of restorative material and the subtle nuances of each brand supplied by the manufacturers. Only then will such materials be scientifically understood and artistically applied to benefit the children.

*Continued*

## Pediatric Dentistry Restorative Materials
## Adhesion Made the Difference—cont'd

### REFERENCES

1. Albers HR: *Tooth-Colored Restoratives.* Santa Rosa, Calif, Alto Books, 1996, pp 4a-3.
2. Croll TP: Restorative dentistry for preschool children. *Dent Clin North Am* 39:737-770, 1995.
3. Croll TP: Permanent molar stainless steel crown restoration. *Quintessence Int* 18:313-321, 1987.
4. Croll TP, Blum JR: The stainless steel crown for a primary canine tooth: a pictorial essay. *J Pedod* 6:301-314, 1982.
5. Croll TP, Castaldi CR: The preformed stainless steel crown for permanent posterior teeth in special cases. *JADA* 97:644-699, 1978.
6. Croll TP, Helpin ML: Preformed resin-veneered stainless steel crowns for restoration of primary incisors. *Quintessence Int* 27:309-313, 1996.
7. Croll TP, Killian CM, Helpin ML: A restorative dentistry renaissance for children: light-hardened glass ionomer/resin cement. *J Dent Child* 60:89-94, 1993.
8. Full CA, Walker JD, Pinkham JR: Stainless steel crowns for deciduous molars. *JADA* 89:360-364, 1974.
9. Pediatric Restorative Dentistry Consensus Conference: *Pediatr Dent* 24:377-516, 2002.
10. Simonsen RJ: Preventive resin restorations (I). *Quintessence Int* 9:69-76, 1978.
11. Simonsen RJ: Preventive resin restorations (II). *Quintessence Int* 9:95-102, 1978.
12. Simonsen RJ: The preventive resin restoration: a minimally invasive, nonmetallic restoration. *Compend Contin Educ Dent* 8:428-432, 1987.

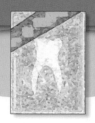

# CHAPTER 21

## Restorative Dentistry for the Primary Dentition

*William F. Waggoner*

Pediatric restorative dentistry is a dynamic combination of ever-improving materials and tried-and-true techniques. Many aspects of primary teeth restoration have not changed for decades. In 1924, G. V. Black outlined several steps for the preparation of carious permanent teeth to receive an amalgam restoration.[6] These steps have been adopted, with slight modification, for the restoration of primary teeth. Restorative techniques for the primary dentition utilizing amalgam and stainless steel crowns (SSCs) have remained relatively consistent for many years (Fig. 21-1). However, with an increased use of adhesive restorative materials and bonding systems, there has been a shift to more conservative preparations and restorations. Materials such as glass ionomers, resin ionomer products, and improved resin-based composite systems have been developed that are having a profound impact on the restoration of primary teeth. Unfortunately, long-term clinical data (i.e., longer than 3 years) regarding many of these materials are limited; but

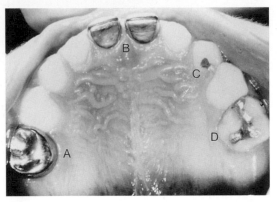

**Figure 21-1**  Restored primary dentition demonstrating stainless steel crown (**A**), open-face steel crowns (**B**), class III amalgam (**C**), and class II amalgam (**D**).

even so, many clinicians are utilizing these materials with increasing frequency. Hence we find ourselves in a transitional age.

The clinician can stay with the proven, successful materials of the past, such as amalgam and stainless steel; or move to newer, more aesthetic materials that offer advantages such as bonding to tooth structure, fluoride release, improved aesthetics, reduction of mercury exposure, and conservation of tooth structure. While none of the aesthetic materials have the track record and proven durability of amalgam or stainless steel, when placed appropriately, they can provide useful restorations for the lifespan of the primary tooth. This chapter will provide information on both the new and the old restorative techniques. For the interested reader, in 2002 the American Academy of Pediatric Dentistry sponsored a Pediatric Dentistry Restorative Consensus Conference. The published proceedings[4] include extensive and up-to-date literature reviews and discussion of pediatric restorative techniques at a greater depth than can be included in this chapter. In addition, a more detailed discussion of dental materials utilized in pediatric restorative dentistry can be found in Chapter 20.

## INSTRUMENTATION

Nearly all instrumentation for restorative procedures is carried out with the high-speed handpiece (100,000 to 300,000 rpm, either electric or air turbine) combined with coolant. The coolant may be water spray or air alone. A water spray coolant is often recommended for high-speed instrumentation; however, there is some evidence

that air coolant alone may be used without creating irreversible pulpal damage.[5,8] There are some instances when a water spray coolant is absolutely necessary. This is especially true when removing old amalgam restorations or using diamond burs. Regardless of the coolant used, intermittent cutting at intervals of a few seconds with light, brushing strokes should be done to prevent excessive heat generation. Protective masks and eyewear should always be worn when using the high-speed air turbine handpiece.

The low-speed handpiece (500 to 15,000 rpm) is most frequently used for caries removal and for polishing and finishing procedures. As with high-speed instrumentation, light pressure and brushing strokes should be used when using the low-speed handpiece. Use of hand instrumentation is minimal in most operative preparations in the primary dentition. It is usually limited to final caries removal or planing of enamel walls.

In recent years another method of instrumentation for preparing teeth has become somewhat popular. This technique, known as air abrasion, uses a stream of purified aluminum oxide particles (27 to 50 μm) that are forced under pressure (40 to 120 psi) through a fine-focused nozzle onto the tooth surface. This cuts through enamel and dentin quickly, and it can also abrade or roughen a tooth surface.[21] Originally introduced in dentistry by R. Black in 1945,[7] air abrasion virtually disappeared from the dental environment by the early 1960s and was reintroduced in the early 1990s. Air abrasion offers several advantages over conventional handpieces. There is an absence of vibration and noise, caries excavation can often be done without the need for local anesthesia, and tooth preparation can be very fast. It is best suited for use with adhesive restorations that require minimal tooth preparation and less rigid classic cavity design than does amalgam. The cost of the air abrasion unit (several thousand dollars), the dust that can be generated during the procedure, and the fact that it does not totally eliminate the need for conventional handpieces are three disadvantages of the system that will probably keep it from gaining widespread use.

## ANATOMIC CONSIDERATIONS OF PRIMARY TEETH

Although some primary teeth resemble their permanent successors, they are not miniature

## BOX 21-1

### Anatomic Differences Between Primary and Permanent Teeth

1. Primary teeth have thinner enamel and dentin thickness than permanent teeth (Fig. 21-2).

2. The pulps of primary teeth are larger in relation to crown size than permanent pulps.

3. The pulp horns of primary teeth are closer to the outer surface of the tooth than permanent pulps. The mesiobuccal pulp horn is the most prominent.

4. In primary teeth, the enamel rods of the gingival third of the crown extend in an occlusal direction from the dentin-enamel junction. This is in contrast to the permanent dentition in which the rods extend in a cervical direction.

5. Primary teeth demonstrate greater constriction of the crown and have a more prominent cervical contour than permanent teeth.

6. Primary teeth have broad, flat proximal contact areas.

7. Primary teeth are whiter than their permanent successors.

8. Primary teeth have relatively narrow occlusal surfaces in comparison with their permanent successors.

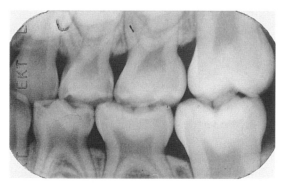

**Figure 21-2** Note the difference in enamel thickness. The enamel of the primary molars is approximately half the thickness of the enamel of the first permanent molars. Also note the interproximal caries requiring restoration on the distal surface of the mandibular first primary molar and between the maxillary first and second primary molars.

## BOX 21-2

### Advantages of Rubber Dam Use

1. Better access and visualization are gained by retracting soft tissues and providing a dark contrasting background to the teeth.

2. Moisture control is superior to other forms of isolation.

3. The safety of the child is improved by preventing aspiration or swallowing of foreign bodies and by protecting the soft tissues.

4. Placement generally results in decreased operating time.

5. Many children tend to become quieter and relaxed with a rubber dam in place. The dam seems to act as a separating barrier, so that movements in and out of the oral cavity are perceived by the child as being less invasive than without the dam in place.

6. With a rubber dam in place, a child becomes primarily a nasal breather. This enhances nitrous oxide administration when it has been deemed necessary from a behavioral standpoint.

permanent teeth. Several anatomic differences must be distinguished before restorative procedures are begun (Box 21-1).

## USE OF THE RUBBER DAM IN PEDIATRIC RESTORATIVE DENTISTRY

The use of the rubber dam is indispensable in pediatric restorative dentistry. Numerous advantages have been listed for its use, all allowing for provision of the highest quality of care (Box 21-2).

Most pediatric restorative procedures can be completed with the rubber dam in place. The few situations in which it may not be used include the following: (1) in the presence of some fixed orthodontic appliances; (2) when a very recently erupted tooth will not retain a clamp; and (3) in a child with an upper respiratory infection, congested nasal passage, or other nasal obstruction. However, even poor nasal breathers may tolerate the rubber dam if a small (2- to 3-cm) hole is cut in the dam in an area away from the operative quadrant. This allows for some mouth breathing.

### Preparing for Placement of the Rubber Dam

The rubber dam is available in an assortment of colors and may even be scented or flavored. Virtually all rubber dams are made of latex, although a latex-free rubber dam material is available (Hygienic Corporation, Akron, Ohio) for use in latex-sensitive patients. A 5 × 5 inch medium-gauge rubber dam is best suited for use in children. Rubber dams are available in which a disposable rubber dam frame is manufactured already attached to the dam (Handidam, Aseptico, Woodinville, Wash.), eliminating the need for a separate dam frame. The darker the dam, the better the contrast between the teeth and dam. The holes should be punched so that the rubber dam is centered horizontally on the face and the upper lip is covered by the upper border of the dam, but the dam does not cover the nostrils. One method of proper hole placement is seen in Figure 21-3, A. Figure 21-3, B demonstrates proper hole size selection for different teeth.

The minimal number of holes necessary for good isolation of all tooth surfaces to be restored is punched in the dam. For single class I or V restorations, only the tooth being restored must be isolated. If interproximal lesions are being restored, at least one tooth anterior and one tooth posterior to the tooth being restored should be isolated. This allows better access, more ease in placing a matrix, and visualization of adjacent marginal ridges for appropriate carving of the restoration.

When isolating several teeth, instead of punching numerous holes in the dam, some clinicians will simply punch two holes approximately ½ inch apart and cut the rubber dam with scissors connecting the two holes. This is called the "slit technique" and allows for very quick placement of the rubber dam. Because there is no rubber dam material interproximally, moisture control is not as dependable with this placement technique, but it is often still adequate, especially for isolation of maxillary quadrants.

Proper clamp selection is one of the most critical aspects of good rubber dam application. Box 21-3 lists the most frequently used clamps and their areas of utilization. Incisors usually require ligation with dental floss for stabilization instead of a clamp.

After selecting an appropriate clamp, place a 12- to 18-inch piece of dental floss on the bow of the clamp as a safety measure (Fig. 21-4). This is necessary for easy retrieval of the clamp if it is dislodged from the tooth and falls into the posterior pharyngeal area.

Before trying the clamp on the tooth, floss the contacts through which the rubber dam will be taken. If floss cannot be passed through the contact because of defective restorations or other factors, modification of the contacts or rubber

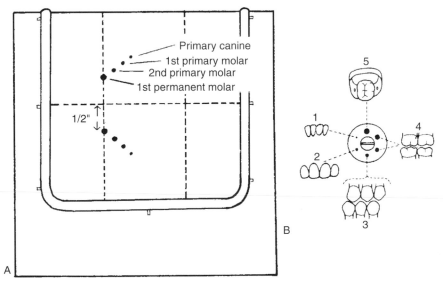

**Figure 21-3** Preparation of the rubber dam. **A,** The Young frame is applied to the rubber dam. The upper limit of the frame coincides with the upper edge of the rubber dam material. The dam is divided vertically into thirds, and the area inside the frame is divided in half horizontally. The holes for each tooth are placed as indicated, at a 45-degree angle 3 to 4 mm apart. **B,** The rubber dam punch table with corresponding teeth and hole sizes. (**B** from *The DAE Project: Instructional Materials for the Dental Health Professions: Rubber Dam.* New York, Teachers College Press © 1982, Teachers College, Columbia University, p 42. )

## BOX 21-3

### Common Rubber Dam Clamps for Pediatric Restorative Dentistry

Partially erupted permanent molars: 14A, 8A*[†‡]

Fully erupted permanent molars: 14, 8*[†‡]

Second primary molars: 26, 27[‡], 3*[†]

First primary molars/bicuspids/permanent canines: 2, 2A*[†] 207, 208[‡]

Primary incisors and canines: 0*, 00[†], 209[‡]

"A" clamps have jaws angled gingivally to seat below subgingival heights of contour.

*Ivory, Miles Inc., Dental Products, South Bend, Ind.
[†]Hygienic Corp, Akron, Ohio.
[‡]HuFriedy, Chicago, Ill.

dam will be necessary before placement. Next, using the rubber dam forceps, place the clamp on the tooth, seating it from a lingual to buccal direction. Be certain that the jaws of the clamp are placed below the height of contour and are not impinging on the gingival tissues. After seating the clamp, remove the forceps and place a finger on the buccal and lingual jaws of the clamp and apply gingival pressure to ensure that the clamp is stable and has been seated as far gingivally as possible.

### Placement of the Rubber Dam

The punched rubber dam should be lightly stretched onto the rubber dam frame prior to placement of the clamp. This holds the corners of the dam out of the line of the operator's vision during placement. If the material is stretched too tightly, tension is too great and the clamp may be dislodged when the material is stretched over the bow of the clamp. Next, pull the floss attached

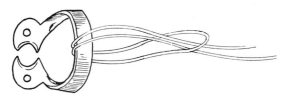

**Figure 21-4** A floss safety through the bow of the rubber dam clamp allows for easy retrieval of the clamp, should it become dislodged from the tooth. (From *The DAE Project: Instructional Materials for the Dental Health Professions: Rubber Dam.* New York, Teachers College Press 1982, Teachers College, Columbia University, p 66.)

to the clamp through the most posterior hole in the dam that has been punched for the clamped tooth. Instruct the child to open the mouth widely, and with the index fingers, stretch the most posterior hole of the rubber dam over the bow and wings of the clamp. Sometimes when isolating the most posterior maxillary molars, the bow of the clamp rests very close to the anterior border of the ramus when the mouth is opened wide. This makes slipping the dam material over the bow difficult, but when one simply asks the child to close the mouth slightly, the ramus will move posteriorly and allow the material to slide between the bow and the ramus.

If necessary, adjust the tension of the rubber dam on the frame. Next, stabilize the rubber dam around the most anterior tooth. This may be done by placing a wooden wedge interproximally, by stretching a small piece of rubber dam through the contact, or by ligating with dental floss. To ligate, place floss (12 to18 inches) around the cervix of the tooth and have the dental assistant hold the floss gingivally on the lingual with a blunt instrument. Draw the floss tightly around the tooth from the buccal and tie a surgical knot below the cervical bulge. Do not cut the ends of the ligature tie as the long ends remind the operator that the ligature is present. After anterior stabilization, all other teeth can be isolated for which holes have been punched. A blunt hand instrument can be used to invert the rubber dam into the gingival sulcus around each isolated tooth.

### Removing the Rubber Dam

To remove the rubber dam, first rinse away all debris and cut and remove any ligatures used for stabilization. Next, stretch the rubber dam so that the dam's interproximal septa may be cut with a pair of scissors. The clamp, frame, and dam are then removed as a unit with the rubber dam forceps. Inspect the dam and the mouth to see that no small pieces of dam material have been left interproximally. Gently massage the tissue around the previously clamped tooth, and rinse and evacuate the oral cavity.

## RESTORATION OF PRIMARY MOLARS

The anatomy of the primary molars, with their fissured occlusal surfaces and broad, flat interproximal contact areas, makes them the most caries-susceptible primary teeth. The importance of primary molars in mastication and as maintainers of space for the succedaneous teeth, coupled with the development of suitable economic restorative materials, has shaped a philosophy of restoring and conserving primary molars. SSCs, amalgam, and, most recently, adhesive materials such as resin-based composites, resin-modified glass ionomers, polyacid-modified resin-based composites (compomers), and, to a small degree, glass ionomers are the materials utilized in the restoration of primary molars. Although the use of adhesive materials for restoring posterior teeth continues to increase, amalgam remains the restorative material of choice for many clinicians. There have, however, been concerns raised about the mercury in amalgam and the exposure of dentists, patients, and the environment to it. This has brought the use of amalgam under recent attack. Current scientific information continues to support the use of amalgam as a restorative material,[43] but for a more detailed discussion of the controversy the reader is referred to Chapter 20. Under conditions of good moisture control, both alloys and adhesive materials can provide very serviceable restorations. Placement procedures for both classes of materials are included in this chapter.

## Class I Amalgam Restorations

### General Considerations

The outline form for class I restorations in primary molars can be seen in Figure 21-5. The outline form should include all retentive fissures and carious areas but should be as conservative as possible. Ideal pulpal floor depth is 0.5 mm into dentin (approximately 1.5 mm from the enamel surface). The length of the cutting end of the no. 330 bur is 1.5 mm, so this becomes a good tool for gauging cavity depth. The cavosurface margin should be placed out of stress-bearing areas and should have no bevel. To help prevent stress concentration, the outline form should be composed of smoothly flowing arcs and curves, and all internal angles should be rounded slightly. When a dovetail is placed in the second primary molars, its buccolingual width should be greater than the width of the isthmus so as to produce a locking form to provide resistance against occlusal torque, which may displace the restoration mesially or distally. The isthmus should be one third of the intercuspal width, and the bucco-

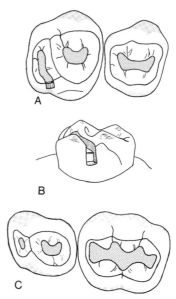

**Figure 21-5** Class I amalgam cavity preparations. **A,** Maxillary right second and first primary molars (occlusal view). **B,** Maxillary second primary molar, lingual view of distolingual groove preparation. **C,** Mandibular right first and second primary molars (occlusal view).

lingual walls should converge slightly in an occlusal direction. The mesial and distal walls should flare at the marginal ridge so as not to undercut ridges. Oblique ridges should not be crossed unless they are undermined with caries or are deeply fissured. Primary mandibular second molars often exhibit buccal developmental pits. When carious, these should be restored with a small teardrop or ovoid-shaped restoration, including all the adjacent susceptible pits and fissures.

Neither liners nor bases are very widely used, but various bases and liners are discussed in Chapter 20. Thin liners such as calcium hydroxide do not provide thermal insulation, and recent evidence suggests that calcium hydroxide may hydrolyze gradually,[46] leaving a small void underneath the restoration and ultimately weakening it.[15] Therefore, use of calcium hydroxide is discouraged. Cavity varnish, though widely used in the past to prevent microleakage, is no longer considered useful. Small amalgam restorations can be placed directly into prepared cavities without any varnish. Placement of bases in primary teeth is also uncommon, but when necessary, use of a glass ionomer material is recommended. Because of the relatively large size of the pulp chamber in primary teeth, preparations that are placed deep enough to require bases are generally found to be in the pulp and hence require other treatment.

The steps of preparation and restoration of class I amalgam restorations are listed in Box 21-4.

### Common Errors with Class I Amalgam Restorations

Some frequent errors made in class I amalgam restorations are (1) preparing the cavity too deep, (2) undercutting the marginal ridges, (3) carving the anatomy of the amalgam too deep, (4) not removing amalgam flash from cavosurface margins, (5) undercarving, which leads to subsequent fracture of amalgam from hyperocclusion, and (6) not including all susceptible fissures. Note that an alternative to including all of the susceptible fissures is to confine the amalgam preparation to the area of decay and seal the rest of the tooth with a pit and fissure sealant.

## Class II Amalgam Restorations

**General Considerations.** The outline form for several class II amalgam preparations is shown in Figure 21-6. The guidelines given for the class I preparation should be followed during the preparation of the occlusal portion of the class II preparation and, additionally, there are several recommendations for the proximal box preparation. The proximal box should be broader at the cervical portion than at the occlusal portion. The buccal, lingual, and gingival walls should all break contact with the adjacent tooth, just enough to allow the tip of an explorer to pass. The buccal and lingual walls should create a 90-degree angle with the enamel. The gingival wall should be flat, not beveled, and all unsupported enamel should be removed. Ideally, the axial wall of the proximal box should be 0.5 mm into dentin and should follow the same contour as the outer proximal contour of the tooth. Because occlusal forces may

---

### BOX 21-4

#### Steps of Preparation and Restoration of Class I Amalgam Restorations

1. Administer appropriate anesthesia and place the rubber dam.

2. Using a no. 330 bur in the high-speed turbine handpiece, penetrate into the tooth parallel to its long axis in the central pit region and extend into all susceptible fissures and pits to a depth 0.5 mm in dentin.

3. Remove all carious dentin. Utilize a large, round bur in the slow-speed handpiece or a sharp spoon excavator.

4. Smooth the enamel walls and refine the final outline form with the no. 330 bur.

5. Rinse and dry the preparation, and inspect for (1) caries removal, (2) sharp cavosurface margins, and (3) removal of all unsupported enamel with hand instruments, as necessary.

6. Triturate the amalgam, and place one carrier load of amalgam into the preparation.

7. Using a small condenser, immediately begin condensation of the amalgam into the preparation, condensing small overlapping increments with a firm pressure until the cavity is slightly overfilled.

8. Following condensation, carving of most of the newer alloys can begin almost immediately. A small cleoid-discoid carver works very well for carving primary restorations. Always keep part of the carving edge of the instrument on the tooth structure so that overcarving of the cavosurface margin does not occur. Remove all amalgam flash from cavosurface margins. Keep the carved anatomy shallow. Placing deep anatomy in primary teeth (i.e., grooves) can weaken the restoration by creating a thin shelf of amalgam at the cavosurface margin and also by reducing the bulk of amalgam in the central stress-bearing areas, both leading to fracture.

9. Burnish the carved amalgam when the amalgam has begun its initial set and resists deformation. Burnishing is done with a small, round burnisher, which is lightly rubbed across the carved amalgam surface to produce a satin-like appearance. Besides smoothing, burnishing creates a substructure with fewer voids and reduces finishing time.

10. A wet cotton pellet can be wiped across the burnished amalgam for a final smoothing (optional).

11. Remove the rubber dam and check the occlusion. Children must be cautioned before the rubber dam is completely removed that they must not close their teeth into occlusion until instructed to do so. With articulating paper, check the restoration for occlusal irregularities, instructing the child to close gently. Make necessary adjustments with the carver.

12. Rinse the oral cavity and massage the soft tissue around the previously clamped tooth.

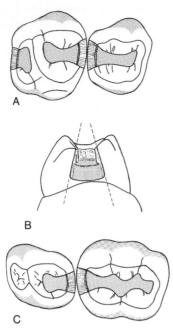

**Figure 21-6** Class II amalgam cavity preparations. **A,** Maxillary right second and first primary molars (occlusal view). **B,** Mandibular second primary molar (proximal view); note occlusal convergence of proximal walls. **C,** Mandibular right first and second primary molars (occlusal view).

permit a concentration of stress within the amalgam around sharp angles, the axiopulpal line angle is routinely beveled or rounded. No buccal or lingual retentive grooves should be placed in the proximal box. The mesiodistal width of the gingival seat should be 1 mm, which is approximately equal to the width of a no. 330 bur.

In primary teeth many practitioners limit class II amalgam restorations to relatively small two-surface restorations. Three-surface (MOD) restorations may be done, but studies have shown that SSCs are a more durable and predictable restoration for large multiple surface restorations in primary teeth.[13,48] Messer and Levering[38] reported that SSCs placed in 4-year-old and younger children showed a success rate approximately twice that of class II amalgams, for each year up to 10 years of service. Roberts and Sherriff[50] reported that after 5 years one third of class II amalgams placed in primary teeth had failed or required replacement, whereas only 8% of SSCs required retreatment. In the preschool child with large proximal carious lesions, SSCs are preferred to amalgams because of their durability. Similar-sized lesions in teeth that are within 2 or 3 years of exfoliation may be restored with amalgam

since the anticipated lifespan is fairly short. Pins for retention of amalgam in primary teeth are contraindicated. Because of the large relative size of the primary pulp, the thin dentin thickness, and the marked cervical constriction of the primary crown, successful placement of the pin is very difficult without pulp exposure or a perforation into the gingival sulcus.

### Matrix Application

Matrices must be placed for interproximal restorations to aid in restoring normal contour and normal contact areas and to prevent extrusion of restorative materials into gingival tissues. Many types of matrix bands are available for use in pediatric dentistry.

1. T band: allows for multiple matrices; no special equipment is needed.
2. Sectional matrix (Strip-T, Denovo, Baldwin Park, Calif.): allows for multiple matrix placement, is very easy to use, is not circumferential, must be held in place by a wedge.
3. AutoMatrix (Caulk, Dentsply, Milford, Del.): allows for multiple matrix placement, is very easy to use, requires special tightening and removal tools.
4. Spot-welded matrix: allows for multiple matrix placement; a spot welder is required at chairside.
5. Tofflemire matrix: is used infrequently because it does not fit primary tooth contour well and is difficult to place as multiple matrices.

T bands are available in different sizes, contours, and materials. A straight, narrow, brass T band will work in almost all pediatric restorative procedures. The T band matrix (Figure 21-7) is formed by folding the band back on itself in the form of a circle and by folding over the extension wings of the "T" to make an adjustable loop. The band is contoured and positioned onto the tooth with the folded extension wings on the buccal surface. The free end of the band is drawn mesially to pull the band snugly against the tooth. The extension folds are then grasped firmly with a pair of Howe no. 110 pliers and removed from the tooth. The band should then be tightened an additional 0.5 to 1.0 mm, and the free end should be bent back over the vertical folds and cut with scissors to a length of 5 to 6 mm. The band is then

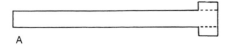

A

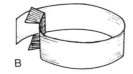

B

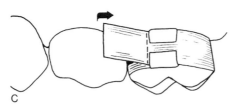

C

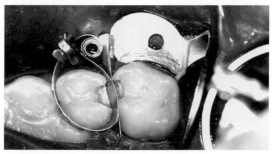

**Figure 21-8**   A sectional matrix (Strip-T, DENOVO) is placed onto a mesioocclusal preparation of the second primary molar. An AutoMatrix (Caulk, Dentsply) is seen placed on the distoocclusal preparation of the first primary molar. The matrix can be tightened to draw the band more closely to the tooth. A wedge secures both in place.

**Figure 21-7**   **A,** The T-band matrix. **B,** The T band is formed into a circle, and the extension wings are folded down to secure the band. **C,** The T band is adapted to fit the tooth tightly and is trimmed with scissors, and the free end is bent back.

reseated onto the tooth and wedged. It must fit below the gingival margin of the preparation and must also be at least 1 mm higher than the marginal ridge of the adjacent tooth. The T band is removed by opening the extension wings with an explorer or spoon excavator and allowing the band to open. Scissors are then used to cut one end of the band close to the restored proximal surface, the wedge is removed, and the band is then drawn buccally or lingually through the contact.

The sectional matrices or "matrix pieces" (Strip-T) are stainless steel matrix strips approximately ½ inch long that do not encircle the prepared tooth but rather only fit in the prepared proximal area (Fig. 21-8). For small class II preparations they are very simple to place and use. After placement they must be firmly wedged to stay in place. They are not recommended for proximal preparations that extend beyond the line angles; a circumferential matrix (or SSC) is more appropriate in that instance.

AutoMatrix (Caulk, Dentsply) is a preformed loop of stainless steel matrix material that is placed on the tooth (see Fig. 21-8) and tightened

with a special tightening tool that comes with the kit. A small pin automatically keeps the tightened matrix tightly bound around the tooth. To remove the matrix, this small pin is clipped (another special tool) and the matrix is easily loosened and removed.

The steps of fabrication and placement of a spot welded matrix retainer are listed in Box 21-5. Steel matrix material of various widths is available in spools. A piece of matrix material approximately 2 inches in length is cut from the spool and the ends of the band are welded together in one spot to form a loop. This loop is then placed around the tooth and adapted snugly by grasping the band with the Howe no. 110 pliers from the buccal surface. The band is removed, and two spot welds are placed at the seam where the band was pinched together on the buccal surface. Excess band material is cut away with scissors. Contouring pliers may be used to contour the cervical and contact areas. The welded band is then placed back onto the tooth and wooden wedges placed interproximally. After the amalgam has been placed, the band may be removed by placing a flat-bladed hand instrument between the tooth's buccal surface and the band and applying a rotational force to the instrument. This should break the spot welds and allow for easy removal of the band.

### Adjacent or Back-to-Back Class II Amalgam Restorations

Adjacent interproximal lesions are not uncommon in the primary dentition. From the standpoint of time and patient management, it is desirable to restore these lesions simultaneously.

## BOX 21-5

### Steps of Preparation and Restoration for Class II Amalgam Restorations

1. Administer appropriate anesthesia and place the rubber dam.

2. Place a wooden wedge in the interproximal area being restored (optional). This retracts the gingival papilla during instrumentation, keeps the operator from cutting the interseptal rubber dam material and underlying gingiva, and creates some prewedging, which helps to ensure a tight proximal contact of the final restoration.

3. Using a no. 330 bur in the high-speed turbine handpiece with a light, brushing motion, prepare the occlusal outline form at ideal depth.

4. To prepare the proximal box, begin at the marginal ridge by brushing the bur buccolingually in a pendulum motion and in a gingival direction at the dentin-enamel junction. Continue until contact is just broken between the adjacent tooth and the gingival wall and the wedge is seen. If the gingival wall is made too deep, the cervical constriction of the primary molar will create a very narrow gingival seat. The widest buccolingual width of the box will be at the gingival margin. Take care not to damage the adjacent proximal surface.

5. Remove any remaining caries with a sharp spoon excavator or with a round bur in the low-speed handpiece.

6. Round the axiopulpal line angle slightly. Because of the shape of the no. 330 bur, all other internal line angles will automatically be gently rounded.

7. Remove any unsupported enamel of the buccal, lingual, or gingival walls with a small enamel hatchet.

8. Remove the wedge placed at the beginning of the treatment and place a matrix band.

9. While holding the matrix band in place, forcefully reinsert the wedge between the matrix band and the adjacent tooth, beneath the gingival seat of the preparation. The wedge is placed with a pair of Howe pliers or cotton forceps from the widest embrasure. The wedge should hold the band tightly against the tooth but should not push the band into the proximal box. It may be necessary to trim the wedge slightly to achieve a proper fit.

10. Triturate the amalgam. With the amalgam carrier, add the amalgam to the preparation in single increments, beginning in the proximal box.

11. Using a small condenser, condense the amalgam into the corners of the proximal box and against the matrix band to ensure the reestablishment of a tight proximal contact. Continue filling and condensing until the entire cavity is overfilled.

12. Carving of the occlusal portion is performed with a small cleoid-discoid carver, as in class I restorations. The marginal ridge can be carved with the tip of an explorer or with a Hollenback carver.

13. Carefully remove the wedge and the matrix band.

14. Remove excess amalgam at the buccal, lingual, and gingival margins with an explorer or Hollenback carver. Check to see that the height of the newly restored marginal ridge is approximately equal to the adjacent marginal ridge.

15. Gently floss the interproximal contact to check the tightness of the contact, to check for gingival overhang, and to remove any loose amalgam particles from the interproximal region.

16. Burnish the restoration, and use a wet cotton pellet held with the cotton pliers for final smoothing if necessary.

17. Remove the rubber dam carefully.

18. Check the occlusion for irregularities with articulating paper and adjust as needed.

---

Preparation for adjacent proximal restorations is identical to those previously described. A matrix is placed on each tooth and is properly wedged. T bands, sectional, or spot-welded matrices are preferable because multiple matrix holders are difficult to place side by side. Condensation of the amalgam should be done in small increments, alternately in each preparation, so that the restorations are filled simultaneously (Fig. 21-9). Condensation pressure toward the matrix will help ensure a tight interproximal contact. Carve the marginal ridges to an equal height, and carefully remove the wedge and matrix bands one at a time. Final carving is similar to that described for solitary class II restorations.

### Problems with Amalgam Restorations

Most restorative problems in pediatric dentistry result from a failure to prepare and restore the teeth in a way that takes into account their anatomic or morphologic structural characteristics and limitations (Fig. 21-10). Fracture of the isthmus of a class II amalgam restoration is a common problem that may result from the restoration being left high in occlusion or from

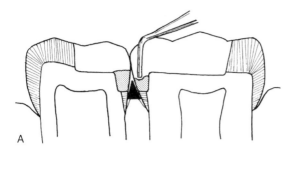

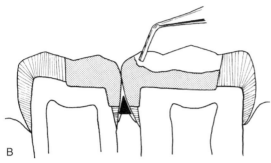

**Figure 21-9** "Back-to-back" amalgam preparations. **A,** After wedging, begin condensing the adjacent proximal boxes alternately. **B,** Continue condensing the amalgams alternately until both preparations are slightly overfilled.

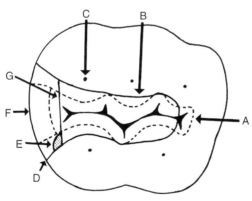

**Figure 21-10** Common errors with class II amalgam cavity preparations. **A,** Failure to extend occlusal outline into all susceptible pits and fissures. **B,** Failure to follow the outline of the cusps. **C,** Isthmus cut too wide. **D,** Flare of proximal walls too great. **E,** Angle formed by the axial, buccal, and lingual walls too great. **F,** Gingival contact with adjacent tooth not broken. **G,** Axial wall not conforming to the proximal contour of the tooth, and the mesiodistal width of the gingival floor is greater than 1 mm. (From Forrester DJ, Wagner M, Fleming J: Restorative procedures. In: Sheldon P, editor. *Pediatric Dental Medicine.* Philadelphia, Lea & Febiger, 1981.)

insufficient bulk of amalgam in the isthmus, because the preparation is too shallow, or because the amalgam has been overcarved. Marginal failure in the proximal box, usually owing to an excessive flare of the cavosurface margin, is another common problem with class II amalgam restorations. Failure to remove all caries or to extend preparations into caries-susceptible fissures is another common cause of restoration failure.[18,39]

### Finishing of Amalgam Restorations

Historically, polishing of amalgams has been advocated to (1) eliminate surface scratches and blemishes, which act as centers of corrosion, (2) remove any remaining amalgam flash not carved away, and (3) refine the anatomy and occlusion. Amalgam polishing is described in a number of textbooks and taught in most, if not all, dental schools. However, anecdotal surveys of practitioners reveal that few dentists routinely polish their amalgams after graduating from dental school. A study by Straffon et al.[59] compared the clinical performance of polished and unpolished amalgams after 3 years. This blinded study demonstrated that there was no significant difference in marginal integrity between carved and burnished-only and polished restorations through 3 years. Polishing of class I amalgam restorations did not result in better adapted margins after 36 months of function. The surface texture of the polished amalgams was significantly smoother than the burnished-only amalgams; however, by 36 months a significant number of the burnished-only restorations had exhibited improvement in surface texture over baseline.

If polishing of amalgam is not going to be done, it is important that the amalgam at least be well burnished and all excess amalgam marginal flash be removed at the time of placement. Burnishing is best accomplished with a rounded instrument. The surface of the amalgam is smoothed by rubbing the burnisher in back-and-forth motion. Burnishing should be done after the amalgam has reached its initial set and is resistant to deformation. Burnishing 10 minutes after the onset of trituration produces the smoothest surface. After burnishing, care should be taken to ensure that all amalgam flash is removed with either a small carver or an explorer. When small overhangs of marginal flash are left, they may fracture under occlusal forces. The fracture may then create a marginal discrepancy.

There are no contraindications to polishing amalgams. Many clinicians do not polish because they feel that it is a time-consuming procedure for which most patients do not care to return or reimburse. However, there is an alternative to a separate polishing appointment. Many restorations could be polished at subsequent restorative visits. Because amalgam polishing does not require anesthesia, a practitioner could anesthetize a child in the area he or she will be restoring that day and then polish previously placed restorations while allowing the anesthesia to take effect. A polishing technique with a simple armamentarium and a low potential for heat production is most desirable. Such a technique is outlined in Box 21-6. Polishing should be delayed for at least 24 hours following amalgam placement.

## Adhesive Materials in Primary Molars

As early as the mid-1960s, composite resins (now referred to as resin-based composites, or RBCs) were suggested as aesthetic replacements for class

---

### BOX 21-6

#### Polishing Technique with Simple Armamentarium and Low Potential for Heat Production

1. If necessary, do gross contouring of the amalgam or flash removal with a tapered green stone.
2. To smooth and shine the surface, use multiple fluted amalgam finishing burs brushed lightly across the restoration at high speeds. For primary teeth, three sizes of round finishing burs, together with a pear-shaped and flame finishing bur, will be sufficient to polish any amalgam restoration.
3. Place a final polish on the restoration using a rotary bristle brush with a pumice slurry to remove small scratches, followed by a polishing agent such as tin oxide for the finish luster. Rubber abrasives may be used for final polishing, but great care should be taken not to generate excessive heat.
4. Proximally, use small sandpaper disks to polish the enamel-amalgam margins. A well-polished amalgam restoration should allow the explorer to pass easily from enamel to amalgam and back again.

---

l and class II amalgam restorations in molars. Initial results were promising, but clinical failures of the resin restorations began to occur after approximately 2 years, with the greatest problem being occlusal wear.[32] However, further improvements in resin-based composite materials, such as smaller filler particles, increases in material strength, and improvement of dentin-bonding agents, have led to improved clinical results. For example, in a 5-year study comparing posterior composites and amalgams, Norman and colleagues[41] reported that both materials were satisfactory over the time period studied and the only significant statistical differences were a poorer marginal integrity for the amalgam and a greater wear rate for the resin. However, the wear rate for the composite was well within the acceptable limits established by the American Dental Association (ADA) Council on Dental Materials. Roberts and associates[51] also found no significant difference in clinical performance or wear of class II amalgam and composite resin restorations evaluated for 3 years. The ADA's Council on Scientific Affairs has concluded that when used correctly in the primary and permanent dentition, the expected lifetimes of resin-based composites can be comparable to that of amalgam in class I, II, and V restorations.[3]

Besides resin-based composites, polyacid-modified resin-based composites (compomers), resin-modified glass ionomers (e.g., Vitremere, 3M ESPE, St. Paul, Minn.), and glass ionomers have all been suggested and studied for use in primary molar restorations. These adhesive restorations in primary molars offer the advantages of improved aesthetics, elimination of mercury, low thermal conductivity, more conservation of tooth structure, and bonding of the restorative material to the tooth. Disadvantages include an exacting technique, increased operator time, potential marginal leakage, possible postoperative sensitivity, and a tendency to open or lose contacts.[1,2,33] The ADA has approved several resin-based composites for use in posterior teeth, and there is no doubt that several more will be approved in the future. Because the use of amalgam will likely continue to be challenged (as mentioned previously in this chapter and in Chapter 20), resin-based composites and resin ionomer products will undoubtedly become more widely used in posterior teeth; therefore, a brief discussion of their use in primary molars is included in this section.

## General Principles for Restoring Primary Posterior Teeth with Resin-Based Composite

Resin-based composite is used increasingly for restoration of defects in posterior teeth. These materials are technique sensitive, and overall clinical performance depends on good case selection and a skilled operator. Proper application of resin-based composites in posterior teeth requires knowledge of adhesives, composites, polymerization kinetics, and the ability to apply those principles to the patient being treated. Adhesive materials are unforgiving in comparison with amalgam.

Several clinical studies have evaluated resin-based composites in primary molars[12,19,49] and found them to perform satisfactorily in comparison with amalgam. In addition, several clinical studies have also evaluated compomer use in primary molars[16,22,36] and likewise found them to provide useful, predictable restorations. Resin-modified glass ionomer cement has also been evaluated in several clinical studies.[10,14,27] It seems that these restorations demonstrate more color change and occlusal wear than resin-based composites or compomers, but still function well in class I, II, III, and V restorations. Glass ionomer cements have also been used in restoring primary molars, but with less satisfactory results than the other adhesive materials.[27,47] Use of glass ionomers for multisurface or large restorations in primary molars, except for teeth with a very limited lifespan, is generally not recommended or indicated.

Some general principles must be remembered when using resin-based composites for restoring posterior primary teeth. (1) Placement of composite resin is highly technique sensitive, and the final restoration is very negatively affected by any moisture contamination. If a dry field cannot be maintained, resin-based composite is probably the worst choice of restorative material. However, a resin-modified ionomer can tolerate some moisture and might be used as an aesthetic material in such a situation. (2) In general, preparations for resin-based composite restorations in primary teeth are more conservative than preparations for amalgam. They do not require as much volume to resist clinical fracture as does amalgam, allowing for smaller, shallower preparations. Noncarious pits and fissures adjacent to caries do not have to be included in the preparation as "extension for prevention"; instead they can simply be sealed as part of the restorative process.[3] (3) Because resin-based composite bonds to tooth structure, the need for mechanical retention in the preparation is lessened. However, remember that the bond strengths of resin to enamel are consistently higher than those of resin to dentin and that reducing mechanical retention in the preparation means a greater reliance on the micromechanical retention of resin to etched enamel. Because primary enamel is approximately one half the thickness of permanent enamel, retention gained solely from acid etching will be similarly reduced, and therefore it is still prudent to include some minor mechanical retention in the preparations. (4) Historically, occlusal wear has been the most common problem with posterior resin-based composites. Wear will be minimized if the preparation can be kept small and out of heavy occlusion. (5) Common sense and knowledge of the dental materials being used dictate final cavity preparation. In the 1980s two studies were conducted to evaluate a conservative, modified preparation for composite resins in primary molars.[42,44] The results from these studies were very discouraging for the modified proximal resin preparations showing high rates of failure. Since those studies were published, however, dentin-bonding agents and resin-based composites and compomers have improved dramatically. In addition, more recent studies have shown conservative proximal box-only preparations to perform as well as classic G. V. Black class II preparations when compomer has been used as the restorative material.[16,34,35,63]

## Sealants and Conservative Adhesive Restorations for Primary Teeth

A thorough discussion of sealants and conservative adhesive restorations for permanent teeth is found in Chapter 32; however, a brief discussion of their use and placement in primary teeth is included here. Pit and fissure sealing is defined as the application and mechanical bonding of a resin material to an acid-etched enamel surface, thereby sealing existing pits and fissures from the oral environment. This prevents bacteria from colonizing in the pits and fissures and nutrients from reaching the bacteria already present. Although sealants are used for the most part on permanent molars and bicuspids, they may be used in primary teeth as well. The indications for sealing a primary molar are essentially the same as those for sealing a permanent tooth. They include (1) deep, retentive pits and fissures that may cause wedging of the explorer; (2) stained pits and fissures with minimal decalcified or opacified appearances; (3) pit-and-fissure caries or restorations in other primary teeth; (4) no radiographic or clinical evidence of interproximal decay; (5) a patient who is receiving other preventive treatment, such as systemic and/or topical fluoride to inhibit interproximal caries formation; (6) a situation in which adequate isolation from salivary contamination is possible.[53]

Sealants are not widely used on primary teeth for a few reasons. One of the main reasons is moisture control. Teeth must be kept absolutely dry during etching and sealant application. Because sealants alone are usually done without anesthesia and preschool children have a low tolerance for the discomfort of a rubber dam clamp on nonanesthetized gingiva, rubber dam placement on primary teeth solely for sealant placement is often avoided. Cotton roll isolation can provide adequate dryness of the tooth in cooperative patients, but poor cooperation makes this isolation extremely difficult. A second reason that sealants are not widely used on primary teeth is due to the limited lifespan of the tooth. If a second primary molar reaches age 6 without caries, it need only go another 4 to 6 years before it is lost to exfoliation. The cost-effectiveness of sealant placement here should be considered. However, if a child has caries on the occlusal surface of one second primary molar, sealing the contralateral molar to prevent caries is probably prudent.

It must be noted that sealant retention on primary molars is similar to that of retention on permanent first molars, that is, 95% after 1 year and 93% after 3 years.[24] Caries development in the pits and fissures is virtually eliminated when the sealant is retained.

Briefly, the technique involves the following steps: (1) Isolate the tooth from salivary contamination. (2) Clean the tooth surface. *Note:* Cleaning the tooth can be done several ways, most often with pumice or prophylaxis paste on a low-speed bristle brush. However, some clinicians use a ¼ round or ½ round bur, or Fissurotomy bur (SS White Burs, Lakewood, N.J.) to "clean out" and widen the fissures in enamel prior to sealant placement. (3) Acid etch for 15 to 20 seconds. (4) Rinse and dry the surface. (5) (Optional) Apply a bonding agent and gently thin with compressed air. (6) Apply the sealant to the etched surface. (6) Polymerize the sealant. (7)

Evaluate the sealant with an explorer. (8) Evaluate and adjust the occlusion.

Conservative adhesive restoration (CAR) is an updated term given to a restoration technique first described by Simonsen and Stallard in 1977,[56] and refined in 1985,[54] as preventive resin restoration (PRR). This restoration combines the preventive approach of sealing susceptible pits and fissures with conservative cavity preparation of caries occurring on the same occlusal surface. Instead of the traditional amalgam cavity preparation's "extension for prevention" beyond the area of decay into the adjacent pits and fissures, the CAR or PRR limits cavity preparation to the discrete areas of decay. These preparations are filled with an adhesive material, usually resin-based composite or compomer, and then the entire occlusal surface is sealed. This results in a restoration that conserves tooth structure and is both therapeutic and preventive. Like sealants, a detailed discussion of CARs is presented in Chapter 32, but a short discussion is included here. Note that "preventive resin restoration" is the nomenclature that has been historically used; however, this terminology has been replaced by "conservative adhesive restoration" to reflect the fact that other adhesive materials, besides resins, may be utilized in these restorations. CARs will be the term used to describe this technique in this chapter.

Originally three types of CARs were described (types A, B, and C,[56] later changed to types 1, 2, and 3).[54] These represented a continuum of tooth preparation and caries activity, with type 1 being the most conservative and type 3 the least.

For many years CARs were considered a distinct entity from an insurance billing standpoint, representing a very conservative restoration. In 2003, however, the insurance code for this procedure was dropped, and rather than being an distinct entity these are now considered "one-surface resin restorations." Regardless of the nomenclature or adhesive material utilized for restoration, the concept described by Simonsen is still useful and recommended for conservatively restoring minor occlusal caries in molars.

The teeth that are suitable for CARs are those that demonstrate small, discrete regions of decay, often limited to a single pit (Fig. 21-11, *A*). As with sealants, the ability to isolate the tooth and keep it dry throughout the procedure is the single most important indication. Amalgam or resin-modified glass ionomers, being less technique

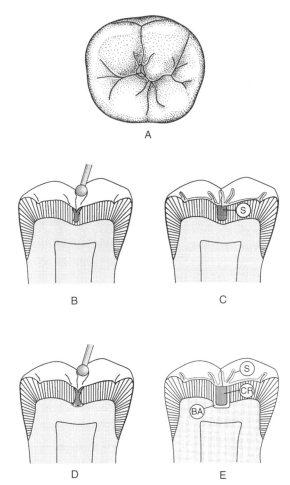

**Figure 21-11** **A,** The occlusal surface of a mandibular second primary molar with a small, discrete area of decay in the central pit. **B,** A small bur (no. 1/4 or 1/2 round or Fissurotomy) is used to remove the decay, which is confined to the enamel. **C,** A filled sealant (S) is applied into the preparation and over all susceptible pits and fissures. This is considered a sealant procedure. **D,** In this diagram, the caries extends into the dentin. Again, a small round bur is used to conservatively remove the decay. **E,** A bonding agent (BA) and resin-based composite (CR) material are placed in the preparation. Then, a sealant (S) is applied over all the remaining susceptible pits and fissures.

and moisture sensitive, would be the restorative materials of choice if the tooth cannot be kept dry. Many CARs do not require anesthesia because of the minimal tooth preparation; however, soft tissue anesthesia may be necessary for comfort in placing the rubber dam.

What Simonsen called the type 1 CAR (PRR) is merely a sealant application with minimal preparation or widening of the pits and fissures with a very small round bur (¼ or ½) or Fissurotomy bur to remove the areas of questionable, incipient decay (Fig. 21-11, *B*, *C*). The preparation is confined to enamel. After selective enameloplasty of the fissures, the tooth is etched and a pit and fissure sealant is applied and polymerized. This is now considered a sealant application, not a restorative technique.

The type 2 CAR (PRR) technique involves a similar ultraconservative preparation with a small round bur in the area of the decay, but is used when the preparation extends to dentin (Fig. 21-11, *D*). Following caries removal the entire preparation and occlusal surface is etched, rinsed, and dried, and a bonding agent placed. Then a wear-resistant resin-based composite or compomer material is placed in the cavity preparation with a brush or plastic instrument. Excess resin is gently agitated into the adjacent pits and fissures to act as a pit and fissure sealant. The entire surface is then polymerized.

The type 3 CAR (PRR) technique is similar to the type 2 CAR, except that a sealant layer forms an integral part of the restoration (Fig. 21-11, *E*). As with the type 2, the preparation extends to dentin, but in a type 3 CAR the wear-resistant resin is used only to restore the cavity preparation. Pit and fissure sealant is then applied to seal the adjacent pits and fissures.

The CAR is ideally suited for minimal carious lesions in teeth that would otherwise lose a considerable amount of tooth structure if the extension for prevention treatment were followed.[55] Houpt et al.[26] reported 79% retention of CARs in permanent molars after 9 years and concluded that the CAR was a successful conservative alternative to treatment of minimal occlusal caries. Although long-term retention studies of CARs in primary teeth are lacking, with retention rates of CARs and sealants in permanent teeth being very similar, it is not unreasonable to believe that retention rates of CARs in primary teeth would also be similar to sealant rates. However, retention studies of primary CARs would be a welcome addition to the literature.

### Class I and II Preparation and Restoration of Primary Molars with Adhesive Restorative Materials

The steps in preparation and restoration of a primary or permanent molar with composite resin are very similar to those followed for restoration with amalgam, but with a few alterations.[9] Particularly for resin-based composites absolute moisture control is a must, making a rubber dam almost mandatory. Tooth preparations for class II resin-based composites have undergone a tremendous evolution over the years, with many peculiar shapes and designs suggested. Unlike amalgam preparations, which have been well defined for years, there is no current consensus about the precise design of a class II preparation for a primary molar to receive an adhesive material. A 2001 survey of pediatric dentistry departments in North American dental schools found that 57% of the dental schools teach a conservative "box-only" preparation (with and without retention grooves), whereas 36% utilize and teach the classical G. V. Black amalgam preparation.[23] Leinfelder[31] recommended that a class II preparation be primarily restricted to the region of the caries, with little to no occlusal extensions. He also states that extending the proximal box line angles in "self-cleansing" areas is not necessary and in fact creates a larger restoration that is more prone to occlusal wear. This type of slot preparation (Fig. 21-12) has been shown in several studies to perform adequately.[16,34,35,63] A short bevel to the cavosurface margin to increase surface area for bonding and to remove the aprismatic layer of enamel is recommended.[20] Prewedging of teeth is highly desirable to achieve a slight separation of teeth and consequently a tighter interproximal contact of the final restoration. The wedge also protects the interproximal gingival tissue during instrumentation and thereby reduces the likelihood of hemorrhage into the proximal box. The preparation should be etched for 15 to 20 seconds with an acid gel. A dentin-bonding agent or glass ionomer liner is placed before placement of a matrix band and the adhesive material. Several self-etching bonding systems are now available that eliminate the separate etching and rinsing steps and may be used if desired. Clear plastic or thin steel matrices may be used. Both may provide acceptable results; however, the steel bands or strips are easier to use and more reliable in producing adequate contact areas. Circumferential matrix bands that are tightly constricted around the tooth may leave open proximal contacts since there will be minimal condensation force against the band to create a tight contact. Circumferential bands should thus be avoided.

Many resin-based composites and compomers are prepackaged in small ampules that can be injected directly into the preparation. A plastic instrument or a condenser can be used to pack

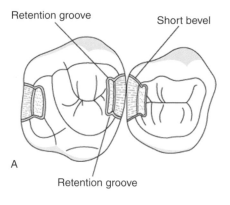

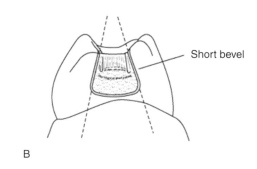

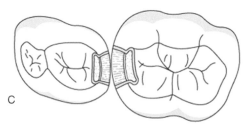

**Figure 21-12**  Modified class II cavity preparations for adhesive restorative materials. Note the short bevel around the preparations and small retention grooves. **A,** Maxillary right second and first primary molars (occlusal view). **B,** Mandibular second primary molar (proximal view); note occlusal convergence of proximal walls. **C,** Mandibular right first and second primary molars (occlusal view).

or condense the composite into the preparation. No more than a 2-mm depth of composite should be polymerized at one time. There is some debate about whether resin-based composites should be placed in bulk or incrementally. It appears that one of the primary concerns is that the curing light must penetrate to the full depth of the material. Limiting the depth of material placed to 2–3 mm per increment should ensure full polymerization and is recommended. Incremental placement may also reduce polymerization shrinkage, a suspected cause of dentin-bonding agent failure. Complete curing or polymerization of the material is very important to the success of the restoration. Undercuring may lead to a weakened restoration prone to failure under masticatory forces. Finishing can begin immediately following polymerization. The occlusal surface is grossly contoured with round, high-speed carbide finishing burs or fine-finishing diamond burs. Gross contouring of proximal surfaces is accomplished with flame-shaped, high-speed carbide finishing burs and with garnet disks, where accessible. Final finishing can be completed with a white stone or with rubber abrasive points to eliminate surface irregularities and final polishing with a composite polish or gloss. Fine abrasive disks or strips are used for final polishing of accessible proximal margins. The application of a surface sealant after polishing may serve to reduce occlusal wear and contraction gaps.[30]

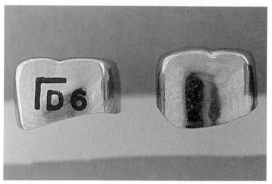

**Figure 21-13**  Buccal view of two types of stainless steel crowns for a mandibular first primary molar. On the left is a Ni-Chro ion crown (3M, St. Paul, Minn). It is a pretrimmed, precontoured crown. On the right is a pretrimmed Unitek (3M) crown. Note how much longer the Unitek crown appears. Also note the straight, noncontoured proximal surfaces of the Unitek crown. The lettering on the crown identifies it as a left mandibular first molar, size 6.

## Use of Stainless Steel Crowns

Preformed metal crowns (PMCs), also referred to as stainless steel crowns (SSCs), were introduced to pediatric dentistry by Humphrey in 1950.[28] Since then they have become an invaluable restorative material in the treatment of badly broken down primary teeth. As mentioned previously, they are generally considered superior to large multisurface amalgam restorations and have a longer clinical lifespan than two- or three-surface amalgam restorations.[13,17,38,48] The crowns are manufactured in different sizes as a metal shell with some preformed anatomy and are trimmed and contoured as necessary to fit individual teeth.

There are two commonly used types of SSCs (Fig. 21-13):

1. Pretrimmed crowns (Unitek [3M] stainless steel crowns and Denovo crowns): These crowns have straight, noncontoured sides but are festooned to follow a line parallel to the gingival crest. They still require contouring and some trimming.
2. Precontoured crowns (Ni-Chro Ion Crowns and Unitek Stainless Steel Crowns [3M]): These crowns are festooned and are also precontoured. Some trimming and contouring may be necessary but usually is minimal. If trimming of these crowns becomes necessary, the precontour will be lost and the crown will fit more loosely than before trimming.

A third type of SSC is available but is not as widely used. These are preveneered SSCs (NuSmile crowns, Orthodontic Technologies, Houston, Tex.). These are SSCs that have resin-based composite bonded to the occlusal and buccal surfaces in a laboratory process to create a more aesthetic posterior crown. These crowns can provide a nice result but are considerably more expensive than regular SSCs, require more tooth reduction, and allow for only minimal crimping for crown adaptation.

Indications for the use of SSCs are listed in Box 21-7. The steps of preparation and placement of SSCs are listed in Box 21-8.

### Two Principles for Obtaining Optimal Adaptation of Stainless Steel Crowns to Primary Molars

With few exceptions most SSCs look good in the mouth. Except in cases of bruxism when crowns may be worn and flattened down, the crowns will continue to appear clinically acceptable for many years. The radiographic appearance of the crowns is usually not as encouraging. Radiographically, margins are noted to be poorly adapted to proximal tooth surfaces. Often they are too long. Proximal contours of crowns are not well reproduced. Fortunately, these deficiencies seem to have little adverse effect on the supporting

## BOX 21-7

### Indications for Use of Stainless Steel Crowns

1. Restoration of primary or young permanent teeth with extensive carious lesions. These include primary teeth with extensive decay, large lesions, or multiple surface lesions. First primary molars with mesial interproximal lesions are included in the category because the morphologic appearance that the tooth exhibits results in inadequate support for mesial interproximal restorations.

2. Restoration of hypoplastic primary or permanent teeth.

3. Restoration of primary teeth following pulpotomy or pulpectomy procedures.

4. Restoration of teeth with hereditary anomalies such as dentinogenesis imperfecta or amelogenesis imperfecta.

5. Restorations in disabled individuals or others in whom oral hygiene is extremely poor and failure of other materials is likely.

6. As an abutment for space maintainers or prosthetic appliances.

7. Strong consideration should be given to the use of SSCs in children who require general anesthesia for dental treatment.[52]

## BOX 21-8

### Steps for Preparation and Placement of Stainless Steel Crowns

Several different preparation designs have been advocated over the years. Only one such preparation, requiring minimal tooth reduction, is discussed here. Either Unitek or Ni-Chro Ion (3M) crowns may be used following these steps.

1. Evaluate the preoperative occlusion. Note the dental midline and the cusp-fossa relationship bilaterally.

2. Administer appropriate local anesthesia, ensuring that all soft tissues surrounding the tooth to be crowned are well anesthetized, and place a rubber dam. Because gingival tissues all around the tooth may be manipulated during crown placement, it is important to obtain lingual or palatal, as well as buccal or facial, anesthesia.

3. Reduction of the occlusal surface is carried out with a no. 169L taper fissure bur or a football diamond in the high-speed handpiece. Make depth cuts by cutting the occlusal grooves to a depth of 1.0 to 1.5 mm, and extend through the buccal, lingual, and proximal surfaces. Next, place the bur on its side and uniformly reduce the remaining occlusal surface by 1.5 mm, maintaining the cuspal inclines of the crown (Fig. 21-14). *Note:* If a preveneered SSC is going to be placed, more occlusal reduction will be necessary to compensate for the thickness of resin on the occlusal surface of the crown.

4. Establish access to decay with a no. 330 or 169L bur in the high-speed handpiece. Then remove decay with a large, round bur in the low-speed handpiece or with a spoon excavator.

5. Proximal reduction is also accomplished with the taper fissure bur or thin, tapered diamond. Contact with the adjacent tooth must be broken gingivally and buccolingually, maintaining vertical walls with only a slight convergence in an occlusal direction. The gingival proximal margin should have a feather-edge finish line. Care must be taken not to damage adjacent tooth structure.

6. Round all line angles, using the side of the bur or diamond. The occlusobuccal and occlusolingual line angles are rounded by holding the bur at a 30- to 45-degree angle to the occlusal surface and sweeping it in a mesiodistal direction. Buccolingual reduction for the stainless steel crown preparation is often limited to this beveling and is confined to the occlusal one third of the crown. If problems are later encountered in selecting an appropriate crown size or in fitting a crown over a large mesiobuccal bulge, more reduction of the buccal and lingual tooth structure may become necessary. *Note:* If a preveneered crown is being placed, circumferential reduction including the buccal and lingual surfaces is definitely necessary. The buccal and lingual proximal line angles are rounded by holding the bur parallel to the tooth's long axis and blending the surfaces together. All angles of the preparation should be rounded to remove corners but not so much as to create a round preparation.

7. Selection of a crown begins as a trial-and-error procedure. The goal is to place the smallest crown that can be seated on the tooth and to establish preexisting proximal contacts. (*Helpful hint:* Size 4 is the most frequently used crown size for molars.) The selected crown is tried on the preparation by seating the lingual first and applying pressure in a buccal direction so that the crown slides over the buccal surface into the gingival sulcus. Friction should be felt as the crown slips over the buccal bulge. Some teeth are an "in-between"

## BOX 21-8

### Steps for Preparation and Placement of Stainless Steel Crowns—cont'd

size, so that one crown size is too small to seat and the next larger size fits very loosely, even after contouring. Further tooth reduction, especially on the buccal and lingual surfaces, may be necessary in these cases to seat the smaller crown.

After seating a crown, establish a preliminary occlusal relationship by comparing adjacent marginal ridge heights. If the crown does not seat to the same level as the adjacent teeth, the occlusal reduction may be inadequate; the crown may be too long; a gingival proximal ledge may exist; or contact may not have been broken with the adjacent tooth, preventing a complete seating of the crown. An extensive area of gingival blanching around the crown indicates that the crown is too long or is grossly overcontoured. Crowns are manufactured longer than necessary for the average tooth, and hence many will require some trimming. A properly trimmed crown will extend approximately 1 mm into the gingival sulcus. The Ni-Chro Ion precontoured crowns usually require the least trimming. Before trimming, place the crown onto the preparation and lightly mark the level of the gingival crest on the crown with a sharp instrument, such as a scaler. The crowns are removed and are trimmed 1 mm below the mark with crown-and-bridge scissors or with a heatless wheel on the low-speed straight handpiece. The crown margins should be trimmed to lie parallel to the contour of the gingival tissue around the tooth and should consist of a series of curves without straight lines or sharp angles.

8. Contour and crimp the crown to form a tightly fitting crown. Contouring involves bending the gingival one third of the crown's margins inward to restore anatomic features of the natural crown and to reduce the marginal circumference of the crown, ensuring a good fit. Contouring is accomplished circumferentially with a no. 114 ball-and-socket pliers (Fig. 21-15, *A*) or with a no. 137 Gordon pliers. Final close adaptation of the crown is achieved by crimping the cervical margin 1 mm circumferentially. The no. 137 pliers may be used for this; special crimping pliers, such as no. 800-417 (Unitek) (Fig. 21-15, *B*), are also available. A tight marginal fit aids in (1) mechanical retention of the crown, (2) protection of the cement from exposure to oral fluids, and (3) maintenance of gingival health. After contouring and crimping, firm resistance should be encountered when the crown is seated. After seating the crown, examine the gingival margins with an explorer for areas of poor fit. Observe the gingival tissue for blanching, and examine the proximal contacts. If proximal contact

is necessary, it can be done with a ball-and-socket pliers after removal of the crown.

When removing the crown, a scaler or amalgam carver can be used to engage the gingival margin and dislodge the crown. A thumb or finger should be kept over the crown during removal so that movement of the crown is controlled.

9. The rubber dam is removed and the crown replaced so that the occlusion may be checked. Examine the occlusion bilaterally with the patient in centric occlusion. Look for movement of the crown occlusogingivally with biting pressure, and check for excessive gingival blanching.

After the rubber dam is removed, special care must be taken when handling the crown in the mouth. A 2 × 2 inch gauze pad should be placed posterior to the tooth being crowned to prevent the crown from dropping into the oropharynx.

10. Final smoothing and polishing of the crown margin should be performed before cementation. Smoothing is begun with the heatless stone to create smooth, flowing curves and to thin the margin of the crown slightly. Rotation of the stone should be toward and at a 45-degree angle to the edge of the crown. A rubber wheel is used to remove surface scratches, using light, brushing strokes. A wire brush can be used to polish the margins to a high shine.

11. Rinse and dry the crown inside and out, and prepare to cement it. A glass ionomer, zinc phosphate, polycarboxylate, or self-curing resin ionomer cement can be used. The crown is filled approximately two thirds with cement, with all inner surfaces covered.

12. Dry the tooth with compressed air and seat the crown completely. Cement should be expressed from all margins. The handle of a mirror or the flat end of a band pusher may be used to ensure complete seating, or the patient may be instructed to bite on a tongue blade. Before the cement sets, have the patient close into centric occlusion and confirm that the occlusion has not been altered.

13. Cement must be removed from the gingival sulcus. Zinc phosphate cement can be easily removed with an explorer or scaler. Polycarboxylate cement, after it has partially set, will reach a rubbery consistency. Excess cement should be removed at this stage with an explorer tip. The interproximal areas can be cleaned by tying a knot in a piece of dental floss and drawing the floss through the interproximal region.

14. Rinse the oral cavity well, and reexamine the occlusion and the soft tissues before dismissing the patient.

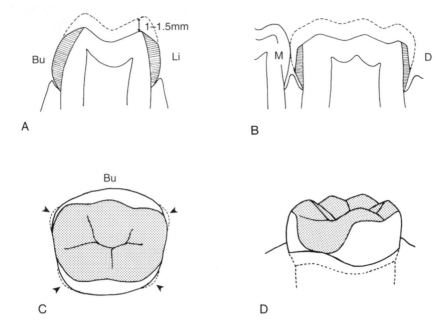

**Figure 21-14**    Stainless steel crown preparation. Mandibular second primary molar. A, Proximal view. Bu, Buccal; Li, lingual. B, Buccal view. Note feather-edge gingival margins. C, Occlusal view. Note rounded line angles. D, Mesiolingual view. Note that lingual and buccal reduction is limited to the beveling of the occlusal third. (From *Stainless Steel Crown Preparation and Restoration*, Project TAPP, Quercus Corporation, 1977.)

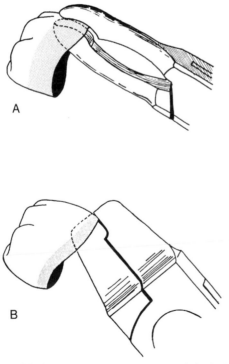

**Figure 21-15**    **A,** Contouring is accomplished with a pair of no. 114 pliers. **B,** Final crimping is accomplished with a pair of no. 800-417 pliers. (From *Stainless Steel Crown Preparation and Restoration*, Project TAPP, Quercus Corporation, 1977.)

periodontal tissues. However, the deficiencies can be largely avoided when attention is paid to two key principles: (1) crown length and (2) shape of the crown's gingival margins.[57]

The length of an SSC should allow the crown to fit just into the gingival sulcus, engaging the natural undercuts. More importantly, the crown length should extend just slightly apical to the tooth's height of contour. For primary teeth the buccal, lingual, and proximal heights of contour happen to be just above the gingival crest. As an SSC is trimmed in length such that its gingival margins come closer to the greatest diameters (heights of contour) of the tooth crown, the spaces between the margins of the crown and tooth surfaces are reduced. Thus, when the margins of the metal crown nearly approximate the greatest diameter of the tooth, the spaces are small enough so that the metal can be adapted closely to the tooth. In other words, crowns that extend well beyond a tooth's height of contour are very difficult to adapt closely to the tooth surface.

The shape or contour of the gingival margins differs from first to second primary molar, as well as from buccal to lingual to proximal. The margins of the trimmed crown should approximate the shape of the gingival crest around the

# Stainless Steel Crowns in Pediatric Dentistry

*N. Sue Seale*

The stainless steel crown (SSC) is an often underused and underappreciated restoration for the primary dentition. It is durable, inexpensive, and easily and quickly placed. However, because it is frequently lumped with cast crowns in the minds of many dentists, it is viewed as an aggressive restorative approach and its indications for use in the primary dentition are poorly understood. For many practitioners, the decision to restore a tooth with a crown denotes excessive tooth removal, great expense, and a general feeling of having compromised the tooth. The weightiness of condemning a permanent tooth to a crown is often transferred to the use of SSCs for the primary teeth. Rarely do dental students have time to assimilate the differences in treatment planning for the developing, changing primary dentition compared with the more static nature of the permanent dentition.

Restorative decisions for the primary dentition are driven by different goals and expectations than for the permanent dentition. The primary teeth are a temporary dentition with known life expectancies of each tooth. By matching the "right" restoration with the expected life span of the tooth, dentists can succeed in providing a "permanent" restoration that will never have to be replaced. This is essentially impossible in the permanent dentition because the life expectancies of the restorations are much shorter than the life expectancies of the teeth. Picking that right restoration involves understanding the limitations of the primary dentition to hold certain types of restorations over time and the durability of the restorative options available. The most commonly used restorative materials available are amalgam, composite, and SSCs.

The strength of the primary tooth itself, rather than the size of the lesion being restored, is often the major limiting factor in the choice of a successful restoration. Primary teeth are small, with correspondingly thin layers of enamel and dentin, and are intended to fit the face and jaws of the 2-year-old child. The removal of even small carious lesions often compromises the structural integrity of the anterior teeth and first molars. In the primary molars, the contact area is broad, and a relatively large truncated box is required to place the margins of an amalgam or composite in self-cleansing areas. The first primary molar is small, and the buccal and lingual retaining walls become thin and weak with little remaining supporting dentin. Therefore, if the restoration is required to last more than 2 years in the first primary molar, shallow preparations combined with weak walls often doom class II restorations to failure.

Studies evaluating the durability and life span of SSCs and class II amalgams demonstrate the superiority of crowns for both parameters.[1] Crowns placed in children 4 years and younger have a success rate approximately twice that of amalgams for each year up to 10 years of service.[1] This trend is also apparent in children older than 4 years, with the success rate of crowns almost twice that of class II amalgams for each year up to 10 years of service. When a choice exists between a class II amalgam and a crown in a child younger than 4 years, the likelihood of failure of the amalgam is approximately twice that of the crown.[1] Where durability is concerned, the SSC is the clear choice.

Two other factors that weigh heavily in the decision to use SSCs are the potential for long-term follow-up and parental compliance in home care. If you will not see the child regularly or home care will not be sufficiently supervised to ensure compliance, an additional advantage of crowns is the preventive aspect that full coverage provides. In the caries-prone child or the child for whom recall and long-term follow-up will be lacking, this restoration provides protection from recurrent caries. Additionally, when a class II restoration fractures and the proximal box is lost before or during active stages of eruption, mesial drifting results in space loss. The SSC is not subject to failure through fracture and improves the chances of successful restoration even without supervision.

The dental school experience rarely prepares the young general dentist to feel confident in placing SSCs. Therefore, even when the class II is not the ideal restoration, many choose it because they are most comfortable with it and are confident they can do it well. When these restorations fail, replacement with another amalgam/composite is usually impossible because recurrent caries removal and redefinition of the preparation further weaken the tooth. A crown (and many times a pulpotomy, depending on recurrent caries involvement) is required for retreatment. Cost comparison studies of restorations in primary teeth have shown that amalgam replaced by a crown is the most costly.[2] Third-party payers are requiring increased accountability for the cost-effectiveness of the outcomes of our treatment. This then becomes part of the multifactorial decision making process dentists use to select a restoration, and the expectation for long-term success must be considered.

*Continued*

## Stainless Steel Crowns in Pediatric Dentistry—cont'd

The dentist treating children should recognize the durability, preventive aspect, and cost-effectiveness of the SSC as a restorative choice for the primary dentition.

### REFERENCES

1. Levering NJ, Messer LB: The durability of primary molar restorations: III. Costs associated with placement and replacement. *Pediatr Dent* 10:86-93, 1988.

2. Messer LB, Levering NJ: The durability of primary molar restorations: II. Observations and predictions of success of stainless steel crowns. *Pediatr Dent* 10:81-85, 1988.

---

tooth. Figure 21-16, A demonstrates the different gingival contours. As you look at the marginal gingiva around the second primary molar you will note that the occlusogingival heights gradually become shorter along the crests of the gingival margins toward both the mesial and distal surfaces. The outline of buccal and lingual gingiva around second primary molars resembles "smiles." The buccal gingiva of the first primary molar has a different outline. Because of the mesiobuccal cervical bulge, the gingival margin dips down as it is traced from distal to mesial. If you can picture the letter S on its side and stretched out somewhat, and if a tooth crown is placed on top of this curved line, the term "stretched-out S" can be used to describe the contour. However, the contours of the lingual marginal gingiva of all first primary molars resemble "smiles." The proximal contours of almost all primary teeth "frown" (Fig. 21-16, B) because the shortest occlusocervical heights are about midpoint buccolingually. By keeping these shapes in mind when trimming the SSCs the close adaptation to the tooth will be made much easier.

The margins of the finished, trimmed steel crown consist of a series of curves or arcs as determined by the marginal gingiva of the tooth being restored. There are no corners, jagged angles, right angles, or straight lines found on these margins. As described in an earlier section, crown and bridge trimming scissors, a heatless stone mounted on the low-speed straight handpiece, and a rubber wheel can be used to neatly trim and smooth an SSC. Contouring and crimping pliers are necessary to apply the appropriate gingival adaptation. Keeping the principles of crown length and marginal shape in mind will ensure

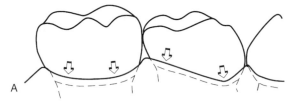

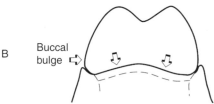

**Figure 21-16    A,** The buccal gingival contour of the second primary molar *(left)* has been described as a smile, and the buccal gingival contour of the first primary molar has been described as a stretched-out S. Note the contour in the region of the mesiobuccal bulge of the first primary molar. The gingival contour of all of the lingual surfaces *(not pictured)* is a smile. **B,** The proximal gingival contour of primary molars has been described as a frown because the shortest occlusocervical heights are about midpoint buccolingually.

optimal adaptation and clinical success of the crown.

### Special Considerations for Stainless Steel Crowns[40]

**Placement of Adjacent Crowns.** When quadrant dentistry is practiced, it often is necessary to place SSCs on adjacent teeth. The tooth preparation and crown selection for placing multiple crowns are similar to that previously described for single crowns. However, there are several areas of consideration as follows:

1. Prepare occlusal reduction of one tooth completely before beginning occlusal reduction of the other tooth. When reduction of two teeth is performed simultaneously, the tendency is to underreduce both.
2. Insufficient proximal reduction is a common problem when adjacent crowns are placed. Contact between adjacent proximal surfaces should be broken, producing an approximately 1.5-mm space at the gingival level.
3. Both crowns should be trimmed, contoured, and prepared for cementation simultaneously. It is generally best to begin placement and cementation of the more distal tooth first. Most importantly, however, the sequence of placement of crowns for cementation should follow the same sequence as that when the crowns were placed for final fitting. Sometimes crowns will seat quite easily in one placement sequence and will seat with great difficulty if the sequence is altered.

### Preparing Crowns in Areas of Space Loss.
Frequently, when the tooth structure is lost as a result of caries, a loss of contact and drifting of adjacent teeth into space normally occupied by the tooth to be restored occur. When this happens, the crown required to fit over the buccolingual dimension will be too wide mesiodistally to be placed and a crown selected to fit the mesiodistal space will be too small in circumference. The larger crown, which will fit over the tooth's greatest convexity, is selected and an adjustment is made to reduce mesiodistal width. This adjustment is accomplished by grasping the marginal ridges of the crown with Howe utility pliers and squeezing it, thereby reducing the mesiodistal dimension. Considerable recontouring of proximal, buccal, and lingual walls of the crown with the no. 137 or no. 114 pliers will be necessary. If difficulty in crown placement is still encountered, additional tooth reduction of the buccal and lingual surfaces and selection of another, smaller crown may be necessary. When the area of space loss is in the region of the distal surface of a mandibular first primary molar and

difficulty is encountered finding the appropriate size crown because of the space loss, another alternative exists. Select a maxillary first primary molar crown for the opposite side of the mouth and try it on the mandibular tooth. Owing to the space loss, often the mandibular tooth preparation resembles a maxillary tooth and therefore is more suited for placement of the maxillary crown. By selecting the maxillary crown for the opposite side of the mouth, the crown's gingival margin contour in the area of the mesiobuccal cervical bulge fits the mandibular mesiobuccal cervical bulge. If several millimeters of space loss have occurred, it may be necessary to extract the tooth and place a space maintainer rather than struggle to place a crown on a compromised tooth preparation.

## RESTORATION OF PRIMARY INCISORS AND CANINES

Indications for restoration of primary incisors and canines are generally based on the presence of (1) caries, (2) trauma, or (3) developmental defects of the tooth's hard tissue. Adhesive materials, usually resin-based composites or resin ionomer products, are placed into class III and class V restorations in primary anterior teeth. Class IV restorations may also be done; however, if a great deal of tooth structure has been lost, full coverage with a crown will provide a superior restoration.

### Class III Adhesive Restorations

Class III adhesive restorations on primary incisors are very challenging to do well (Fig. 21-17). Caries often extend subgingivally, making good isolation and hemorrhage control difficult. Because of the large size of the pulps of these teeth, the preparations must be kept very small. But in spite of trying to keep the restoration small and conservative, experience has found that retention of class III restorations solely with acid etching is often inadequate and additional mechanical retention is required. Retention can be gained with retentive locks on the facial or lingual surface and by beveling the cavosurface margin to increase the surface area of the enamel etched.[11,37] It has been suggested that preparing the entire facial surface by 0.5 mm and veneering the surface

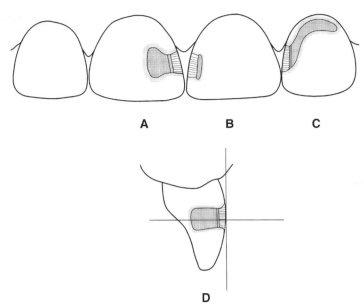

**Figure 21-17**    Class III cavity preparations (A, B, C: labial view). Note that a short bevel is placed on the cavosurface margin of all three preparations. **A,** Slot preparation with a dovetail (the most frequently used class III preparation). The dovetail provides additional retention. **B,** Slot preparation, used for very small class III carious lesions. **C,** Modified slot preparation, used when extensive gingival decalcification is evident adjacent to interproximal caries. **D,** The interproximal box is placed perpendicular to a line tangent to the labial surface.

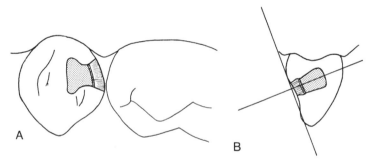

**Figure 21-18**    Class III preparation for primary canines. **A,** The dovetail is usually placed on the lingual surface of maxillary canines and on the labial surface of mandibular canines. A short bevel *(not shown)* is placed on the cavosurface margin of preparations to be restored with resin-based composite. **B,** The proximal box is placed perpendicular to a line tangent to the surface on which the dovetail is placed.

for additional bonding can significantly improve retention of class III restorations.[45]

Restoring the distal surface of primary canines (Fig. 21-18) requires a preparation slightly different from that for incisors. The proximal box is directed at a different angle toward the gingiva. Either amalgam or adhesive materials may be used as the restorative material in this location. The preparation, with the exception of a short cavosurface bevel for resin materials, is identical regardless of the restorative material chosen. A dovetail may be placed on the facial surface, except when amalgam is chosen for a maxillary canine; in that situation, the dovetail is placed on the palatal surface. The steps in preparation and placement of a class III composite restoration are listed in Box 21-9.

## Class V Restorations for Incisors and Canines

Class V restorations may be adhesive materials (most frequently) or amalgams. They are most often needed on the facial surface of canines. To prepare these restorations, penetrate the tooth in

## BOX 21-9

### Steps in Preparation and Placement of a Class III Adhesive Restoration

1. Administer appropriate anesthesia, and place the rubber dam. Ligation of individual teeth with dental floss provides the best stability.

2. Place a wooden wedge interproximally to minimize gingival hemorrhage by depressing the papilla and protecting it from the bur.

3. Create access, and remove caries with a no. 330 bur or a no. 2 round bur in the high-speed handpiece, utilizing a facial access. The axial wall is ideally placed 0.5 mm into dentin. A round bur in the low-speed handpiece can be used to remove deep decay. The gingival and lingual walls should just break contact with the adjacent tooth. It is not necessary to break contact with the incisal wall of the preparation to maintain adequate tooth structure.

4. To enhance retention, a dovetail or lock is placed on the labial or lingual surface. The lock should not extend more than halfway across the labial surface and is kept in the middle horizontal third of the tooth.

5. Place a short bevel (0.5 mm) at the cavo-surface margin. This may be accomplished with a fine, tapered diamond or with a flame-shaped composite finishing bur.

6. Clean and dry the preparation with water and compressed air.

7. Place a plastic or sectional metal matrix. Most plastic matrices will first have to be cut in half horizontally because they are manufactured for permanent teeth and are too wide for primary teeth. The matrix is placed interproximally and a wedge is reinserted. Note: A resin strip crown form can be trimmed to cover the preparation only (not the entire crown) to create a custom matrix, which often is easier to use than a matrix strip.

8. Etch the preparation for 15 to 20 seconds. An acid gel is preferable. Etching aids in retention and ensures improved marginal integrity and reduced marginal leakage. After etching, rinse and dry the preparation well. If a self-etching bonding agent is used, this step is eliminated.

9. Place a dentin-bonding agent in the preparation with a small brush. Gently blow compressed air into the preparation to disperse a thin layer of bonding agent evenly over both dentin and enamel. Polymerize the bonding agent.

10. With a plastic instrument or a pressure syringe, place the composite in the preparation. Pull the matrix tightly around the cavity preparation with finger pressure and hold until cured. Visible-light-cured composites provide a controlled polymerization time and are recommended over autopolymerizing materials. Hold the visible light as closely as possible to the composite and polymerize according to the manufacturer's instructions. The light should be directed from both the facial and the lingual surfaces to ensure complete polymerization. Avoid looking directly at the polymerization light when it is turned on.

11. Finishing and polishing can be performed immediately following polymerization. The smoothest and most desirable surface of a composite is that which remains after a properly adapted matrix is removed; however, it is difficult to adapt a matrix so accurately that additional adjustment to the margins is unnecessary. Gross finishing or contouring can be performed with fine-grit diamonds or with carbide finishing burs. A flame carbide finishing bur (12 to 20 flutes) is excellent for finishing the facial and interproximal surfaces. A scalpel with a curved blade may be used to remove gingival flash. The lingual surface is best finished with a round or pear-shaped carbide finishing bur. A lubricated, pointed white stone may also be used for smoothing. Composite polishing gloss may be used for final polishing to create a luster-like appearance.

Final interproximal polishing of the restoration is completed with sandpaper strips. These strips will be best used if they are cut into thin strips 2 to 3 mm in width. Mounted abrasive disks can be used to finish the facial and lingual surfaces.

As an optional step, after polishing is completed, an unfilled resin glaze may be added to the polished restoration. The glaze provides a better marginal seal and a smooth, finished surface. Before adding the glaze, the restoration and surrounding enamel should first be etched for 15 to 20 seconds to remove surface debris. After rinsing and drying, the resin is painted onto the restoration and is polymerized. Care should be taken not to bond adjacent teeth together with the resin glaze.

12. When finishing is completed, remove the rubber dam and floss the interproximal areas to check for overhangs and to remove excess glaze material.

the area of caries with a no. 330 bur until dentin is reached (approximately 1 mm from the outer enamel surface). Move the bur laterally into sound dentin and enamel, thus establishing the walls of the cavity. The pulpal wall should be convex, parallel to the outer enamel surface. The lateral walls are slightly flared near the proximal surfaces to prevent undermining of enamel. The final external outline is determined by the extent of caries. Mechanical retention in the preparation can be achieved with a no. 35 inverted cone bur or a no. ½ round bur, creating small undercuts in the gingivoaxial and incisoaxial line angles. For resin-based composites, a short bevel is placed around the entire cavosurface margin. Etching, bonding, material placement, and finishing are similar to that described for class III adhesive restorations, except that no matrix is used.

## Full Coronal Coverage of Incisors

### Indications
The indications for full coverage of incisors are as follows:

1. Incisors with large interproximal lesions
2. Incisors that have received pulp therapy
3. Incisors that have been fractured and have lost an appreciable amount of tooth structure
4. Incisors with multiple hypoplastic defects or developmental disturbances (e.g., ectodermal dysplasia)
5. Discolored incisors that are aesthetically unpleasing
6. Incisors with small interproximal lesions that also demonstrate large areas of cervical decalcification

It is a challenging task to repair extensively destroyed anterior teeth with restorations that are durable, retentive, and aesthetic (Fig. 21-19). There are several methods of providing full coronal coverage to primary incisors: adhesive resin–based composite crowns (Fig. 21-19, *B*), SSCs, and veneered or open-face SSCs (Fig. 21-19, *C*). Each has shortcomings (Table 21-1), but each may be used at some time. The most aesthetic, and a frequently placed crown, is the adhesive resin–based composite crown or "strip" crown. Open-face crowns are popular with many operators because their retention is superior to that of adhesive resin crowns; however, aesthetic results are

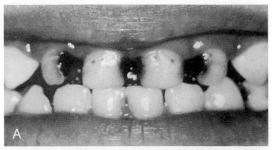
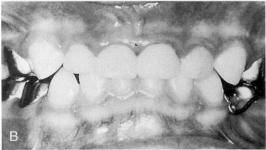
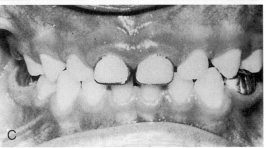

**Figure 21-19** Full coronal coverage of primary incisors. **A,** Extensive caries in primary incisors. **B,** Same incisors after restoration with adhesive resin–based composite crowns (strip crowns). **C,** Open-face stainless steel crowns on maxillary central incisors (see Fig. 21-1 for lingual view).

compromised. Plain SSCs provide a very durable restoration but are aesthetically unpleasing to most parents. SSCs with a resin veneer prebonded to the facial surface are commercially available. These crowns provide a one-step aesthetic restoration that, unlike resin-based composite crowns or open-face crowns, can be placed in the presence of hemorrhage without affecting the final aesthetic result.[61]

The steps for preparation and placement of resin crowns are listed in Box 21-10.

### Preparation and Placement of an Open-Face (Chairside-Veneered) Steel Crown
Nonveneered SSCs are not frequently used on maxillary primary incisors because of the poor aesthetics. However, they are often used on severely decayed canines and mandibular incisors,

## TABLE 21-1

### Comparison of Full Coverage Techniques for Primary Incisors

| Technique | Aesthetics | Durability | Time for Placement | Selection Criteria |
|---|---|---|---|---|
| Resin (strip) crowns* | Very good initially; may discolor over time | Retention dependent on amount of tooth structure present and quality of acid etch. Can be dislodged fairly easily if traumatized | Time required for optimum isolation, etching, placement, finishing | When aesthetics are a great concern. Adequate tooth structure remains for etching/bonding. Child is not highly prone to trauma. Gingival hemorrhage is controllable. |
| Steel crowns[†] | Poor | Very good; a well-crimped, cemented crown is very retentive and wears well. | Fastest crown to place | Severely decayed teeth. Aesthetics of little concern. Unable to adequately control gingival hemorrhage. Need to place a restoration quickly because of inadequate cooperation or time. |
| Open-face steel crowns | Good; however, usually some metal shows. | Good; like steel crowns, are very retentive; however, facings may be dislodged. | Takes longest to place because of two-step procedure: - Crown placement - Composite placement | Severely decayed teeth. Durability needed: active, accident-prone child or severe bruxism evident. |
| Prefabricated veneered steel crowns | Good | Good; however, facings occasionally break. | Not as fast as the plain steel crown; must make tooth fit the crown. | Aesthetics are a concern. Hemorrhage difficult to control. |

*Restoration of choice aesthetically.
[†]Avoid using because of aesthetics.

where aesthetics are less noticeable. Steps for preparation and placement of both veneered[25] and nonveneered crowns are discussed in this section.

The preparation for a steel crown is identical to that of a resin crown, except that no facial undercut is made for the steel crown. After the preparation is completed, select a crown and try it on the tooth. Anterior steel crowns often must have their cervical shapes changed before placement. When manufactured, the crowns have an ovoid shape with a small faciolingual dimension. This must often be changed to allow the crown to slip onto the tooth. This is done by simply squeezing the crown slightly mesiodistally with a pair of Howe no. 110 utility pliers, thereby increasing the faciolingual dimension. The fit of the crown should be snug, and difficulty may be encountered seating the crown with finger pressure only. A gentle rocking of the crown faciolingually facilitates its seating. An orthodontic band pusher or tongue blade may be used to aid in seating, but care should be used not to apply too much pressure. Anterior steel crowns do not generally require much trimming. If trimming is necessary, it is best done with a heatless stone on a straight low-speed handpiece.

Contouring and crimping are necessary to ensure a good marginal fit. Number 137 Gordon

## BOX 21-10

### Preparation and Placement of Adhesive Resin–Based Composite Crowns (Strip Crowns, 3M Company, St. Paul, Minnesota)

1. Administer appropriate anesthesia.

2. Select the shade of composite resin to be used. Then place and ligate the rubber dam.

3. Select a primary incisor celluloid crown form (Unitek Strip Crown, 3M, St. Paul, Minn) with a mesiodistal width approximately equal to the tooth to be restored.

4. Remove decay with a large round bur in the low-speed handpiece. If pulp therapy is required, do it at this time.

5. Reduce the incisal edge by 1.5 mm using a fine, tapered diamond or a no. 169L bur.

6. Reduce the interproximal surfaces by 0.5 to 1.0 mm (Fig. 21-20). This reduction should allow a crown form to slip over the tooth. The interproximal walls should be parallel, and the gingival margin should have a feather edge.

7. Reduce the facial surface by at least 1.0 mm and the lingual surface by at least 0.5 mm. Create a feather-edge gingival margin. Round all line angles.

8. Place a small undercut on the facial surface in the gingival one third of the tooth with a no. 330 bur or a no. 35 inverted cone. When the resin material polymerizes, engaging the undercut, this serves as a mechanical lock.

9. Trim the selected crown form by cutting away excess material gingivally with crown-and-bridge scissors, and trial fit the crown form. A properly trimmed crown form should fit 1 mm below the gingival crest and should be of comparable height to adjacent teeth. Remember that maxillary lateral incisor crowns are usually 0.5 to 1.0 mm shorter than those of central incisors.

10. After the celluloid crown is adequately trimmed, punch a small hole in the lingual surface with an explorer to act as a vent for the escape of trapped air as the crown is placed with resin onto the preparation.

11. If a self-etching bonding agent is not used, etch the tooth with acid gel for 15 to 20 seconds. Rinse and dry the tooth; then apply a dentin bonding agent to the entire tooth and polymerize.

12. Fill the crown form approximately two thirds full with a resin-based composite material, and seat onto the tooth. Excess material should flow from the gingival margin and the vent hole. While holding the crown in place, remove the gingival excess with an explorer.

13. Polymerize the material. Be certain to direct the curing light from both the facial and lingual directions.

14. Remove the celluloid form by using a composite finishing bur or a curved scalpel blade to cut the material on the lingual surface, and then peel the form from the tooth.

15. Remove the rubber dam and evaluate the occlusion.

16. Little finishing should be required on the facial surface. A flame carbide finishing bur can be used to finish the gingival margin should any irregularities be noted upon tactile examination with an explorer. A round or pear-shaped finishing bur may be used for final contouring of the lingual surface. Abrasive disks are used for final polishing of areas of the crown that require contouring.

---

pliers are best suited for this task. Check the final marginal adaptation with an explorer. Polishing and cementation procedures are identical to those for posterior steel crowns. These procedures complete the nonveneered SSC placement. For placement of the open-face or veneered steel crown, the cement must be allowed to set completely; then a labial window is cut in the crown, using a no. 330 or no. 35 bur. The window extends just short of the incisal edge— gingivally, to the height of the gingival crest; and mesiodistally, to the line angles. It is desirable that very little metal be seen from the facial aspect. With a no. 35 inverted cone bur remove the cement to a depth of 1 mm. Undercuts must be placed at each margin. This can be performed with the no. 35 bur or with a no. $\frac{1}{2}$ round bur. Mechanical retention is necessary because there is usually little enamel to etch. Smooth the cut margins of the crown with a fine green or white finishing stone.

Use of a glass ionomer liner to mask any differences in color between remaining tooth structure and remaining cement will provide for a more aesthetic veneer. A thin layer of dentin-bonding agent and then resin-based composite is placed into the cut window, engaging the undercuts. Resin is added with a plastic instrument. Polymerize the material, and finish with abrasive disks. Always run the disks from resin to metal at the margins. Disks running from metal to resin will discolor the resin with metal particles.

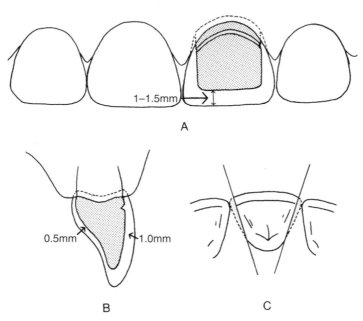

**Figure 21-20** Adhesive resin–based composite crown (strip) preparation. **A,** Labial view. **B,** Proximal view. **C,** Incisal view. The proximal slice should be parallel to the natural external contours of the tooth.

As mentioned previously, preveneered SSCs for primary incisors and canines are now commercially available (Kinder Krowns, Mayclin Dental Studios, Minneapolis, Minn.; Dura Crowns, Space Maintainers Laboratory, Van Nuys, Calif.; NuSmile Primary Crowns, Houston, Tex.; Cheng Crowns, Peter Cheng Orthodontic Laboratories, Philadelphia, Penn.) (Fig. 21-21). The advantages of these crowns are that an aesthetically pleasing result can be obtained with relatively short operating time, and the durability of the steel crown is obtained. In addition, when moisture control is difficult and the resin crowns cannot be placed, these crowns, being less moisture sensitive, may offer a good alternative. The preparation of the teeth for these crowns is similar to the preparation just described for the nonveneered and the open-face crown with one important distinction. These preveneered crowns allow for very little recontouring or reshaping, and therefore the operator must prepare and adjust the tooth to fit the crown, rather than adjusting the crown to fit the tooth. In general more tooth reduction, especially on the buccal and lingual surfaces, is necessary to fit these crowns. When fitting these crowns it is important that a "snap" fit not be achieved. Forcing these crowns onto a prepared tooth under a lot of pressure often leads to microfractures of the veneer and ultimate veneer loss. A snug, sleeve-like fit of the crown over the tooth is recommended.[60]

These crowns have at least three limitations: (1) crimping is limited primarily to the lingual surfaces, not allowing as close an adaptation; (2)

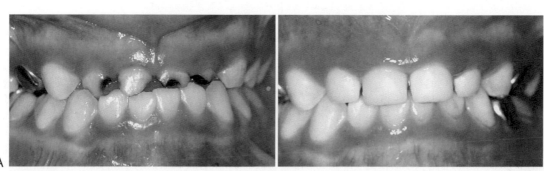

**Figure 21-21** **A,** Extensive caries in primary incisors. **B,** Preveneered crowns (NuSmile, Orthodontic Technologies, Houston, Tex.) restoring the four incisors.

they cost approximately $17 to $18 apiece, compared to approximately $5 for plain stainless steel, making an inventory much more costly; and (3) there are few published clinical data available as to the durability of these crowns. However, anecdotal information indicates that these crowns can provide aesthetically pleasing results for several years. The most common problem seen with these crowns is that occasionally part of the veneer may chip off. This is usually a result of trauma or of forcing the crown onto the tooth with excessive pressure during cementation. If part of the veneer is lost it can be repaired by cutting a small window in the stainless steel, as done for an open-face crown, and new composite can be added. If the veneer fracture is large, simply replacing the crown may provide a faster, more aesthetically pleasing result.

## PROSTHETIC REPLACEMENT OF PRIMARY ANTERIOR TEETH

Premature loss of maxillary primary incisors as a result of extensive caries, trauma, or congenital absence requires consideration for providing a prosthetic tooth replacement for the child.[58] In most instances, prosthetic replacement of primary incisors is considered an elective procedure. Space maintenance in this region is not generally necessary. The most common reason for placement of a prosthetic appliance is parental concern about aesthetics.

Lack of compliance in appliance wear and care by the young child is the greatest limitation of and contraindication for these appliances. If a young child decides that he or she does not like the appliance, he will find a way to remove it from his mouth and will usually discard it. Education of the parents regarding this fact is essential before the decision to construct an appliance is made. Another contraindication for prosthetic replacement is the presence of an anterior deep bite.

Prosthetic appliances may be either fixed or removable (Fig. 21-22), and many different designs are utilized for both. A fixed appliance will almost always be preferred to a removable appliance in preschool children because of compliance issues. When constructing either type, it is best to allow at least 6 to 8 weeks following the tooth loss before fabrication. This allows for good healing and gingival shrinkage. Appliances

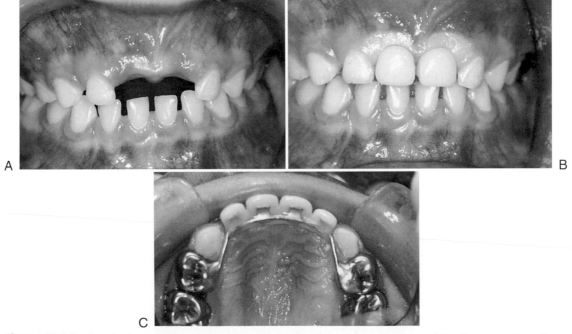

**Figure 21-22**   Prosthetic replacement of primary anterior teeth. **A,** Edentulous space following extraction of two primary incisors. **B,** Fixed prosthetic appliance replacing the two incisors in place. **C,** Example of a fixed prosthetic appliance replacing four incisors. *Note:* Stainless steel crowns are used on the first primary molars as abutments. These provide better retention and durability than orthodontic bands.

can be placed the same day the extractions are done, however, and gingival tissue seems to heal and adapt very well around the prosthetic teeth.

One fixed appliance design is a Nance-like device, constructed with two bands or, preferably, steel crowns on primary molars that are connected by a palatal wire to which the replacement teeth are attached. These prosthetic appliances can be fabricated by any laboratory but are commercially available through Space Maintainers Laboratory of Van Nuys, California. This appliance is cemented onto the molars and is not easily removed by the child. It requires minimal adjustment.[62] The teeth can be made to sit directly on the ridge of the edentulous space (preferred), or acrylic gingiva can be added. Disadvantages of

this appliance include (1) possible decalcification around the bands, (2) more difficulty in home cleaning, and (3) bending of the wires with fingers or sticky foods, which may create occlusal interferences and the need for adjustments. Potential loosening of the bands resulting from continual torquing of bands by the movement of the wire during normal chewing may necessitate frequent recementation.

The removable appliance is a Hawley-like device that replaces the teeth and utilizes circumferential and ball clasps on the molars. These appliances require the most compliance of any of the prosthetic replacements. They are not indicated in children younger than 3 years. Clasps will need adjustment, the frequency of which depends on the child's handling of the appliances. The

## Alternative Restorative Treatment
*Michael J. Kanellis*

Alternative restorative treatment (ART), formerly known as atraumatic restorative treatment, is a minimally invasive treatment technique for restoring teeth by means of hand instrumentation for decay removal and fluoride-releasing adhesive materials (glass ionomer) for filling.[1] ART has been promoted by the World Health Organization as a means of delivering care in underdeveloped countries that do not have electricity or access to sophisticated dental equipment.[2,4] In 2001 the American Academy of Pediatric Dentistry (AAPD) adopted a policy on ART, referring to it as "alternative restorative treatment." The AAPD policy acknowledges that "not all dental disease can be treated by 'traditional' restorative techniques" and recognizes ART as "a useful and beneficial technique in the treatment and manage-

ment of dental caries where traditional cavity preparation and placement of traditional dental restorations are not possible."[3]

There are several potential advantages to ART when used with young children. Because hand instrumentation is used, the noise and vibration of dental handpieces is eliminated. Also eliminated is the need for acid etching, water coolant, and the accompanying high-velocity suction. Caries removal using hand instrumentation also often eliminates the need for local anesthesia. Because instrumentation is kept to a minimum, treatment can easily be carried out in the knee-to-knee position. The use of a fluoride-releasing restorative material helps prevent further decay.

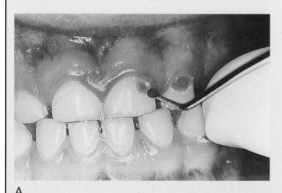

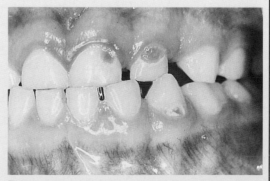

A                                              B

**A,** Facial caries evident on incisors and cuspid. **B,** Spoon excavator positioned for decay removal.        *Continued*

## Alternative Restorative Treatment—cont'd

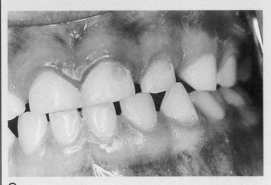

C

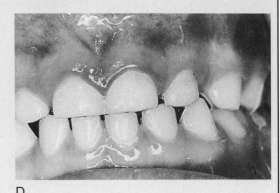

D

C, Appearance after caries removal with spoon excavator. D, Teeth restored with glass ionomer restorative material.

### REFERENCES

1. Frencken JE, Pilot T, Songpaisan Y, Phantumvanit P: Atraumatic restorative treatment (ART): rationale, technique, and development. *J Public Health Dent* 56(3):135-140, 1996.
2. Phantumvanit P, Songpaisan Y, Pilot T, Frencken JE: Atraumatic restorative treatment (ART): a three-year community field trial in Thailand— survival of one-surface restorations in the permanent dentition. *J Public Health Dent* 56(3):141-145, 1996.
3. Policy on Alternative Restorative Treatment (ART): *Pediatr Dent* 25(7 suppl):23, 2003–04.
4. World Health Organization: "Revolutionary new procedure for treating dental caries." Press release WHO/28, April 7, 1994.

greatest advantages of these appliances are the ability to remove the appliance for daily cleaning and the fact that adjustments are easily made by the dentist without having to remove and recement bands.

## REFERENCES

1. ADA Council on Dental Materials, Instruments, and Equipment: Posterior composite resins. *JADA* 112(5):707-709, 1986.
2. ADA Council on Dental Materials, Instruments, and Equipment: Posterior composite resins: an update. *JADA* 113(6):950, 1986.
3. ADA Council on Scientific Affairs: Statement on posterior resin-based composites. *JADA* 129(11): 1627-1628, 1998.
4. AAPD: Pediatric Restorative Dentistry Consensus Conference. *Pediatr Dent* 24(5):377-516, 2002.
5. Bhaskar SN, Lilly GE: Intrapulpal temperature during cavity preparation. *J Dent Res* 44(4):644-647, 1965.
6. Black GV: *A Work on Operative Dentistry*, Vol 11, 5th ed. Chicago, Medico-Dental Publishing, 1924.
7. Black R: Technique for nonmechanical preparation of cavities and prophylaxis. *JADA* 39:953-965, 1945.
8. Bouschor CF, Matthews JL: A four-year clinical study of teeth restored after preparation with an air turbine handpiece with air coolant. *J Prosthet Dent* 16(2):306-309, 1966.
9. Christensen GJ: Don't underestimate the class II resin. *JADA* 123(3):103-104, 1992.
10. Croll TP, Bar-Zion Y, Segura A, Donly KJ: Clinical performance of resin-modified glass ionomer cement restorations in primary teeth. *JADA* 132(8):1110-1115, 2001.
11. Croll TP, Berg J: Simplified primary incisor proximal restorations. *Pediatr Dent* 25(1):67-70, 2003.
12. Cunha RF: A thirty months clinical evaluation of a posterior composite resin in primary molars. *J Clin Pediatr Dent* 24(2):113-115, 2000.
13. Dawson LR, Simon JF, Taylor PP: Use of amalgam and stainless steel restorations for primary molars. *J Dent Child* 48(6):420-422, 1981.
14. Donly KJ, Segura A, Kanellis M, Erickson RL: Clinical performance and caries inhibition of resin-modified glass ionomer cement and amalgam restorations. *JADA* 130(10):1459-1466, 1999.
15. Donly KJ, Wild TW, Jensen ME: Posterior composite class II restorations: in vitro comparison of preparation designs and restorative techniques. *Dent Mater* 6:88-93, 1990.
16. Duggal MS, Toumba KJ, Sharma NK: Clinical

performance of a compomer and amalgam for the interproximal restoration of primary molars: a 24-month evaluation. *Br Dent J* 193(6):339-342, 2002.

17. Einwag J, Dunninger P: Stainless steel crown versus multisurface amalgam restorations: an 8 year longitudinal study. *Quintessence Int* 22(5):321-323, 1996.

18. Fuks AB: The use of amalgam in pediatric dentistry. *Pediatr Dent* 24(5):448-455, 2002.

19. Fuks AB, Araujo FB, Osorio LB et al: Clinical and radiographic assessment of class II esthetic restorations in primary molars. *Pediatr Dent* 22(6):479-485, 2000.

20. Garcia-Godoy F. Resin-based composites and compomers in primary molars. *Dent Clin North Am* 44(3):541-570, 2000.

21. Goldstein RE, Parkins FM: Air abrasive technology: its new role in restorative dentistry. *JADA* 125:551-57, 1994.

22. Gross LC, Griffen Al, Casamassimo PS: Compomers as class II restorations in primary molars. *Pediatr Dent* 23(1):24-27, 2001.

23. Guelmann M, Mjor IA, Jerrel GR: The teaching of class I and II restorations in primary molars: a survey of North American dental schools. *Pediatr Dent* 23(5):410-414, 2001.

24. Hardison JR, Collier OR, Sprouse CW et al: Retention of pit and fissure sealants on the primary molars of 3- and 4- year old children after 1 year. *JADA* 114(4):613-615, 1987.

25. Helpin ML: The open-face steel crown restoration in children. *J Dent Child* 50(1):34-38, 1983.

26. Houpt M, Fuks A, Eidelman E: The preventive resin (composite/sealant) restoration: nine year results. *Quintessence Int* 25(3):155-159, 1994.

27. Hubel S, Mejare I: Conventional versus resin-modified glass ionomer cement for class II restorations in primary molars. A 3 year clinical study. *Int J Pediatr Dent* 13(1):2-8, 2003.

28. Humphrey WP: Use of chromic steel in children's dentistry. *Dent Surv* 26:945-947,1950.

29. Kupietzky A: Bonded resin composite strip crowns for primary incisors: clinical tips for a successful outcome. *Pediatr Dent* 24(2):145-148, 2002.

30. Lacy AM, Young DA: Modern concepts and materials for the pediatric dentist. Pediatr Dent 18(7): 469-475, 1996.

31. Leinfelder KF: A conservative approach to placing posterior composite resin restorations. *JADA* 127(6):743-748, 1996.

32. Leinfelder KF, Sluder TB, Santos JR, Wall JT: Five-year clinical evaluation of anterior and posterior restorations of composite resin. *Oper Dent* 5:57-65, 1980.

33. Leinfelder KF, Vann WF: The use of composite resins on primary molars. *Pediatr Dent* 4(1):27-31, 1982.

34. Marks LAM, Weerheijm LK, van Amerongen WE et

al: Dyract versus Tytin class II restorations in primary molars: 36 months evaluation. *Caries Res* 33(5):387-392, 1999.

35. Marks LAM, van Amerogen WE, Kreulen CM et al: Conservative interproximal box-only polyacid modified composite restorations in primary molars, twelve-month clinical results. *J Dent Child* 66(1):23-29, 1999.

36. Mass E, Gordon M, Fuks AB: Assessment of compomer proximal restorations in primary molars: a retrospective study in children. *J Dent Child* 66(2):93-97, 1999.

37. McAvoy SA: A modified class III cavity preparation and composite resin filling technique for primary incisors. *Dent Clin North Am* 28(1):145-155, 1984.

38. Messer LB and Levering NJ: The durability of primary molar restorations: II. Observations and predictions of success of stainless steel crowns. *Pediatr Dent* 10(2):81-85, 1988.

39. Myers DR: Factors producing failure of class Il silver amalgam restorations in primary molars. *J Dent Child* 44(3):226-229, 1977.

40. Nash DA: The nickel-chromium crown for restoring posterior primary teeth. *JADA* 102(1):44-49, 1981.

41. Norman RD, Wright JS, Rydberg RJ, Felkner LL: A 5-year study comparing a posterior composite resin and an amalgam. *J Prosthet Dent* 64(5):523-529, 1990.

42. Oldenburg TR, Vann WF, Dilley DC: Composite restorations for primary molars: results after four years. *Pediatr Dent* 9(2):136-143, 1987.

43. Osborne JW, Summitt JB, Roberts HW: The use of dental amalgam in pediatric dentistry: review of the literature. *Pediatr Dent* 24(5):439-447, 2002.

44. Paquette DE, Vann WF, Oldenburg TR, Leinfelder K: Modified cavity preparations for composite resins in primary molars. *Pediatr Dent* 5(4):246-251, 1983.

45. Piyapinyo S, White GE. Class III cavity preparation in primary anterior teeth: in vitro retention comparison of conventional and modified forms. *J Clin Pediatr Dent* 22(2):107-112, 1998.

46. Pereira JC, Manfio AP, Franco EB, Lopes ES: Clinical evaluation of Dycal under amalgam restorations. *Am J Dent* 3:67-70, 1990.

47. Qvist V, Laurberg L, Poulsen A, Teglers PT: Longevity and cariostatic effects of everyday conventional glass ionomer and amalgam restorations in primary teeth: three year results. *J Dent Res* 76:387-1396, 1997.

48. Randall RC. Preformed metal crowns for primary and permanent molar teeth: review of the literature. *Pediatr Dent* 24(5):489-500, 2002.

49. Rastelli FP, Vieira RS, Rastelli MCS. Posterior composite restorations in primary molars: an in vivo comparison of three restorative techniques. *J Clin Pediatr Dent* 25(3):227-230, 2001.

50. Roberts JF, Sherriff M: The fate and survival of amalgam and preformed crown molar restorations placed in a specialist pediatric dental practice. *Br Dent J* 169(10):237-239, 1990.

51. Roberts MW, Folio J, Moffa JP, Guckes AD: Clinical evaluation of a composite resin system with a dental bonding agent for restoration of permanent posterior teeth: a 3-year study. *J Prosthet Dent* 67:301-306, 1992.

52. Seale NS: The use of stainless steel crowns. *Pediatr Dent* 24(5):501-505, 2002.

53. Siegal MD, Kumar JV: Workshop on guidelines for sealant use: recommendations. *J Public Health Dent* 55(special issue):263-273, 1995.

54. Simonsen RJ: Conservation of tooth structure in restorative dentistry. *Quintessence Int* 16(1):15-24, 1985.

55. Simonsen RJ: The preventive resin restoration: a minimally invasive, nonmetallic restoration. *Compend Cont Educ Dent* 8(6):428-435, 1987.

56. Simonsen RJ, Stallard RE: Sealant-restorations utilizing a dilute filled resin: one year results. *Quintessence Int* 8(6):77-84, 1977.

57. Spedding RH: Two principles for improving the adaptation of stainless steel crowns to primary molars. *Dent Clin North Am* 28(1):157-175, 1984.

58. Steffen JM, Miller JB, Johnson R: An esthetic method of anterior space maintenance. *J Dent Child* 38(3):154-157, 1971.

59. Straffon LH, Corpron RE, Dennison JB et al: A clinical evaluation of polished and unpolished amalgams: 36 month results. *Pediatr Dent* 6(4):220-225, 1984.

60. Waggoner WF: Clinical tips for restoration of primary anterior teeth with preveneered anterior stainless steel crowns. *J Pediatr Dent Care* 9(3):25-29, 2003.

61. Waggoner WF: Restoring primary anterior teeth. *Pediatr Dent* 24(5):511-516, 2002.

62. Waggoner WF, Kupietzky A: Anterior esthetic fixed appliances for the preschooler: considerations and a technique for placement. *Pediatr Dent* 23(2):147-150, 2001.

63. Welbury RR, Shaw AJ, Murray JJ et al: Clinical evaluation of paired compomer and glass ionomer restorations in primary molars: final results after 42 months. *Br Dent J* 189(2):93-97, 2000.

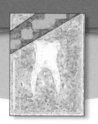

# CHAPTER 22

## Pulp Therapy for the Primary Dentition

*Anna B. Fuks*

Despite modern advances in the prevention of dental caries and an increased understanding of the importance of maintaining the natural dentition, many teeth are still lost prematurely. This can lead to malocclusion or to aesthetic, phonetic, or functional problems that may be transient or permanent.[34,35,52] Maintaining the integrity and health of the oral tissues is the primary objective of pulp treatment. It is desirable to attempt to maintain pulp vitality whenever possible. However, pulp autolysis can be stabilized, or the pulp can be entirely eliminated without significantly compromising the function of the tooth.

This chapter provides a brief review of the normal histologic characteristics of the primary pulp as well as of the dentinogenesis process in health and in response to injury, and discusses the basis for the different forms of pulpal treatment for the primary dentition.

## THE PULP-DENTIN COMPLEX

### Histology

The pulp of a primary tooth is histologically similar to that of a permanent tooth. The odontoblasts have been described traditionally as cells that line the periphery of the pulp space and extend their cytoplasmic processes into the dentinal tubules. These cells have several junctions, which provide a means for intercellular communication and help to maintain the relative position of one cell to another. The cell-free zone is located just below the odontoblastic layer and contains an extensive plexus of unmyelinated nerves and blood capillaries. The core of the dental pulp contains larger blood vessels and nerves, which are surrounded by loose connective tissue.[95] Although this description is correct during active dentinogenesis, it is now accepted that the size of the odontoblasts and the content of their cytoplasmic organelles vary throughout their life cycle and are closely related to their functional activity. The relationship between the size of the odontoblasts and their secretory activity can be demonstrated by differences in their size in the crown and in the root, and may express different dentinogenic rates in these two areas of the tooth.[89]

The odontoblasts are highly specialized cells and are responsible for the formation of dentin. Owing to the extension of their cytoplasmic processes into the dentinal tubules, these cells compose the main part of the pulp-dentin complex. When this complex is damaged by disease or attrition or is affected by operative procedures, it reacts in an attempt to defend the pulp.

Recent progress in understanding the molecular and cellular changes during tooth development and how they are mimicked during tissue repair offers the opportunity to assess the biological validity of the various vital pulp treatments. For this purpose, the dentinogenesis process during tooth formation, throughout life, and in response to injury will be briefly described.

## Dentinogenesis in Healthy State

The inner enamel epithelium and its associated basement membrane have an important role in direct odontoblastic cytodifferentiation. They present bioactive molecules, including growth factors immobilized on the basement membrane, that send signals to the cells of the dental papilla, inducing differentiation.[97] Thus, the odontoblasts are cells derived from the ectomesenchymal cells of the dental papilla.

During the postmitotic state the odontoblasts line the formative surface of the matrix and start secreting primary dentin. At the initiation of the dentinogenesis, during mantle dentin formation, mineralization is achieved through the mediation of matrix vesicles.[18] When mantle dentin formation is completed and the odontoblasts form a tightly packed layer of cells, the matrix of dentin is produced exclusively by the odontoblasts. The

other cells of the pulp (in the subodontoblastic layer and in the pulp core), although supporting dentinogenesis, do not have a direct role in primary dentin secretion.[53] As the matrix is secreted the odontoblasts move pulpally, leaving a single cytoplasmic process embedded in a dentinal tubule in the matrix. These tubules, which increase in density near to the pulp, confer the property of permeability on the dentin, a feature that has significant clinical importance.[89]

After secretion of the bulk of dentin during primary dentinogenesis, physiologic secondary dentin is secreted at a much slower rate throughout the life of the tooth, leading to a slow reduction in the size of the pulp chamber.[4] The original postmitotic odontoblasts, responsible for primary dentinogenesis, survive for the life of the tooth, unless subjected to injury. These cells remain in a resting stage after primary dentinogenesis, and the physiologic secondary dentin formation represents a basal level of cell activity in the resting stage.[53]

## Dentinogenic Response to Injury

The pulp-dentin complex responds to injury by formation of new hard tissue, mainly tertiary dentin, increasing the distance between the injury and the pulp and sometimes by decreasing the dentin permeability (sclerotic dentin).[97]

The nature and quality of the tertiary dentin is dependent on its tubular structure and influences the dentin permeability of the area. Thus, in case of a mild injury, the odontoblasts responsible for the primary odontogenesis can frequently survive the challenge and are stimulated to secrete reactionary dentin beneath the injury site.[87] Since the original odontoblasts are responsible for this matrix secretion, there will be tubular continuity and communication with the primary dentin matrix[61] (Fig. 22-1, A). Reactionary dentin might be considered as an extension of physiologic dentinogenesis. However, since it is a pathologic response to injury, it should be regarded as distinct from the primary and secondary dentinogenesis.

When the injury is severe, the odontoblasts beneath the injury may die; however, if suitable conditions exist in the pulp, a new generation of odontoblast-like cells may differentiate from underlying pulp cells, secreting a reparative dentin matrix. Since this dentin is formed by a new generation of cells, there will be discontinuity

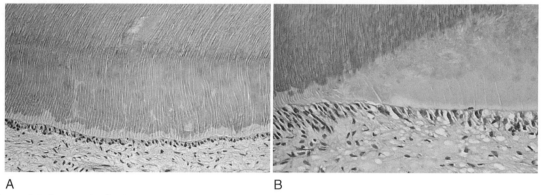

**Figure 22-1**   **A,** Histologic section showing tubular continuity in reactionary dentin. **B,** Histologic section showing lack of continuity in the reparative dentin. (Courtesy of Carlos Alberto S. Costa, DMD, PhD.)

in the tubular structure, with a subsequent reduction in permeability[9] (Fig. 22-1, *B*).

A critical question concerns the factors responsible for triggering the stimulation of odontoblastic activity. Although there is still much to learn regarding the molecular control of cell activity in general and of odontoblastic activity in particular, one family of growth factors, the transforming growth factors (i.e., TGF-β) superfamily, has been reported to have extensive effects on the mesenchymal cells of many connective tissues.[60]

During tooth development, the odontoblasts secrete TGF-β, and some remains sequestrated in the dentin matrix. The sequestrated TGF-β may be released during any process leading to tissue dissolution, like dental caries or the use of acid etching, for example.[97] Thus, dentin matrix should be considered not as an inert dental hard tissue but rather as a potential tissue store of a cocktail of bioactive molecules (particularly growth factors) waiting to be released, if appropriate tissue conditions prevail.[97]

In contrast to reactionary responses, reparative dentinogenesis represents a more complex sequence of biological processes. Migration and differentiation of pulpal progenitor cells must take place, creating a new generation of odontoblast-like cells, prior to matrix secretion. A series of stereotypic wound healing reactions occurs in the pulpal connective tissue, including vascular and cellular inflammatory reactions.

In vitro and in vivo experiments on reparative odontogenesis demonstrate that the noninflamed pulp constitutes an appropriate environment where competent pulp cells (potential preodontoblasts) can differentiate into new odontoblast-like cells, forming reparative dentin.[56,65,72]

### Reactions to Dental Caries

When the carious process advances from the enamel into the dentin, sclerotic dentin is formed by the apposition of minerals into and between the tubules (intra- and intertubular dentin), and reactionary tertiary dentin is secreted. Sclerotic dentin can be seen in radiographs as a radiopaque area, as the mentioned apposition of minerals increases the radiopacity of this dentin.

The quality and amount of tertiary dentin is contingent on the depth and rate of progression of the carious lesion. The faster the lesion progresses, the poorer and more irregular will be the reactionary dentin. In addition, if the noxious irritant is too intense, the cytoplasmic processes of the odontoblasts degenerate and "dead tracts" are formed.

When the carious process advances more rapidly than the elaboration of reactionary dentin, the blood vessels of the pulp dilate, and scattered inflammatory cells become evident, particularly subjacent to the area of the involved dentinal tubules (transitional stage). If the carious lesion remains untreated, a frank exposure will eventually occur. The pulp will react with an infiltration of acute inflammatory cells, and the chronic pulpitis will become acute. A small abscess may develop under the region of the exposure, and cells of the chronic inflammatory series may be formed further away from the central area of irritation. The remainder of the pulp may be uninflamed (chronic partial pulpitis with acute exacerbation). As the exposure progresses, the pulp may undergo partial necrosis, followed in some instances by total necrosis.

Drainage is apparently the factor determining whether or not partial or total necrosis will occur.

If the pulp is open and drainage can occur, the apical tissue may remain uninflamed or chronically inflamed. If drainage is impeded by food packing or a restoration, the entire pulp may become necrotic more rapidly. Figure 22-2 describes the reaction of the pulp to dental caries.[86]

### Reactions to Operative Procedures

The factors affecting the dentin-pulp complex during operative procedures (cavity and crown preparations) are mainly the cutting of the dentin per se, the generation of heat, and the desiccation of tissue. When uninvolved dentin is operated on, as in extension for prevention or in crown preparation, tubules that are not protected by reactionary dentin are cut. The tissue reaction that occurs is similar to that occurring with caries: intra- and intertubular mineralization takes place, resulting in sclerotic dentin, followed by the formation of tertiary dentin. The amount and regularity of the tertiary dentin are related to the depth of the cavity preparation: As cavity depth is increased and the remaining dentin is smaller than 0.5 mm, the regularity and quality of the reactionary dentin are compromised. Also, dead tracts may result from damage done to the odontoblastic processes. The effect of cutting the dentin can be observed histologically as a calciotraumatic band, which represents an interruption of the apposition between the secondary and tertiary dentin.

Pulp reactions to operative procedures can be mild or severe, depending on the technique used. When the technique is gentle, the reaction will be mild, and minor alterations in the odontoblastic layer can be observed as a result of fluid accumulation. In a severe reaction, the nuclei of the odontoblasts may be aspirated into the dentinal tubules, hemorrhage may be present, and inflammation is extensive, sometimes resulting in cell necrosis. Figure 22-3 summarizes the sequence of pulp reaction to irritation resulting from operative procedures as related to the state of the pulp.[86] A gentle technique implies use of appropriate cooling and minimal pressure. Cutting a cavity without using water cooling might lead to irreversible changes in the pulp owing to the heat generated at the tip of the bur. The application of pressure increases the damage. Prolonged air blasts are also deleterious to the pulp. Thus, in order to prevent the generation of heat and damage to the pulp, the following measures should be taken: (1) the cavity should be prepared as shallowly as possible, respecting the principles of cavity preparation; (2) small and sharp burs should be used; (3) appropriate cooling should be employed and minimal pressure exerted; and (4) excessive drying of dentin by air syringe should be avoided.[34]

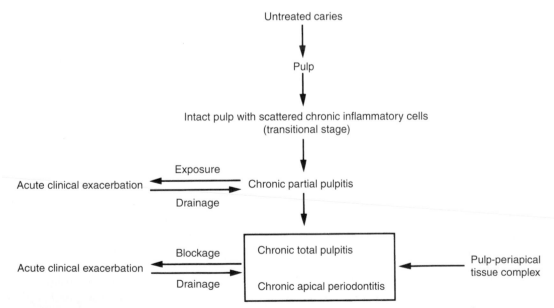

**Figure 22-2**  Pulp reactions to dental caries. (From Seltzer S, Bender IB: *The Dental Pulp*, 3rd ed. Philadelphia, Lippincott, 1984, p 188.)

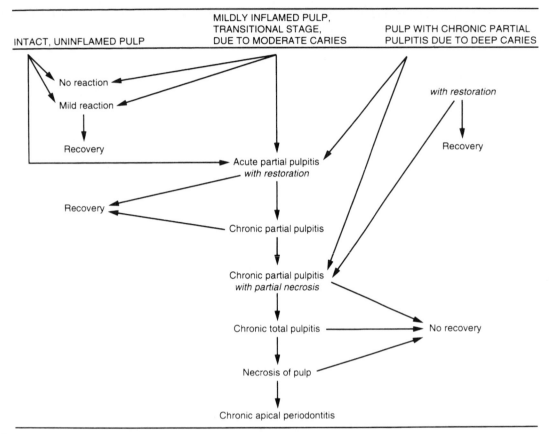

**Figure 22-3**   Sequence of pulp reaction to irritation from operative procedures. (From Seltzer S, Bender IB: *The Dental Pulp,* 3<sup>rd</sup> ed. Philadelphia, Lippincott, 1984, p 256.)

## CLINICAL PULPAL DIAGNOSIS

It is difficult if not impossible to determine clinically the histologic status of the pulp. However, with thorough clinical and radiographic assessment, it is possible to determine whether the tooth pulp is treatable. Selection of the appropriate treatment for a tooth is essential to its long-term prognosis. To make the most accurate diagnosis, information must be obtained from several sources, including a careful medical history and notation of the characteristics of the pain, and thorough clinical and radiographic examinations.

### History and Characteristics of Pain

The history and characteristics of pain are often important in determining whether the pulp is in a treatable condition. However, children may have extensive carious lesions, often with draining paruli, with no apparent history of pain or, if dental problems developed early (such as with nursing bottle decay), the child may have no experience of the teeth feeling any other way.[5] Being aware of these limitations, the dentist should distinguish between two main types of dental pain: provoked and spontaneous. Provoked pain is stimulated by thermal, chemical, or mechanical irritants, and is reduced or eliminated when the noxious stimulus is removed. This sign frequently indicates dentin sensitivity due to a deep carious lesion or a faulty restoration. The pulp is in a transitional state in most cases (see Fig. 22-2), and the condition is usually reversible.

Spontaneous pain is a throbbing, constant pain that may keep the patient awake at night. This type of pain usually indicates advanced pulpal damage, and the pulp is usually nontreatable. However, a final diagnosis can only be made based on clinical tests in conjunction with radiographic assessment. Spontaneous, throbbing pain simulating an irreversible pulp condition can be observed when the dental papilla is inflamed owing to food impaction. This condition may cause bone destruction, and the pulp in these teeth may be treatable. The symptoms disappear with proper restoration of the tooth and reestablishment of an adequate contact point (Fig. 22-4).

The chief complaint and the history of pain are important factors to be considered when establishing a diagnosis. In addition, obtaining an accurate medical history is imperative. A child with a systemic disease may require an alternative treatment approach than that used for a healthy child.

## Clinical Examination

A careful extraoral and intraoral examination can be of extreme importance in detecting the presence of a pulpally involved tooth. Several signs,

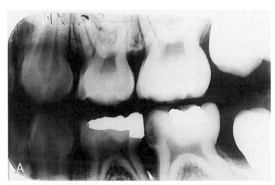
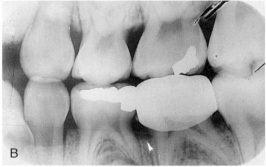

**Figure 22-4  A,** Mandibular second primary molar with extensive mesial caries and alveolar bone resorption *(arrow)* due to food impaction. The history of spontaneous pain associated with tenderness to percussion may suggest pulp involvement. **B,** The same tooth after restoration of the contact point with a stainless steel crown. The symptoms disappeared and bone regeneration is evident *(arrow).* (Courtesy Enrique Bimstein, CD.)

such as redness and swelling of the vestibulum or grossly decayed teeth with draining paruli, are definitely indicative of pulpal pathoses. In addition, attention should be paid for missing or fractured restorations or to those with carious marginal breakdown because these may also be indicators of pulp involvement.

Palpation, assessment of tooth mobility, and sensitivity to percussion are helpful diagnostic tools. Fluctuation, felt by palpating a swollen mucobuccal fold, may be the expression of an acute dentoalveolar abscess prior to exteriorization. Bone destruction following a chronic dentoalveolar abscess can be also detected by palpation. Comparing the mobility of a suspicious tooth with its contralateral tooth is of particular importance. If a significant difference is observed, pulpal inflammation might be suspected. Care should be taken not to misinterpret as pathologic the mobility present during the normal time of exfoliation. Sensitivity to percussion may reveal a painful tooth in which inflammation has progressed to involve the periodontal ligament (acute apical periodontitis). However, care should be taken in interpreting these tests (see Fig. 22-4, *A*). Belanger[5] suggests that percussion should be done very gently with the tip of a finger and not with the end of a dental mirror to prevent exposing the child to unnecessary uncomfortable stimuli.

Other classic vitality tests, such as sensitivity to heat or cold or electric pulp testing, are of a little value because they seldom provide accurate data in primary teeth. False-positive results may be obtained from stimulation of the gingiva or of the periodontal ligament. In addition, because a child might be apprehensive, use of this type of stimulation by the dentist might result in loss of the child's confidence, causing disruptive behavior.

## Radiographic Examination

Following the clinical examination the clinician should obtain a high-quality bitewing radiograph. Interradicular radiolucencies, a common finding in primary teeth with pulpal pathoses, can be better observed in bitewing radiographs. If the apical area cannot be clearly observed in such a film, a periapical view of the affected side should be obtained. The integrity of the lamina dura of the affected tooth should be compared with that of adjacent or contralateral teeth. Radiographs are valuable as aids in visualizing the presence or absence of the following:

1. Deep caries with possible or definite pulp involvement.
2. Deep restorations close to a pulp horn.
3. Successful or failing pulpotomy or pulpectomy.
4. Pulpal changes, such as pulp calcifications (denticles) and pulp obliteration.
5. Pathologic root resorption, which may be internal (within the root canal) or external (affecting the root or the surrounding bone). Internal resorption indicates inflammation of a vital pulp, whereas external resorption demonstrates a nonvital pulp with extensive inflammation, including resorption of the adjacent bone.
6. Periapical and interradicular radiolucencies of bone. In primary teeth, any radiolucency associated with a nonvital tooth is usually located in the furcation area, not at the apices. This is because of the presence of accessory canals on the pulpal floor area. Thus, a bitewing film is frequently a useful diagnostic aid, particularly in maxillary molars where the developing premolar obscures the furca in a periapical radiograph.

Belanger[5] emphasizes that the dentist should be familiar with the normal factors that complicate the interpretation of radiographs in children, that is, largest bone marrow spaces, superimposition of developing tooth buds, and normal resorption patterns of the teeth.

## Operative Diagnosis

There are instances when a final diagnosis can only be reached by direct evaluation of the pulp tissue and a decision about treatment is made accordingly. For example, if a formocresol pulpotomy is planned, the nature of the bleeding from the amputation site should be normal (red color and hemostasis evident in less than 5 minutes with mild cotton pellet pressure). If bleeding persists, a more radical treatment should be undertaken (pulpectomy or extraction) because excessive bleeding is an indication that the inflammation has reached the radicular pulp. Conversely, if a pulp polyp is present and bleeding stops normally after coronal pulp amputation, a formocresol pulpotomy may be performed instead of a more radical procedure.[34]

## PULP TREATMENT PROCEDURES

The most important and also the most difficult aspect of pulp therapy is determining the health of the pulp or its stage of inflammation so that an appropriate decision can be made regarding the best form of treatment. Several different types of pulp treatment have been recommended for primary teeth. They can be classified into two categories: conservative (those that aim to maintain pulp vitality) and radical (consisting of pulpectomy and root filling). When the infection cannot be arrested by any of the methods listed and bony support cannot be regained, the tooth must be extracted.

### Conservative Treatment

*Protective Base*

The American Academy of Pediatric Dentistry recommends placement of a protective base or liner on the pulpal and axial walls of a cavity preparation to act as a protective barrier between the restorative material and the tooth.[1] Dentin is permeable and allows the movement of materials from the oral cavity to the pulp and vice versa. It was believed for several years that pulp inflammation was caused by the toxic effects from dental materials.[90] Today, however, there is sufficient evidence to show that pulpal inflammation resulting from dental materials is mild and transitory, with adverse reactions occurring as the result of pulpal invasion by bacteria or their toxins.[8,12] Continued marginal leakage with secondary recurrent caries is probably the most common cause of pulp degeneration under restorations; this pulpal irritation is often related to the permeability of the dentin. In deep cavities the dentin covering the pulp is thin, and the tubules are large in diameter and packed close together. This dentin is extremely permeable and should be covered with a material that seals dentin well, usually glass ionomer cement.[76]

Copal varnish had been utilized to seal the amalgam tooth interface until corrosion products formed to eliminate the gap and to provide a barrier against the passage of irritants.[13] The materials most recently used as cavity sealers are those that have demonstrated multisubstrate bonding ability to bond the restorative material to the tooth. These include resin cements, glass ionomers, and dentin-bonding agents. The benefits of utilizing these materials to bond composite to tooth structure is a well-documented and accepted procedure.[41] However, employing them in conjunction with amalgam is more controversial. The insoluble adhesive layer may act as a barrier to prevent amalgam corrosion products from ultimately sealing the gap. Thus, the dentin-bonding agents may potentially put the patient at a greater risk for marginal leakage and recurrent caries in the long term.[41] Mahler et al.[57] observed no difference between amalgam restorations placed with and without bonding after 2 year and concluded that the use of bonding agents under traditional amalgam fillings should not be recommended. Thus, protective liners or bases should only be placed in deep cavities approaching the pulp.

### Indirect Pulp Treatment

Indirect pulp treatment (IPT) is recommended for teeth that have deep carious lesions approximating the pulp but no signs or symptoms of pulp degeneration. In this procedure, the deepest layer of the remaining carious dentin is covered with a biocompatible material to prevent pulp exposure and additional trauma to the tooth. This results in the deposition of tertiary dentin, which increases the distance between the affected dentin and the pulp, and in the deposition of peritubular (sclerotic) dentin, which decreases dentin permeability. It is important to remove the carious tissue completely from the dentinoenamel junction and from the lateral walls of the cavity in order to achieve optimal interfacial seal between the tooth and the restorative material, so preventing microleakage.

The dilemma that clinicians face lies in the assessment of how much caries to leave at the pulpal or axial floor. The carious tissue that should remain at the end of the cavity preparation is the quantity that, if removed, would result in overt exposure. It is difficult to determine whether an area is an infected carious lesion or a bacteria-free demineralized zone. The best clinical marker is the quality of the dentin: soft, mushy dentin should be removed, and hard discolored dentin can be indirectly capped. The ultimate objective of this treatment is to maintain pulp vitality[16] by (1) arresting the carious process, (2) promoting dentin sclerosis (reducing

permeability), (3) stimulating the formation of tertiary dentin, and (4) remineralizing the carious dentin.

Clinical experience and a good understanding of the process of caries progression can allow for better control of the "partial removal caries step"; the use of a large round bur (no. 6 or 8) can provide better results than the use of spoon excavators.[22] In the last decade, a chemical-mechanical approach to caries excavation known as Carisolv (Medi Team Dental, Savedalen, Sweden) has been developed. This method consists of a gel, made of three amino acids and a low concentration of sodium hypochlorite rubbed into the carious dentin with specially designed hand instruments. With Carisolv, sound and carious dentins are clinically separated, and only carious dentin is removed, resulting in a more conservative preparation. When a bur is used, healthy tissue is frequently removed. The main drawback in this technique is the time needed to complete the procedure, as it is much slower than with the use of a bur.[20]

Two materials are most commonly used in IPT: calcium hydroxide and zinc oxide–eugenol (ZOE) paste. The rationale for IPT is that few viable bacteria remain in the deeper dentin layers and that after the cavity has been sealed properly they will be inactivated. These facts argue against a two-step procedure, in which the tooth is reentered for the purpose of excavating the previously carious dentin and to confirm the formation of reactionary dentin. The procedure risks creation of a pulp exposure and further insult to the pulp.[15]

Atraumatic restorative treatment, an approach for managing caries of dentin with hand instruments without local anesthesia, has been considered a form of IPT. Massara et al.[59] demonstrated that use of glass ionomer creates conditions that lead to remineralization and suggest that it can be recommended as a good base for indirect pulp capping.

Dentin-bonding agents have been recommended for use in direct and indirect pulp capping.[46] However, there are some concerns regarding an IPT with these materials. Nakajima and coworkers[67] found a significant loss of bond strength to human carious dentin when compared with sound dentin. This finding leads one to question even further the integrity of the bond and subsequent ability to prevent bacterial invasion of a carious substrate.

Success rates of IPT have been reported to be higher than 90% in primary teeth, and thus its use is recommended in patients in whom a preoperative diagnosis suggests no signs of pulp degeneration.[22,23,69,91,92] The value of taking a good history complemented by a careful clinical and radiographic examination cannot be overestimated when trying to reach an accurate diagnosis. However, sometimes this cannot be achieved and the prognosis of the tooth will be affected. Figure 22-5 shows the treatment outcome of two mandibular first primary molars in the same patient. The tooth treated with a mineral trioxide aggregate (MTA) pulpotomy presents internal root resorption, whereas its antimere, restored conservatively with a composite over an IPT, looks normal. These findings were probably attributable to the preoperative status of the pulp. The radicular pulp of the pulpotomized tooth was probably chronically inflamed at the time of treatment but could not be disclosed even by operative diagnosis.

The overall success of IPT has been reported to be higher than the success rates of direct pulp capping or pulpotomy, the alternative pulp treatments for primary molars with deep dentinal caries.[22,23,78,91,92]

New strategies utilizing bioactive molecules such as enamel matrix protein (Emdogain) or TGF-β have been utilized experimentally to stimulate tertiary dentin formation and decrease dentin permeability.[68] However, these are not yet in clinical use.[97]

### Direct Pulp Capping

Direct pulp capping is carried out when a healthy pulp has been inadvertently exposed during an operative procedure. The tooth must be asymptomatic, and the exposure site must be pinpoint in diameter and free of oral contaminants. A calcium hydroxide medicament is placed over the exposure site to stimulate dentin formation and thus "heal" the wound and maintain the vitality of the pulp.[52] The effectiveness of TGF-β and bone morphogenetic proteins in inducing reparative dentinogenesis in pulp capping situations in vivo[44,66,84,85,96] provides the basis for development of a possible new generation of biomaterials. Since the specificity of these growth factors to induce reparative processes is not clear, more studies are required to fully explain the kinetics of growth factor release and the sequence of growth factor–induced reparative dentinogenesis.

Direct pulp capping of a carious pulp exposure in a primary tooth is not recommended but can be used with success on immature permanent teeth. The direct pulp cap is indicated for small mechanical or traumatic exposures when conditions for a favorable response are optimal. Even in these cases the success rate is not particularly high in primary teeth. Failure of treatment may result in internal resorption (Fig. 22-6) or acute dentoalveolar abscess. Kennedy and Kapala[48] claim that the high cellular content of the primary pulp tissue may be responsible for the increased failure rate of direct pulp capping in primary teeth. These authors believe that undifferentiated mesenchymal cells may differentiate into odontoclasts, leading to internal resorption, a principal sign of failure of direct pulp capping in primary teeth.

Some investigators advocate the use of dentin-bonding agents for direct pulp capping.[46,47] The rationale for this is based on the belief that if an effective, permanent seal against bacterial inva-

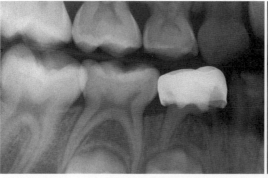
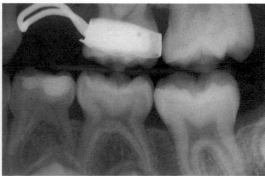

A                                                    B

**Figure 22-5** Mandibular first primary molars of the same patient three years after treatment of deep caries. **A,** Tooth treated with mineral trioxide aggregate pulpotomy. Internal resorption is evident. **B,** Contralateral tooth treated conservatively with indirect pulp treatment and a composite restoration. The pulp looks normal.

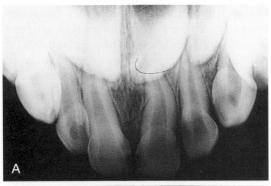

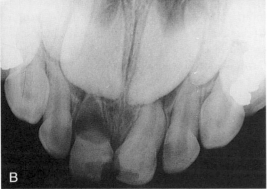

**Figure 22-6** **A,** Maxillary primary central incisor treated by direct pulp capping with CaOH following pinpoint iatrogenic pulp exposure. **B,** Extensive internal resorption was evident 6 months later.

sion is provided, pulp healing will occur. Animal research has shown good compatibility of mechanically exposed pulps to visible-light-activated composite when bacteria are excluded.[12] Araujo et al.[2] reported good clinical and radiographic results in cariously exposed primary teeth 1 year after acid etch and capping with a bonding agent and restoration with a composite resin. Based on these reports, Kopel[49] proposed a "revisitation" of the direct pulp capping technique in primary teeth. He suggested "gently wiping the dentin floor and the exposed pulp with an antibacterial solution such as chlorhexidine or a fixative such as formocresol or a weak glutaraldehyde solution," replacing calcium hydroxide with dentin-bonding agents. In another publication a year later, Araujo et al.[3] examined histologically primary molars with microexposures that were successfully treated with a composite acid etch technique and then extracted or exfoliated. These authors observed microabscesses adjacent to the exposure site, and no dentin bridge was formed in any specimen. These results were confirmed by Pameijer and Stanley,[73,74] who concluded that "the

belief that any material placed on an exposed pulp will allow bridge formation as long as the cavity is disinfected is a fallacy." Costa et al.,[11] in a review on pulp capping with dentin-adhesive systems, reported that self-etching adhesive systems led to inflammatory reactions, delay in pulpal healing, and failure of dentin bridging in human pulps capped with bonding agents. They state that vital pulp therapy using acidic agents and adhesive resins seems to be contraindicated.

Presently, direct pulp capping should still be looked on with some reservations in primary teeth. However, this treatment could be recommended for exposed pulps in older children 1 or 2 years prior to normal exfoliation. In these children, a failure of treatment would not imply the need for space maintainer following extraction, as it would in younger children.

### Pulpotomy

The pulpotomy procedure is based on the rationale that the radicular pulp tissue is healthy or is capable of healing after surgical amputation of the affected or infected coronal pulp.[34,35] The presence of any signs or symptoms of inflammation extending beyond the coronal pulp is a contraindication for a pulpotomy. Thus, a pulpotomy is contraindicated when any of the following are present: swelling (of pulpal origin), fistula, pathologic mobility, pathologic external root resorption, internal root resorption, periapical or interradicular radiolucency, pulp calcifications, or excessive bleeding from the amputated radicular stumps. Other signs, such as a history of spontaneous or nocturnal pain or tenderness to percussion or palpation, should be interpreted carefully (see Fig. 22-4, *A*).

The ideal dressing material for the radicular pulp should (1) be bactericidal, (2) be harmless to the pulp and surrounding structures, (3) promote healing of the radicular pulp, and (4) not interfere with the physiologic process of root resorption. A good deal of controversy surrounds the issue of pulpotomy agents, and, unfortunately, the "ideal" pulp dressing material has not yet been identified. The most commonly used pulp dressing material is formocresol (Buckley's solution: formaldehyde, cresol, glycerol, and water). Primosch et al.[79] reported in 1997 that the majority of the predoctoral pediatric dental programs in the United States advocate the use of either full-strength formocresol (22.6%) or a one-fifth dilution (71.7%) of formocresol as the preferred pulpotomy medicament for vital primary teeth. Issues regarding the selection of pulpotomy medicaments will be discussed later in this chapter.

**Pulpotomy Technique.** After local anesthesia has been given and the rubber dam placed, all superficial caries should be removed before pulpal exposure to minimize bacterial contamination following exposure. The roof of the pulp chamber should be removed by joining the pulp horns with bur cuts. This procedure is usually accomplished using a no. 330 bur mounted in a water-cooled high-speed turbine. The coronal pulp is then amputated using either a sharp excavator or a slowly revolving round bur. This procedure should be done carefully to prevent further damage to the pulp and perforation of the pulpal floor (Fig. 22-7). Care must be taken to ensure that all the coronal pulp tissue has been removed. Tags of tissue remaining under ledges of dentin may continue to bleed, masking the actual status of the radicular pulp stumps and thus obscuring a correct diagnosis.

Following coronal pulp amputation, one or more cotton pellets should be placed over each amputation site, and pressure should be applied for a few minutes. When the cotton pellets are removed, hemostasis should be apparent, although a minor amount of wound bleeding may be evident. Excessive bleeding that persists in spite of cotton pellet pressure and a deep purple color of the tissue may indicate that the inflammation has extended to the radicular pulp. Such signs indicate that the tooth is not a good candidate for formocresol pulpotomy, and pulpectomy or extraction should be done. No intrapulpal local anesthesia or other hemostatic agent should be

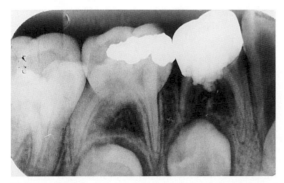

**Figure 22-7** Zinc oxide–eugenol paste extruded through a perforated pulpal floor due to improper use of a bur.

used to minimize hemorrhage because bleeding is a clinical indicator of the radicular pulp status. Following hemostasis, a cotton pellet moistened with Buckley's solution (full concentration or one-fifth solution) is placed over the pulp stumps for 5 minutes. When the pellet is removed, the amputation site should appear dark brown (when a full concentration of formocresol is utilized) or dark red (when the one-fifth dilution is employed). In both cases, very little or no hemorrhage is present. A base of ZOE (either plain or reinforced) is placed over the amputation site and lightly condensed to cover the pulpal floor. A second layer is then condensed to fill the access opening completely. The final restoration is preferably a stainless steel crown, which should be placed at the same appointment. Holan and coworkers[43] observed that pulpotomized primary molars could be successfully restored with one-surface amalgams if their natural exfoliation is expected within 2 years or less. However, if placing the final restoration is not possible, the ZOE base will serve as an acceptable interim restoration until the stainless steel crown can be placed. Guelmann et al.[40] analyzed the success rates of emergency pulpotomies in primary molars. They concluded that the low success rate (53%) of the pulpotomies during the first 3 months could be attributed to undiagnosed subclinical inflammation of pulps, whereas long-term failures might be associated with microleakage of the temporary restorations.

Clinical and radiographic studies have demonstrated that formocresol pulpotomies have success rates ranging from 70% to 97%.[6,26,62,81,83] The use of a one-fifth dilution of formocresol has been advocated by several authors[26,62] because of its reportedly equal effectiveness and potential for less toxicity. This solution is prepared by making a diluent of three parts glycerin and one part water. Four parts of this diluent are then mixed with one part Buckley's solution to make the one-fifth dilution.

Although many studies have reported the clinical success of formocresol pulpotomies, an increasing body of literature has questioned the use of formocresol. Rolling and Thylstrup[83] demonstrated that its clinical success rate decreased as follow-up time increased. Furthermore, the histologic response of the primary radicular pulp to formocresol appears to be unfavorable. Some investigators claim that, subsequent to formocresol application, fixation occurs in the coronal third of the radicular pulp, chronic inflammation in the middle third, and vital tissue in the apical third.[6] Others report that the remaining pulp tissue is partially or totally necrotic.[51] Several reports have questioned the safety and efficacy of formocresol,[27,63] and most authorities now agree that formocresol is at least potentially immunogenic and mutagenic. For these reasons, efforts have increased to find a substitute medicament.

**Potential Substitutes for Formocresol.** Glutaraldehyde (GA) has been proposed as an alternative to formocresol because it is a mild fixative and is potentially less toxic. Due to its cross-linking properties, penetration into the tissue is more limited with less effect on periapical tissues. The short-term success of 2% GA as a pulpotomy agent has been demonstrated in several studies.[14,30,31,38,80,93]

However, longer term success rates matching those of formocresol have not been reported. Fuks et al.[29] reported a failure rate of 18% in human primary molars 25 months after pulpotomy using a 2% concentration of GA. In the same study sample at 42 months follow-up, the authors noted that 45% of the teeth that underwent pulpotomy with GA resorbed faster than their controls.[31]

Some biological materials have been proposed as pulp dressings on the theoretical basis that they would promote physiologic healing of the pulpotomy wound. Varying levels of success in early experimental states have been reported with freeze-dried bone[21]; autolyzed, antigen-extracted, allogenic dentin matrix[64]; allogenic bone morphogenetic protein64; and enriched collagen solutions.[7,28] Clinical studies have reported promising results using ferric sulfate (FS), a hemostatic agent, in pulpotomized human primary teeth.[24,32] Fuks et al.[33] reported a success rate of 93% in teeth treated with FS and 84% in those where dilute formocresol (DFC) was employed. These teeth were followed-up between 6 to 35 months. In a preliminary report of the same study, a much lower success rate was described (77.5% for the FC group and 81% for the DFC teeth), with internal resorption evident in 5 teeth treated with FC and 4 teeth fixed with DFC.[32] This discrepancy can be explained by an excessively severe interpretation of the initial findings. Areas listed initially as internal resorption on the preliminary report remained unchanged after 30 months, and therefore were reassessed as normal in the last evaluation[33] (Fig. 22-8). Success rates comparable

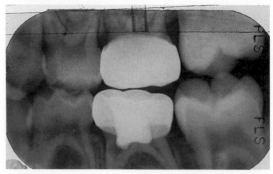

**Figure 22-8** Mandibular second primary molar presenting internal root resorption following pulpotomy with ferric sulfate. The area remained unchanged for 2 years.

to those of formocresol were also reported by Smith et al.[88] A higher percentage of internal resorption using ferric sulfate and formocresol was reported by Papagiannoulis[75] after a longer follow-up time; comparable results were seen in shorter postoperative examinations.

More recently, considerably better results have been obtained with MTA, and statistically significant differences were reported in comparison with formocresol.[17] None of the MTA-treated teeth showed a clinical or radiographic pathologic process. Pulp canal obliteration was detected in 13% of the teeth treated with formocresol and in 41% of those treated with MTA. Radiograph of two primary molars treated with MTA is presented in Figure 22-9. Internal root resorption, a finding seen both in FS- and DFC-treated teeth in other studies,[33,75] was not observed in MTA-treated teeth on the preliminary report.[16] This finding could be observed in one tooth at a later

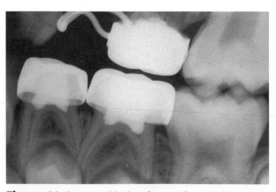

**Figure 22-9** Mandibular first and second primary molars 36 months after pulpotomy with mineral trioxide aggregate. Pulp canal obliteration is evident in the distal root of the second molar; both procedures were rated as successful.

follow-up time (unpublished results) and is presented in Figure 22-5, A.

MTA is commercially available as Proroot MTA (Dentsply, Paris), but its price is very high. Since the material cannot be kept once the envelope is opened, its clinical use in pediatric dentistry practice becomes almost prohibitive. Thus, FS can still be an appropriate and inexpensive solution for pulpotomies in primary teeth.

Nonpharmacotherapeutic approaches to pulpotomy include the treatment of radicular pulp tissue by electrocautery or laser to eliminate residual infectious processes. Although these techniques are being currently used by a number of practitioners, no long-term controlled clinical studies are available to evaluate their success.[19,45,54]

In summary, the search for alternatives to formocresol as a pulp dressing in primary tooth pulpotomies has yet to reveal an agent or technique that has long-term clinical success rates better than those of formocresol. Until such an agent is found, formocresol (either in a one-fifth dilution or full strength), FS, or MTA can be used as capping agents in primary tooth pulpotomies.[37]

## Radical Treatment

### Pulpectomy and Root Filling

The pulpectomy procedure is indicated in teeth that show evidence of chronic inflammation or necrosis in the radicular pulp. Conversely, pulpectomy is contraindicated in teeth with gross loss of root structure, advanced internal or external resorption, or periapical infection involving the crypt of the succedaneous tooth.[1] The goal of pulpectomy is to maintain primary teeth that would otherwise be lost. However, disagreement exists among clinicians about the utility of pulpectomy procedures in primary teeth. Difficulty in the preparation of primary root canals that have complex and variable morphologic features and the uncertainty about the effects of instrumentation, medication, and filling materials on developing succedaneous teeth dissuade some clinicians from using the technique. The behavior management problems that sometimes occur in pediatric patients have surely added to the reluctance among some dentists to perform root canal treatments in primary teeth. These problems notwithstanding, the success of pulpectomies in primary teeth has led most pediatric dentists to prefer them to the alternative of extractions and space maintenance.

Certain clinical situations may justify pulpectomy even with the knowledge that the prognosis may not be ideal. An example of such a case is pulp destruction of a primary second molar that occurs before the first permanent molar erupts. A premature extraction of the primary second molar without placement of a space maintainer usually results in mesial eruption of the first permanent molar with subsequent loss of space for the second premolar (Fig. 22-10). Although a distal shoe space maintainer could be used, maintaining the natural tooth is definitely the treatment of choice. Therefore, a pulpectomy in a primary second molar is preferable, even if that tooth is maintained only until the first permanent molar has adequately erupted and is followed eventually by extraction of the primary second molar and placement of a space maintainer (Fig. 22-11).

**Root Filling Materials.** Developmental, anatomic, and physiologic differences between primary and permanent teeth call for differences

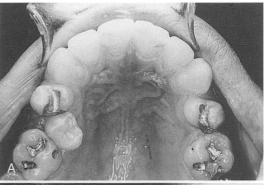
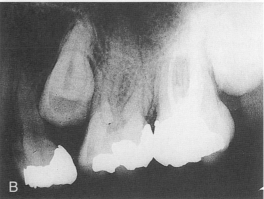

**Figure 22-10** **A,** Occlusal view of the permanent dentition following bilateral premature extractions of the maxillary primary second molars. The right second bicuspid erupted ectopically, and the left is impacted. **B,** Radiograph of the area showing the impacted left premolar. (Courtesy Ilana Brin, DMD.)

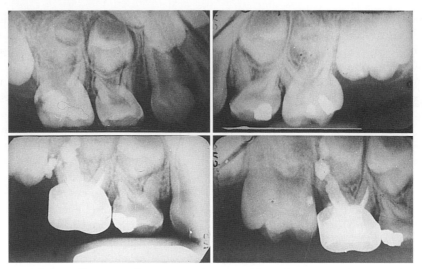

**Figure 22-11**    Nonvital maxillary second primary molar, treated by pulpectomy with zinc oxide–eugenol (ZOE). *Top left,* Prior to pulpectomy. *Top right,* Contralateral vital tooth. Bottom left, Excess of ZOE in palatal and distobuccal canals. *Bottom right,* Primary tooth successfully retained until eruption of first permanent molar.

in the criteria for root canal filling materials. The ideal root canal filling material for primary teeth should resorb at a similar rate as the primary root, be harmless to the periapical tissues and to the permanent tooth germ, resorb readily if pressed beyond the apex, be antiseptic, fill the root canals easily, adhere to their walls, not shrink, be easily removed if necessary, be radiopaque, and not discolor the tooth.[55] No material currently available meets all these criteria. The filling materials most commonly used for primary pulp canals are ZOE paste, iodoform paste, and calcium hydroxide.

*Zinc Oxide-Eugenol Paste.* ZOE is probably the most commonly used filling material for primary teeth in the United States. Camp[10] introduced the endodontic pressure syringe to overcome the problem of underfilling, a relatively common finding when thick mixes of ZOE are employed. However, underfilling is frequently clinically acceptable. Primary teeth frequently present with interradicular radiolucent areas but without periapical lesions and sometimes even have some vital pulp at the apex (Fig. 22-12). Overfilling, on the other hand, may cause a mild foreign body reaction. Another disadvantage of ZOE paste is the difference between its rate of resorption and that of the tooth root.[34] Although particles of ZOE may remain in the alveolar bone for a long time, it is not certain that this has a clinically significant effect (Fig. 22-13).

*Iodoform Paste.* Several authors have reported the use of Kri paste (Pharmachemie, Zurich),

which is a mixture of iodoform, camphor, para-chlorophenol, and menthol.[82] It resorbs rapidly and has no undesirable effects on succedaneous teeth when used as a pulp canal medicament in abscessed primary teeth. Further, Kri paste that extrudes into periapical tissue is rapidly replaced

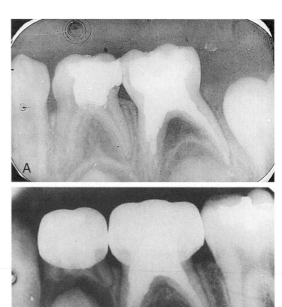

**Figure 22-12**    **A,** Mandibular second primary molar immediately after completion of root canal treatment with ZOE. Note the interradicular radiolucent area and the underfill of the mesial canals. **B,** The same tooth 5 years later showing healing of the lesion. (Courtesy Gideon Holan, DMD.)

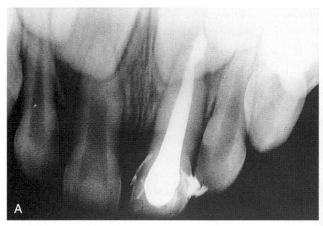
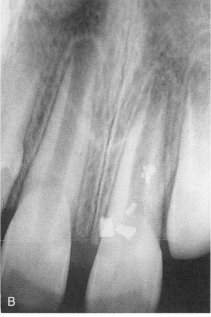

**Figure 22-13** **A,** Maxillary primary central incisor with excessive zinc oxide–eugenol (ZOE) immediately after pulpectomy. **B,** Permanent successor of the root-treated primary tooth showing remnants of ZOE in the alveolar bone. (From Fuks AB, Eidelman E: Pulp therapy in the primary dentition. *Curr Opin Dent* 1:556-563, 1991.)

with normal tissue.[42] Sometimes the material is also resorbed inside the root canal (Fig. 22-14).

A paste developed by Maisto has been used clinically for many years, with good results reported.[58,94] This paste has the same components as the Kri paste with the addition of zinc oxide, thymol, and lanolin.

*Calcium Hydroxide.* Calcium hydroxide is generally not used in pulp therapy for primary teeth. However, several clinical and histopathologic investigations of a calcium hydroxide and iodoform mixture (Vitapex, Neo Dental Chemical Products, Tokyo) have been published in Japan.[25,70] These authors found that this material is easy to apply, resorbs at a slightly faster rate than that of the roots, has no toxic effects on the permanent successor, and is radiopaque. For these reasons, Machida[55] considers the calcium hydroxide–iodoform mixture to be a nearly ideal primary tooth filling material. Another preparation with similar composition is available in the United States under the trade name Endoflas (Sanlor Laboratories, Colombia, South America). The results of root canal treatments using Endoflas in a student's clinic reported similar results to those observed with Kri paste.[36] A complete review of filling materials for primary root canals has been published by Kubota et al.[50]

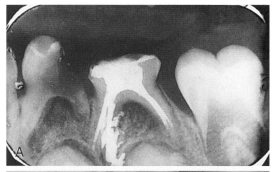
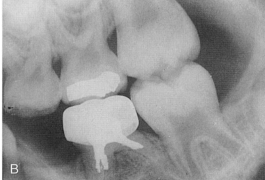

**Figure 22-14** **A,** Mandibular second primary molar pulpectomy with Kri paste. Note the excess of material immediately after treatment. **B,** Nine months after treatment the material has resorbed considerably and the lamina dura appears normal. (Courtesy Gideon Holan, DMD.)

**Pulpectomy Technique.** The pulpectomy procedure should be performed as follows. An access opening should be prepared similar to the methods used in a pulpotomy, but the walls may need flaring more to facilitate access of the canal openings for broaches and files.[10] Each canal orifice of the roots should be located and a properly sized barbed broach selected. The broach is used gently to remove as much organic material as possible from each canal. Endodontic files are selected and adjusted to stop 1 or 2 mm short of the radiographic apex of each canal as determined by a radiograph (Fig. 22-15). This is an arbitrary length but is intended to minimize the chance of overinstrumenting apically and causing periapical damage. The removal of organic debris is the main purpose for filing.[5]

The canal should be periodically irrigated to aid in removing debris. A sodium hypochlorite solution may be used because it helps dissolve organic material; however, because of concern about forcing it into the periapical tissues, the solution should be used very carefully and with no excessive irrigation pressure. Sterile saline may be used as an alternative solution. The canal is dried with appropriately sized paper points.

When a ZOE mixture is used, several filling techniques may be employed.[5] For large canals, as in primary anterior teeth, a thin mixture can be used to coat the walls of the canal, followed by a thick mixture that can be manually condensed into the remainder of the lumen. An endodontic plugger or a small amalgam condenser is useful for compacting the paste at the level of the canal orifice. Care should be taken not to overfill the canal. In primary molars, some of the canals may be quite small and difficult to fill. Commercial pressure syringes have been developed for this purpose. An alternative technique is to use a disposable tuberculin syringe or a local anesthetic syringe, in which the anesthetic capsule is emptied, after which the canal is dried and filled with ZOE paste.

When the root canal is filled with a resorbable paste such as Kri, Maisto, or Endoflas, a spiral lentulo mounted on a low-speed turbine can be used, facilitating introduction of the material into the canal. When the canal is completely filled, the material is compressed with a cotton pellet. Excessive material is rapidly resorbed (see Fig. 22-14).

Vitapex is packed in a very convenient and sterile syringe, and the paste is injected into the canal with disposable plastic needles. This technique is particularly easy to use for primary incisors but less practical for narrow canals of primary molars.[71]

## Criteria for Radiographic Success

Another point to consider is the criteria for radiographic assessment. Traditionally, root treatments were considered successful when no pathologic resorption associated with bone rarefaction is present.[39,42] Payne et al.[77] claim that most clinicians are prepared to accept pulp-treated primary teeth that have a limited degree of radiolucency or pathologic root resorption (Po), in the absence of clinical signs and symptoms. This is contingent on the assurance that the parent will contact the dentist if there is an acute problem and the patient will return for recall in 6 months. According to Payne et al.,[77] most of the pulp therapy studies in the existing literature have considered such teeth to be "successfully treated." These criteria seem to be more suitable for pediatric dentist practices and have been adopted clinically by Fuks et al.[36] These authors, despite describing a low overall success rate (69%) because it did not include teeth in which the pathologic lesion was not completely healed (Po), extracted only one tooth (Px), whereas the remaining (Po) teeth were left for follow-up.

## SUMMARY

Pulp therapy for the primary dentition includes a variety of treatment options, depending on the vitality of the pulp. Conservative treatment is performed when vital pulp remains because

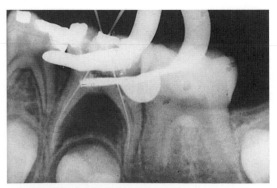

**Figure 22-15** Radiographic determination of the length of the canals.

the potential for recovery exists once the irritation has been removed. Pulpectomy is indicated in teeth showing evidence of chronic, irreversible inflammation or necrosis in the radicular pulp.

# REFERENCES

1. American Academy of Pediatric Dentistry: Reference manual. Guideline for pulp therapy for primary and young permanent teeth. *Pediatr Dent* 24:86, 2002–2003.

2. Araujo FB, Barata JS, Garcia-Godoy F: Clinical and radiographic evaluation of the use of an adhesive system over primary dental pulps. *J Dent Res*(special issue) 75:280(Abstr 2101), 1996.

3. Araujo FB, Barata JS, Costa CAS et al: Clinical, radiographical and histological evaluation of direct pulp capping with a resin in primary teeth. *J Dent Res*(special issue) 76:179(Abstr 1327), 1997.

4. Baume LJ: The biology of pulp and dentin. In: Myers HM, editor. *Monographs in Oral Science,* Vol 8. Basel, Karger, 1980.

5. Belanger GK: Pulp therapy for the primary dentition. In: Pinkham JR, editor: *Pediatric Dentistry: Infancy Through Adolescence.* Philadelphia, Saunders, 1988.

6. Berger JE: Pulp tissue reaction to formocresol and zinc oxide–eugenol. *J Dent Child* 32:13, 1965.

7. Bimstein E, Shoshan S: Enhanced healing of tooth pulp wounds in the dog by enriched collagen solution as a capping agent. *Arch Oral Biol* 26:97, 1981.

8. Brannstrom M: Communication between the oral cavity and the dental pulp associated with restorative treatment. *Oper Dent* 9:57, 1984.

9. Byers M, Narchi M: The dental injury model: experimental tools for understanding neuro-inflammatory interactions and polymodal nociceptors functions. *Crit Rev Oral Biol Med* 10:4, 1999.

10. Camp JH: Pulp therapy for primary and young permanent teeth. *Dent Clin North Am* 28:651, 1984.

11. Costa CA, Hebling J, Hanks CT: Current status of pulp capping with dentin adhesive systems: a review. *Dent Mater* 16:188, 2000.

12. Cox CF, Keall CL, Keall HJ et al: Biocompatibility of surface-sealed dental materials against exposed pulps. *J Prosthet Dent* 57:1, 1987.

13. Craig RG: Restorative Dental Materials, 9th ed. St Louis, Mosby, 1993, pp 203.

14. Davis MJ, Myers R, Switkes MD: Glutaraldehyde: an alternative to formocresol for vital pulp therapy. *J Dent Child* 49:176, 1982.

15. Dumsha T, Hovland E: Considerations and treatment of direct and indirect pulp capping. *Dent Clin North Am* 29:251, 1985.

16. Eidelman E, Finn SB, Koulourides T: Remineralization of carious dentin treated with calcium hydroxide. *J Dent Child* 32:218, 1965.

17. Eidelman E, Holan G, Fuks AB: Mineral trioxide aggregate vs. formocresol in pulpotomized primary molars: a preliminary report. *Pediatr Dent* 23:15, 2001.

18. Eisenmann DR, Glick PI: Ultrastructure of initial crystal formation in dentin. *J Ultrastruct Res* 41:18, 1972

19. Elliott RD, Roberts MW, Burkes J et al: Evaluation of the carbon dioxide laser on vital human primary pulp tissue. *Pediatr Dent* 21:327, 1999.

20. Ericson D, Zimmerman M, Raber H et al: Clinical evaluation of efficacy and safety of a new method for chemo-mechanical removal of caries: a multicentre study. *Caries Res* 33:171, 1999.

21. Fadavi S, Anderson AW, Punwani IC: Freeze-dried bone in pulpotomy procedures in monkey. *J Pedod* 13:108, 1989.

22. Falster CA, Araujo FB, Straffon LH et al: Indirect pulp treatment: in vivo outcomes of an adhesive resin system vs calcium hydroxide for protection of the dentin-pulp complex. *Pediatr Dent* 24:241, 2002.

23. Farooq NS, Coll JA, Kuwabara A: Success rates of formocresol pulpotomy and indirect pulp therapy in the treatment of deep dentinal caries in primary teeth. *Pediatr Dent* 22:278, 2000.

24. Fei AL, Udin RD, Johnson R: A clinical study of ferric sulfate as a pulpotomy agent in primary teeth. *Pediatr Dent* 13:327, 1991.

25. Fuchino T: Clinical and histopathological studies of pulpectomy in deciduous teeth. *Shikwa Gakubo* 80:971, 1980.

26. Fuks AB, Bimstein E: Clinical evaluation of diluted formocresol pulpotomies in primary teeth of school children. *Pediatr Dent* 3:321, 1981.

27. Fuks AB, Bimstein E, Bruchim A: Radiographic and histologic evaluation of the effect of two concentrations of formocresol on pulpotomized primary and young permanent teeth in monkeys. *Pediatr Dent* 5:9, 1983.

28. Fuks AB, Michaeli Y, Sofer-Saks B et al: Enriched collagen solution as a pulp dressing in pulpotomized teeth in monkeys. *Pediatr Dent* 6:243, 1984.

29. Fuks AB, Bimstein E, Guelmann M et al: Assessment of a 2% buffered glutaraldehyde solution in pulpotomized primary teeth of school children. *J Dent Child* 57:371, 1990.

30. Fuks AB, Cleaton-Jones P, Michaeli Y et al: Pulp response to collagen and glutaraldehyde in pulpotomized primary teeth of baboons. *Pediatr Dent* 13:142, 1991.

31. Fuks AB, Bimstein E: Glutaraldehyde pulpotomies in primary teeth of school children: 42 month results. *J Dent Res*(special issue) 70:473(Abstr 1654), 1991.

32. Fuks AB, Holan G, Davis J et al: Ferric sulfate versus

formocresol in pulpotomized primary molars: preliminary report. *J Dent Res*(special issue), 73:885(Abstr 27), 1994.

33. Fuks AB, Holan G, Davis JM et al: Ferric sulfate versus diluted formocresol in pulpotomized primary molars: long term follow-up. *Pediatr Dent* 19:327, 1997.

34. Fuks AB: Pulp therapy for the primary dentition. In: Pinkham JR, editor: *Pediatric Dentistry: Infancy Through Adolescence.* Philadelphia, Saunders, 1999.

35. Fuks AB: Pulp therapy in the primary and young permanent dentitions. *Dent Clin North Am* 44:571, 2000.

36. Fuks AB, Eidelman E, Pauker N: Root fillings with Endoflas in primary teeth: a retrospective study. *J Clin Pediatr Dent* 27:41, 2002.

37. Fuks AB: Current concepts in vital primary pulp therapy. *Eur J Paediatr Dent* 3:115, 2002.

38. Garcia-Godoy F: A 42-month clinical evaluation of glutaraldehyde pulpotomies in primary teeth. *J Pedod* 10:148, 1986.

39. Garcia-Godoy F: Evaluation of an iodoform paste in root canal therapy for infected primary teeth. *J Dent Child* 54:30, 1987.

40. Guelmann M, Fair J, Turner C et al: The success of emergency pulpotomies in primary molars. *Pediatr Dent* 24:217, 2002

41. Hilton TJ: Cavity sealers, liners, and bases: current philosophies and indications for use. *Oper Dent* 21:134, 1996.

42. Holan G, Fuks AB: Root canal treatment with ZOE and KRI paste in primary molars: a retrospective study. *Pediatr Dent* 15: 403, 1993.

43. Holan G, Fuks AB, Keltz N: Success of formocresol pulpotomy in primary molars restored with crown vs. amalgam. *Pediatr Dent* 24:212, 2002.

44. Hu CC, Zhang C, Qian Q et al: Reparative dentin formation in rat molars after direct pulp capping with growth factors. *J Endod* 24:744, 1998

45. Jukic S, Anic I, Koba K et al: The effect of pulpotomy using CO2 and Nd:YAG lasers on dental pulp tissue. *Int Endod J* 30:175, 1997.

46. Kanca J III: Replacement of a fractured incisor fragment over pulpal exposure: a case-report, *Quintessence Int* 24:81, 1993.

47. Kashiwada T, Takagi M: New restoration and direct pulp capping systems using adhesive composite resin. *Bull Tokyo Med Dent Univ* 38:45, 1991.

48. Kennedy DB, Kapala JT: The dental pulp: biological considerations of protection and treatment. In: Braham RL, Morris E, editors. *Textbook of Pediatric Dentistry.* Baltimore, Williams & Wilkins, 1985.

49. Kopel HM: The pulp capping procedure in primary teeth "revisited." *J Dent Child* 64:327, 1997.

50. Kubota K, Golden BE, Penugonda B: Root canal filling materials for primary teeth: a review of the literature. *J Dent Child* 59:225, 1992.

51. Langeland LK, Dowden W, Langeland K: Formo-

52. Levine N, Pulver F, Torneck CD: Pulpal therapy in primary and young permanent teeth. In: Wei SHY, editor. *Pediatric Dentistry: Total Patient Care.* Philadelphia, Lea & Febiger, 1988.

53. Linde A, Goldberg M: Dentinogenesis. *Crit Rev Oral Biol Med* 4:679, 1993.

54. Liu JF, Chen LR, Chau SY: Laser pulpotomy of primary teeth. *Pediatr Dent* 21:128, 1999.

55. Machida Y: Root canal therapy in deciduous teeth. *Jap Dent Assoc J* 36:796, 1983.

56. Magloire H, Joffre A, Bleicher F: An in vitro model of human dental pulp repair. *J Dent Res* 75:1971, 1996.

57. Mahler DB, Engle JH, Simms LE et al: One year clinical evaluation of bonded amalgam restorations. *JADA* 127:345, 1996.

58. Mass E, Zilberman U: Endodontic treatment of infected primary teeth, using Maisto's paste. *J Dent Child* 56:117, 1989.

59. Massara MLA, Alves JB, Brandão PRG: Atraumatic restorative treatment: clinical, ultrastructural and chemical analysis. *Caries Res* 36:430, 2002.

60. Messagne J: The transforming growth factor-β family. *Annu Rev Cell Biol* 6:597, 1990.

61. Mjor IA: *Dentin and Pulp: Reaction Patterns in Human Teeth.* Boca Raton: CRC Press, 1986.

62. Morawa A, Straffon LH, Han SS et al: Clinical evaluation of pulpotomies using dilute formocresol. *J Dent Child* 42:28, 1975.

63. Myers DR, Pashley DH, Whitford GM et al: Tissue changes induced by the absorption of formocresol from pulpotomy sites in dogs. *Pediatr Dent* 5:6, 1983.

64. Nakashima M: Dentin induction of implants of autolyzed antigen extracted allogeneic dentin in amputated pulp in dogs. *Endod Dent Traumatol* 5:279, 1989.

65. Nakashima M, Nagasawa H, Yamada Y et al: Regulatory roll of transforming growth factor-β bone morphogenetic protein-2 and protein-4 on gene expression of extracellular matrix proteins and differentiation on dental pulp cells. *Dev Biol* 162:18, 1994.

66. Nakashima M: Induction of dentine in amputated pulp of dogs by recombinant human bone morphogenetic proteins 2 and 4 with collagen matrix. *Arch Oral Biol* 39:1085, 1994.

67. Nakajima M, Sano H, Burrow MF et al: Bonding to caries affected dentin. *J Dent Res*(special issue): 36(Abstr 74):194, 1995.

68. Nakamura Y, Hammarstrom L, Lundberg E et al: Enamel matrix derivative promotes reparative process in the dental pulp. *Adv Dent Res* 15:105, 2001.

69. Nirschl RF, Avery DR: Evaluation of a new pulp

capping agent in indirect pulp therapy. *J Dent Child* 50:25, 1983.

70. Nishino M et al: Clinico-roentgenographical study of iodoform-calcium hydroxide root canal filling material Vitapex in deciduous teeth. *Jap J Pedod* 18:20, 1980.

71. Nurko C, Ranly DM, Garcia-Godoy F et al: Resorption of a calcium hydroxide/iodoform paste (Vitapex) in root canal therapy for primary teeth: a case report. *Pediatr Dent* 22:517, 2000.

72. O'Kane S, Ferguson MWJ: Transforming growth factor βs and wound healing. *Int J Biochem Cell Biol* 29:63, 1997.

73. Pameijer CH, Stanley HR: The disastrous effects of the "Total Etch" technique in vital pulp capping in primates. *Am J Dent* 11:545, 1998.

74. Pameijer CH, Stanley HR: Pulp capping with "Total Etch" and other experimental methods. *J Dent Res* 78: 219(Abstr 911), 1999.

75. Papagiannoulis L: Clinical studies on ferric sulfate as a pulpotomy medicament in primary teeth. *Eur J Paediatr Dent* 3:126, 2002.

76. Pashley DL: Clinical consideration of microleakage. *J Endod* 16:70, 1990.

77. Payne RG, Kenny DJ, Johnston D H et al: Two-year outcome study of zinc oxide-eugenol root canal treatment for vital primary teeth. *J Can Dent Assoc* 59:528, 1993.

78. Perdigão J, Swift EJJR, Denehy GE et al: In vitro bond strengths and SEM evaluation of dentin bonding systems to different dentin substrates. *J Dent Res* 73:44, 1994.

79. Primosch RE, Glomb TA, Jerrell RG: Primary tooth pulp therapy as taught in predoctoral pediatric dental programs in the United States. *Pediatr Dent* 19:118, 1997.

80. Ranly DM, Lazzari EP: A biochemical study of two bifunctional reagents as alternatives to formocresol. *J Dent Res* 62:1054, 1983.

81. Ranly DM, Garcia-Godoy F: Current and potential pulp therapies for primary and young permanent teeth. *J Dent* 28:153, 2000.

82. Rifkin A: The root canal treatment of abscessed primary teeth: a three to four year follow-up. *J Dent Child* 49:428, 1982.

83. Rolling I, Thylstrup A: A three year clinical follow-up study of pulpotomized primary molars treated with the formocresol technique. *Scand J Dent Res* 83:47, 1975.

84. Rutheford RB, Wahle J, Tucker M et al: Induction of reparative dentine formation in monkeys by recombinant human osteogenic protein-1. *Arch Oral Biol* 38:571, 1993

85. Rutheford RB, Spanberg L, Tucker M et al: The time-course of the induction of reparative dentine formation in monkeys by recombinant human osteogenic protein-1. *Arch Oral Biol* 39:833, 1994

86. Seltzer S, Bender IB: *The Dental Pulp*, 3rd ed. Philadelphia, Lippincott, 1984.

87. Smith AJ, Cassidy N, Perry H et al: Reactionary dentinogenesis. *Int J Dev Biol* 39:273, 1995.

88. Smith NL, Seale NS, Nunn ME: Ferric sulfate pulpotomy in primary molars: a retrospective study. *Pediatr Dent* 22:192, 2000.

89. Smith AJ: Dentin formation and repair. In: Hargreaves KM, Goodies HE, editor. *Seltzer and Bender's dental pulp*. Chicago, Quintessence Int, 2002.

90. Stanley HR: Pulpal responses to ionomer cements-biological characteristics. *JADA* 120:25, 1990.

91. Straffon LH, Corpron RL, Bruner FW et al: Twenty-four-month clinical trial of visible-light-activated cavity liner in young permanent teeth. *J Dent Child* 58:124, 1991.

92. Straffon LH, Loos P: The indirect pulp cap: a review and commentary. *J Israel Dent Assoc* 17:7, 2000.

93. Tagger E, Tagger M: Pulpal and periapical reactions to glutaraldehyde and paraformaldehyde pulpotomy dressing in monkeys. *J Endod* 10:364, 1984.

94. Tagger E, Sarnat H: Root canal therapy of infected primary teeth. *Acta Odontol Pediatr* 5:63, 1984.

95. Torneck CD: Dentin-pulp complex. In: Ten Cate AR, editor. *Oral Histology, Development, Structure and Function*, 2nd ed. St Louis, Mosby, 1985.

96. Tziafas D, Alvanou A, Komnenou A et al: Effects of basic fibroblasts growth factor, insulin-like growth factor-II and transforming growth factor β1 on dental pulp cells after implantation in dog teeth. *Arch Oral Biol* 43:431, 1998.

97. Tziafas D, Smith AJ, Lesot H: Designing new treatment strategies in vital pulp therapy. *J Dent* 28:77, 2000.

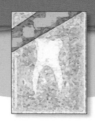

# CHAPTER 23

## Patient Management

*Jimmy R. Pinkham*

As has been mentioned several times in this book so far, the usual and customary age of children entering a dentist's office for the first time has been around the third birthday. The authors and editors believe that this is *no longer a reasonable entry time*. Strategies for effective prevention of dental disease simply must be implemented much earlier in life.

Before dentistry became prevention oriented, entry at age 3 years made sense from a patient treatment standpoint. As reviewed in the first section on the dynamics of change (Chapter 12), it is not until around the third birthday that the majority of children have acquired the communication skills and are sufficiently socialized to comply with the demands of a dental appointment. Also, it is not until the age of 3 years that most children have the language and communication skills to learn from the dentist the essential things about what the dentist is doing that allow them to dismiss their fears about a new, unknown, and potentially threatening person and environment.

Obviously, some children as young as 2 years can go to a dentist and learn to be good patients. Conversely, some youngsters as old as 4 years reliably have a difficult time because of their slow development. However, it is relatively safe to assert that the vast bulk of behavior management techniques practiced, discussed in the literature, and taught in dental schools today are geared primarily to the preschool-aged child of 3 to 6 years. Most dentists agree that the preschool child clearly requires the most energy and talent for effective management.

## THE IMPORTANCE OF CONVICTION, EXPERIENCE, AND GOOD INTENTIONS

Although dentistry for children is doable, not all dentists enjoy working with children. Any dentist who regularly treats preschool children sees some crying, wiggling and kicking, tantrums, and a variety of other avoidance behaviors. Coping with and devoting energy to intercepting these behaviors exasperates some dentists. Other dentists feel guilty or anxious. Still others feel uncomfortable around the involved parents, and some may dread treating the next child scheduled in the appointment book.

One aspect of the dental treatment of children (barring burnout) seems to be predictive of those who can work with children and those who cannot. That aspect is experience.[26,27] Dental students and young practitioners may be discouraged by the anxiety they feel and the insecurity they experience when certain children start to misbehave. However, with time and dedication to the techniques taught in dental school and outlined in this book, a practitioner's skills in managing child patients become refined, and with this refinement comes self-confidence in this area of dentistry. The self-confidence of the dentist in his or her management skills is essential to successful interchanges with potentially unruly children.

## AN EMBARRASSMENT OF RICHES

In 1977, Dr. David Chambers, a psychologist with extensive interest in dentistry for children and considerable input into the literature on how dentists should manage children, labeled the available ways dentists can handle situations with children as an "embarrassment of riches."[10] Anyone knowledgeable about dentistry for children will concur with Dr. Chambers. So many ways of dealing with children's behavior have been described in journals and textbooks that few if any dentists can master them all.

There is, however, a basic inventory of skills that remains critical. Some of these management techniques are nice and polite, some have reasonable elegance in psychological terms, and some, on first inspection by a layperson (and perhaps by sophomore dental students, too), may appear rigorous and authoritative.

## PATIENT MANAGEMENT BY DOMAIN

There are five basic domains for securing the cooperation of children during the dental experience. These are the physical domain, the pharmacologic domain, the aversive domain, the reward-oriented domain, and the linguistic domain.[27]

For most practitioners the most reasonable domain is the linguistic domain. The importance of this particular domain is discussed later in the chapter. However, the practitioner should be knowledgeable about certain particulars of the other four domains.

### Physical Domain

The physical domain ranges from the use of hand restraint by a dental assistant to the use of tools such as the Papoose Board (Olympic Medical, Seattle, Wash.) and Pedi-Wrap (Clark Associates, Worcester, Mass.). Other restraint systems include tape, sheets with tape, cloth wraps, and belts (Fig. 23-1). The use of mouth props also belongs in the physical domain for child patient management (Fig. 23-2). Obviously, these techniques, when used for the duration of an appointment, are reserved for basically unmanageable children. An alternative to physical restraint usually involves management by drugs or general anesthesia.

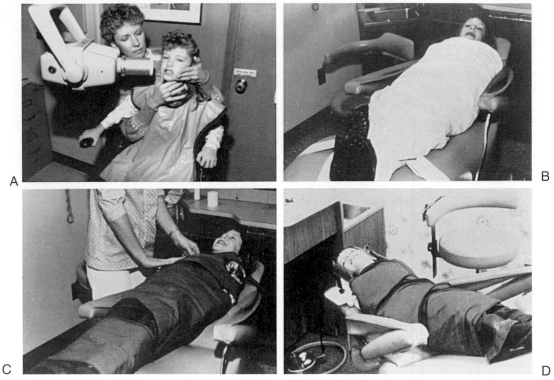

**Figure 23-1**    Patient stabilization. **A,** Parental restraint. **B,** Sheet and ties. **C,** Papoose board (Olympic Medical Corporation, Seattle, Wash.). **D,** Papoose board with head stability attachment.

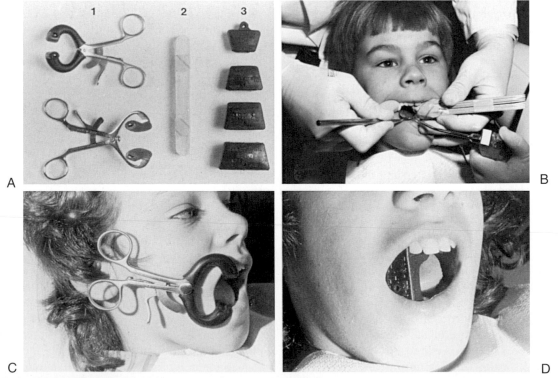

**Figure 23-2**    Jaw stabilization devices. **A,** *1,* Molt mouth gags; *2,* taped tongue blades (sizes can be varied according to size of patient); *3,* McKesson mouth props. **B–D,** Clinical uses of devices.

These techniques can be expensive and are sometimes dangerous.

The physical domain has proven to be useful in treating emergencies on hysterical children and children who cannot be reached in language because of their age. Developmentally disabled children and children who for whatever reason cannot cooperate with the dentist may also need management in this domain. The use of many techniques in the physical domain necessitates explanations to parents, guardians, or caretakers. For instance, the use of a papoose board on a normal child demands informed consent.

## Pharmacologic Domain

Pain and anxiety control by way of pharmacologic methods is discussed in Chapters 7 and 8. This domain includes modalities as safe and easy to deliver as nitrous oxide/oxygen to the profound management provided by general anesthesia in a hospital setting.

Obviously, any drug that has the capability of decreasing respiration, depressing the gag reflex, or making the child sleepy or causing sleep is potentially dangerous. The smaller the child, the more dramatic the danger. Dentists wishing to work with medications need to have training in such techniques, appropriate monitoring equipment, and a protocol that ensures safety for the child. Again, this domain requires parental understanding of the techniques, risks, and alternatives.

## Aversive Domain

A technique can be described as aversive if its use on a child is objectionable enough that the child will cooperate in order to avoid the technique. Parental spanking is an example of aversive management. Generally speaking, dentists who work with children generally refrain or wish to refrain in introducing any aversion to the dental appointment at all.

Some physical techniques can be regarded as aversive if they are used or seem to be used as a punishment. Such practices of these techniques should be avoided: they are unwarranted; they are legally dangerous; and they probably will be ineffective.

Hand-over-mouth (HOM), sometimes described as hand-over-the-mouth exercise or HOME, is regarded by many to be an aversive technique. It can be practiced as such, although, as will be discussed later, it can be practiced as a linguistic technique as well. However, if it is practiced aversively to quiet a crying or screaming child, the clinician must secure informed consent from the parent or guardian. Use of HOM as well as other techniques is covered in guidelines developed by the American Academy of Pediatric Dentistry.[4] Any dentist active in the treatment of children should be aware of these guidelines.

## Reward-Oriented Domain

Rewards can be used to secure a child's cooperation. The reward can be arranged by the dentist, the parent, or the two in concert. The use of rewards by parents may have a negative effect on the appointment. The child may misread the intentions of the parents as their offering a reward because they think the dental appointment will be difficult, frightening, or scary for the child. Certain children who see that they are getting an unusual reward may also conclude that the more anxiety that they develop about the forthcoming dental appointment, the greater the reward may be. As a rule, I request that parents not promise things like ice cream or toys as a reward for going to the dentist *before the dental appointment*. Afterward it can come as a surprise, and the surprise will have no ramifications on what has already transpired during the dental appointment.

## Linguistic Domain: The Linguistic Advantage to Child Patient Behavior Management

Linguistic techniques are those communication techniques that involve the conversation of the dentist with the child and the child with the dentist.[27] Therefore, maturity in language is important for the child patient.[2,6,7] For the almost complete majority of normally developed and normally socialized children who have no mental or emotional handicaps, the process of coming into maturity in language by way of conversation occurs between 2 and 4 years of age. The vast majority of children are competent in language by their third birthday. Few children are competent to cooperate through language during a complicated dental appointment such as an operative session before 30 months of age, and almost all (normal) children are competent at 42 months of age. Therefore, as a general rule, no child is competent in language before the second birthday and all normal children are competent in language after the fourth birthday.

The linguistic domain demands that the dentist be a communicator. The dentist will be a teacher, a coach, a rewarder, a psychologist, a distracter, and an authority figure when using linguistic techniques.

### Requests and Promises

Of all the speech acts that are appropriate to human collaboration and the securing of cooperation, the constitutive speech acts of requests and promises are the most important.[16,25] Cooperation in the human community happens when two or more individuals take effective actions together. With human beings this can only be done in language. Therefore the basic dental experience of a child is a communication experience of the child with his or her dentist.

To be effective, the dentist must make effective requests of the child and sometimes effective re-requests. For the child to be a good patient, the child must make effective commitments to take responsible actions at the reasonable requests of the dentist. These actions are best described as *promises*. It is when a child declines a request that a behavior management strategy must be initiated. This strategy will ultimately reframe the original request. The essence of this reframing is that it convinces the child that the dentist is serious about the request.

### The Dentist as an Ontological Coach

Ontology means our way of being. The best way for the child to be during the dental appointment is quiet, listening for requests, and cooperating with these requests. Obviously, a hysterical, screaming child does not have a way of being that works well for the linguistic domain. Therefore, the dentist becomes not just an educator or a requester but an ontologic coach in trying to make the child's way of being during the dental appointment appropriate for linguistic techniques.[27] This can be enhanced with nonverbal techniques as well.

## BASICS IN MANAGING CHILDREN IN THE DENTAL EXPERIENCE

### Preappointment Experience

The preappointment experience entails bringing the child to the dental office for a tour and orientation. The child is made aware beforehand that *absolutely nothing* will be done that day. The child meets the receptionist, dental assistant, and dentist. If things go well, certain dental equipment can be shown and explained in "childese," such as "Mr. Wind" and "Mr. Water" for the triplex or "Mr. Buzzer" for the handpiece.

*Comments*

The preappointment experience provides two offerings that make it powerful for the dentist. First, it eliminates for the child any unfavorable imaginings as to the realities of the dentist's office and its personnel. Today's dental offices are not frightening. The child's experience in the reception area, if appropriately furnished and stocked with toys, can be delightful. If the child sees other children who are in the dental setting and having fun, the entire visit is enhanced.

Second, linguistically, the experience sets up a greater likelihood that the requests of the dentist at the first real appointment will be objectively dealt with by appropriate promises of action by the child. People, including children, react more favorably to the requests of familiar persons than with strangers.

Preappointment experiences are not used much anymore owing to the time constraints of both the dentist and the parents. This approach is somewhat different from an observation appointment, in which a child watches the dentist treat his or her parent or sibling or someone else. Observation appointments can be useful, but common sense also tells one that they may backfire if children see something that frightens them.

Common sense also dictates that a young child's first appointment should be kept as pleasant and simple as possible. For most children 3 years old or older, an examination and prophylaxis and fluoride treatment can be made a pleasant and even enjoyable experience.

### Tell-Show-Do

The tell-show-do method is the backbone of the educational phase of developing an accepting, relaxed child dental patient. The technique is simple and usually works. The technique dictates that before anything is done (except the injection of a local anesthetic or other procedures that defy explanation, such as pulp extirpation), the child be told what will be done and then shown by some sort of simulation exactly what will happen before the procedure is started. For example:

> Matt, I'm going to clean your teeth with this special dental toothbrush (prophy angle and rubber cup). You see this soft rubber cup? Well, when I step on this gas pedal this cup turns, and when it is full of toothpaste it can really make your teeth shine. Now, Matt, pinch the cup and you will see how soft it is. Now, let me run it on your fingernail so you can feel how it works. Okay, Matt, please open your mouth for me. Thank you.

*Comments*

Choice of words is important in the tell-show-do technique. Achieving the desired result requires that the dentist have a substitute vocabulary for his or her tools and procedures that the child can understand. At least four of five children who are older than 3 years and have a normal social history and emotional status can be guided through a new technique successfully by the use of the tell-show-do method.

Tell-show-do is an educational technique. As the child receives information about an experience, a technique, or piece of equipment, his or her fears of the unknown or the anticipation of pain quickly go away. Again, this technique linguistically enhances the chances that the appropriate request by the dentist will be met by an appropriate, effective action on the part of the child.

## Voice Control

Voice control requires the dentist to interject more authority into his or her communication with the child. There is no question that, to be practiced successfully, voice control requires an attitude of confidence by the practitioner.[11,20] The tone of voice is important. It must have an "I'm in charge here" ring to it. The facial expression of the dentist must also mirror this attitude of confidence.[9] In fact, a dentist can use "voice control" with facial expressions alone. Voice control can be used with deaf children.

*Comments*

Voice control is an essential technique for managing the behavior of preschool children. It is extremely effective at intercepting inappropriate behaviors as they start to happen and is moderately effective at intercepting them after they are full blown. In other words, voice control is a

useful way of reframing a request that has been refused by the child.

As a purely linguistic technique, voice control relies on tonality, cadence, and other aspects of the quality of the dentist's communication with the child. It seems likely that voice control is probably a misnomer, however, and should be understood by the practicing dentist to have nonverbal components. This ramification is discussed further in the nonverbal advantage discussion later in this chapter.

## Hand-Over-Mouth

The HOM technique calls for the dentist to place a hand over the mouth of a hysterically crying child.[17] It is used to intercept tantrums or other fits of rage. It has to be paired with voice control. This technique works reliably with a variety of child personality types.[17] The technique is not intended to scare the child. As said before, it should not be practiced aversively. It is intended to get the child's attention and quiet the child so that he or she can hear what the dentist is saying. Obviously, it reframes the seriousness of a previous request. The practice of HOM requires informed consent.

*Comments*

The American Academy of Pediatric Dentistry recognizes HOM as a legitimate technique with certain indications and contraindications.[3] The technique is indicated in the normal child who is old enough to understand the directions of the dentist and to cooperate with the expectations of the appointment but who exhibits "defiant, obstreperous, or hysterical avoidance behaviors to dental treatment." Contraindications include practice on disabled, immature, or medicated children whose understanding of the desires of the dentist is compromised. Prevention of the child from breathing is a second basic contraindication.

The HOM technique has remained somewhat controversial for obvious reasons. Critics have suggested that it may be psychologically aggravating to the child. There is no formal study that verifies this suspicion. The technique remains in many dentists' repertoire of management techniques simply because it works. It works fast and therefore is cost effective. Patients who qualify for this technique usually would require management with medication, physical restraint, hospitalization, or significant further social and psychological maturation if the technique were not used.

It should be pointed out that most experienced practitioners who practice this technique note that they very seldom need to do it.

The way that HOM can be regarded as a linguistic technique is when it is not used aversively but rather is practiced as a tap on the lips to remind the child that crying is not appreciated during the dental appointment. Used this way, in which there is no airway restraint intended at all, it becomes a coaching technique and a way of reframing earlier requests to be quiet and cooperative.

## Physical Restraint

Physical restraint is its own domain; however, the touching of a child's hands during the injection procedure by a dental assistant, stabilization of a leg that was starting to lift from the chair by a dental assistant, or stabilization of a shoulder by a dentist as a child starts to roll over, when paired with language, becomes part of the entire linguistic management of the child. This is ontologic coaching.

### Comments
Gentle physical restraint allows the dentist to reframe a previous request.

## Praise and Communication

Praise and communication are self-explanatory. All people, including children, react favorably to praise. Furthermore, effective dentistry for children means effective communication of the dentist with the child and vice versa. Both allow for distraction of the anxious child. Language obviously needs to be age appropriate. Knowing how to talk to children of different ages comes with experience.

### Comments
Praise and effective communication combined with tell-show-do form an unbeatable linguistic combination for managing the dental experience for the majority of children 3 years or older.

## Other Methods

There are other management techniques that are readily available to the dentist and are taught in at least some dental schools in North America. Among these are maternal anxiety reduction techniques. (Paternal anxiety reduction has not been studied, but such study probably would lead to similar conclusions.) It has been shown that as a mother's anxiety about her child's dental appointment lessens, so does her child's anxiety. Pairing a frightened child with a "brave" child in the clinic has had some success. Hypnosis and relaxation techniques have some devotees. Play therapy, "time out" to listen to music or "white sound," other distraction techniques, desensitization sessions, gift giving, and observation appointments all have been advocated to some degree at one time or another.

# THE NONVERBAL ADVANTAGE TO CHILD PATIENT MANAGEMENT

In 1964, Dr. John Brauer, one of the founders of the specialty of pediatric dentistry, noted the following pertaining to the technique called "voice control of the child patient":

> Voice control by the practitioners is an all-important factor in management of the patient.[8] The tone and the emphasis employed in talking with the child produce favorable or unfavorable reactions. While many dentists have recognized the value of voice control and have mastered satisfactory voice techniques, additional research is warranted in this area.

In the same chapter of his textbook, Dr. Brauer offered another conclusion about voice control:

> The voice, with certain qualities under control, has motivated nations in peace as well as war; has captured audiences at all age levels; and it can have a profound influence in the behavior pattern of the individual. It is a powerful instrument employed in too few instances in child behavior problems. The profession must learn more of the positive value of this technique.

The article "Voice Control: An Old Technique Reexamined" concluded that facial expression was just as important as the voice (if not more important) during the phenomenon that has been traditionally called "voice control of the child patient."[20] It was noted that facial expression of the dentist conveys to the child that the practitioner is serious and in control. It is the voice and the face that make the dentist powerful in management of the child's behavior. A variety of authorities on nonverbal communication from other disciplines were cited to verify this conclusion.[2,5,6,7,12,14,18,19]

Since that paper, the linguistic phenomena of requests and promises and their importance for the child during the dental experience have been described. In fact, these papers portrayed the entire dental experience as being a social interaction based on two constituent speech acts: that of requests made by the dentist and that of promises by the child patient to take effective actions in response to those requests. What this discussion describes is that the request or re-request of the dentist in the domain called "voice control" implies that there is a body posture that may or may not be entirely visible to the child but that takes the dentist to "a place" from which the dentist can speak with authority, command, and self-confidence. This place allows the experience of the nonverbal advantage. This means the clinician is in a posture and state of body control that empowers his or her coaching of the child patient.

Effectiveness in the nonverbal management of children, even those who display or develop recalcitrant behavior during their dental appointment, is demonstrated by clinicians who not only make the verbal request to stop such behavior but are able to re-request when needed with more verbal determination, with appropriate facial expression, and from a bodily posture in which they know that they are competent. The power of re-requesting is the essence of being competent in managing misbehaving children. This ability is both mental (the words) and physical (the face and body). The body is important to both the voice and the face. This body dimension is described, for lack of a better word, as "a place" but it is to be interpreted as total body posture. Feet, hands, and head are in a relationship to the torso, spine, and breathing pattern such that the total posture energizes the clinician and simultaneously (with or without conscious recognition) allows the clinician to adopt a posture and motion from which his or her most powerful articulations and self-expressions can emanate.

The HOM exercise is also favorably enhanced by the nonverbal advantage. In fact, effective voice control either precedes or is concomitant with effective HOM. I argue that effective HOM would be impossible without effective voice control, and effective voice control is probably impossible without the nonverbal advantage.

## Where Is "The Place?"

There is no formal research in pediatric dentistry describing the most effective posture in which to practice the nonverbal advantage. It is my observation in watching veteran clinicians intercept the misbehaviors of preschool children that they do so by looking at the child in a downward and forward position of their bodies. Clinicians who notice the deterioration of behavior while in a posture in which they are largely behind the child generally move to a position from which there is frontal facial posture available for the child to see expressions and to have eye contact. The leaning downward and forward dramatizes to the child nonverbally that the original requests of the clinician are important.

This posture also offers the possibility of having a profound positive effect on the confidence of the clinician. This confidence shift is the nonverbal advantage. It could be argued that leaning away or adjusting to a higher posture might be contraindicated when the clinician is seeking the nonverbal advantage with a misbehaving child. Importantly, once it is mastered, the clinician will reflexively go to the posture of downward and forward; it does not have to be re-remembered. It is like stepping on the brakes of your car when a red light appears. It occurs in your body. It is because the nonverbal advantage is so reflexive that clinicians who have mastered it are reticent to abandon it. It is also obvious for practitioners who have never mastered the approach that when they try to practice it consciously it is not as effective as when it is reflexively practiced.

Nowhere is this philosophy of body affecting confidence so well described in contemporary Western literature as in the book *Retooling on the Run* by Stuart Heller and David Surrenda.[15] The book addresses the origins of self-confidence as they relate to the body, and is intended for the business world and its executives; however, the issues involved with posture, centered presence, and changing one's experience through motion have direct implications for the dental clinician who works with children as well. Anyone interested in a more thorough description is encouraged to read and study this book.

Figure 23-3, entitled "Your Attitude and Postural Dynamics," is a copyrighted portrayal by Dr. Heller that summarizes how body position affects attitude. Dr. Heller draws on the research

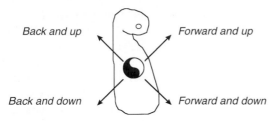

**Attitude:** grounded, decisive, and powerful
**Posture:** *forward and down*

**Attitude:** supportive, caring, and adaptable
**Posture:** *back and down*

**Attitude:** dynamic, inspiring, and friendly
**Posture:** *forward and up*

**Attitude:** thoughtful, peaceful, and perceptive
**Posture:** *back and up*

**Figure 23-3** Attitude and postural dynamics. (Adapted from artwork copyrighted by Dr. Stuart Heller.)

of Dr. Albert Mehrabian, who found that during the communication experience, 7% of one's impact comes from the words that are chosen, 38% from how those words are spoken (tone, volume, pacing), and 55% from nonverbal expressions, including such features as movement, posture, gesture, and timing.[18,19] Dr. Heller also offers that attitude is a function of the interactions between state of mind, feeling, and how one carries oneself.[16] Therefore, an attitude of confidence by a clinician has a great deal to do with the way he or she postures.

From the figure it can be seen that the forward and down position conveys a grounded, direct, and powerful attitude. This is what is needed to intercept misbehavior or potential misbehavior of the child patient. It should be noted that this is not the only posture that a clinician needs to adopt. In fact, there are times for all four postures. For the domain that has previously been called voice control, however, there seems to be no question that the forward and down posture is the one that is relevant to the clinician who requests and re-requests appropriate behaviors from a misbehaving or possibly misbehaving child patient.

This posture is important in the performance of the HOM exercise. In fact, HOM often requires that the practitioner whisper to the child his or her desires for a better behavior and the promise to remove the hand once behavior is acceptable. This forces the clinician into that downward and forward posture in which, I contend, the non-

verbal advantage lies. Being forced into this posture may be one of the reasons *why* those practitioners who effectively use HOM *are* effective. Unknown to them is the fact that the posture they need to succeed with the technique is the very posture that is most empowering for them.

## An Explanation for Body Affecting Mind

Until recently, Western science has been dominated by the Cartesian notion of the duality of mind and body. This theory has been attacked by a number of disciplines ranging from medicine to philosophy and from biology to linguistics. A recent and popular book, *Descartes' Error,* presents a vivid and convincing argument about the mistakes in this theory.[11]

What is emerging is that clearly there is no duality. Mind belongs to body and body belongs to mind. There is no seam between them. Mental processes such as worry, anxiety, and anger have profound physiologic effects on the body. Moreover, motion, movement, posture, and breathing have dynamic impacts on attitudes, emotions, and moods. In fact, training the body can sometimes alter mental characteristics and processes faster than information absorbed directly by reading or hearing.

I submit that the power of the requests and re-requests of a competent clinician is enhanced by the clinician's control of his or her body. This control favorably affects such factors as facial expression and tonality of voice. This is a distinct nonverbal advantage and a useful predictor that distinguishes those clinicians who have the "knack" of working with children. They have the knack even though their dialogue may be identical to someone who does not have the knack. They may have smaller frames and less muscle mass than their less competent colleagues. They may have a higher voice, be less articulate, or even suffer from a speech impediment and still be more effective than others who have outstanding voice qualities. The nonverbal advantage is a bodily advantage that empowers these clinicians during the communication process of making requests of the child patient.

## Categories of Nonverbal Advantage Competency

Clinicians can experience various levels of competency in their practice of the nonverbal advantage. I think that no one comes into dentistry having mastered the nonverbal advantage with children even though they may be parents or older siblings or have had educational experiences with children. Simply said, most American adults today have little opportunity to interact with children in ways that demand they learn to make bodily adjustments to empower their requests and re-requests with the children in their lives. The one exception might be people who have coached children in domains in which fear was an issue to be overcome through the coaching. For instance, swimming and diving coaches of young children may have unconsciously experienced a nonverbal advantage as they encouraged children to overcome fear of water and heights.

### Beginners

Dental students come to their dental education as beginners in the domain of the nonverbal advantage. The effectiveness of the curriculum, handouts, textbook assignments, and clinical challenges sets the stage for whether a dental student wishes to master the nonverbal advantage or not. Obviously, if the educators do not recognize the nonverbal advantage and do not practice from a nonverbal advantage point of view, the students will probably not even be aware of this phenomenon. However, if the pediatric dentistry faculty believe in it, practice it, and serve as role models, some students may initially intellectually accept that this does work and, because of curiosity and enthusiasm, try to develop this talent while in dental school.

It should be noted that this is a difficult technique to teach because it comes from a level of self-awareness that is reached by each individual in his or her own fashion and time. It is difficult to structure appointments and recruit patients so as to allow realization of the nonverbal advantage. Therefore, it is submitted that, except for those students that have a significant amount of clinical pediatric dentistry, often in extramural clinics in which misbehavior is present, most dental students have no opportunity to develop this advantage until after dental school. Also, the nonverbal advantage is difficult to learn in the presence of parents because some degree of experimentation with body, tonality of voice, and facial expression is required while learning. The presence of a parent may arouse enough anxiety in the young clinician to thwart experimentation in these dimensions of the nonverbal advantage.

It is also obvious that there are clinicians who, from the beginning of their dental education, do not want a nonverbal advantage. Students of pediatric dentistry who believe that children are psychologically delicate or who think that the practice of such aspects of the nonverbal advantage as raising one's voice could compromise the child's self-esteem or promote anxiety manifesting after the dental appointment will probably not wish to master the nonverbal advantage. Furthermore, students who do not believe the nonverbal advantage to be more effective than other techniques will probably not put much effort into mastering it during the course of their career.

Last, there is evidence that clinicians who have the nonverbal advantage may sometimes lose it. Some offices that routinely opened their operatories to parents have reported that some clinicians who practice the nonverbal advantage when unobserved by anyone other than dental staff feel uncomfortable practicing it in the presence of nondental observers, particularly parents and guardians. Other clinicians may have sought other solutions: mastery of sedative methods, referral of misbehaving children to other clinicians, willingness to delay treatment, and willingness to work on a crying child stabilized by a papoose board. A clinician may, through lack of practice, eventually lose the nonverbal advantage after having practiced it for years.

### Experimental Mastery

Experimental mastery relates to the person who has with conviction tried to find the nonverbal advantage. This clinician has looked for that "place" in which his or her request or re-request has the strongest design and the greatest impact on the child. Generally speaking, any person who has experienced the positive effects of the nonverbal advantage will enthusiastically try to practice it more. But until a clinician can access this place spontaneously and reflexively, the nonverbal advantage may not be relied on each and every time a child starts to misbehave. There is a time of trial and error that some clinicians can bear until they master the technique. Increasingly, however, the climate of today's dental practice, complete with risk management, informed consent, litigation, parental presence, and other societal issues that inhibit dentists from being as aggressive in the management of children's behavior as they were in past decades, may preclude any possibility of obtaining the nonverbal advantage as a reflexive behavior.

*Mastery*

Most dentists who reflexively practice with a nonverbal advantage do so because they initially believed in that approach. They have experienced the power of the technique. They have obtained great rewards from it, and they do not think it has long-term side effects. These clinicians are mostly older and were educated in an era when the nonverbal advantage was a technique of choice and when sedative techniques were not necessarily a part of the curriculum of an advanced training program in pediatric dentistry. For younger clinicians who have not seen the nonverbal advantage practiced but who want to, competent clinicians exist in virtually all regions of the country who could serve as role models for young clinicians wishing to develop their skills.

## Mastering the Nonverbal Advantage

Figure 23-4, labeled "Stages of Learning Child Patient Management," portrays the process of mastering the nonverbal advantage.

The beginning point for most student clinicians as they seek to become adept at managing children's behavior is a change in the clinician's "story" and movement patterns. The story is one of gaining confidence that managing difficult behavior is possible and that the student's own confidence will increase, that is, "This is doable; I can do it." As the story evolves, the clinician's movement patterns, encompassing posture, breathing, action of limbs, walking, concentration, and emotion, will begin to change. The story begins as didactic knowledge is gained in the classroom and in homework assignments and evolves into experience based on clinical contact with children. That is why there is an "x" between the top two ovals on the figure. In other words, didactic information alone will not produce an effective clinician in the domain of child patient management.

The second step is a perception by the clinician that his or her story is appropriate and that the body and the story are in harmony. In other words, the clinician is starting to have confidence about his or her competence in the behavior management domain and is starting to feel comfortable around children, including those who are misbehaving. In the early stages only the clinician will know that this is happening. Most observers will not be aware that this process is going on. However, at some point the confidence of the clinician becomes apparent and the movement patterns more sophisticated. At this point an informed observer can see the approach being used. In the clinical training of a dental student who is likely to treat children in a general practice, this step is critical.

The refinement attained in the third step is what allows for the fourth step: the clinician's movement and body patterns become appropriate for the challenges at hand. The clinician now can take even more effective actions with the child that were impossible before. It is absolutely verifiable when dental students and practitioners arrive at this level of mastery. They will feel their arrival. Again, informed observers can see it.

Fifth and finally, the shift in possible actions allows the clinician to work with maximal effi-

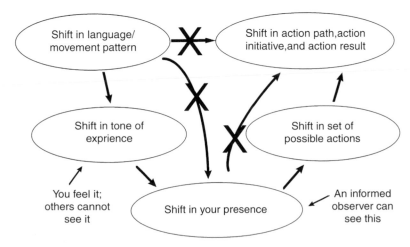

**Figure 23-4** Stages of learning child patient management. (Adapted from artwork copyrighted by Dr. Stuart Heller.)

ciency allowed by the nonverbal advantage. The clinician has a variety of actions and directions from which to choose that will reinforce the power of his requests to the child. Linguistically he or she has gained the advantage of making powerful requests and re-requests. This is the culmination of the nonverbal advantage.

This whole five-step process can happen quickly, and some dentists can remember learning it on a particular day with a particular patient. The other side of the story is that a dentist may realize that a shift in his or her ability to influence a child patient's behavior has occurred and that he or she can take more effective actions with child patients in the nonverbal dimension but was not aware of acquiring such skill.

## Summary: Nonverbal Advantage

The nonverbal advantage has been and still is a powerful technique for behavioral management of children. Paradoxically, it has been referred to as "voice control" over the years. It belongs in the domain of nonpharmacologic management. It is a linguistic technique because it is an enhancement to requests. It can generally be called a psychological technique. Most importantly, it has to affect the clinician before it can have any advantageous effect on the child.

The nonverbal advantage affects the voice: its tonality, cadence, and other qualities. It affects facial expression, a powerful part of nonverbal communication. It affects the self-talk of the clinician and therefore the self-confidence about the distinctions the clinician is making about his or her ability to successfully treat the child. There is a distinct and important postural aspect to this. It is my observation that for most clinicians, assuming a downward and forward position in front of the child while simultaneously establishing eye contact is how most clinicians find the nonverbal advantage.

## PROFILE OF THE GOOD CHILD DENTAL PATIENT

When new acquaintances find out that a dentist treats children, they often conclude that he or she must be a remarkably patient person. But that conclusion is not necessarily correct. The reason that people make this false assumption stems in part from a misconception about what it takes to treat children successfully in a dental clinic. These people probably imagine the dentist sitting in the clinic, patiently holding the hand of every child patient, and searching for words and phrases that will persuade the child to cooperate.

Such a perception is generally wrong. The fact remains that the great majority of children older than 36 to 40 months are astonishingly well behaved and compliant dental patients when handled correctly. In fact, they may be the easiest of all patients to treat. They don't demand exceptional patience from the dentist. They don't need it.

Performing dentistry for these kids is a pleasant, rewarding professional experience. In many cases, the dentist develops a personal attachment to his young patients. It's fun to talk to children, ask them questions, find out what they will wear at Halloween or want for Christmas, know their favorite television show or food, or find out how they feel about their new baby brother. Conversing with children is refreshing and should be, overall, a relaxing part of a general practitioner's day.

The good child dental patient reacts to "critical moments" of the dental appointment appropriately. This means that he or she reacts *as well as he or she can*. The most common critical moments in dentistry for children and how the good child dental patient manages them are described as follows.

## CRITICAL MOMENTS IN THE DENTAL APPOINTMENT AND THE GOOD CHILD DENTAL PATIENT

### Separation from the Parent

As already discussed, separation from the parent is not always imposed. Children under 36 to 40 months of age often behave better if the parent accompanies them to the dental operatory. Often the parent of a child younger than 3 years has an opinion about whether the youngster's behavior will be better or worse if a parent is present. After this age, most children do not need a parent to accompany them, but the dentist may prefer to have a parent present during the appointment. The parent and child should be made aware of the dentist's preference *at least* before the first treatment appointment (e.g., fillings, extractions).

If the parent of a child older than 3 years does accompany the child to the operatory, he or she should be prepared to leave if the youngster does not behave. This agreement between parent and dentist about leaving should be made *before* the child is seated in the dental chair. It is important for the child to know about the agreement.

The good child dental patient, as a general rule, separates easily from the parent. This is not to say that the separation is easy for the child emotionally, but it does mean that the child has the wherewithal to do it. At his or her best, the child looks eager to get started, shows no observable fear, and talks freely with the dental assistant who escorts him or her from the reception room. At the worst the child acts as a victim so the parent can become the rescuer.[23,24] The dental appointment is a perfect time for this last scenario to take place. Every dentist who treats children should expect this on some recurring and perhaps even predictable basis.

### Getting into the Chair

As simple as it sounds, some kids have difficulty getting into the dental chair. This may stem from natural fears and the perceived vulnerability that goes along with being off one's feet. Some kids need assistance and have to be guided by the hand or even picked up and placed in the chair.

The good child dental patient gets right into the chair. It is really pleasant when this happens because it provides the first real opportunity to praise the child for his good behavior and ability to do the things asked of him. ("Wow, John, look at you. I bet your daddy couldn't have gotten into this chair any faster.")

### Dentist Seated at Chair

The dentist approaching the chair indicates to the child that treatment is imminent. The well-adjusted child can handle this and responds to his or her name (most dentists have learned the value of nicknames), answer questions, and accept and react to praise. ("What a pretty dress." "Thank you, Mommy got it for me.")

The dentist also represents the most authoritative figure in the dental office, and the good child patient realizes that his or her directives must be followed. Directives such as "Hands on your tummy and open wide-tall" are obeyed by the child, and obeyed quickly.

### The Injection

Without question, the injection is the most universally feared procedure in dentistry for children and maybe in dentistry in general. However,

it is not a major obstacle for most children. A large percentage of children do not react at all to the injection. The technique is now so painless that many little kids never even know that they received a "shot" when the dentist gave them "sleepy water." A good-tasting topical anesthetic is usually indicated. However, it is not indicated in the obviously agitated child who appears to be getting worse.

A small percentage of young children have learned from siblings, parents, and peers that they will receive an injection. Unfortunately, many youngsters have heard frightening descriptions of the needle. They expect pain. Fortunately, many of these kids still accept the procedure with only a few tears and with virtually no avoidance behaviors. They learn that the "shot" isn't bad at all, and at later appointments the "pinch" is experienced as just that, a little pinching feeling in the mouth. The dentist must not lie about the needle. If asked whether the injection will hurt, he or she should say, "You will feel a little pinch."

If the child starts to show avoidance behaviors, firm voice control is needed. Seldom does delaying the injection result in better behavior. Few dentists have found any benefit in showing the syringe to the child who "wants to see what it looks like." Therefore, clinicians are encouraged not to be hesitant with this procedure. In fact, not using a topical anesthetic may, in certain situations, be wise because of the additional waiting time involved.

A child can cry during the injection and perhaps even need some momentary restraint of arms and body by a dental assistant and yet still qualify as a good dental patient. The test is whether the crying and squirming stop when the needle disappears.

Figure 23-5 shows a recommended method for the dental assistant to pass the needle from the tray to the dentist. Obviously, the use of needles around wiggling, thrashing children must be done with caution.

### The Dental Procedure

Nine times out of ten, the dental procedure is restorative treatment if an injection for anesthesia has been given. Fortunately, dentists do not have to extract many teeth in children anymore. For the good child patient, the procedure itself (i.e., the drilling) is easy compared with the injection. Many youngsters fall asleep during the procedure. This may come as a surprise, but most children,

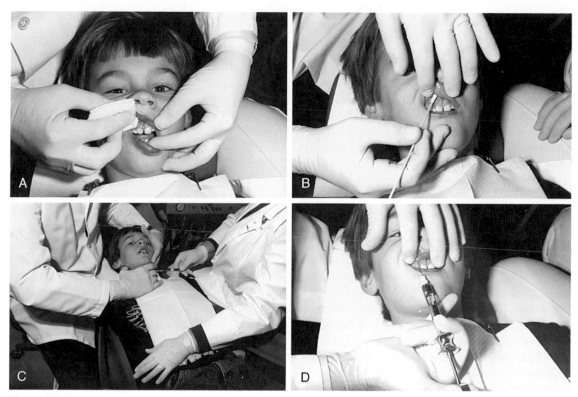

**Figure 23-5** **A,** Drying of mucosa prior to using an acceptable-tasting topical anesthetic. **B,** Application of topical anesthetic. This step can be eliminated for very apprehensive children. **C,** Under-the-chin transfer of syringe. Note that the dental assistant is prepared to restrain the child's arms. **D,** Introduction of syringe to oral cavity. Note how the syringe is stabilized by a finger touching the patient's chin.

even 3-year-olds, can tolerate a fairly long dental appointment without becoming restless. As stated earlier, most kids are great dental patients.

There is still some need for extractions. Here again, most kids do well, but clinical experience still leads many dentists to believe that this can be a scary procedure for little ones. Some authors have assigned Freudian castration implications to this fear. I think that it is the force and torquing applied to the tooth that arouses anxiety. Luckily, most extractions in children are quick and simple.

## End of the Appointment

It may seem silly to label the end of the appointment a crisis, but sometimes people spend all their emotional reserves during the heat of battle and then become unglued afterward. A good child dental patient ends his or her appointment on a high note. He or she is eager to leave yet is patient enough and human enough to want to stay around to be congratulated and praised for good behavior in the chair.

## Return to the Parent

The return of the child to the parent also may not seem like a crisis event. When one understands how some misbehaving child dental patients handle this aspect of their dental appointment, however, this time and its importance become clearer. Some children want their parents to feel guilty about making them go to the dentist and portray themselves as victims. This dramatization can often be intercepted if the dentist or auxiliary is present.

Good child dental patients return to their parents beaming with pride. They know that they have done well and have pleased their parents. They are pleased with themselves. The dentist's compliments to their parents about them are returned by way of smiles and bright eyes. For the dentist, this is a happy occasion.

In summary, most kids turn out to be good, accepting dental patients. However, there are exceptions, and these exceptions need to be understood.

## PARENTAL ATTENDANCE IN THE DENTAL OPERATORY

The issue of whether a parent (or parents) should be present in the dental operatory during a child's dental appointment is one that inspires divergent opinions among practitioners of dentistry for children. Parents have varying opinions on this issue also.[23,24]

Certainly, it can be said that for most of the twentieth century, many dentists as a general rule did not want the parents in attendance during treatment. This was particularly true if the child was older than 3 years and had normal social, psychological, and emotional development. A study in 1971 of 120 American Association of Pedodontics diplomates would seem to have verified these facts, at least among specialists. In this study, only 5 always had the parents back; 18 never did; and 97 did in selected cases. Age of the child was the most cited reason for allowing parents in attendance. A total of 90 dentists responded to a question about the appropriateness of the parent's attendance compared with the child's age: 71 thought it was appropriate at birth to 1 year; 76 at 1 to 2 years; 35 at 2 to 4 years; and 8 at 4 to 6 years.

However, the changing times of the 1990s affected the number of dentists who reconsidered their policy about admitting parents.[23] It should be noted that in a litigious society when risk management is an important feature in running a practice that involves children's behavior, allowing parental attendance during difficult management circumstances may be a safer approach legally than denying such attendance. Attendance also may foster a more secure feeling in certain parents because they know that, in observing the entire appointment, they can act as an advocate for their child and verify his or her safety.[24]

It seems reasonable to encourage dentists to think through their own policy regarding parental attendance and to be flexible about the arrangements they have made regarding this presence. It can be argued that there are parents who want to be in attendance and may not remain with the practice or may be anxious about staying in the practice if they are eliminated as a matter of routine procedure because of the philosophy of the dental office. Conversely, there are definite instances when the presence of the parent may actually heighten the alarm of the child; when being accompanied by the parent allows the child to portray himself or herself as a victim and thereby, it is hoped, recruiting the parent into the role of rescuer; or when the parents frankly are so anxious about dentistry themselves that they heighten the fear responses of the child.

## MISBEHAVING CHILD DENTAL PATIENTS

It is now appropriate to explore the types of children who reliably misbehave at the dental office. These are children who just can't cope or, importantly, just *won't* cope with the stimuli and behavioral demands of the dental experience.

The first group are special children who are emotionally compromised. This is not a large group of children, but they do exist. Dental procedures, as well as many other challenges of life, are difficult for these children to endure because of their psychological or emotional problems. It is important to realize that a psychological or emotional disorder may be undiagnosed.

The next largest group are the "shy birds." These are introverted, poorly socialized children who are afraid of the social challenges associated with going to the dentist. The best management technique with these children is to break the barrier of shyness with friendship.

The third group is composed of children who have a hard time with dentistry because they are frightened. (Fear of dentistry is discussed later.) It is my opinion that fear of needles accounts for 90% of cases involving fear of dentistry.

Another group of misbehaving children is those who do not like authority. These children don't like dental appointments, and their dislike is based on an aversion to complying with adult directives.

### Category I: The Emotionally Compromised Child

A common finding in patients with emotional illness is anxiety. When the anxiety of an emotional illness is compounded by the anxiety associated with a dental appointment, a behavioral explosion often occurs. Emotionally compromised children are generally poor dental patients. At best, they are no fun.

Often a problem with emotionally compromised patients is that there is no confirmed diagnosis. Parents, even intelligent, well-informed parents, may have no idea that anything is wrong. Because they have grown accustomed to their child's behaviors, they often overlook the abnormalities or rationalize an explanation for why their child behaves in certain ways. This situation is extremely unfortunate because most emotional illnesses are diagnosable and manageable, and, as is often the case, the earlier the upset is addressed, the faster and more effective is the therapy.

Emotional illness can also be a problem for children from broken homes and other unfortunate parenting circumstances. The children of poverty probably suffer more from emotional upsets in their families than do children from more privileged classes.[22] As a group, abused and neglected children exhibit a high incidence of emotional dysfunction.[22]

The author has had little success in convincing parents that their child's misbehavior during a dental appointment might be attributable to an unknown emotional problem. However, it is good professional behavior for a dentist to share with parents any matters that have bearing on their child's welfare. Of course, if abuse and neglect are suspected, the dentist is legally obligated to issue a report to the appropriate authorities.

## Category II: The Shy, Introverted Child

Introversion or shyness is a problem for many people, including children, especially very young children. Because the dental experience for children is a fairly intense human encounter that demands rapport and communication between the adult dentist and the child patient, it is obvious that a very shy child will find the experience stressful. This stress can cause the child to exhibit avoidance behavior such as crying. Usually the crying takes the form of compensatory whimpering. Rarely does the introverted child display aggressive avoidance behavior such as a tantrum. These children can be likened to puppies in some respects. When threatened, they go limp and tremble.

The dental profession has long recognized that shy children have a hard time adjusting to the expectations of a dental appointment. As with all children, the dentist's first objective is to establish rapport, trust, and communication. With shy children this requires patience because they are unskilled at "feeling people out" and they

are categorically paralyzed by the challenge of communicating.

However, as formidable as the challenge may seem, the various approaches to talking to these children at their own level, using praise and the tell-show-do technique, reliably enable the clinician to penetrate the shell that these youngsters have erected around their personalities and in time, sometimes startlingly fast, they open up. When they open up, they usually become fantastic patients because the dental appointment becomes a social event wherein somebody knows their name, is interested in them, and is willing and ready to talk to them. This opening up happens often, but not always.

## Category III: The Frightened Child

A child who is frightened is a formidable challenge to the dentist as well as to teachers, physicians, parents, and everyone else who encounters him or her. In treating such a child, the dentist has a particular problem in that even though the dental encounter is not very long, it is intense and requires, ideally, enormous cooperation from the child. The dentist also contends with the problem of fear to perhaps a greater degree than that encountered by most other adults who come in contact with the child. Such fear ranges from fear of needles to fear of bodily harm to general fear of the unknown. If someone really wanted to make a complete and specific list of all the possible sights, sounds, smells, and expectations that are reasonably unique to the dental experience, it would probably fill up a legal pad. The handheld instruments alone would provide an extensive list of possibilities.

The answer to the question of whether a child may misbehave in the dental office because of fear is definitely affirmative. Determining whether a child's misbehavior is motivated by fear or another cause is, as one would expect, a more challenging proposition. Yet information paired with experience and common sense reliably allows the dentist to determine what motivates the child's behavior.

Some common causes of fear of dentistry are as follows:

- A child is intellectually unable, even when educated by a parent or dentist, to arrest his or her fears about the dental appointment either because of his or her chronologic age (generally speaking, 36 to 40 months is the age when most normal children are intellectually able to arrest their fears when given information about what will ensue) or because of slow development (such as mental retardation).

- A child is overreacting to fears because of other emotional upsets in his or her life.[22] This category includes children who come from homes that are in acute chaos because of an impending divorce or parental separation, children who are abused, and children who are grieving the death of a relative or friend. Children who are coping with other health problems are also included in this category. These circumstances often yield self-limiting emotional disturbances. The problems resolve in time, but when present they make dentistry, particularly some of the more rigorous procedures such as tooth extraction, difficult for these children to endure.
- A child has been "sold" a set of fears by peers, siblings, or parents. Such fears are called *acquired fears*.
- A child has had a previous difficult or painful experience at a physician's or dentist's office or at a hospital. These are called *learned fears*.
- A child is emotionally ill.

All of these categories of children, with perhaps the exception of the emotionally ill, are easily identified. Emotional illness, as discussed previously, is something parents may not address at home, and the real clues to emotional disturbances often do not emerge until these youngsters are enrolled in a formal educational process and are observed by a teacher on a daily basis.

One major point is in order here. If the misbehavior occurs because of an intense dread or fear of dentistry, it is important for the parent and the dentist to establish this fact in no uncertain terms. If a child is so frightened of dentistry that good behavior is impossible, it is the obligation of both adults to do everything possible to avoid increasing the child's anxieties. This may mean postponing dental work, or using drugs, or even mean performing dental procedures under general anesthesia. Whatever is required, it is important to take the most appropriate measures regardless of cost, inconvenience, and loss of efficiency. That is the only humane course to take.

As stated earlier, children who are extremely fearful usually can be identified before dentistry begins. The only gray zone concerns the child who may have an emotional illness. When there is a high suspicion of emotional illness (no one can explain why the youngster is so frightened), it is the most professional and humane course for the dentist to refer the child to a psychiatrist, psychologist, or other counselor. The parent should accept this referral in the spirit in which it is given—that is, the best thing that can be done for this child at this time is to establish whether he or she is emotionally healthy enough to go through a dental appointment without resorting to maladaptive behavior and its sequelae.

## Category IV: The Child Who Is Averse to Authority

The Duke of Windsor, during one of his visits to the United States, noted tongue-in-cheek that one of the things that he liked about America was how well American parents minded their children. Much has been written in the dental literature over the years about children who are difficult because they cannot or will not follow adult directives.[21] Labels that have been applied to such youngsters include "spoiled," "incorrigible," "overindulged," and "defiant." Certainly, even the most casual observer can verify that children exhibit a variety of misbehaviors. One trip to a grocery store, a fast food restaurant, or even a public swimming pool where parents and children congregate will reliably show misbehaving children. If children misbehave in a shopping mall, in their parents' automobile, and even in their own homes, why should they not misbehave at the dentist's office?

What is the nature of this misbehavior? Why does it happen? There are children for whom emotional illness, introversion, or fear simply is not the reason for inappropriate behavior at the dentist's office. These children have an aversion to authority. On analysis, it is easy to see that a dentist is a strong authoritative figure in his or her own office and therefore a prime candidate for bringing out the worst behavior of such children.

Where did the aversion to authority come from? Dr. Alfred Adler, who was a contemporary of Freud and Jung, and Dr. Rudolph Dreikurs, a student and devotee of Adler, pointed out that there are four potential misdirected goals in the life of a child.[1,13] These goals influence the personality repertoire of the child, where they subtly satisfy the strong human craving for superiority, believed by Adler to be the main force that drives all human behavior. Noting that one potential way of feeling superior is achieved by manipulating other people, both authors warn parents that their child may adopt a style of behavior with the parents that will carry over to other authority figures whom the child encounters in life, such as the dentist. These misdirected goals and what they mean to the involved children are as follows:[1,13,23]

1. *Undue attention:* "In order to satisfy my need to feel superior, I will, through manipulative behavior, make sure that my parents pay attention to me anytime I want them to. Because their paying attention to me quickly relieves my insecurities about my being superior, I am likely to want much more attention than is reasonable."
   *Behavioral characteristics:* Annoying, irritating, teasing, disruptive.
2. *Struggle for power:* "In order to satisfy my need to feel superior, I am prepared to have a power struggle with my parents about getting attention. This is a challenge and I intend to win. They will pay attention to me or else."
   *Behavioral characteristics:* Argues and contradicts, does the opposite of instructions, makes people angry, throws temper tantrums.
3. *Retaliation and revenge:* "In order to satisfy my need to feel superior, if I do not get what I want, which in a nutshell is attention, I will get even with my parents and I will punish them. I will not let them do this to me without hurting them back."
   *Behavioral characteristics:* Displays violent temper, says things that hurt people, seeks revenge, gets even.
4. *Inadequacy:* "In order to satisfy my need to feel superior, I have convinced myself that I am special in the worst sort of way. I am totally unable to grow up, unable to achieve, and in fact I plan to do nothing at all for myself, my parents, or anyone else on the face of this earth."
   *Behavioral characteristics:* Gives up easily, rarely participates, acts as if he or she is incapable, displays inadequacy.

Space does not permit a detailed discussion about misdirected children. It seems obvious that each of the four misdirected goals becomes more serious from one level to the next. The child who simply wants some attention may find dentistry a nice experience in that it is such a personal one-on-one occasion. The child who engages in a power struggle has a bully's attitude and may have no reservations about arguing with a dentist or challenging a dentist's authority. The child who engages in retaliation and revenge can frankly be dangerous. This is the type of child who may bite. He or she is not warm and fun and probably will not respond to praise. The child who thinks about himself in a defeated, inadequate way is likely to show a variety of misbehaviors when the dentist requests his cooperation. Overcoming the challenges of the dental appointment is beyond the grasp of this child. When challenges arise, this child tells himself that he is inferior and can't possibly measure up.

I think that misdirected children can often also be described as prefigurative children. The terms *prefigurative, postfigurative,* and *configurative* were introduced by Margaret Mead.[23,24] Basically, prefigurative describes a person raised outside of any consistent cultural tradition. This is a phenomenon that started in the United States after World War II and that Dr. Mead predicted would eventually spread throughout the world. It has also been noted that children of prefigurative parents are not well rehearsed in handling adults' requests. Obviously, with dentistry being such an intense communication experience that relies heavily on requests and promises, this lack of rehearsal predicts potential problems for the dentist who works with such children.

A parallel concern for dentists treating today's children is the phenomenon of learned helplessness. Because contemporary parents are so busy, often with two parents working full time, some children may find that a strategy of helplessness is a predictable way of getting attention from their parents in their home setting. Because the misdirected behavior of some parents sets the stage on which their child wishes to act as a helpless victim so the parents will come to the rescue, the dental experience can easily precipitate this behavior.

It should also be noted that severely misdirected children present problems in a variety of social circumstances and generally have trouble in school. Fortunately, most of these children eventually outgrow their maladaptive behavior. One may find only remnants or subtle manifestations of their misdirected behavior during adolescence and young adulthood.

### Summary: Misbehaving Children

The four categories of misbehaving children have been outlined based on the relative frequency with which a dentist encounters them. In other words, there are fewer emotionally disturbed children than there are introverted children, fewer introverted children than frightened children, and fewer frightened children than children who just do not like to comply with authoritative adults. Blends of the four problem groups obviously exist. In fact, a blend is probably the norm.

I think that dental students and clinicians with little experience in dentistry for children and certainly in dealing with the parents of misbehaving children often attribute the majority of misbehavior in the dental office to a fear of dentistry. Conversely, older and more experienced clinicians do not endorse the fear theory as much but assert that inappropriate behavior really has little to do with the dental appointment. They note that these children do not cope well with any sort of stress and that they dislike cooperating with any adults who make demands on them. Authority, not dentistry, is what these children dread.

The child who has a genuine dreadful fear of dentistry must be handled carefully, and such handling should represent, whenever possible, a cooperative effort on the part of the dentist and the parents. Mild to modest fear of dentistry, particularly fear of the needle, is normal. Importantly, for normal children older than 3 years who have a competent dentist who takes the time to educate them with tell-show-do as the primary technique, these fears can be arrested or made manageable.

In summary, the dental experience is a complex social/psychological arena for the three main participants: the dental team, the parent/guardian, and the child. The practice of effective contemporary pediatric dentistry in the linguistic domain demands sophisticated understanding of all the psychosocial themes that can come into play in the course of a child's dental visit.

## THE BOTTOM LINE

It can be offered that the bottom line in employing behavioral management in dentistry for children today is based in part on first dealing with the parents, their expectations, dreads, uncertainties, and so on. To some extent this is new ground. So is the keen interest in risk management and informed consent, especially in the area of managing the child's behavior assertively or pharmacotherapeutically. There is no evidence that the importance of these concepts will diminish in the foreseeable future.

The most important recommendation for the dental clinician is to *talk* to the parents of the young children treated in your office, especially if your management style may be an issue. The ability to create a healthy dialogue with the parents is the skill needed here. The process of articulating your options and your limits is not only informative for them but good for you. Such communication helps to develop your practice and refine your own convictions about child patient management. It also can be helpful for some parents and their children.

In the final analysis, if everyone, including you, understands your intent, then a more satisfactory outcome is likely for all involved.

## REFERENCES

1. Adler A: *What Life Should Mean to You.* New York, Capricorn Books, 1958.
2. Allport GW: *Pattern and Growth in Personality.* New York, Holt, Rinehart and Winston, 1961, p 41.
3. American Academy of Pediatric Dentistry: Guidelines for behavior management. *Pediatr Dent* 16(7):41-45, 2001–2002.
4. American Academy of Pediatric Dentistry: Reference manual. Quality assurance criteria for pediatric dentistry: behavior management. *Pediatr Dent* 16(7):84-87, 1994–1995.
5. Baker S: *Visual Persuasion.* New York, McGraw-Hill, 1961.
6. Birdwhistell RL: Background to kinesics, etc. *A Review of General Semantics* 13:0-18, 1955.
7. Brandt HF: *The Psychology of Seeing.* New York, Philosophical Library, 1945, pp 32, 107.

8. Brauer JC: Applied psychology in pedodontics. In: Lindahl RL, editor. *Dentistry for Children,* 5th ed. New York, McGraw-Hill, 1964, pp 33-68.

9. Byrnes G: *A Complete Guide to Cartooning.* New York, Grosset and Dunlap, 1950, p 46.

10. Chambers DW: Behavior management techniques for pediatric dentists: an embarrassment of riches. *J Dent Child* 44(1):30-34, 1977.

11. Damasio AR: *Descartes' Error.* New York, G. P. Putnam, 1994.

12. Darwin C: *The Expression of the Emotions in Man and Animals.* London, John Murray, 1904, pp 143, 372-373.

13. Dreikurs R, Soltz RN: *Children, the Challenge.* New York, Hawthorn Books, 1964.

14. Goodenough FL: The expression of the emotions in infancy. *Child Dev* 2:96-101, 1931.

15. Heller S, Surrenda DS: *Retooling on the Run.* Berkeley, Frog, 1994.

16. Heller S: The non-verbal advantage from the Art of Coaching Course. A joint presentation of the Education for Life Seminars, Inc. and the Institute for Movement Psychology, 1996.

17. Levitas TC: HOME: hand over mouth exercise. *J Dent Child* 41(3):23-25, 1974.

18. Mehrabian A: Communication without words. *Psychol Today* 11:53, 1968.

19. Mehrabian A: *Nonverbal Communication.* New York, Aldine-Atherton, 1972, pp 1-2.

20. Pinkham JR: Voice control: an old technique reexamined. *J Dent Child* 52:199-202, 1985.

21. Pinkham JR: Classifying and managing child dental patients' misbehaviors: a three-step Adlerian approach. *J Dent Child* 5(4):437-441, 1983.

22. Pinkham JR, Casamassimo P, Levy S: Dentistry and the children of poverty. *J Dent Child* 55(1):17-23, 1988.

23. Pinkham JR: Behavioral themes in dentistry for children: 1968–1990. *J Dent Child* 57(1):38-45, 1990.

24. Pinkham JR: An analysis of the phenomenon of increased parental participation during the child's dental experience. *J Dent Child* 58(6):458-463, 1991.

25. Pinkham JR: The roles of requests and promises in child patient management. *J Dent Child* 60:169-174, 1993.

26. Pinkham JR: Personality development: managing behavior of the cooperative preschool child. *Dent Clin North Am* 39:771-788, 1995.

27. Pinkham JR: Behavior management of children in the dental office. *Dent Clin North Am* 44:471-486, 2000.

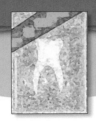

# CHAPTER 24
## Periodontal Problems in Children and Adolescents
### *Ann L. Griffen*

Children and adolescents are affected by a variety of periodontal diseases and conditions. Gingivitis is common, especially around puberty. Significant loss of periodontal attachment or alveolar bone is more unusual in young patients but can result from systemic disease or occur as isolated dental disease. In addition, gingival anatomic problems, such as lack of attached gingiva, can arise during development and may necessitate early management.

## GINGIVITIS

Simple gingivitis is characterized by inflammation of the gingival tissues with no loss of attachment or bone. It occurs in response to the bacteria that live in biofilms at the gingival margin and in the sulcus. The clinical signs of gingivitis include erythema, bleeding on probing, and edema. In the early primary dentition, gingivitis is uncommon. Younger children have less plaque than adults do and appear to be less reactive to the same amount of plaque. This can be explained both by differences in bacterial composition of plaque and by developmental changes in the inflammatory response. Gingivitis occurs in half the population by the age of 4 or 5 years, and the incidence continues to increase with age. The prevalence of gingivitis peaks at close to 100% at puberty, but after puberty it declines slightly and stays constant into adulthood.[9] Some children exhibit severe gingivitis at puberty, as shown in Figure 24-1. Puberty-associated gingivitis is believed to be related to increases in steroid hormones. The

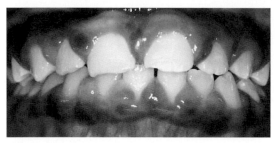

**Figure 24-1**  Puberty-associated gingivitis in a 13-year-old black boy. The dark pigmentation of the gingiva is a normal racial characteristic.

gingiva may be enlarged with granulomatous changes similar to those occurring in pregnancy. The peak prevalence of puberty-associated gingivitis is at age 10 years in girls and age 13 years in boys.

Certain local factors may be important contributors to gingivitis in children. Crowded teeth and orthodontic appliances may make oral hygiene more difficult and predispose to gingivitis. Mouth breathing may cause chronically dehydrated gingiva in the maxillary labial area and lead to a characteristic localized gingivitis as shown in Figure 24-2. Inflammation, especially erythema, often occurs around erupting primary and permanent teeth.

Gingivitis is reversible and can be managed with improved oral hygiene. Appropriately sized toothbrushes and toothpaste and floss flavored to appeal to children may enhance compliance. Young children, especially those younger than 8 to 10 years, are not capable of performing effective oral hygiene measures and require assistance. Older children and even adolescents probably need at least some parental supervision.

## GINGIVAL ENLARGEMENT

### Chronic Inflammatory Gingival Enlargement

Long-standing gingivitis in young patients sometimes results in chronic inflammatory gingival enlargement, which may be localized or generalized. It commonly occurs when plaque is allowed to accumulate around orthodontic appliances as shown in Figure 24-3 or in areas chronically dried by mouth breathing. The interdental papillae and the marginal gingiva become enlarged, and the tissue is usually erythematous and bleeds easily. It may be soft and friable with a smooth, shiny surface. Inflammatory gingival enlargement often slowly resolves when adequate plaque control is instituted, so gingivectomy is rarely required.

### Drug-Induced Gingival Enlargement

Long-term therapy with certain systemic medications can produce an overgrowth of gingival tissue (Fig. 24-4).[7] It can occur after therapy with the anticonvulsant phenytoin (Dilantin), the immunosuppressant cyclosporine, or a calcium channel blocker. Cyclosporine is used to control host rejection of transplanted organs and to manage autoimmune diseases. The calcium channel blockers such as nifedipine and nitrendipine are cardiac drugs that are sometimes prescribed for children to control hypertension. The overgrowth is painless and differs from chronic inflammatory enlargement in that it is fibrous, firm, and pale pink, often with little tendency to bleed. The enlargement occurs first in the interdental region and may appear lobular. It gradually spreads to the gingival margin. The condition can

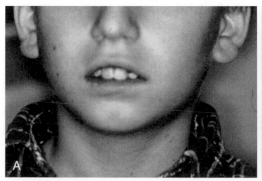
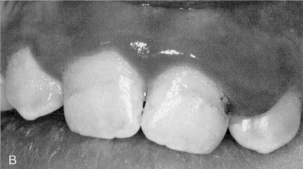

**Figure 24-2**  **A,** The typical oral posture of mouth breathing. **B,** The resultant gingivitis of the upper facial gingiva.

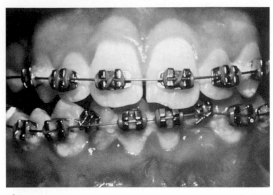

**Figure 24-3** Gingival enlargement that occurred in response to long-standing plaque accumulation on the lower incisors secondary to orthodontic appliances.

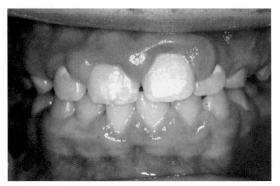

**Figure 24-4** Mild gingival enlargement secondary to phenytoin therapy.

become extreme, sometimes covering the crowns of the teeth and interfering with eruption or occlusion.

Drug-influenced gingival enlargement occurs slowly and may resolve to some degree when medication is discontinued. There appears to be a genetic component to susceptibility to gingival enlargement. The severity of the enlargement is also affected by both the adequacy of oral hygiene and the gingival concentration of the medication. If medication cannot be discontinued or changed, the enlargement can be surgically removed, but it will recur. The tissue can be removed either by gingivectomy or by a flap with an internal bevel. Surgery is indicated when the appearance of the gingiva is unacceptable to the patient, when the enlargement interferes with comfortable functioning, or when the enlargement has produced a periodontal pocket that cannot be maintained in a healthy state. The most severe cases of gingival enlargement usually occur in mentally retarded patients, in part because of poor oral hygiene. Postoperative discomfort after gingivectomy can be considerable and should be carefully weighed against potential benefits for patients who may not be able to give fully informed consent.

## ANATOMIC PROBLEMS

### Development and Defects of the Attached Gingiva

When teeth erupt they pierce through an existing band of keratinized gingiva, and the width of this band and its relationship to the teeth change very little during subsequent growth and development. Deflections in the path of eruption, such as those due to crowding or overretention of primary teeth, may result in a narrowed band of attached gingiva.[2] This is particularly common when mandibular incisors erupt labial to the alveolar ridge as shown in Figure 24-5, *A*. If the

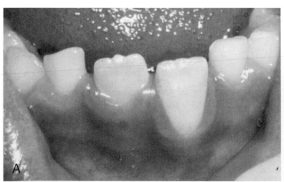
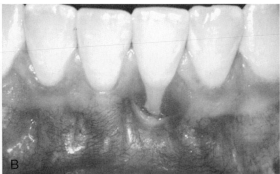

**Figure 24-5**   **A,** A reduction in the width of keratinized gingiva resulting from labial eruption of the left central incisor. **B,** After orthodontic alignment of the labially positioned left central incisor, a gingival defect was observed. Localized recession occurred as the result of plaque accumulation in an area that was difficult to clean and had inadequate attached gingiva.

band of attached gingiva is very narrow, even a small subsequent loss of attachment can result in a mucogingival defect (which occurs when the pocket depth exceeds the width of keratinized gingiva) and recession may occur rapidly as shown in Figure 24-5, *B*. The gingival architecture often makes labially erupted teeth difficult to clean, particularly once recession has occurred, leaving them even more vulnerable to periodontitis and attachment loss. The loss of attachment and recession that occurs with a labially malpositioned tooth is sometimes called *stripping*. Other factors that may contribute to recession are the use of smokeless tobacco and habit-related self-induced injury.

A gingival graft is indicated to stabilize and repair the labial attachment of teeth with significant recession. A free gingival graft using donor tissue from the palate is commonly performed. Orthodontic movement of a labially malpositioned tooth in the direction of the alveolar ridge may produce a small increase in attached gingiva and place the tooth in a periodontally more stable position. Particularly when defects are not severe, it is desirable to postpone grafting until after orthodontic treatment.

### Frena

A prominent maxillary frenum, often accompanied by a large midline diastema, is a common finding in children. It is often a cause for concern by parents and health care providers. Unless the frenum attachment exerts traumatic force on the facial attached gingiva of a permanent tooth (an uncommon situation), immediate treatment is unnecessary. Instead, treatment should be delayed until the permanent incisors and cuspids have erupted to allow natural closure of the diastema. If orthodontic treatment is planned, surgical treatment should generally be postponed until the diastema has been closed. If the appearance is unacceptable after closure, frenectomy is indicated.

A restrictive lingual frenum ("tongue tie") is not uncommon in children (Fig. 24-6). If the attachment limits normal tongue mobility, treatment may be indicated. Children generally accommodate well to the restriction, but if the child cannot protrude the tongue from the mouth or touch the tip of the tongue to the upper alveolar process, a simple frenotomy in which the attachment is released will make oral functioning, including speech, easier.

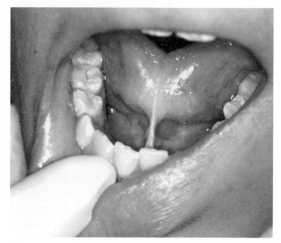

**Figure 24-6**   Restrictive lingual frenum in a teenaged patient.

## PERIODONTITIS

Significant loss of periodontal attachment is common in adults, with chronic periodontitis (formerly called "adult onset" periodontitis) affecting the majority of the population. When careful measurements are made, 20% of 14- to 17-year-olds in the United States are found to have attachment loss of at least 2 mm at one or more sites.[3] The number and severity of affected sites increase steadily with age, demonstrating that chronic periodontitis often begins in adolescence. Chronic periodontitis responds well to oral hygiene measures and can more easily be arrested in its early stages when attachment loss is minimal and deep pockets have not developed.

Smoking is a major risk factor for periodontitis, and smoking is increasing among adolescents, particularly females. Smoking status should be determined as part of a periodontal assessment for young patients and appropriate counseling provided.

### Aggressive Periodontitis

Rare, rapidly progressing forms of periodontitis also affect children and adolescents. Both periodontitis as a manifestation of systemic disease and aggressive periodontitis affecting children who are otherwise healthy occur in the pediatric population. Because of their rarity, it has been difficult to study these diseases. For this reason our understanding is often incomplete, and further research is needed on both the causes and the management of early-onset disease forms. Classification and nomenclature for these diseases was changed in 1999,[3] but since much of the literature contains the older terminology, both terms are given here.

## Localized Aggressive Periodontitis in the Permanent Dentition

Localized aggressive periodontitis (LAP), formerly called localized juvenile periodontitis (LJP), is characterized by the loss of attachment and bone around the permanent incisors and first permanent molars. The radiographic appearance is distinctive (Fig. 24-7). The attachment loss is rapid, occurring at three times the rate of chronic disease. Inflammation in LAP is not as extreme as that occurring in periodontitis associated with systemic disease such as neutropenia, but both inflammation and plaque accumulation are often greater than that found in the typical teenager. The disease is usually detected in early adolescence, but retrospective examination of earlier radiographs has sometimes revealed undetected disease in the primary dentition. This suggests that LAP of the permanent dentition and LAP of the primary dentition (discussed later) are the same disease entity, differing only in age of onset or detection. The prevalence of LAP is estimated to be about 1%, and in the United States it most commonly occurs in the African-American population. In at least some cases the disease appears to be inherited as an autosomal dominant trait, and LJP has been linked to a neutrophil chemotactic defect.

Despite the genetic component, LAP is clearly linked to the presence of high numbers of *Actinobacillus actinomycetemcomitans*, and successful treatment outcomes correlate well with eradication of the bacteria. Treatment consists of local measures in combination with systemic antibiotic therapy and microbiological monitoring. Systemic tetracyclines have been used with some success, but metronidazole alone or in combination with amoxicillin appears to be more effective in arresting disease progression.[11] Some reattachment and resolution of the periodontal defects can occur after antibiotic therapy, but localized surgical intervention is often necessary to manage the residual defects.

## Generalized Aggressive Periodontitis

Generalized aggressive periodontitis (GAP) sometimes occurs in adolescents and teenagers. In young adults the same disease was formerly called rapidly progressive periodontitis.[1] Unlike LAP, GAP may affect the entire dentition and is not self-limiting. Heavy accumulations of plaque and calculus are found in GAP, and inflammation may be severe. GAP is not associated with the high levels of *A. actinomycetemcomitans* that occur in

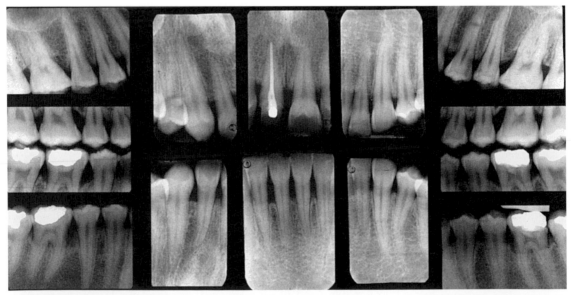

**Figure 24-7** Radiographic appearance of localized aggressive periodontitis showing the typical bone loss pattern around first permanent molars and central incisors. Note the root canal treatment of the central incisor. Luxation injuries are common in these patients because of mobility of the incisors.

LAP but instead has a microbiological profile closer to that of chronic disease. It should be managed aggressively with local therapy as well as systemic antibiotics.

### Localized Aggressive Periodontitis in the Primary Dentition

LAP in the primary dentition (formerly called localized prepubertal periodontitis [LPP]) is characterized by localized loss of attachment in the primary dentition. It occurs in children without evidence of systemic disease. The disease is most commonly manifested in the molar area, where localized, usually bilaterally symmetric loss of attachment occurs (Fig. 24-8). In the United States, LAP of the primary dentition occurs most commonly in the African-American population. It is usually accompanied by mild to moderate inflammation, and heavier than average plaque deposits may be visible. Calculus may also be present. It is commonly first diagnosed during the late primary dentition or early transitional dentition. LAP of the primary dentition may progress to LAP in the permanent dentition and is probably the same disease entity, differing only in the age of onset or diagnosis.

LAP in the primary dentition is believed to be the result of a bacterial infection combined with specific, but minor, host immunologic deficits. LAP in the primary dentition has not been as extensively studied as has LAP of the permanent dentition, and a causative bacterial species has not been identified. Antibiotic therapy combined with local debridement appears to be effective. Tetracyclines, commonly used to manage LAP in the permanent dentition, are contraindicated in the primary dentition because of the potential for staining developing permanent teeth. Metronidazole is the antibiotic of choice for LAP of the primary dentition.

### Necrotizing Ulcerative Gingivitis/Periodontitis

Necrotizing ulcerative gingivitis/periodontitis is characterized by the rapid onset of painful gingivitis with interproximal and marginal necrosis and ulceration. The incidence peaks in the late teens and early twenties in North America and Europe, but in less developed countries it is common in young children. Malnutrition, viral infections, stress, and lack of sleep have been reported as predisposing factors. Necrotizing ulcerative gingivitis/periodontitis is associated with high levels of spirochetes and *Prevotella intermedia*. Local debridement usually produces rapid resolution of the disease, but antibiotic therapy with penicillin or metronidazole may be indicated when elevated temperature occurs.

## SYSTEMIC DISEASES AND CONDITIONS WITH ASSOCIATED PERIODONTAL PROBLEMS

Early loss of periodontal attachment in children often is a sign of systemic disease. Periodontitis may occur in the presence of defects in the immune system that result in susceptibility to infection, such as leukocyte adhesion deficiency or neutropenia. Early loss of attachment may also occur because of developmental defects in the attachment apparatus as in hypophosphatasia. Periodontal defects and gingival lesions may also

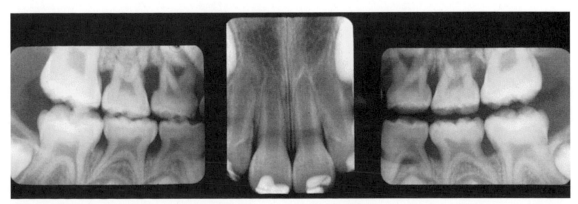

**Figure 24-8**  Radiographic appearance of localized aggressive periodontitis showing the characteristic loss of bone around the primary molars. In this patient the disease has not progressed to include the permanent teeth, as sometimes occurs.

result from the invasion of neoplastic cells as in leukemia.

## Diabetes

An increased risk and earlier onset of periodontitis occur in both insulin-dependent and non–insulin-dependent diabetes mellitus,[6] probably because of impaired immune function. As many as 10% to 15% of teenagers with insulin-dependent diabetes mellitus have significant periodontal disease. Poor metabolic control increases the risk of periodontitis, and untreated periodontitis in turn worsens metabolic control of diabetes. Effective preventive regimens and early diagnosis and treatment of periodontitis are important for the overall health of patients with diabetes.

## Down Syndrome

Down syndrome, a genetic form of mental retardation resulting from the presence of three copies of chromosome 21, is accompanied by an increased susceptibility to periodontitis. Most patients develop periodontitis by 30 years of age, and it may first occur in the primary dentition.[10] Plaque levels are high in these patients, but the severity of periodontal destruction exceeds that attributable to local factors alone. Various minor immune deficits, particularly in neutrophil function, have been identified in patients with Down syndrome and may be responsible for the increased susceptibility to periodontitis. Severe recession in the mandibular anterior region

associated with a high frenum attachment is also common in Down syndrome.

## Hypophosphatasia

Hypophosphatasia is a genetic disorder in which the enzyme bone alkaline phosphatase is deficient or defective. Phenotypes of hypophosphatasia can vary from premature loss of deciduous teeth to severe bone abnormalities leading to neonatal death.[5] In general, the earlier the presentation of symptoms, the more severe the disease. In mild forms the early loss of primary teeth may be the first and only clinical sign, as shown in Figure 24-9. The early loss of teeth is the result of defective cementum formation, which in turn results in a weakened attachment of tooth to bone. The teeth are affected in the order of formation, so that those that form the earliest are most likely to be involved and the most severely affected. There currently is no treatment for the disease, but the dental prognosis for the permanent teeth is good. Typically the primary incisors are exfoliated before the age of 4 years, the other primary teeth are affected to varying degrees, and the permanent dentition is normal. Hypophosphatasia can be diagnosed by a finding of low alkaline phosphatase levels in a serum sample.

## Leukocyte Adhesion Deficiency

Leukocyte adhesion deficiency (LAD) is a rare, recessive genetic disease. In LAD, the CD18 surface protein on leukocytes is defective or absent,

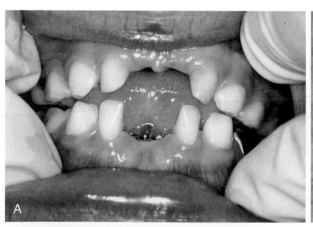
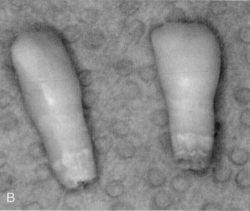

**Figure 24-9    A,** The dentition of a child 4 years of age with early loss of upper and lower central incisors due to hypophosphatasia. **B,** The lower incisors, exfoliated at 13 months of age. Note the incomplete root development at the time the teeth were exfoliated.

resulting in poor migration to infection sites and impaired phagocytic function. This leaves patients susceptible to bacterial infections, including periodontitis. Due to the high incidence of skin abscesses, recurrent otitis media, pneumonitis, and other bacterial infections of soft tissues, a diagnosis is usually made before dental symptoms appear. Dental symptoms are manifested early in the primary dentition. Bone loss is rapid around nearly all teeth, and inflammation is marked. In the dental literature LAD has sometimes been called generalized prepubertal periodontitis.[13] Scrupulous oral hygiene measures are necessary to control the periodontitis associated with LAD, but in part because of these patients' chronic problems with illness, adequate compliance may be difficult to achieve.

## Neutropenia

Neutropenia is a hematologic disorder characterized by reduced numbers or complete disappearance of neutrophils from the blood and bone marrow. In addition to increased susceptibility to recurrent infections such as otitis media and respiratory and skin infections, patients with neutropenia generally suffer from severe gingivitis and pronounced alveolar bone loss. Several different forms of neutropenia, including cyclic neutropenia, have been associated with oral symptoms in children. Neutropenia can be diagnosed by a finding of depressed neutrophils on a differential blood count. Periodontal therapy consists of rigorous local measures to control plaque, but patients are seldom able to maintain the level of oral hygiene necessary to prevent disease.

## Papillon-Lefèvre Syndrome

Papillon-Lefèvre syndrome is a rare disease that has as a symptom the onset of severe periodontitis in the primary or transitional dentition. It is a genetic disorder that is easily identified on clinical examination by the finding of hyperkeratosis of the palms of the hands and soles of the feet. Severe inflammation and rapid bone loss are characteristic of the periodontitis. Therapy consists of aggressive local measures to control plaque formation. Successful treatment outcomes in children have been reported with antibiotic therapy.[8]

## Histiocytosis

Langerhans cell histiocytosis (LCH), previously known as histiocytosis X, is a rare disorder of childhood with typical presentation as infiltration of bones, skin, liver, and other organs by histiocytes. In 10% to 20% of cases, the initial infiltrates occur in the oral cavity, usually in the mandible. Typical findings are gingival enlargement, ulceration, mobility of teeth with alveolar expansion, and discrete, destructive lesions of bone that can be observed on radiographs. Teeth may be left "floating in air" and eventually exfoliated. The lesions of histiocytosis may initially be mistaken for localized aggressive periodontitis. LCH may be diagnosed by biopsy. Therapy consists of local measures such as radiation and surgery to remove lesions and systemic chemotherapy for disseminated disease. The prognosis for disseminated early-onset disease is poor, with mortality rates exceeding 60%. Mild localized LCH, on the other hand, has an excellent prognosis. The lesions of LCH and the local therapy used to remove them may result in the loss or arrested development of teeth.

## Leukemia

Leukemia is the most common form of childhood cancer. Acute lymphoblastic leukemia (ALL) is the most common and has the best prognosis. Acute myeloid leukemia (AML) accounts for about 20% of childhood leukemias and has a poorer long-term survival rate. AML, but not usually ALL, may present with gingival enlargement caused by infiltrates of leukemic cells. The lesions are bluish red and may sometimes invade bone. In addition to the gingival lesions, the patient may have fever, malaise, gingival or other bleeding, and bone or joint pain. AML may be diagnosed by a blood cell count. Anemia, abnormal leukocyte and differential counts, and thrombocytopenia are usually observed.

## PERIODONTAL EXAMINATION OF CHILDREN

The periodontal health of children and adolescents should be assessed at each examination. The gingival tissues should be examined for redness, edema, bleeding, or enlargement. Oral hygiene may be assessed via a plaque index. Use of a disclosant provides an excellent oral hygiene instruction tool, and a plaque index provides a method for monitoring and documenting oral hygiene practices. Calculus is not as common in young patients as it is in adults, but it is found in about 10% of children and approximately one third of teenagers. The most common areas in which it occurs are the lingual surfaces of the mandibular incisors followed by the buccal surfaces of the maxillary molars. Patients' teeth should always be checked for calculus at the periodic examinations and deposits removed.

Particularly after the eruption of permanent teeth, attachment levels should be determined by periodontal probing, at least of selected sites. Probing of the permanent incisors and first permanent molars provides a diagnostic screening for LJP. Because erupting teeth can be probed all the way to the cementoenamel junction, transient deep pockets are a normal finding in the transitional dentition and must be distinguished from true attachment loss by locating the cementoenamel junction.

When radiographs are available, bone levels should be examined. Normal crestal height should be within 1 to 2 mm of the cementoenamel junction.[12] Once permanent teeth have erupted, the patient should also be examined for deficiencies in the width of attached gingiva and areas of recession noted.

# REFERENCES

1. American Academy of Periodontology. Position paper: epidemiology of periodontal diseases. *J Periodontol* 67:935-945, 1996.

2. Andlin-Sobocki A, Bodin L: Dimensional alterations of the gingiva related to changes of facial/lingual tooth position in permanent anterior teeth of children. A 2-year longitudinal study. *J Clin Periodontol* 20:219-224, 1993.

3. Armitage GC: Development of a classification system for periodontal diseases and conditions. *Ann Periodontol* 4:1-6, 1999.

4. Bhat M: Periodontal health of 14-17-year-old US schoolchildren. *J Public Health Dent* 51:5-11, 1991.

5. Chapple IL: Hypophosphatasia: dental aspects and mode of inheritance. *J Clin Periodontol* 20:615-622.

6. de Pommereau V, Dargent-Pare C, Robert JJ, Brion M: Periodontal status in insulin-dependent diabetic adolescents. *J Clin Periodontol* 19:628-632, 1992.

7. Dongari A, McDonnell HT, Langlais RP: Drug-induced gingival overgrowth. *Oral Surg Oral Med Oral Pathol* 76:543-548, 1993.

8. Ishikawa I, Umeda M, Laosrisin N: Clinical, bacteriological, and immunological examinations and the treatment process of two Papillon-Lefèvre syndrome patients. *J Periodontol* 65:364-371, 1994.

9. Matsson L: Factors influencing the susceptibility to gingivitis during childhood: a review. *Int J Paediatr Dent* 3:119-127, 1993.

10. Reuland-Bosma W, van Dijk J: Periodontal disease in Down's syndrome: a review. *J Clin Periodontol* 13:64-73, 1986.

11. Saxen L, Asikainen S: Metronidazole in the treatment of localized juvenile periodontitis. *J Clin Periodontol* 20:166-171, 1993.

12. Sjodin B, Matsson L: Marginal bone level in the normal primary dentition. *J Clin Periodontol* 19:672-678, 1992.

13. Watanabe K: Prepubertal periodontitis: a review of diagnostic criteria, pathogenesis, and differential diagnosis. *J Periodontal Res* 25:31-48, 1990.

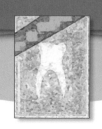

# CHAPTER 25

## Space Maintenance in the Primary Dentition

*John R. Christensen and Henry W. Fields, Jr.*

## GENERAL CONSIDERATIONS

Management of premature tooth loss in the primary dentition requires careful thought by the clinician because the consequences of proper or improper space management may influence dental development well into adolescence.[6] Early loss of primary teeth may compromise the eruption of succedaneous teeth if there is a reduction in the arch length. On the other hand, timely intervention may save space for the eruption of the permanent dentition. The key to space maintenance in the primary dentition is in knowing which problems to treat.[4]

Premature tooth loss in this age group is best thought of in terms of anterior (incisors and canines) and posterior (molars) teeth. The causes and treatment of missing teeth differ in these two regions. Anterior tooth loss is due primarily to trauma and tooth decay. Injuries to the primary incisors are common because a child of this age is learning to crawl, walk, and run. Although the prevalence of dental decay appears to be declining, a small number of children still suffer from early childhood caries and rampant decay and experience most of the dental disease.[1] These decay patterns result in tooth loss in both the anterior and posterior regions. The majority of posterior tooth loss is due to dental caries; rarely are primary molars lost to trauma. If no space loss has occurred immediately after tooth loss, space maintenance is appropriate because the permanent successor will not erupt for several years. If space loss has occurred, a comprehensive evaluation is required to determine whether space maintenance, space regaining, or no treatment is indicated. This type of evaluation and decision making is described in the discussions of mixed dentition (Chapters 30 and 35) because most attempts at regaining space are made at that time.

Missing primary incisors are usually replaced for four reasons: space maintenance, function, speech, and aesthetics. Some dentists think that early removal of a primary incisor results in space loss because the adjacent teeth drift into the space formerly occupied by the lost incisor. However, this does not seem to be true in most clinical situations. There may be some rearrangement of space between the remaining incisors, but there is no net loss of space. Intuitively, this makes sense because there is no apparent movement or drifting of teeth when developmental spacing is present in the primary dentition.

Poor masticatory function has also been proposed as a reason for replacing missing primary incisors. Concerns have been expressed about a child's ability to eat after four maxillary incisors have been removed as a result of early childhood caries. Feeding is not a problem, and when given a proper diet, the child continues to grow normally.

Some investigators have cited slowed or altered speech development as a justification for replacing missing maxillary incisors. This may be valid if the child has lost a number of teeth very early and is just beginning to develop speech. Many sounds are made with the tongue touching the lingual side of the maxillary incisors, and inappropriate speech compensations may develop if these teeth are missing. However, if the child has already acquired speech skills, the loss of an incisor is not particularly important.[7]

Probably the most valid reason for replacing missing incisors is aesthetics. Aesthetic concerns are voiced by some parents but not by others. If parents do not indicate a desire to replace missing anterior teeth, certainly no treatment is appropriate. If the parents do wish to replace the missing teeth, either a fixed lingual arch or a removable partial denture with attached primary teeth can serve as a prosthetic replacement (Fig. 25-1). The dentist should present both alternatives and let the parents make an educated decision.

Loss of a primary canine as a result of either trauma or decay is rare. Because it is so rare, there is some debate about whether space loss will occur if the tooth is not replaced. From a

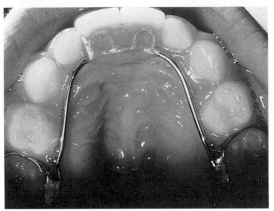

**Figure 25-1** A fixed (as shown here) or removable partial denture can be used to replace missing anterior teeth in the primary dentition. In most cases the partial denture is placed for aesthetic reasons rather than to prevent space loss in the anterior dental arch.

conservative point of view, a band-and-loop space maintainer (see later discussion in this chapter) or a removable partial denture may be placed if the patient is cooperative. Either of these appliances will have to be remade when the permanent lateral incisor erupts because the permanent lateral incisor will require more space than the primary lateral incisor and will interfere with space maintenance. If a space maintainer is not placed in the maxilla, a midline shift to the affected side should be anticipated when the permanent incisors erupt. In the mandible, lingual movement of the incisors and movement of the midline to the affected side will occur. A lingual arch may be appropriate after the permanent incisors erupt to prevent the midline shift.

Therefore, space maintenance during the primary dentition years is aimed primarily at the replacement of primary molars. Loss of interproximal contact as a result of decay, extraction, or ankylosis of an adjacent tooth results in space loss because of mesial and occlusal drift of the tooth distal to the newly created space. There is also evidence that the tooth mesial to the affected molar will drift distally into the space.[5] Therefore, loss of space or arch length can occur from both directions (Fig. 25-2).

Space maintenance begins with good restorative dentistry. The dentist should strive for ideal restoration of all interproximal contours. Early restoration of interproximal caries ensures that no space loss occurs. In some instances, however, large carious lesions may make ideal restoration of the tooth impossible, and space loss is inevit-

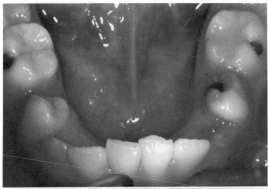

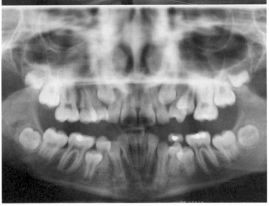

A

B

**Figure 25-2** Premature loss of the primary first molar results in loss of space from both directions. The primary mandibular second molar drifts mesially, and the primary canine drifts distally, but predominantly there is movement from the anterior in the posterior direction for the mandibular arch. **A,** Arch perimeter has been lost on both sides. **B,** Panoramic radiograph shows the canine and two premolars attempting to erupt into the limited space.

able. Even if the pulpal tissues have been compromised, pulp therapy should be initiated and the tooth maintained, if at all possible, because the natural tooth is still superior to the best space maintainer available; it is functional, is the correct size, and exfoliates appropriately. In cases of ankylosis, the tooth should be maintained until space loss is imminent; it is then extracted and the space maintained. Ankylosed teeth usually show limited vertical change in the primary dentition years.

Teeth lost during the primary dentition years will cause later-than-normal eruption of the succedaneous teeth. This means that the appliances should be monitored, adjusted, and possibly replaced over a longer period of time. Abutment teeth for appliances may exfoliate or interfere with adjacent erupting teeth, and decay and decalcification are more likely. These aspects of

care should be considered during treatment planning.

## APPLIANCE THERAPY

Four appliances generally are used to maintain space in the primary dentition: the band and loop, the lingual arch, the distal shoe, and the removable appliance.

### Band and Loop

The first appliance, the band and loop, is used to maintain the space of a single tooth. This appliance is inexpensive and easy to fabricate. Its use requires continuous supervision and care, however, and it does not restore the occlusal function of the missing tooth. In the majority of patients requiring space maintenance in the primary and mixed dentitions, the band-and-loop appliance is used. The appliance is indicated in the following situations:

1. Unilateral loss of the primary first molar before or after eruption of the permanent first molar (Fig. 25-3)

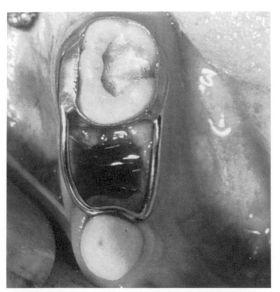

**Figure 25-3** The band and loop appliance is used to maintain the space after the premature loss of a single tooth. The band and loop appliance is indicated when there is unilateral loss of a primary first molar before or after the eruption of the permanent first molar. The loop is constructed of 36-mil round wire and is soldered to the band.

2. Bilateral loss of a primary molar before the eruption of the permanent incisors (Fig. 25-4)

The initial step in constructing a band-and-loop appliance is to select and fit a band on the abutment tooth. Band selection is a trial-and-error affair, and bands are fitted until one can be nearly seated on the tooth with finger pressure (Fig. 25-5, *A*). A band pusher and band biter are used to achieve the final occlusogingival position (Fig. 25-5, *B* and *C*). A properly placed band is seated approximately 1 mm below the mesial and distal marginal ridges (Fig. 25-5, *D*). If a band cannot be easily fitted, orthodontic separators should be placed to create space for the band material (Fig. 25-5, *E*). This same technique is used to place orthodontic bands on the posterior teeth when fixed orthodontic therapy is indicated. The next step is to make a quarter-arch impression of the band and edentulous area with either compound or alginate impression material. If alginate impression material is used, the tray should be perforated so that the material can flow through the perforations and prevent the impression from becoming distorted when it is removed. After the impression is made, the band is gently removed with a band remover and is placed and stabilized in the impression in the correct position.

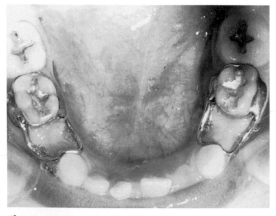

**Figure 25-4** If both primary first molars are lost prematurely in the mandibular arch and the permanent incisors have not erupted, bilateral band and loop appliances are used to maintain space. A lingual arch is not indicated in this situation because it may interfere with the subsequent eruption of the permanent mandibular incisors.

The impression is poured in stone with the band in place. The cast is separated, and a 36-mil wire is formed into a loop and contoured to fit the band and alveolar ridge. The loop should parallel the edentulous ridge 1 mm off the gingival tissue and should rest against the adjacent tooth at the contact point. The faciolingual dimension of the loop should be approximately 8 mm. This dimension should allow the permanent tooth to erupt freely but not impinge on the buccal mucosa or tongue. The loop should not restrict any physiologic tooth movement, such as the increase in intercanine width that occurs during eruption of the permanent lateral incisors. When the band-and-loop appliance is returned from the laboratory, it should be fitted and adjusted if necessary. Following that, the band should be cemented onto a clean, dry abutment tooth with zinc phosphate or glass ionomer cement. The patient should be recalled every 6 months to check that the appliance still fits properly, the cement has not washed out, and the abutment teeth are firm. The eruption of the permanent tooth is an easily recognized indication for removal.

Two modifications of the band-and-loop appliance are not recommended for use in space maintenance therapy. The bonded band and loop is a contoured wire similar to the loop portion of the band-and-loop appliance that is bonded to the abutment tooth with composite resin. There are two reasons why the bonded band and loop is not recommended. First, it is difficult to keep the wire bonded to the tooth because of the shearing force of occlusion. If the bond breaks, there is a potential for space loss and the added danger of aspiration of the wire. Second, the bonded band and loop is nearly impossible to adjust. The other band-and-loop variation that is not recommended is the crown-and-loop appliance. The crown-and-loop technique requires preparation of the abutment tooth for a stainless steel crown followed by soldering of a space-maintaining wire directly to the crown. Care and maintenance of the band-and-loop appliance also are easier than that needed for the crown and loop if the appliance is damaged or has to be modified. If the soldered joint fails and the wire breaks loose, there is no way to repair the crown-and-loop appliance intraorally. The crown must be cut off, a new crown fitted, and the wire resoldered. It is much easier to restore the abutment tooth with a stainless steel crown and then make a band and loop that fits the crown.

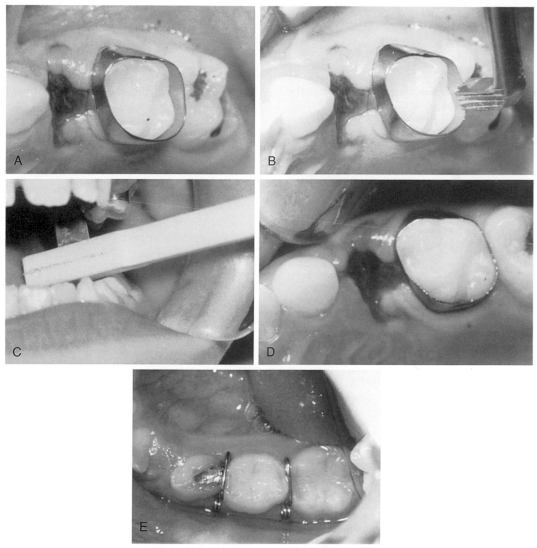

**Figure 25-5**   **A,** The initial step in fabricating a band and loop device is to fit a band on the abutment tooth. Band selection is a trial-and-error procedure and continues until a band can be nearly seated on the tooth with finger pressure. **B,** A band pusher is used to seat the band to a nearly ideal position. The dentist should maintain a good finger rest because soft and hard tissue injury can occur if the pusher slips without proper support. **C,** Final occlusogingival position is achieved with a band biter. In the maxillary arch, the band biter should be placed on the distolingual portion of the band for final positioning. In the mandibular arch, the band biter should be placed on the distofacial portion of the band. **D,** A properly fitted band is seated approximately 1 mm below the mesial and distal marginal ridges. **E,** If a tight interproximal contact prevents the band from seating properly, orthodontic separators are placed to create space for the band material. The separators are removed within 7 to 10 days, and the band is fitted.

## Lingual Arch

The second type of appliance used to maintain posterior space in the primary dentition is the lingual arch. The lingual arch is often suggested when teeth are lost in both quadrants of the same arch. Because the permanent incisor tooth buds develop and erupt somewhat lingual to their primary precursors in the lower arch, a conventional mandibular lingual arch is not recommended in the primary dentition; the wire resting adjacent to the primary incisors might interfere with the eruption of the permanent dentition (Fig. 25-6). Instead, two band-and-loop appliances are recommended when there is bilateral tooth loss in the mandibular arch.

Use of the maxillary lingual arch is feasible in the primary dentition because it can be constructed to rest away from the incisors. Two types

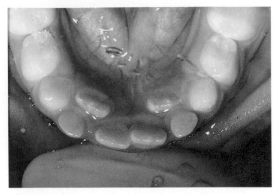

**Figure 25-6** Lingual eruption of the permanent mandibular incisors is not uncommon. A mandibular lingual arch is not recommended as a space maintainer in the primary dentition because it may interfere with the eruption of these incisors. Bilateral band and loop appliances are recommended when both primary mandibular first molars are lost prematurely.

of lingual arch designs are used to maintain maxillary space: the Nance arch and the transpalatal arch (TPA). These appliances use a large wire (36 mil) to connect the banded primary teeth on both sides of the arch that are distal to the extraction site. The difference between the two appliances has to do with where the wire is placed in the palate. The Nance arch incorporates an acrylic button that rests directly on the palatal rugae. The TPA is made from a wire that traverses the palate directly without touching it (Fig. 25-7). Although the TPA is a cleaner appliance and is easier to

construct, many clinicians think that it allows the teeth to move and tip mesially, resulting in space loss.

## Distal Shoe

The distal shoe appliance is used to maintain the space of a primary second molar that has been lost before the eruption of the permanent first molar (Fig. 25-8). An unerupted permanent first molar drifts mesially within the alveolar bone if the primary second molar is lost prematurely. The result of the mesial drift is loss of arch length and possible impaction of the second premolar.

The appliance can be constructed from an impression taken after removal of the primary second molar or from an impression taken before the tooth is extracted. In the former situation, the gingiva must be incised when the appliance is placed because of healing in the extraction site. In the latter situation, the construction cast must be modified to simulate loss of the primary second molar, but placement in the extraction site at the time of surgery is straightforward.

The appliance is constructed very much like the band and loop. The primary first molar is banded and the loop extended to the former distal contact of the primary second molar. A piece of stainless steel is soldered to the distal end of the loop and placed in the extraction site. The stainless steel extension acts as a guide plane for

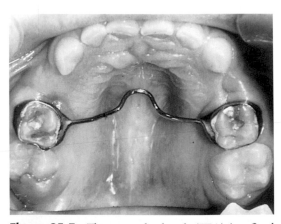

**Figure 25-7** The transpalatal arch (TPA) is a fixed lingual arch appliance used to maintain space following bilateral loss of maxillary teeth. The TPA is more hygienic than the Nance appliance because it consists of only the 36-mil palatal wire, but it can allow the abutment teeth to tip mesially in some cases, resulting in space loss.

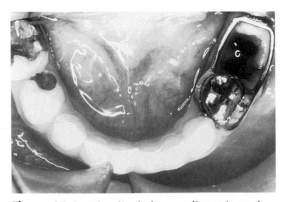

**Figure 25-8** The distal shoe appliance is used to maintain the space of a primary second molar that has been lost prematurely before the eruption of the permanent first molar. A stainless steel extension is soldered to the distal end of the band and 36-mil loop; this extension is positioned 1 mm below the mesial marginal ridge of the unerupted permanent first molar. The extension serves to guide the eruption of the permanent first molar.

the permanent first molar to erupt into proper position and should be positioned 1 mm below the mesial marginal ridge of the unerupted molar in the alveolar bone. After the permanent molar has erupted, the extension can be cut off or a new band-and-loop appliance can be constructed. To ensure that the stainless steel extension is in the proper position and in close proximity to the permanent first molar, a periapical radiograph is recommended before the appliance is cemented (Fig. 25-9).

There are many problems associated with the distal shoe appliance. Because of its cantilever design and the fact it is anchored on the occlusally convergent crown of the primary first molar, the appliance can replace only a single tooth and is somewhat fragile. No occlusal function is restored because of this lack of strength. In addition, histologic examination shows that complete epithelialization does not occur after placement of the appliance.[3] Because the epithelium is not intact, the distal shoe appliance is contraindicated in medically compromised patients and in patients who require subacute bacterial endocarditis coverage.

Some clinicians advocate an appliance with a wire simply resting on the soft tissue (or resting with some pressure) approximately where the distal surface of the lost primary second molar was located to control space and movement of the nonerupted permanent first molar. To date, there are no data to support this recommendation. Another modification of this appliance is the crown and distal shoe. Although feasible, it, like the crown and loop, is difficult to modify and

repair. Finally, some clinicians use the prefabricated band and loops and distal shoes. These can be fabricated intraorally and save laboratory expense. These are a practical alternative[2] but may lack durability.

## Removable Appliances

Removable appliances also can be used to maintain space in the primary dentition (Fig. 25-10). The appliance is typically used when more than one tooth has been lost in a quadrant. The removable appliance is often the only alternative because there are no suitable abutment teeth and because the cantilever design of the distal shoe or the band-and-loop appliance is too weak to withstand occlusal forces over a two-tooth span. Not only can the partial denture replace more than one tooth, but it also can replace occlusal function.

Two drawbacks of the appliance are retention and compliance. Retention is a problem because primary canines do not have large undercuts for clasp engagement. If multiple tooth loss is unilateral, retention problems can be overcome by placing sturdy retention clasps on the opposite side of the arch. However, if multiple teeth are lost bilaterally, retention problems are almost inevitable. The problem of compliance is closely related to that of retention. Three- to six-year-old children will not tolerate an ill-fitting appliance and

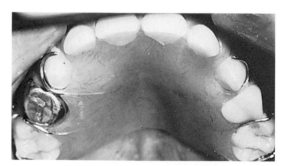

**Figure 25-10** A removable partial denture is used to maintain posterior space in the primary dentition when more than one tooth in a quadrant is lost. This appliance is the only suitable space maintainer because the canine is a poor abutment and the cantilever design of the band and loop or distal shoe is too weak to withstand occlusal forces. In the patient portrayed here, both anterior and posterior teeth have been replaced. (From Fields HW, Proffit WR: Orthodontics in general practice. In: Morris AL, Bohannan HM, Casullo DP, editors. *The Dental Specialties in General Practice.* Philadelphia, Saunders, 1983, p 299.)

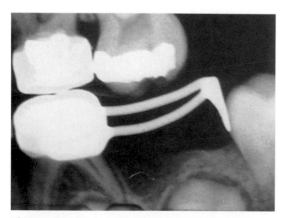

**Figure 25-9** A periapical radiograph is recommended prior to cementing the distal shoe appliance to ensure that it is properly positioned in relation to the unerupted permanent first molar.

will not use it. In fact, some children will not tolerate a retentive appliance. The dentist is then resigned to waiting until the permanent teeth (molars) erupt so that they can be used as abutments for a conventional lingual arch appliance. Partial dentures occasionally require clasp adjustment and acrylic modification to maintain good retention and allow eruption of the underlying or adjacent permanent teeth. Some children are compliant in wearing an appliance but not in cleaning the appliance and the underlying tissue. This can result in tissue decay, tissue irritation, and hyperplasia.

## SUMMARY

Space maintenance in the primary dentition should be considered in terms of anterior and posterior space loss. Space maintenance is not required for missing primary incisors. Primary incisors should be replaced only if aesthetic concerns are a factor. Posterior space maintenance is a necessity in this age group and should be undertaken when primary molars are lost prematurely and the space is adequate. The band-and-loop appliance is used most often; other appliances can be employed as different situations dictate. Judicious space maintenance benefits the child patient and may prevent future alignment and crowding problems.

## REFERENCES

1. American Association of Dental Schools: In: Walachovic RW, editor. *Trends in Dental Education 2000: The Past, Present and Future of the Dental Profession and the People It Serves.* Washington, DC, The Association, 2000.
2. Brill WA: The distal shoe space maintainer: chairside fabrication and clinical performance. *Pediatr Dent* 24:561-565, 2002.
3. Mayhew MJ, Dilley GJ, Dilley DCH et al: Tissue response to appliances in monkeys. *Pediatr Dent* 6:148-152, 1984.
4. Ngan P, Fields HW: Orthodontic diagnosis and treatment planning in the primary dentition. *J Dent Child* 62:25-33, 1995.
5. Owen DG: The incidence and nature of space closure following the premature extraction of deciduous teeth: a literature survey. *Am J Orthod* 59:37-48, 1971.
6. Proffit WR, Fields HW: Treatment of moderate nonskeletal problems in preadolescent children. In: *Contemporary Orthodontics,* 3rd ed. St Louis, Mosby, 1999.
7. Rieckman GA, ElBadrawy HE: Effect of premature loss of primary maxillary incisors on speech. *Pediatr Dent* 7:119-122, 1985.

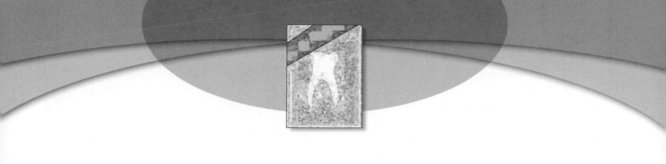

# CHAPTER 26

## Oral Habits

*John R. Christensen, Henry W. Fields, Jr., and Steven M. Adair*

The presence of an oral habit in a 3- to 6-year-old child is an important finding during the clinical examination. An oral habit is not usually present in children near the end of this age group. Preferably, a habit that has resulted in movement of the primary incisors or has inhibited eruption will have been eliminated before the permanent incisors erupt. If a habit that causes dental changes is not eliminated before the permanent incisors erupt, they too will be affected. On the other hand, these are not irreversible changes. If the habit is stopped during the mixed-dentition years, the adverse dental changes will begin to reverse naturally. Some appliance therapy may be required, but generally the teeth will move toward a more neutral position with the absence of the forces of the habit.

If no dental changes have occurred, no treatment can be advocated on the grounds of dental health, but some patients and parents may want treatment because digit or pacifier habits become less socially acceptable as the child becomes older. One study has shown that school-aged children consider thumb suckers significantly less intelligent, less attractive, and less desirable as friends.[8] Efforts to discourage the habit may involve as little as a conversation between the dentist and the child, or they may involve more complex appliance therapy. The most important point to remember about any intervention is that the child must want to discontinue the habit for treatment to be successful.

## THUMB AND FINGER HABITS

Thumb and finger habits make up the majority of oral habits. About two thirds of such habits are ended by 5 years of age.[11] Dentists are often questioned about the kinds of problems these habits may cause if they are prolonged. The malocclusions caused by nonnutritive sucking may be more of an individual response than a highly specific cause-and-effect relationship.[4] The types of dental changes that a digit habit may cause vary with the intensity, duration, and frequency of the habit as well as the manner in which the digit is positioned in the mouth. Intensity is the amount of force that is applied to the teeth during sucking. Duration is defined as the amount of time spent sucking a digit. Frequency is the number of times the habit is practiced throughout the day. Duration plays the most critical role in tooth movement caused by a digit habit. Clinical and experimental evidence suggests that 4 to 6 hours of force per day is probably the minimum necessary to cause tooth movement. Therefore, a child who sucks intermittently with high intensity may not produce much tooth movement at all, whereas a child who sucks continuously (for more than 6 hours) can cause significant dental change. The duration of digit sucking habits (months or years) is positively related to an increased prevalence of anterior open bite or reduced overbite, increased overjet, greater maxillary arch depth, and decreased maxillary arch width.[17] The most frequently reported dental signs of an active habit are the following:

1. Anterior open bite
2. Facial movement of the upper incisors and lingual movement of the lower incisors
3. Maxillary constriction

Anterior open bite, or the lack of vertical overlap of the upper and lower incisors when the teeth are in occlusion, develops because the digit rests directly on the incisors (Fig. 26-1). This prevents complete or continued eruption of the incisors, whereas the posterior teeth are free to erupt. Anterior open bite may also be caused by intrusion of the incisors. However, inhibition of eruption is easier to accomplish than true intrusion, which would be the result of a habit of great duration.

Faciolingual movement of the incisors depends on how the thumb or finger is placed and how

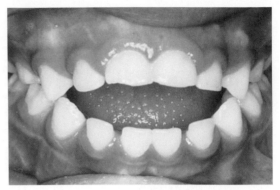

**Figure 26-1**  This patient's anterior open bite is a direct result of an active thumb sucking habit. An open bite results when the thumb impedes eruption of the anterior teeth, moves them facially, and allows the posterior teeth to erupt passively. Actual intrusion of the anterior teeth is possible but unlikely.

many fingers are placed in the mouth. Some consider this positional variable to be a confounding factor related to intensity, duration, and frequency. Usually, the thumb is placed so that it exerts pressure on the lingual surface of the maxillary incisors and on the labial surface of the mandibular incisors (Fig. 26-2). A child who actively sucks can create enough force to tip the upper incisors facially and the lower incisors lingually. The result is an increased overjet and, by virtue of the tipping, decreased overbite.

Maxillary arch constriction is probably due to the change in equilibrium balance between the oral musculature and the tongue. When the thumb is placed in the mouth, the tongue is

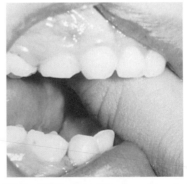

**Figure 26-2**  With most thumb sucking habits, the thumb exerts pressure on the lingual surface of the maxillary incisors and on the facial surface of the mandibular incisors. This causes the maxillary incisors to tip facially and the mandibular incisors to tip lingually, resulting in increased overjet.

forced down and away from the palate. The orbicularis oris and buccinator muscles continue to exert a force on the buccal surfaces of the maxillary dentition, especially when these muscles are contracted during sucking. Because the tongue no longer exerts a counterbalancing force from the lingual surface, the posterior maxillary arch collapses into crossbite.

Data on the amount of skeletal change are not clear. Some believe the maxilla and its alveolar process are moved anteriorly and superiorly.[14] Certainly, if the teeth are moved, some alveolar change is made. Whether this is translated to the skeletal maxilla is not as well known. In one study a significantly higher percentage of distal step molar relationships in 5-year-olds was noted among digit suckers compared with children with no sucking habit.[9]

## Treatment

Timing of treatment must be gauged carefully. If parents or the child do not want to engage in treatment, it should not be attempted. The child should be given an opportunity to stop the habit spontaneously before the permanent teeth erupt. If treatment is selected as an alternative, it is generally undertaken between the ages of 4 and 6 years. Delay until the early school age years allows for spontaneous discontinuation of the habit by many children, often through peer pressure at school. As long as the habit is eliminated prior to full eruption of the permanent incisors, the eruption process will spontaneously reduce the overjet and open bite as the permanent teeth occupy new positions. It is generally agreed that interception of a digit sucking habit does no harm to the child's emotional development, nor does it result in habit substitution. However, the dentist should evaluate the child for psychological overtones prior to embarking on habit elimination. Such procedures might best be postponed for children who have recently undergone stressful changes in their lives, such as separation or divorce of parents, moving to a new community, or changing schools. Four different approaches to treatment have been advocated, depending on the willingness of the child to stop the habit.

### Counseling

The simplest yet least widely applicable approach is counseling with the patient. This involves discussion between the dentist and the patient of the problems created by nonnutritive sucking. These adult-like discussions focus on the changes that have occurred because of the sucking and their impact on aesthetics. Usually an appeal is made to the children on the basis of their maturity and responsibility. Clearly, this approach is best aimed at older children who can conceptually grasp the issue and who may be feeling social pressure to stop the habit. Some children are captured by this approach and successfully eliminate their habit.

### Reminder Therapy

The second approach, reminder therapy, is appropriate for those who desire to stop the habit but need some help. The purpose of any treatment should be thoroughly explained to the child. An adhesive bandage secured with waterproof tape on the offending finger can serve as a constant reminder not to place the finger in the mouth (Fig. 26-3). The bandage remains in place until the habit is extinguished. Some clinicians have used a mitten or sock to cover the fingers of the hand. This is especially useful during sleeping hours. Another approach is to paint a commercially available bitter substance on the fingers that are sucked. All these methods are aimed at reminding the child not to place the fingers in the mouth. However, sometimes this type of therapy is perceived as punishment and may not be as effective as a neutral reminder.

### Reward System

A third treatment for oral habits is a reward system. A contract is drawn up between the child and the parent or between the child and the

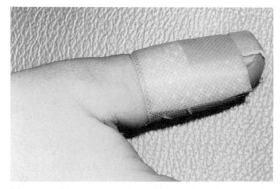

**Figure 26-3** One or two adhesive bandages can be taped to a child's finger to serve as a reminder not to place the finger in the mouth. The Band-Aid is worn until the child stops sucking the finger.

dentist. The contract simply states that the child will discontinue the habit within a specified period of time and in return will receive a reward. The reward does not need to be extravagant but must be special enough to motivate the child. Praise from the parents and the dentist has a large role. The more involvement the child takes in the project, the more likely it is that the project will succeed. Involvement may include placing stick-on stars on a homemade calendar when the child has successfully avoided the habit for an entire day. At the end of the specified time period, the reward is presented with verbal praise for meeting the conditions of the contract (Fig. 26-4). Reward systems and reminder therapy can be combined to improve the likelihood of success.

*Adjunctive Therapy*

If the habit persists after reminder and reward therapy and the child truly wants to eliminate the habit, adjunctive therapy that includes a method to physically interrupt the habit and remind the patient can be used. This type of treatment usually involves either wrapping the patient's arm in an elastic bandage so it cannot be flexed and the hand inserted in the mouth,[3] or placing an appliance in the mouth that physically discourages the habit by making it difficult to suck a thumb or finger. The dentist should explain to the patient

and parent that the appliance is not a punishment but rather a permanent reminder not to place the finger in the mouth.

The elastic bandage method is usually applied only at night. The bandage is loosely wrapped over the arm extending from below the elbow to above it. The sheer mass of elastic material (not the tightness) prohibits the child from sucking the fingers. Success over several weeks should be rewarded. The total program may take 6 to 8 weeks (anecdotally noted by success in children who have stopped habits while arms were casted for broken bones).

An intraoral appliance approach can also be employed in the adjunct method. The two appliances used most often to discourage the sucking habit are the quad helix and the palatal crib. The quad helix is a fixed appliance commonly used to expand a constricted maxillary arch—a common finding accompanied by posterior crossbite in patients who practice nonnutritive sucking (Fig. 26-5). The helices of the appliance serve to remind the child not to place the finger in the mouth. The quad helix is a versatile appliance because it can correct a posterior crossbite and discourage a finger habit at the same time.

The palatal crib is designed to interrupt a digit habit by interfering with finger placement and sucking satisfaction. The palatal crib is generally used in children in whom no posterior crossbite exists. It may, however, also be used as a retainer after maxillary expansion with a quad helix in a

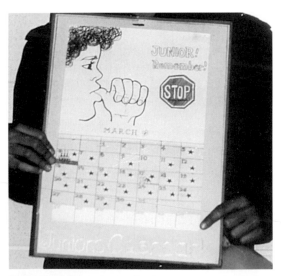

**Figure 26-4**  A personalized calendar can be used to motivate a child to stop a thumb sucking habit. Stick-on stars are applied to the calendar on days when the child has successfully avoided the habit. At the end of a month or a specified period of time, a reward and verbal praise can be provided for discontinuing the habit.

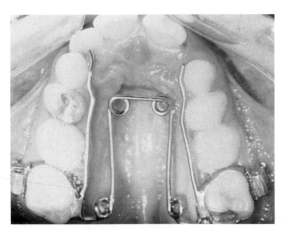

**Figure 26-5**  The quad helix is a fixed appliance used to expand a constricted maxillary arch. The anterior helices also discourage a sucking habit by reminding the child not to place a finger in the mouth. This appliance is often used in children in whom there is an active sucking habit and a posterior crossbite.

child who has not stopped sucking with the quad helix. For a palatal crib, bands are fitted on the permanent first molars or primary second molars. A heavy lingual arch wire (38 mil) is bent to fit passively in the palate and is soldered to the molar bands. Additional wire is soldered onto this base wire to form a crib or mechanical obstruction for the digit. It is advisable to make a lower cast at the time the appliance is constructed so that the occlusion can be checked for interferences (Fig. 26-6). The parent and child should be informed that certain side effects appear temporarily after the palatal crib is cemented. Eating, speaking, and sleeping patterns may be altered during the first few days after appliance delivery. These difficulties usually subside within 3 days to 2 weeks.[10] An imprint of the appliance usually appears on the tongue as an indentation. This imprint disappears soon after the appliance is removed. The major problem with the palatal crib and, to a lesser degree, the quad helix is the difficulty of maintaining good oral hygiene. The appliance traps food and is difficult to clean thoroughly. Oral malodor and tissue inflammation can result.

Adjunctive habit discouragement appliances should be left in the mouth for 6 to 12 months as a retainer. The palatal crib usually stops the child from sucking immediately but requires at least another 6 months of wear to extinguish the habit completely.[10] The quad helix also requires a minimum of 6 months of treatment. Three months is needed to correct the crossbite, and 3 months is required to stabilize the movement.

## PACIFIER HABITS

Dental changes created by pacifier habits are largely similar to changes created by thumb habits, and no clear consensus indicates a therapeutic difference (Fig. 26-7). Anterior open bite and maxillary constriction (with posterior crossbite) occur consistently in children who suck pacifiers. Labial movement of the maxillary incisors may not be as pronounced as that accompanying a digit habit. Manufacturers have developed pacifiers that they claim are more like a mother's nipple and not as deleterious to the dentition as a thumb or conventional pacifier. Research results have not substantiated this statement.[1,2,5] Increased duration of pacifier habits is related to an increased prevalence of anterior open bite and reduced overbite and posterior crossbite.[17]

Pacifier habits appear to end earlier than digit habits. More than 90% were reported ended before 5 years of age and 100% by age 8.[11] Pacifier habits theoretically are easier to stop than digit habits because the pacifier can be discontinued gradually or completely withdrawn with discussion and explanation to the child. This type of control is obviously not possible with digit habits, which makes a notable difference in the degree of patient compliance required to eliminate the two types of habits. In a few cases, the child may stop the pacifier habit and then start sucking a digit. Elimination of the subsequent finger habit may be necessary.

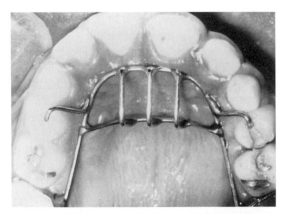

**Figure 26-6** A palatal crib is a fixed appliance designed to stop a digit habit by mechanically interfering with digit placement and sucking satisfaction. The parent of the child should expect temporary disturbances in eating, speaking, and sleeping patterns during the first few days after use of the appliance.

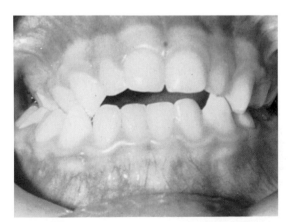

**Figure 26-7** A pacifier can create dental changes that are nearly identical to those of a digit habit. The labiolingual movement of the incisors is usually not as pronounced as that associated with a digit habit.

## LIP HABITS

Habits that involve manipulation of the lips and perioral structures are called lip habits. A number of lip habits exist, and their influence on the dentition is varied. Lip licking and lip pulling are relatively benign habits as far as dental effects are concerned. Red, inflamed, and chapped lips and perioral tissues during cool weather are the most apparent signs associated with these habits (Fig. 26-8). Little can be done to stop these habits effectively. Treatment is usually palliative and limited to moisturizing the lips, although some clinicians have used appliances to interrupt the habits.

Although most lip habits do not cause dental problems, lip sucking and lip biting certainly can maintain an existing malocclusion if the child engages in them with adequate intensity, frequency, and duration. Whether these habits can create a malocclusion is a question that is not easily answered. The most common presentation of lip sucking is the lower lip tucked behind the maxillary incisors (Fig. 26-9). This places a lingually directed force on the mandibular teeth and a facial force on the maxillary teeth. The result is a proclination of the maxillary incisors, a retroclination of the mandibular incisors, and increased overjet. This problem is most common in the mixed and permanent dentitions. Treatment depends on the skeletal relationship of the child and on the presence or absence of space in the arch. If the child has a class I skeletal relationship and an increased overjet that is solely the result of tipped teeth, the clinician can tip the teeth to their original or a more normal position with either a fixed or a removable appliance. If a class II skeletal relationship exists, a more involved growth modification procedure is needed to manage the malocclusion.

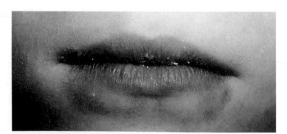

**Figure 26-8**   Red, inflamed, chapped lips and perioral tissues are often indicative of a lip sucking or licking habit. These problems are more common and severe during the winter months.

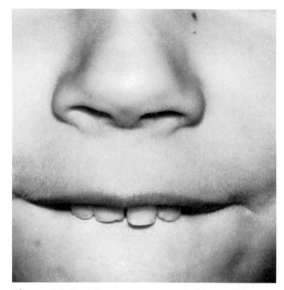

**Figure 26-9**   The most common habit involving the lips is tucking the lower lip behind the maxillary incisors. The lower lip forces the maxillary teeth facially and the mandibular teeth lingually, resulting in an increased overjet. In addition, the lower lip and other perioral tissues can become chapped and inflamed as a result of constant wetting.

## TONGUE THRUST AND MOUTH BREATHING HABITS

Recently, a great deal of attention has been given to tongue thrust and mouth breathing habits as sources of malocclusion. Tongue thrust is characteristic of the infantile and transitional swallows, both considered normal for the neonate. Epidemiologic data indicate that the percentage of persons with infantile and transitional swallowing patterns is greater than the percentage of persons with open bite.[12] This indicates there is no simple cause-and-effect relationship between tongue thrusting and open bite. Furthermore, data measuring the duration, intensity, and frequency of force associated with tongue thrust suggest that the habit may sustain an open bite but not create one.[15] Therefore, tongue thrusting should be considered a finding and not a problem to be treated.

Mouth breathing and its association with malocclusion is a complex issue. Research designed to answer questions about this association has not been well controlled. The major problem with this research has been the unreliable identification of mouth breathers. Some persons may appear to be mouth breathers because of their mandibular

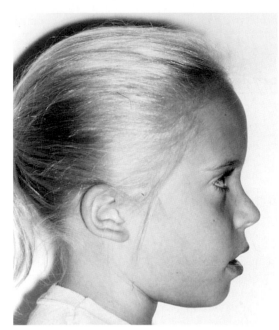

**Figure 26-10** The normal relaxed lip posture in the 3- to 6-year-old child is for the lips to be slightly apart or incompetent. These children are often labeled mouth breathers because of this posture, but they may in fact be completely nasal breathers.

posture or incompetent lips. It is normal for a 3- to 6-year-old to be slightly lip incompetent (Fig. 26-10). Other children have been labeled mouth breathers because of a suspected nasal airway obstruction. Two locations have been suggested consistently as sites of obstruction: the nasal turbinates and the nasopharyngeal adenoidal tissues. Clinical judgment is not accurate enough to confirm a diagnosis of nasal airway impairment. The only reliable method for determining the mode of respiratory function is to use a plethysmograph and airflow transducers to ascertain total nasal and oral air flow. One cross-sectional study used the plethysmograph on normal children and reported that prior to age 8 there were as many oral or predominantly oral breathers as nasal or predominantly nasal breathers. After age 8, the majority of the children were nasal or predominantly nasal breathers.[16] Despite the difficulties encountered in identifying mouth-breathing persons, there is some indication of a weak relationship between mouth breathing and malocclusion characterized by a long lower face and maxillary constriction. However, it should be noted that this relationship is very weak and does not imply that turbinec-tomy or adenoidectomy is required to clear the nasal airway.[6,18]

## NAIL BITING

Nail biting is a rare habit in persons younger than 3 to 6 years. The number of persons who bite their nails is reported to increase until adolescence, but there are very few data on this subject. It has been suggested that the habit is a manifestation of increased stress. There is no evidence that nail biting can cause malocclusion or dental change other than minor enamel fractures; therefore, there is no recommended treatment. Nail biting may damage the fingernail beds, however, and it may be necessary to use appropriate nail care products to protect the nails.

## BRUXISM

Bruxism is grinding of the teeth and is usually reported to occur while a child is sleeping. However, some children grind their teeth when awake. Most children engage in some bruxism that results in moderate wear of the primary canines and molars. Rarely, with the exception of handicapped persons, does the wear endanger the pulp by proceeding faster than secondary dentin is produced (Fig. 26-11). Masticatory muscle soreness and temporomandibular joint pain have also been attributed to bruxism. The exact cause of significant bruxism is unknown, although most explanations center on local, systemic, and psychological factors.[13] The local theory suggests that

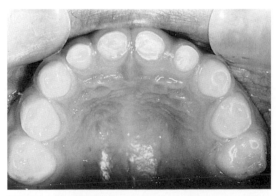

**Figure 26-11** This patient's primary maxillary incisors and canines were worn more rapidly than normal owing to a habit of bruxism.

bruxism is a reaction to an occlusal interference, high restoration, or some irritating dental condition. Systemic factors implicated in bruxism include intestinal parasites, subclinical nutritional deficiencies, allergies, and endocrine disorders. The psychological theory submits that bruxism is the manifestation of a personality disorder or increased stress. Children with musculoskeletal disorders (cerebral palsy) and severely mentally retarded children commonly grind their teeth. These patients' bruxism is the result of their underlying physical and mental condition and is difficult to manage dentally.

Treatment should begin with simple measures. Occlusal interferences should be identified and equilibrated if necessary. If occlusal interferences are not located or equilibration is not successful, referral to appropriate medical personnel should be considered to rule out any systemic problems. If neither of these two steps is successful, a mouthguard-like appliance can be constructed of soft plastic to protect the teeth and discourage the grinding habit. If the habit is thought to be due to psychological factors, which is unlikely, referral to a child development expert is warranted. Rarely, occlusal wear is so extensive that stainless steel crowns are needed to prevent pulpal exposure or eliminate tooth sensitivity.

## SELF-MUTILATION

Self-mutilation, repetitive acts that result in physical damage to the person, is extremely rare in normal children. However, the incidence of self-mutilation in the mentally retarded population is between 10% and 20%.[7] It has been suggested that self-mutilation is a learned behavior. This may be the case because it is one of the few behaviors that are reliably reinforced; that is, attention is always gained. A frequent manifestation of self-mutilation is biting of the lips, tongue, and oral mucosa. Any child who willfully inflicts pain or damage on himself or herself should be considered psychologically abnormal. Such children should be referred for psychological evaluation and treatment. Self-mutilation has also been associated with biochemical disorders, such as Lesch-Nyhan and de Lange's syndromes. Besides behavior modification, treatment for self-mutilation includes use of restraints, protective padding, and sedation. If use of restraints and protective padding is unsuccessful, extraction of selected teeth may be necessary.

## REFERENCES

1. Adair SM, Milano M, Dushku JC: Evaluation of the effects of orthodontic pacifiers on the primary dentitions of 24- to 59-month-old children: preliminary study. *Pediatr Dent* 14:13-18, 1992.
2. Adair SM, Milano M, Lorenzo I, Russell C: Effects of current and former pacifier use on the dentition of 24- to 59-month old children. *Pediatr Dent* 17:437-444, 1995.
3. Adair SM. The Ace bandage approach to digit-sucking habits. *Pediatr Dent* 21:451-452, 1999.
4. Baril C, Moyers RE: An electromyographic analysis of the temporalis muscles and certain facial muscles in thumb- and finger-sucking patients. *J Dent Res* 39:536-553, 1960.
5. Bishara SE, Nowak AJ, Kohout FJ et al: Influence of feeding and non-nutritive sucking methods on the development of the dental arches: longitudinal study of the first 18 months of life. *Pediatr Dent* 9:13-21, 1987.
6. Bresolin D, Shapiro CC, Shapiro PA et al: Facial characteristics of children who breathe through the mouth. *Pediatrics* 73:622-625, 1984.
7. DenBesten PK, McIver FT: Oral self-mutilation in a child with congenital toxoplasmosis: a clinical report. *Pediatr Dent* 6:98-101, 1984.
8. Friman PC, McPherson KM, Warzak WJ, Evans J: Influence of thumb sucking on peer social acceptance in first-grade children. *Pediatrics* 91:784-786, 1993.
9. Fukata O, Braham RL, Yokoi K, Kurosu K: Damage to the primary dentition resulting from thumb and finger (digit) sucking. *J Dent Child* 63:403-408, 1996.
10. Haryett RD, Hansen FC, Davidson PO: Chronic thumb-sucking: a second report on treatment and its psychological effects. *Am J Orthod Dentofacial Orthop* 57:164-178, 1970.
11. Helle A, Haavikko K: Prevalence of earlier sucking habits revealed by anamnestic data and their consequences for occlusion at the age of eleven. *Proc Finn Dent Soc* 70:191-196, 1974.
12. Kelly JE, Sanchez M, Van Kirk LE: An assessment of the occlusion of teeth of children. National Center for Health Statistics, US Public Health Service, DHEW Publication No. HRA 74-1612, 1973.
13. Kuch EV, Till MJ, Messer LB: Bruxing and non-bruxing children: a comparison of their personality traits. *Pediatr Dent* 1:182-187, 1979.
14. Larsson E: Dummy- and finger-sucking habits with special attention to their significance for facial

growth and occlusion: 4. Effect on facial growth and occlusion. *Swed Dent J* 65:605-634, 1972.

15. Proffit WR, Mason RM: Myofunctional therapy for tongue-thrusting: background and recommendations. *JADA* 90:403-411, 1975.

16. Warren DW, Hairfield WM, Dalston ET: Effect of age on nasal cross-sectional area and respiratory mode in children. *Laryngoscope* 100:89-93, 1990.

17. Warren JJ, Bishara SE: Duration of nutritive and nonnutritive sucking behaviors and their effects on the dental arches in the primary dentition. *Am J Orthod Dentofacial Orthop* 121: 347-356, 2002.

18. Wenzel A, Hojensgaard E, Henriksen JM: Craniofacial morphology and head posture in children with asthma and perennial rhinitis. *Eur J Orthod* 7:83-92, 1985.

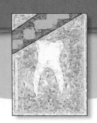

# CHAPTER 27

## Orthodontic Treatment in the Primary Dentition

*John R. Christensen and Henry W. Fields, Jr.*

The goals of orthodontic care in the primary dentition should be either intervention for conditions that predispose one to develop a malocclusion in the permanent dentition or monitoring of conditions that are best treated later.[8] Some conditions can be effectively managed, and the result provides a long-term benefit. With other conditions, treatment should be deferred.

The clinician needs to differentiate skeletal problems from dental problems in order to fulfill these goals. Treatment of skeletal malocclusions in this age group is ordinarily deferred until a later age, not because skeletal change cannot be effected but for more practical reasons. Three general reasons are offered for delaying treatment. First, the diagnosis of skeletal malocclusion is difficult in this age group. Subtle gradations of skeletal problems and immature soft tissue development make clinical diagnosis of all but the most obvious cases difficult. Second, although the child is growing at this stage, the amount of facial growth remaining when the child enters the mixed dentition years is sufficient to aid in the correction of most skeletal malocclusions. Third, any skeletal treatment at this age requires prolonged retention because the initial growth pattern tends to reestablish itself when treatment is discontinued.

On the other hand, several dental problems merit attention during the primary dentition years. This chapter is devoted largely to these issues.

## SKELETAL PROBLEMS

Skeletal problems are addressed only if there is progressive asymmetry as a result of a functional disturbance.[9] The reason for treating these patients early is that treatment at a later time may be more difficult and complex if the child continues to grow asymmetrically and if dental compensation increases. The goal of early treatment is to prevent the asymmetry from becoming worse or to alter growth so that the asymmetry improves. The majority of progressive asymmetry patients are treated first with removable functional appliances that are designed to alter growth by manipulating skeletal and soft tissue relationships and allowing differential eruption of teeth. Orthognathic surgery is a second treatment for progressive asymmetry but is reserved for patients with the most severe asymmetry or those whose condition does not respond to functional appliance therapy. It may be necessary to operate a second time when the child is older because growth often tends to remain asymmetric even after surgical correction. Because diagnosis and treatment of progressive asymmetry are difficult, it is recommended that these cases be referred to a specialist for evaluation and treatment.

Early treatment of patients with dentofacial anomalies is also advocated. Dentofacial anomalies include a number of environmentally and genetically induced conditions that alter the relationship of the facial structures. Examples of such anomalies include cleft lip and palate, hemifacial microsomia, Crouzon's and Apert's syndromes, and mandibulofacial dysostosis (Treacher Collins syndrome). A specialist or specialty team works to minimize the facial disfigurement through early surgical and orthodontic intervention.

## DENTAL PROBLEMS

Selected dental malocclusion in the primary dentition is readily managed by the practitioner who has a knowledge of fixed and removable appliances. The key to successful orthodontic management is careful diagnosis and treatment planning, which depend on the database obtained at the initial examination. In this age group, tooth movement usually is restricted to tipping teeth into the proper position, such as anterior crossbite correction. Rarely are orthodontic appliances designed to move teeth bodily indicated, but posterior crossbite correction is one of those.

Before specific treatment problems are discussed, the biology of tooth movement should be reviewed briefly. A force applied to a tooth causes alterations in the periodontal ligament and surrounding alveolar bone. Recent reviews of bone cell biology show that the osteoblast plays a significant role in tooth movement. Studies have indicated that the osteoblast dictates both the resorptive and formative phases of bone remodeling. In addition, the osteoblast is a receptor for many of the resorptive agents in bone. Prostaglandin production and cyclic adenosine monophosphate elevation are thought to be the primary mediators associated with tooth movement and bone remodeling. These messengers interact with the cell membranes. Change in shape of individual cells through mechanical stress in the biological system may also have a role in initiating metabolic activity.[11]

After the bone remodeling process begins, the tooth starts to move. When the tooth has moved a certain distance, the force exerted by the orthodontic appliance diminishes to an amount below that necessary for tooth movement. During this time, remodeling is completed and the periodontal ligament and alveolar bone cells begin to return to their normal state. This reorganization period is necessary to prevent injury to the tooth and supporting structures. The clinical implication of cellular change, tooth movement, and cellular reorganization is that orthodontic appliances should be reactivated only at 4- to 6-week intervals with a light, continuous force to avoid injury to the periodontium. Therefore, there is some biological basis for the recommendation of monthly visits during orthodontic treatment After tooth movement is complete, the patient enters the retention phase of treatment. Retention is the period of time that the teeth are held in their new position. Retention is necessary because teeth that have been moved orthodontically tend to move back or relapse into their original position after the appliance has been removed. Relapse may be due to many factors; however, gingival changes are a factor. The gingival tissue does not regain its pretreatment shape like bone and periodontal ligament. The gingiva contains a network of gingival fibers that are compressed or stretched during tooth movement. The genes of both collagen and elastin are activated, and tissue collagenase is inhibited. This causes the extracellular matrix of the gingiva to become more elastic and at greater risk for relapse. Surgical treatment such as a gingival fibrotomy has been shown to overcome instability indicating the role of gingival fibers in relapse.[10] If surgical treatment is not performed, long-term retention is indicated to prevent relapse.[5]

## ARCH LENGTH PROBLEMS

The most common arch length problem in the primary dentition is tooth loss. This is managed as outlined in Chapter 25 with space maintenance if the space is adequate. If space has been lost, which can occur in the posterior sextants because of the tooth loss, space regaining can be instituted. A notable situation in which to use space regaining is when the primary first molar is lost prematurely. If the second primary molar is lost, timely placement of the distal shoe is required and space loss will not be evident if it occurs until eruption of the permanent first molar. Thus, the only realistic space regaining in the primary dentition is repositioning of the primary second molar prior to permanent first molar eruption. A removable appliance is best used for this purpose. A primary second molar can be repositioned approximately 1 mm per month using a removable appliance with multiple clasps and a finger spring. Three millimeters of molar movement is a realistic extent of the treatment. This appliance is similar to the appliance used to reposition a permanent first molar.

Although inviting and seemingly intuitive, there is little relationship between the arch length (arch perimeter) in the primary and permanent dentitions.[2] This means that weak correlations do not support early interventions described below. Some have advocated early expansion of the primary arches with either a fixed or a removable appliance. This treatment is provided to ensure space for the permanent teeth.[7] The expansion provides variable increases in arch width and arch perimeter and is associated with little long-term benefit.[6] This early approach to potential crowding remains controversial and unsubstantiated. This type of treatment is especially troublesome when studies have shown that up to 4.5 mm of crowding can be treated in the late mixed

dentition simply with the use of a passive lower lingual arch.[3]

## INCISOR PROTRUSION AND RETRUSION

In addressing the anteroposterior plane of space, the clinician is mainly concerned with the position of the incisors, particularly the maxillary incisors. The majority of anteroposterior problems involve anterior crossbite, a condition in which the maxillary incisors occlude lingual to the mandibular incisors. A fixed lingual arch or a removable appliance can be used to correct the crossbite. Several things should be kept in mind when moving primary anterior teeth. First, the crowns are extremely short incisogingivally. This means that overly aggressive activation of springs will cause them to slip past the lingual surface and not engage the crowns of the teeth. Gentle activation and springs directed gingivally are usually best in these cases. Second, the crowns of some primary first molars converge toward the occlusal surface. This makes banding or clasp retention challenging. Third, there are few or no undercuts on the anterior teeth that will engage a labial bow for retention. For this reason, if a labial bow in the primary dentition is not used for tooth movement, it probably should be discarded. Finally, because the primary teeth will be exfoliated near 6 to 7 years of age, it is probably not wise to consider moving a primary incisor much after 4 years of age.

The lingual arch can be designed in one of two ways. The arch can be activated to tip maxillary teeth into proper position, or auxiliary wires can be soldered onto it to exert the tipping forces. The lingual arch (36-mil wire) is activated approximately 1 mm per visit because it is a heavy-gauge wire that exerts a heavy force. The auxiliary wires can be activated 2 mm, which is the normal amount for a 22-mil wire (Fig. 27-1). Generally, a tooth moves 1 mm per month during treatment. Therefore, if a tooth requires 3 mm of movement to be properly aligned, 3 months of treatment is necessary.

With a removable appliance, wire finger springs are incorporated into the palatal acrylic to move the teeth facially. Placing retentive clasps on the posterior teeth stabilizes the appliance. The finger springs are activated 1.5 to 2.0 mm per month. If the patient exhibits a positive overbite and overjet after treatment, retention is probably not neces-

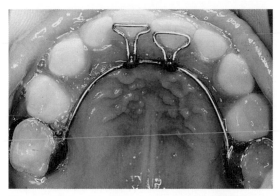

**Figure 27-1**   This patient's anterior crossbite involving the primary maxillary central incisors is being treated with a T spring soldered to a lingual arch. The spring is activated 1 to 2 mm per month until the incisors are tipped out of crossbite.

sary because the occlusion generally holds the tipped incisor in its new position. If there is no overbite, the appliance should be maintained until overbite is established to ensure that relapse does not occur.

One further point should be made about anterior crossbite. In some cases of posterior crossbite or occlusal interference, a child positions the jaw forward (known as a mandibular shift) to achieve maximal intercuspation and an anterior crossbite results (usually called a pseudo class III malocclusion because the patient is not really class III but some other type, often class I). In this situation, the patient only positions the lower jaw forward to obtain comfortable intercuspation as needed to function. This type of anterior crossbite is due to jaw posturing rather than tooth or jaw malposition. In these cases, treatment is directed to the posterior crossbite or the occlusal interference and not to the anterior crossbite. In some cases, the interfering tooth is the one in crossbite.

Excessive overjet in the primary dentition is usually due to a nonnutritive sucking habit or to a skeletal mismatch between the upper and lower jaws. As mentioned previously, because of the tendency for abnormal growth patterns to recur, most skeletal problems should not be treated at this time. However, incisor protrusion as a result of a sucking habit can be addressed. Treatment is usually directed at eliminating the habit rather than at correcting the incisor protrusion if the patient and the parents both want to have the patient stop the habit. Incisor protrusion usually corrects itself or is significantly reduced if the habit is discontinued and if the equilibrium

between the tongue, lips, and perioral musculature is reestablished. The quad helix and palatal crib are discussed in Chapter 26 and are the appliances of choice for habit therapy (see Figs. 26-5 and 26-6). Studies designed to determine how long the appliance must remain in place to terminate the habit effectively suggest a 6-month minimum.[4]

## POSTERIOR CROSSBITE

Posterior crossbite in the primary dentition is usually a result of constriction of the maxillary arch. Constriction often results from an active digit or pacifier habit, although there are many cases in which the origin of the crossbite is undetermined. The first step in managing a posterior crossbite is to establish whether there is an associated mandibular shift. If a mandibular shift is present, treatment should be implemented to correct the crossbite. Some authors have implicated a mandibular shift as the cause of asymmetric growth of the mandible (although few human data exist). The asymmetry is thought to occur because the condyles are positioned differently within each fossa. Muscle and soft tissue stretch exert forces on the underlying skeletal and dental structures that may alter normal growth and arch development. If no shift is detected, the mandible should grow symmetrically.

When there is no shift, treatment is usually delayed until the permanent first molars erupt, unless gross crowding is present. In this situation, expansion of the arch should result in more room for the primary and permanent teeth. If the permanent molars erupt into crossbite, treatment can be initiated if no other malocclusion exists. When the permanent molars erupt normally and there is no mandibular shift, treatment may not be indicated for the crossbite of the primary molars until the premolars erupt. Correction of the crossbite in the primary molar region during the period of mixed dentition increases the chance that the premolars will not erupt in crossbite.[12]

There are three basic approaches to the management of posterior crossbite in children: (1) equilibration to eliminate mandibular shift, (2) expansion of the constricted maxillary arch, and (3) repositioning of specific teeth to correct intraarch alignment. In a few cases, the mandibular shift is due to interference caused by the primary canines. These cases can be diagnosed by repositioning the mandible and noting the interference. Selective removal of enamel with a diamond bur in both arches eliminates the interference and the lateral shift into crossbite.

In cases of bilateral maxillary constriction, expansion is needed to correct the crossbite and sometimes the lateral shift. This situation should be managed as soon as it is diagnosed unless the permanent first molar is expected to erupt within 6 months. In this situation, it is better to allow the permanent molars to erupt and to incorporate these teeth into treatment if necessary. Both fixed and removable appliances can be designed to correct maxillary constriction, although fixed appliances are reliable and require little patient cooperation.

Fixed appliances are variations of a lingual arch bent into the shape of a "W." In fact, one of the most popular appliances used to treat crossbites is named the "W arch" (Fig. 27-2). Another popular appliance is the quad helix (see Fig. 26-5). The W arch is constructed of 36-mil wire that rests 1.0 to 1.5 mm off the palate to prevent soft tissue irritation. The W arch is expanded approximately 4 mm wider than its passive width or so that one arm of the "W" is resting over the central grooves of the teeth when the other arm is in the proper position. To move teeth preferentially in the anterior region of the mouth, the appliance is activated by bending the palatal portion of the arm near the solder joint, as demonstrated in Figure 27-3. If more correction is needed in the molar region, the appliance is activated via bending of the anterior palatal por-

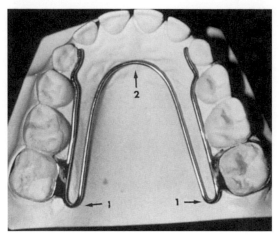

**Figure 27-3**  The preferred way to move teeth in the anterior region of the mouth is to activate the W arch by bending the arm of the "W" in the area marked location 1. If the clinician wants to obtain more movement in the molar region, he or she can activate the appliance by bending the anterior portion of the "W" in the area marked location 2.

tion. The appliance expands the arch approximately 1 mm per side per month.

The patient should return monthly to allow the dentist to check the progress of treatment and to reactivate the W arch if needed. The appliance can be activated intraorally, although the force and direction of activation may be difficult to approximate and unwanted tooth movement can result. Usually it is easier and more accurate to remove, activate, and recement the appliance. Expansion should continue until the crossbite is slightly overcorrected and the lingual cusps of the maxillary teeth occlude on the lingual inclines of the buccal cusps of the mandibular teeth. Most crossbites are corrected in 3 months, and the teeth are retained for an additional 3 months.

The quad helix is designed much like the W arch but incorporates more wire into the appliance, making it more flexible. It is constructed of 38-mil wire with two helices in the anterior palate and two helices near the solder joint in the posterior palate. The helices are wound away from the palate and can serve to remind the digit-sucking patient to refrain from the habit if they are positioned correctly where the patient places the finger or thumb. Therefore, this is the preferred appliance for a patient with a finger habit and posterior crossbite. Because the quad helix has more wire than the W arch, it has a greater range of action and can be activated farther than the W arch while delivering an equivalent amount

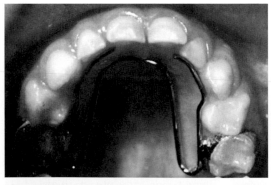

**Figure 27-2**  The W arch is a fixed appliance used to correct posterior crossbites in the primary dentition. The appliance is activated 3 to 4 mm beyond its passive width or to such an extent that one arm of the W extends over the central grooves of the teeth when the other arm is in the proper position.

of force. Overcorrection and retention are required for the quad helix as well.

Despite activation of the W arch or quad helix on one side only, teeth on both sides of the arch react to equivalent force. In other words, the teeth should all move the same distance. This is desirable when there is bilateral maxillary constriction. If, however, the crossbite is due to a true unilateral maxillary constriction, it would be more appropriate to move only the teeth at fault. One way to accomplish this with a fixed appliance is to construct an unequal W arch or quad helix that has long and short arms (Fig. 27-4). The short arm touches only the teeth that have to be moved, and the long arm touches as many contralateral teeth as possible. The idea behind the unequal W arch is to pit movement of a large number of teeth against movement of a small number of teeth. The side with the smaller number of teeth tends to have more movement than the side with the larger number, although there will be expansion on both sides of the arch. An alternative method of unilateral treatment is to place a mandibular lingual arch to stabilize the lower arch and attach cross-elastics to the constricted maxillary teeth. This results in true unilateral movement of the maxillary teeth. This alternative requires more cooperation from the patient and is technically

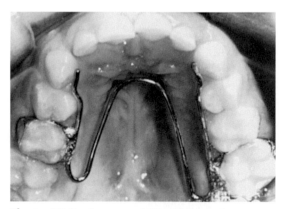

**Figure 27-4** An unequal W arch is used to treat a true unilateral crossbite in the primary dentition. The short arm is placed on the constricted side of the arch against the teeth that are to be moved out of the crossbite. The long arm of the arch is placed on the opposite side of the arch, resting against as many teeth as possible to resist tooth movement on that side. In theory, the constricted side of the arch will move more than the opposite side. (From Fields HW, Proffit WR: Orthodontics in general practice. In: Morris AL, Bohannan HM, Casullo DP, editors. *The Dental Specialists in General Practice*. Philadelphia, Saunders, 1983, p 315.)

more difficult. These types of fixed lingual arch type appliances have been shown to produce both skeletal and dental changes in the primary and mixed dentitions.[1]

### Case Study

M.C., a 6-year-old white boy, presented to the dental office for a 6-month dental examination. His mother reported that he still sucked his thumb every night while falling asleep but had stopped sucking during the day. A dental examination revealed a bilateral maxillary constriction in centric relation with a mandibular shift into a left posterior crossbite in centric occlusion. The overjet was 5 mm, and there was a 2-mm open bite in the left central incisor region (Fig. 27-5, *A*).

M.C.'s parents had instituted reminder therapy and a reward system after the last 6-month dental examination. A bandage was placed on his thumb, and M.C. was asked to place stars on a calendar on days when he did not suck. The combination of reminder therapy and reward system was effective enough to help M.C. eliminate the sucking habit during the daytime hours.

A treatment plan was offered to M.C. and his parents to correct the maxillary constriction and stop the bedtime habit. The plan called for a fixed quad helix appliance. The quad helix would be activated monthly to correct the crossbite and then made passive to serve as a retainer. The helices in the appliance would serve as a physical reminder not to suck the thumb.

After three activations over a 3-month period, the crossbite was overcorrected. The appliance was made passive and recemented. The quad helix now served as a retainer. Both M.C. and his parents reported that the habit was extinguished (Fig. 27-5, *B*). On M.C.'s subsequent 6-month examination, the crossbite correction was found to be stable and the habit had not returned (Fig. 27-5, *C*).

### OPEN BITE

Vertical problems in the primary dentition usually are due to a finger or pacifier habit and result in an anterior open bite. Treatment for an anterior open bite that is due to a sucking habit is discussed in Chapter 26. Deep bite in the primary dentition is generally not corrected at this time. The depth of bite usually improves with the erup-

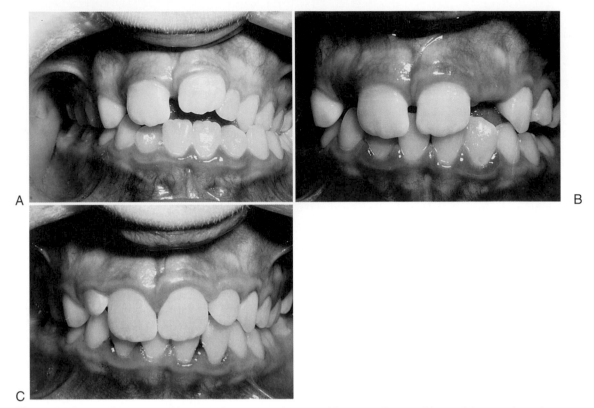

**Figure 27-5    A,** This 6-year-old patient has an anterior open bite, posterior crossbite, and increased overjet as a result of a thumb sucking habit that is still present. **B,** A quad helix appliance was used to correct the posterior crossbite and extinguish the thumb sucking habit. Note the overcorrection of the patient's left buccal segment. **C,** At the subsequent recall examination, the posterior crossbite correction is stable, reasonable occlusion has been established, and the habit has not returned.

tion of the permanent first molars if the problem is the result of dental malocclusion.

## REFERENCES

1. Bell R, LeCompte E: The effects of maxillary expansion using a quad helix appliance during the deciduous and mixed detentions. *Am J Orthod Dentofacial Orthop* 79:152-161, 1981.
2. Bishara SE, Khadivi P, Jakobsen JR: Changes in tooth size–arch length relationships from the deciduous to the permanent dentition: a longitudinal study. *Am J Orthod Dentofacial Orthop* 108:607-613, 1995.
3. Gianelly AA. Treatment of crowding in the mixed dentition. *Am J Orthod Dentofacial Orthop* 121:569-571, 2002.
4. Haryett RD, Hansen FC, Davidson PO: Chronic thumbsucking: a second report on treatment and its psychological effects. *Am J Orthod Dentofacial Orthop* 57:164-178, 1970.
5. Lang G, Alfter G, Goz G, Lang GH: Retention and stability: taking various treatment parameters into account. *J Orofacial Orthop* 63:26-41, 2002.
6. Lutz HD, Poulton D: Stability of dental arch expansion in the deciduous dentition. *Angle Orthod* 55:299-315, 1985.
7. McInaney JB, Adams RM, Freeman M: A nonextraction approach to crowded dentitions in young children: early recognition and treatment. *JADA* 101:251-257, 1980.
8. Ngan P, Fields HW: Orthodontic diagnosis and treatment planning in the primary dentition. *J Dent Child* 62:25-33, 1995.
9. Proffit WR, Fields HW: Treatment of moderate nonskeletal problems in preadolescent children. *Contemporary Orthodontics*, 3rd ed. St Louis, Mosby, 1999, Chapter 13.
10. Redlich M, Shoshan S, Palmon A: Gingival response to orthodontic force. *Am J Orthod Dentofacial Orthop* 116:152-157, 1999.
11. Sandy J, Farndale R, Meikle M: Recent advances in understanding mechanically induced bone remodeling and their relevance to orthodontic theory and practice. *Am J Orthod Dentofacial Orthop* 103:212-222, 1993.
12. Thilander B, Wahlund S, Lennartsson B: The effect of early interceptive treatment in children with posterior crossbite. *Eur J Orthod* 6:25-34, 1984.

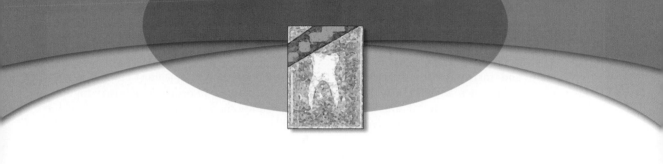

# CHAPTER 28

# Local Anesthesia and Oral Surgery in Children

*Stephen Wilson and R. Denny Montgomery*

Successful treatment of patients, especially pediatric patients, in terms of allaying their anxiety and discomfort during restorative and surgical procedures is facilitated by profound local anesthesia.

Good operator technique in obtaining local anesthesia in pediatric patients is essential and requires mastery of the following areas: (1) child growth and development (physical and mental); (2) behavior management; (3) physiologic pain modulation; and (4) pharmacology of local anesthetics.

Oral surgery procedures in children are similar to and possibly easier than those in adults. There are some important differences as well. This chapter presents an overview of the principles of local anesthesia and oral surgery in children.

## LOCAL ANESTHESIA IN CHILDREN

### Topical Anesthesia

Topical anesthesia is used to obtund the discomfort associated with the insertion of the needle into the mucosal membrane. The usefulness of topical anesthesia has been debated. For instance, the taste of the anesthetic, the period during which the patient anticipates the needle, and the establishment of a conditioned patient response from the needle immediately following the application of topical anesthetic have been considered to be detrimental factors. However, the operator's effectiveness in interacting with children to distract them and increase their suggestibility about managing their own anxieties may supersede the disadvantages of topical anesthesia. Therefore, we recommend the use of a benzocaine topical anesthetic that is good tasting and that is available in an easy-to-control gel. The best results behaviorally and physiologically is to use the gel sparingly and apply to a very dry mucosal surface for at least 2 minutes.

A small amount of topical anesthetic should be applied with a cotton-tipped applicator to a mucosa that has been adequately dried and isolated with a $2 \times 2$ inch cotton gauze pad (Fig. 28-1). The time required for the topical anesthetic to reach its full effectiveness may vary from 30 seconds to 5 minutes. Although a toxic response to topical anesthesia is rare, excessive amounts should be avoided.

A relatively new delivery system involving "lidocaine patches" (small flat applicators similar in shape to a miniature adhesive strip impregnated with a relatively high concentration of lidocaine) has been available in recent years. An example of this type of patch is DentiPatch (Noven Pharmaceuticals, Miami, Fla.), which

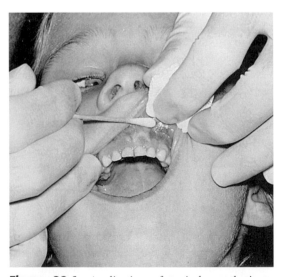

**Figure 28-1** Application of topical anesthetic to vestibular tissues for buccal infiltration of incisors. Note a minimal amount of anesthetic on the cotton-tipped applicator. *Technique:* 1. Reflect tissue to expose injection site. 2. Dry soft tissue with $2 \times 2$ gauze pad. 3. Apply topical gel with cotton-tipped applicator. 4. Maintain applicator on tissue site for at least 30 seconds (see manufacturer's recommendations). 5. Remove applicator and proceed with injection.

contains 46.1 mg of lidocaine. The patches are especially effective in pediatric dentistry for analgesic conditioning of the surface mucosa of the maxillary anterior segment of the mouth or the hard palate prior to local anesthetic infiltration; however, it is extremely important that the patch be used according to the manufacturer's instruction for maximal benefit (i.e., placement of the patch for a minimum of 10 minutes on a very dry mucosa prior to needle insertion).

## General Considerations for Local Anesthesia

The mechanism of action of local anesthetics has been further elucidated in recent years. The evidence supports the notion that through attachment and subsequent configurable changes of sodium receptors of neural members, local anesthetics block sodium channels. The net result is inhibition of neuronal excitability, which reduces the likelihood of action potential transmission. Therefore, local anesthetics alter the reactivity of neural membranes to propagated action potentials that may be generated in tissues distal to the anesthetic block. Action potentials that enter an area of adequately anesthetized nervous tissue are blocked and fail to transmit information to the central nervous system (CNS).[3]

The efficacy of local anesthesia depends on the concentration of the anesthetic on a segment of the nerve. Beyond a fixed amount of local anesthetic necessary for blockage of neuronal impulses, any excess is wasteful and potentially dangerous. Failure to obtain anesthesia is most likely due either to operator error in depositing the solution sufficiently close to the nerve or to anatomic aberrations (e.g., accessory innervation).

Local infection and inflammation can modify the normal local physiology of tissue by causing the release of neuroactive substances (e.g., histamine, leukotrienes, kinins, and prostaglandins) and by lowering the pH. These changes reduce the lipid solubility of the anesthetic and interfere with its ability to penetrate the nervous tissue. Blocking the nerve at a more proximal site distant from the infected area may be a viable alternative. This may include the deposition of local anesthesia in intraligamental or intrapulpal sites. Antibiotic administration may reduce the extent of infection and permit definitive treatment under local anesthesia that would otherwise be impossible.

Local anesthesia may be obtained anatomically by one of three means:

1. *The nerve block,* which is the placement of anesthetic on or near a main nerve trunk. This results in a wide area of tissue anesthesia.
2. *The field block,* which is the placement of anesthetic on secondary branches of a main nerve.
3. *Local infiltration,* which is the deposition of the anesthetic on terminal branches of a nerve. Adequate diffusion of local anesthetic from local infiltration readily occurs in children because their bones are less dense than those of adults.

Local anesthetics used in dentistry are classified as esters or amides. Amides are used more frequently because of their reduced allergenic characteristics and greater potency at lower concentrations. The concentration of the different agents varies, and care must be taken to prevent overdose (Table 28-1). As an example, two full cartridges (carpules) of 2% lidocaine (Xylocaine) without vasoconstrictor may be easily tolerated by an adult, but the same amount exceeds the maximal allowable dosage (2 mg/lb body weight) for a 20-pound child.

Local anesthetic carpules (1.8 ml) also contain preservatives, organic salts, and sometimes vasoconstrictors. The preservatives (e.g., methylparaben) may be a source of allergic reactions. Concern about rubber products in local anesthetic cartridges as a source of allergic reactions has not been supported by any studies or case reports.[14] The vasoconstrictors (e.g., epinephrine) are used to constrict blood vessels, counteract the vasodilatory effects of the local anesthetic, and prolong the duration of the anesthetic.

## Operator Technique

Communication in language the child can understand is necessary in a pediatric dentistry practice. The dentist may have to modify his or her wording to accommodate the level of the child's understanding when discussing the injection. For instance, the child may be told that the tooth will be "going to sleep" after a "little pinch" is felt

### TABLE 28-1
#### Maximum Recommended Doses of Local Anesthetics for Children

| DRUG | MAXIMUM DOSE (MG/KG) | MILLIGRAMS/CARTRIDGE* |
|------|----------------------|------------------------|
| Lidocaine (2%) w/wo epinephrine | 4.4 (300 mg max) | 36.4 |
| Mepivacaine (2%) w/wo levonordefrin | 4.4 (300 mg max) | 36.4 |

| PATIENT WEIGHT (KG/LB)[†] | MAXIMUM DOSAGE | |
| | MILLIGRAMS | NO. OF CARTRIDGES |
|---------------------------|------------|--------------------|
| 10/23 | 44 | 1.2 |
| 15/34.5 | 66 | 1.8 |
| 20/46 | 88 | 2.4 |
| 25/57.5 | 100 | 2.7 |
| 30/69 | 132 | 3.6 |
| 40/92 | 176 | 4.8 |
| 50/115 | 220 | 6.1 |
| 60/138 | 264 | 7.3 |
| 70/161 | 300 | 8.3 |

Data from Malamed SF: *Handbook of Local Anesthesia,* ed 5, St Louis, 2004, Mosby.
*2% = 20 mg/ml × 1.8 ml/cartridge = 36.
[†]1 kg = 2.3 lbs.

near his tooth. The dentist should not deny that the injection might hurt because this denial may cause the child to lose trust in the dentist and confidence about the procedure. The dentist should minimize but not reinforce the child's anxieties and fears about the "pinch."

The discomfort of the injection may be lessened by counterirritation, distraction, and a slow rate of administration. Counterirritation is the application of vibratory stimuli (e.g., rapid displacement of loose alveolar tissue) or of moderate pressure (e.g., with a cotton-tipped applicator) to the area adjacent to the site of injection. These stimuli have a physical and psychological basis for modifying noxious input. Distraction can be accomplished by continuing a constant monologue with the child and by maintaining his or her attention away from the syringe. The operator should always aspirate and alter the depth of the needle if necessary prior to slowly injecting the anesthetic. The deposition of a single Carpule should take at least 1 minute. Rapid injections tend to be more painful because of rapid tissue expansion. They also potentiate the possibility of a toxic reaction if the solution is inadvertently deposited in a blood vessel.

The role of the dental assistant is important during transfer of the syringe and in anticipation of patient movement. During the transfer of the syringe from the assistant to the dentist, the child's eyes tend to follow the dentist's. The eyes of the dentist should be focused on the face of the patient (Fig. 28-2). The hand of the dentist that is to receive the syringe is extended close to the head or body of the child. The body of the syringe is placed between the index and middle finger, with the ring of the plunger slipped over the dentist's thumb by the assistant. The plastic sheath protecting the needle is then removed by the assistant. The dentist's peripheral vision guides the syringe to the mouth in a slow, smooth movement.

Reflexive movements of the child's head and body should be anticipated.[13] The head can be stabilized by being held firmly but gently between the body and arm or hand of the dentist. The assistant passively extends his or her arm across the child's chest so that potential arm and body movements can be intercepted. The area of soft tissue that is to receive the injection is reflected by the free hand of the dentist. The hand can also be used to block the vision of the child as the syringe approaches the mouth. Once tissue penetration by the needle has occurred, the needle should not be retracted in response to the child's reactions. Otherwise, the child's behavior may deteriorate significantly if he or she anticipates reinjection. Use of finger rests is strongly advocated.

A short (20 mm) or long (32 mm), 27- or 30-gauge needle may be used for most intraoral injections in children, including mandibular blocks. There apparently is little difference in discomfort level between the 25-gauge and 30-gauge needles for inferior alveolar injections; thus, the 27-gauge needle would seem less likely to break or bend during injections and is preferred.[5] An extrashort (10 mm), 30-gauge needle is appropriate for maxillary anterior injections.

Because of the concern for inadvertent needle sticks, retractable needle delivery systems are becoming popular and in some cases required in hospital settings. Injection delivery systems now have needles covered by a needle sheath and a retractable cover preventing needle sticks associated with resheathing needles after injection.

## Maxillary Primary and Permanent Molar Anesthesia

The innervation of maxillary primary and permanent molars arises from the posterior superior alveolar nerve (permanent molars) and middle superior alveolar nerve (mesiobuccal root of the first permanent molar, primary molars, and premolars).

In anesthetizing the maxillary primary molars or permanent premolars, the needle should penetrate the mucobuccal fold and be inserted to a depth that approximates that of the apices of the buccal roots of the teeth (Fig. 28-3). The solution should be deposited adjacent to the bone. The

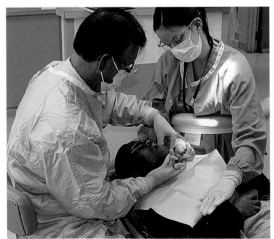

**Figure 28-2** Preparing for the injection. Note the hand positions of the dentist and assistant to stabilize the child's head and body during the injection.

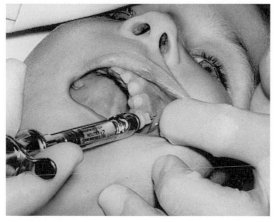

**Figure 28-3** Buccal infiltration for anesthetizing maxillary primary molars. *Technique:* 1. Reflect tissue to expose injection site. 2. Orient bevel of needle to be parallel to the bone. 3. Insert needle in mucobuccal fold. 4. Proceed to depth that approximates the apices of the buccal roots of the molar(s). 5. The bevel of the needle should be adjacent to the periosteum of the bone. Aspirate. 6. Deposit the bolus of anesthetic slowly. 7. Remove needle and apply pressure with 2 × 2 gauze for 1 minute to obtain hemostasis.

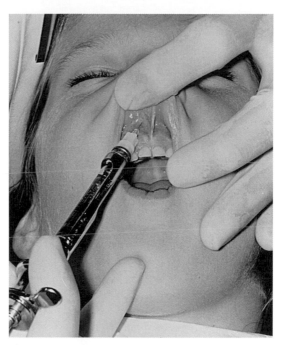

**Figure 28-4** Labial infiltration of maxillary incisor area. *Technique for maxillary primary and permanent incisors and canines:* 1. Reflect tissue to expose injection site. 2. Orient bevel of needle to be parallel to the bone. 3. Insert needle in mucobuccal fold. 4. Proceed to depth approximating that of root apices. This depth is less in the primary dentition than in the permanent dentition. 5. The bevel of the needle should be adjacent to the periosteum of the bone. Aspirate. 6. Inject the bolus of anesthetic very slowly. 6. Remove needle and apply pressure to area with 2 × 2 gauze for hemostasis.

maxillary permanent molars may be anesthetized with a posterior superior alveolar nerve block or by local infiltration.

## Maxillary Primary and Permanent Incisor and Canine Anesthesia

The innervation of maxillary primary and permanent incisors and canines is by the anterosuperior alveolar branch of the maxillary nerve. Labial infiltration commonly is used to anesthetize the primary anterior teeth. The needle is inserted in the mucobuccal fold to a depth that approximates that of the apices of the buccal roots of the teeth (Fig. 28-4). Rapid deposition of the solution in this area is contraindicated because it produces discomfort during rapid expansion of the tissue. The innervation of the anterior teeth may arise from the opposite side of the midline. Thus, it may be necessary to deposit some solution adjacent to the apex of the contralateral central incisor.

Infraorbital block injection is an excellent technique that may be used in place of local infiltration of the anterior teeth. All ipsilateral anterior maxillary teeth are anesthetized by this block. The needle is inserted anywhere in the mucobuccal fold from the lateral incisor to the first primary molar and is advanced next to bone to a depth that approximates the infraorbital foramen. The foramen is readily palpated as a notch on the infraorbital rim of the bony orbit. The solution is deposited slowly.

## Palatal Tissue Anesthesia

The tissues of the hard palate are innervated by the anterior palatine and nasal palatine nerves. Surgical procedures involving palatal tissues usually require a nasal palatine nerve block (Fig. 28-5) or anterior palatine anesthesia (Fig. 28-6). These nerve blocks are painful, and care should be taken to prepare the child adequately. These injections are not usually required for normal restorative procedures. However, if it is anticipated that the rubber dam clamp will impinge on the palatal tissue, a drop of anesthetic solution should be deposited into the marginal tissue adjacent to the lingual aspect of the tooth. Blanching of the tissue will be observed.

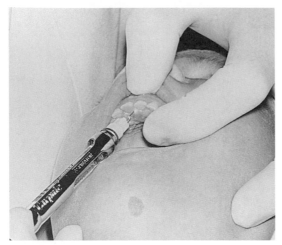

**Figure 28-5** Nasal palatine block. The needle is inserted to the left or right side of the papilla. Note the blanching of tissue at the injection site.

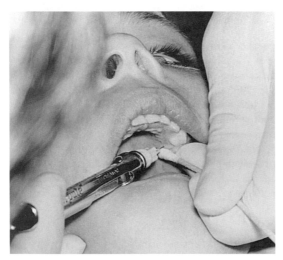

**Figure 28-6** Palatal infiltration of primary molars anesthetizing the anterior palatine nerve. The cotton-tipped applicator is held firmly against the palatal tissue. The needle is inserted in the area between the applicator and tooth. The applicator may provide a masking or distracting effect. *Technique:* 1. Apply pressure with cotton-tipped applicator to site that is to receive the needle. 2. Insert needle with bevel oriented parallel to the bone immediately adjacent to the applicator. 3. Proceed to depth at which the bevel of the needle is adjacent to the periosteum and aspirate. 4. Inject the bolus of anesthetic very slowly. 5. Remove needle and apply pressure to area with 2 × 2 gauze for hemostasis.

## Mandibular Tooth Anesthesia

The inferior alveolar nerve innervates the mandibular primary and permanent teeth. This nerve enters the mandibular foramen on the lingual aspect of the mandible. The position of the

foramen changes by remodeling more superiorly from the occlusal plane as the child matures into adulthood. The foramen is at or slightly above the occlusal plane during the period of the primary dentition.[2] In adults, it averages 7 mm above the occlusal plane. The foramen is approximately midway between the anterior and posterior borders of the ramus of the mandible.

For the inferior alveolar nerve block, the child is requested to open his or her mouth as far as possible. Mouth props may aid in maintaining this position for the child. The ball of the thumb is positioned on the coronoid notch of the anterior border of the ramus, and the fingers are placed on the posterior border of the ramus. The needle is inserted between the internal oblique ridge and the pterygomandibular raphe (Fig. 28-7). The barrel of the syringe overlies the two primary mandibular molars on the opposite side of the arch and parallels the occlusal plane. The needle is advanced until it contacts bone, aspiration is completed, and the solution is slowly deposited.

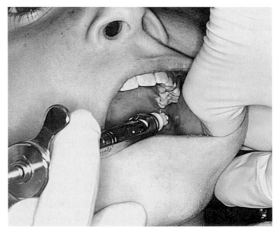

**Figure 28-7** Inferior alveolar block. *Technique:* 1. With patient's mouth opened as wide as possible, place the ball of the thumb on the coronoid notch on the anterior border of the mandible. 2. Position the index and middle fingers on the external posterior border of the mandible. 3. Insert the needle with bevel oriented parallel to the bone and at the level of the occlusal plane between the internal oblique ridge and the pterygomandibular raphe. The barrel of the syringe will be exiting the mouth adjacent to the lip commissure contralateral to the side that is to be anesthetized. 4. Insert the needle to a depth that is adjacent to the bone. Aspirate. 5. Slowly inject the bolus of anesthetic. 6. Remove the needle and apply pressure to area with 2 × 2 gauze for hemostasis.

Occasionally, the inferior alveolar nerve block is not successful. A second try may be attempted; however, the needle should be inserted at a level higher than that of the first injection. Care must be taken to prevent an overdose of anesthetic (see Table 28-1).

The long buccal nerve supplies the molar buccal gingivae and may provide accessory innervation to the teeth. It should be anesthetized along with the inferior alveolar block. A small quantity of solution is deposited in the mucobuccal fold at a point distal and buccal to the most posterior molar (Fig. 28-8).

Some operators advocate the use of a periodontal ligament injection for anesthetizing singular teeth.[10] An advantage of this method is that soft tissue is not anesthetized, which may prevent inadvertent tissue damage resulting from chewing after dental procedures. However, there is some evidence that this type of injection may produce areas of hypoplasia or decalcification on succedaneous teeth.[4]

## Complications of Local Anesthesia

The complications of local anesthesia may include local and systemic effects.[11] Local complications may include masticatory trauma (Fig. 28-9),

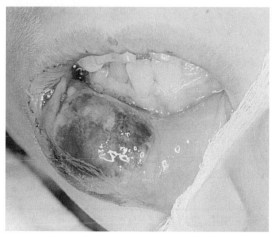

**Figure 28-9** Masticatory trauma to lower lip that has been anesthetized with an inferior alveolar block.

hematomas, infections, nerve damage by the needle, trismus, and, rarely, needle breakage in the soft tissue. These types of complications may be minimized by aspirating, decreasing needle deflection, and warning the parent and child that the soft tissue will be anesthetized for a period of up to 1 to 2 hours after the restorative procedure.

Systemic complications include allergic reactions and cardiovascular and CNS dysfunctions. The CNS responses to local anesthetics are complex and depend on plasma concentrations. These responses range from dizziness, blurred vision, and anxiety to tremors, convulsions, CNS depression, and death.[8] The primary effect of local anesthetics on the heart is that of myocardial depression.

Management of overdoses varies, depending on the presenting symptoms and signs. Mild reactions require little more than patient reassurance and, if necessary, termination of the planned treatment. Severe reactions require oxygen supplementation, ventilatory support, and possible hospitalization.

## Alternative Anesthesia Systems

In recent years, alternative delivery systems of dental anesthesia have been available including a computer-controlled system called the Wand (Milestone Scientific, Livingston, N.J.). The advantage of the Wand is the thin, wand-like syringe that appears similar to and is held like a pen. A foot control delivers the anesthetic at a relatively slow rate and constant pressure by a microprocessor-controlled regulator. Some evi-

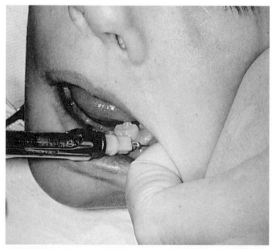

**Figure 28-8** Long buccal nerve block. *Technique:* 1. Reflect tissue to expose site of injection. 2. Insert needle in the mucobuccal fold at a point distal and buccal to the most posterior molar. The bevel of the needle should be oriented parallel to the bone. 3. Insert needle to a depth that is adjacent to the bone. Aspirate. 4. Slowly inject the bolus of anesthetic. 5. Remove the needle and apply pressure to the area with 2 × 2 gauze for hemostasis.

dence suggests this system may appear less threatening to a young child.[1]

Another system used primarily for topical anesthesia associated with injections or for minor gingival procedures is electronic dental anesthesia. Electronic dental anesthesia is based primarily on the concept of hyperpolarization of excitable tissue; however, it has not been well accepted in pediatric dentistry despite evidence that children may prefer electronic dental anesthesia to traditionally delivered local anesthesia.[15]

# ORAL SURGERY IN CHILDREN

In many ways, oral surgical procedures for children are similar to and possibly easier than those performed for adults. There are some important differences as well. The purpose of this section is to present basic techniques and surgical principles needed to perform oral surgical procedures safely and competently on children and adolescents. This section discusses the extraction of teeth, minor soft tissue procedures (i.e., biopsies and frenectomies), odontogenic infections, and the recognition and initial management of facial injuries and fractures.

## Preoperative Evaluation

The dentist treating the child patient must be careful to consider the entire patient and not focus only on the oral cavity. Important considerations in caring for the child patient include the following:

1. Obtaining a good medical history
2. Obtaining appropriate medical and dental consultations
3. Anticipating and preventing emergency situations
4. Being fully capable of managing emergency situations when they occur

In addition to the medical preoperative evaluation, it is important to perform a thorough dental preoperative evaluation, which includes taking appropriate preoperative radiographs. These often include two or more periapical radiographs of the same area in order to determine buccal, lingual, facial, or palatal relationships of impacted teeth. Another preoperative consideration is the future need for space main-

tenance as a result of the premature loss of primary teeth. Failure to provide immediate space maintenance may allow for the mesial migration of permanent first molars after premature primary molar loss.

## Tooth Extractions

### Armamentarium

Many dentists choose to use the same surgical instruments for child patients as they routinely use for adult patients. However, most pediatric dentists and oral and maxillofacial surgeons prefer the smaller pediatric extraction forceps, such as the no. 150S and 151S (Fig. 28-10), for the following reasons:

1. Their reduced size more easily allows placement in the smaller oral cavity of the child patient.
2. The smaller pediatric forceps are more easily concealed by the operator's hand.
3. The smaller working ends (beaks) more closely adapt to the anatomy of the primary teeth.

The choice of the proper instrumentation can also depend on special considerations unique to

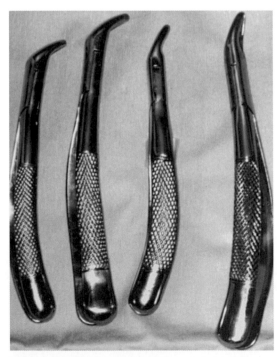

**Figure 28-10**  Extraction forceps: left to right, no. 151S, no. 151, no. 150S, no. 150.

the child and the adolescent. The use of cow horn mandibular forceps is contraindicated for primary teeth, owing to the potential for injury to the developing premolars. Great care must also be given to the routine use of elevators and forceps adjacent to large restorations such as chrome crowns and especially restorations adjacent to erupting single-rooted teeth that may easily become dislodged with the slightest force.

### General Considerations

The manual technique used to perform extractions in the child patient is similar to the manual extraction technique used in the adult. The greatest difference is in patient management. It is essential that the dentist take the time to describe the ensuing procedure completely and accurately to the child. The extraction appointment should always begin with proper topical and local anesthesia, with consideration given to oral, intravenous, or nitrous oxide sedation on an individual basis (see Chapter 8). A few children require general anesthesia for the surgical procedure. The choice of proper local anesthesia/sedation/general anesthesia technique depends on the psychological constitution of the child and the extent and nature of the surgical procedure. The appropriate local anesthetic technique for each type of tooth is described earlier in this chapter.

Several steps of the extraction procedure should be performed with every extraction. The dentist should consult with the child and the parents prior to surgery in order to prepare them for the upcoming procedure. The dentist should provide any preoperative needs, such as prescriptions or any dietary restrictions that might be necessary as a result of the planned sedative techniques. The entire surgical procedure and the expected postoperative recovery course should also be described. This allows the parents to make special postoperative arrangements, such as the need for a soft diet or child care support. As noted before, the dentist should perform a thorough review of the patient's medical history, with special emphasis on medical conditions that might complicate treatment.

There is no other type of dental treatment in which the principles of tell-show-do are more important than during extractions. The dentist should be sure to obtain profound anesthesia because once the patient has felt pain, it may be difficult to regain the child's confidence to a level

in which he or she will behave in a manner that allows completion of the procedure.

Just prior to the actual extraction, the dentist should place the balls of the index finger and thumb in the area of the extraction and demonstrate to the child the types of pressures and movements that he or she will encounter during the extraction. This digital pressure should be firm enough to rock the child's head from side to side in the headrest.

Several factors make it possible for the child patient to aspirate or swallow foreign objects during dental treatment. These factors include (1) the common practice of treating the child patient in a reclining position, (2) poor visibility as a result of the smaller opening into the oral cavity and the proportionately larger tongue of the child, and (3) the increased likelihood of unexpected movements by the child patient. To prevent this from happening, the patient should be positioned in the chair so that the upper jaw is at no more than a 45-degree angle with the floor (Fig. 28-11). If an angle greater than 45 degrees is preferred by the operator, consideration should be given to either placing a light gauze pack in the

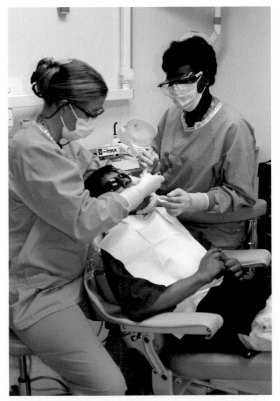

**Figure 28-11** To help prevent aspiration of extracted teeth, the child is positioned so that the upper jaw is at a 45-degree angle to the floor.

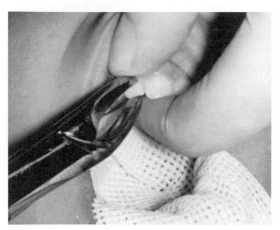

**Figure 28-12**   A gauze screen in the oral cavity helps prevent aspiration of extracted teeth.

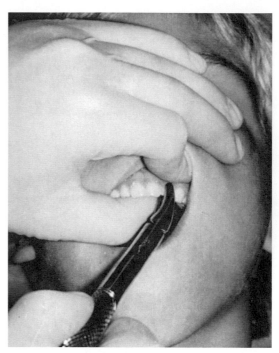

**Figure 28-13**   The dentist's nondominant hand helps control the child's head, supports the jaw being treated, retracts adjacent soft tissues, and palpates the alveolar process and adjacent teeth during extraction.

posterior oral cavity (Fig. 28-12) or performing the extraction with the use of a rubber dam.

The dentist should be placed in the position in which he or she can easily control the instrumentation, have good visual access to the surgical site, and control the child's head. The nondominant hand of the dentist in then placed in the patient's mouth. The role of the nondominant hand is to help control the patient's head; to support the jaw being treated; to help retract the cheek, lips, and tongue from the surgical field; and to palpate the alveolar process and adjacent teeth during the extraction (Fig. 28-13).

Once the proper operator and nondominant hand positions are established, the actual extraction technique may begin. Variations in technique for individual teeth are discussed later in this chapter, but the following general principles apply to all extractions.[9] An instrument such as a dental curette or periosteal elevator is used to separate the epithelial attachment of the tooth to be extracted (Fig. 28-14). Then appropriate elevators may be used to luxate the tooth to be extracted, but great care must be used not to damage adjacent or underlying teeth. The appropriate forceps are then placed on the tooth to be extracted, usually seating the lingual or palatal beak first and then rotating the facial beak into proper position. During the entire extraction technique, firm apical pressure should be placed on the forceps. The extraction is then performed via the proper forceps technique.

After the tooth is removed from its socket, the surgical site is evaluated visually and with the use of a curette. The curette should be used as an extension of the dentist's finger to palpate and

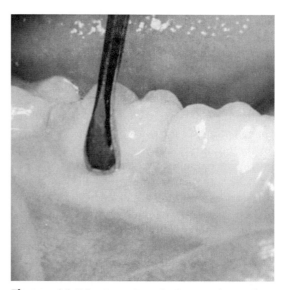

**Figure 28-14**   A periosteal elevator is used to separate the epithelial attachment of the tooth prior to extraction.

evaluate the extraction site. No attempt should be made to scrape the extraction site. If a pathologic lesion such as a cyst or periapical granuloma is present at the apex of a permanent tooth socket, it should be gently enucleated. Aggressive manipulation of a curette in a primary tooth socket is contraindicated owing to the potential for damage to the succeeding tooth bud. The operator should palpate both the facial and palatal or buccal and lingual aspects of the surgical site to feel for any bone irregularities or alveolar expansion. Any bone sharpness should be conservatively removed with the use of either a rongeur or a bone file. Digital pressure should be sufficient to return the alveolus to its presurgical configuration if gross expansion has occurred.

The extraction site should now be evaluated for the need for sutures, although they are rarely indicated after extraction of primary teeth. The first postoperative concern is that of obtaining initial hemostasis by way of an intraoral gauze pack. In the anesthetized, deeply sedated, or very young child, a pack that extends out of the oral cavity should be used to prevent swallowing of the gauze. Before the patient is dismissed, a written list of postoperative instructions should be given and explained to both the patient and the parents (Box 28-1). The postoperative instruction list should explain how to contact the dentist after hours in case of an emergency.

### Maxillary Molar Extractions

Primary maxillary molars differ from their permanent counterparts in that the height of contour is closer to the cementoenamel junction and their roots tend to be more divergent and smaller in diameter. Because of the root structure and potential weakening of the roots during the eruption of the permanent tooth, root fracture in primary maxillary molars is not uncommon.

Another important consideration is the relationship of the primary molar roots to the succeeding premolar crown. If the roots encircle the crown, the premolar can be inadvertently extracted with the primary molar (Fig. 28-15).

After the epithelial attachment is separated, a no. 301 straight elevator is used to luxate the tooth (Fig. 28-16). The extraction is completed using a maxillary universal forceps (no. 150S). Palatal movement is initiated first, followed by alternating buccal and palatal motions with slow continuous force applied to the forceps. This allows expansion of the alveolar bone so that the primary molar with its divergent roots can be extracted without fracture.

### Extraction of Maxillary Anterior Teeth

The maxillary primary and permanent central incisors, lateral incisors, and canines all have

---

## BOX 28-1
### Postoperative Instruction List for Patients

1. Bite on gauze for 30 minutes. Don't chew on the gauze.
2. Do not use a straw to drink for 24 hours.
3. Brush remaining teeth daily, but don't rinse or use a mouthwash on the day of the surgery.
4. Take pain pills and any other medication as directed.
5. If pain increases after 48 hours or if abnormal bleeding continues, call our office.
6. To prevent bleeding and swelling, keep your head elevated on two or three pillows while you rest or sleep.
7. Do not spit. Spitting will cause bleeding. Excess saliva and a little bit of blood looks like a lot of bleeding.
8. If bleeding starts again, put a gauze pad, a clean white cloth, or a damp tea bag over the bleeding area and bite on it with firm steady pressure for 1 hour. Do not chew on it.
9. Ice packs can be used immediately after surgery and for the next 24 hours to reduce swelling. Keep ice packs on for 10 minutes and off for 10 minutes.
10. Black and blue marks are bruises that often occur after surgery. Usually they are barely noticeable. Sometimes the skin is discolored. Do not worry about this.
11. Drink lots of liquid and eat anything you can swallow.

Call our office about any complications or if you need to change your appointment.

Dr. E. X. Traction. Office no: 555-0123. After hours, call 555-3210.

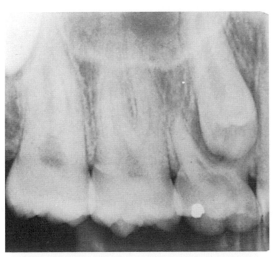

**Figure 28-15** Primary molars with roots encircling the developing premolar may have to be sectioned to prevent accidental extraction of the premolar.

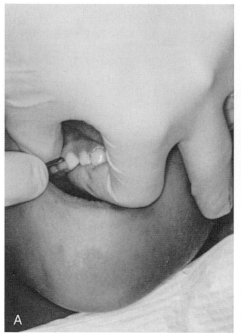
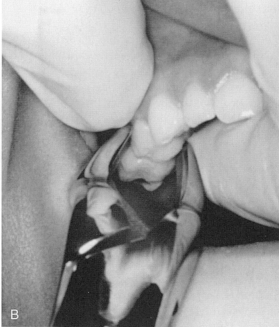

**Figure 28-16**   **A,** A no. 301 straight elevator is used to luxate the tooth. Extreme care is taken to prevent accidental luxation of adjacent teeth. **B,** The molar is extracted using slow continuous force in alternating buccal and palatal directions.

single roots that are usually conical. This makes them much less likely to fracture and allows for more rotational movement during extraction than is possible with multirooted teeth. A no. 1 forceps is useful in the extraction of maxillary anterior teeth (Fig. 28-17).

*Mandibular Molar Extractions*

When extracting mandibular molars, the dentist must pay special attention to the support of the mandible with the nonextraction hand so that no injury to the temporomandibular joints is inflicted (Fig. 28-18). After luxation with a no. 301 straight elevator, a no. 151S forceps is used to extract the tooth with the same alternating buccal and palatal motions used to extract maxillary primary molars.

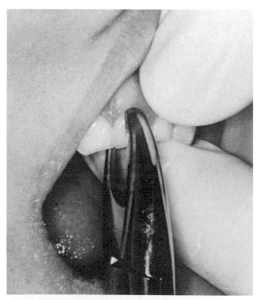

**Figure 28-17**   Rotational movements and buccolingual motions are used to extract primary incisors.

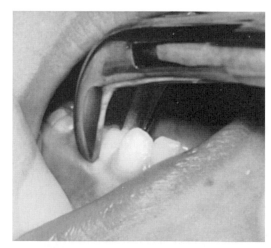

**Figure 28-18**   The nonextraction hand supports the mandible during extraction of mandibular molars.

*Extraction of Mandibular Anterior Teeth*

The mandibular incisors, canines, and premolars are all single rooted. Therefore one must take great care that the forceps does not place any force on adjacent teeth because they can become easily dislodged. This also enables the dentist to use rotational movements in the extraction process. Then slow, continuous force applied in alternating labial and lingual movements facilitates easy removal of these teeth.

*Management of Fractured Primary Tooth Roots*

Any dentist who extracts deciduous molars occasionally has the opportunity to treat root fractures. Once the root has fractured, the dentist must consider the following factors. Aggressive surgical removal of all root tips may cause damage to the succedaneous teeth. On the other hand, leaving the root may increase the chance for postoperative infection and may increase the theoretical potential of delaying permanent tooth eruption, although most primary root tips will resorb. A common-sense approach is best. If the tooth root is clearly visible and can be removed easily with an elevator or root tip pick, the root should be removed. If several attempts fail or if the root tip is very small or is situated very deep within the alveolus, the root is best left to be resorbed, most probably by the erupting permanent tooth. In some cases, the root tips do not resorb but are situated mesially and distally to the succeeding premolar and do not impede its eruption (Fig. 28-19). The patient and parents should be notified that a root fragment has been retained, and they should be assured that the chance of unfavorable sequelae is remote.

If the preoperative evaluation indicates that a root fracture is likely or that the developing succedaneous tooth may be dislodged during the extraction, an alternative extraction technique should be used. In these cases, the crown should be sectioned with a fissure bur in a buccolingual direction so that the detached portions of the crown and roots can be elevated separately.[13]

## Soft Tissue Surgical Procedures

A number of soft tissue procedures occasionally must be performed for the child patient. Careful presurgical consideration should be given to the following:

1. Expected change in the condition with maturation
2. Optimal time (or age) for the procedure
3. Type of anesthetic or sedation required

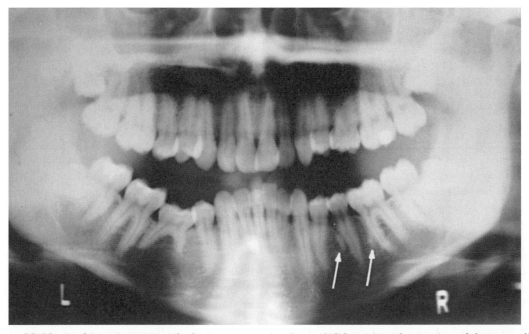

**Figure 28-19**   In this patient unresorbed primary root tips *(arrows)* did not impede eruption of the succeeding premolar. Also note that the congenitally missing primary molar roots are not resorbing and the occlusal surface of this tooth is well below the occlusal plane.

4. Postoperative complications or sequelae
5. Expected results

### Biopsies

Biopsy techniques in children are similar to those in adults. A very small lesion is probably best managed with an excisional biopsy, whereas lesions 0.5 cm or larger should probably have an incisional biopsy, especially if there is any doubt regarding the diagnosis of the lesion. Before performing a biopsy on a lesion, the dentist should consider the possibility that the lesion is vascular. Any such area should be palpated for intravascular turbulence (thrill), auscultated with a stethoscope for the presence of a bruit, and checked by needle aspiration for the presence of blood within the lesion. Biopsies should not be performed on vascular lesions until a thorough workup has been completed.[7]

Some areas of the oral cavity, such as the mucosa and lips, are easily accessible, whereas other areas, such as the tongue, can be difficult and may require sedation or general anesthesia in order to accomplish the biopsy. The biopsy area should be carefully evaluated for proximity to important anatomic structures, such as the mental nerve or salivary ducts or their orifices. Resorbable sutures are preferred to prevent the necessity of removing sutures in the child patient. The disadvantage of some resorbable sutures is that the knot can be very hard and stiff and irritating to the child. Soaking gut sutures in glycerin prior to their use softens them considerably.

### Frenectomies

**Maxillary Labial Frenectomies.** Recent trends justify significantly fewer maxillary labial frenectomies. These procedures should only be performed after it has been shown that the frenum is a causative factor in maintaining a diastema between the maxillary central incisors. This cannot be determined until after the permanent canines have erupted. Therefore, a maxillary labial frenectomy prior to the age of 11 or 12 is probably not indicated.

**Lingual Frenectomies.** Evidence from speech pathologists indicates that only the most severe ankyloglossia (tongue-tied) conditions significantly affect speech. Therefore, lingual frenectomies should not be performed until after an evaluation and therapy by a qualified speech therapist.

## Dentoalveolar Surgery

More difficult dentoalveolar procedures may involve the use of mucoperiosteal flaps and bone openings of the maxilla or mandible. These are indicated for procedures such as retained roots, bone cysts, impacted teeth (e.g., canines, supernumerary teeth), or intrabony pathologic lesions. Basic technique involves the preparation of an adequate mucoperiosteal flap as well as an adequate bone opening. At the same time, the operator must be cautious to avoid injury to such structures as the mental or inferior alveolar nerves, developing or erupting teeth, and maxillary sinus.

Procedures to uncover impacted maxillary canines have been associated with a high rate of success.[6] Preoperative radiographs are taken to accurately locate the canine in the alveolus. It is often necessary to take two or more periapical radiographs, using the buccal object rule to predict the labiopalatal position of an impacted tooth. The appropriate soft tissue approach (either labial or palatal) is used in a conservative bone uncovering of the crown. Great care is taken not to disturb the root of the impacted canine because it is thought that the chance of ankylosis increases if the cementum is disturbed. If root development has not been complete, the exposed canine may be allowed to erupt passively. If the impacted canine has complete root development or is poorly positioned, an orthodontic bracket may be bonded to the exposed portion of the crown with autopolymerized resin. The exposed canine can now be orthodontically positioned in the maxillary arch.

## Facial Injuries

The dentist may be the first health care professional consulted for injuries to the teeth, lips, jaws, or soft tissues of the face. The dentist should be aware of potential problems with each type of injury and either treat the patient appropriately or refer him or her to a qualified specialist.

Initial care should be directed to pain control, hemorrhage control, patient reassurance, wound toiletry if possible, and tetanus prophylaxis. Care should be taken to account for all teeth. Chest or abdominal radiographs may be needed to locate swallowed or aspirated teeth. Traumatic injuries to the teeth are discussed in Chapters 15 and 34.

Facial trauma is rarely life threatening. A significant number of patients who present with facial trauma may also have acute life-threatening injuries such as chest or abdominal trauma or, more commonly, serious head or neck injury. The dentist must be sure that there are no other serious injuries before treating the facial injuries.

Soft tissue injuries of the face or oral cavity can usually be managed with primary closure. Great care must be taken to be certain that no foreign objects are left hidden within the wound. Gravel or dirt left embedded in soft tissue may leave a permanent tattoo on the face.

Puncture-type wounds often carry glass or debris deep within the wound. When there is doubt about the presence or absence of a foreign body in the soft tissue, a soft tissue radiograph may be helpful in identifying the presence of embedded material (see Fig. 15-9).

Small lacerations of the wet portion of the lips, gingivae, alveolar mucosa, or tongue usually heal very well even if left unsutured. Large lacerations should be closed, regardless of their location. A resorbable suture is most commonly used intra-orally, although some practitioners prefer using silk suture material because it has a softer texture. The disadvantage of silk suture is that it requires removal in 5 to 7 days and the patient is still generally tender to manipulation of that area. Lacerations that extend from the face into the oral cavity (through-and-through lacerations) require a layered closure. Principles of a layered closure include a watertight mucosal closure, followed by closure of the muscular, facial, subcutaneous, and skin layers as necessary. Facial lacerations are always reapproximated first at significant anatomic structures, such as the vermilion border, columella of the nose, or eyebrows. Malalignment of these structures produces a noticeable cosmetic defect.

**Facial Fractures.**   The definitive treatment of facial fractures is best handled by an experienced dental practitioner, such as an oromaxillofacial surgeon. Often the patient presents to the dentist with an unsuspected fracture.

Patients with maxillary or midface fractures may present with any or all of the signs and symptoms listed in Box 28-2. Patients with mandibular fractures may present with any or all of the signs or symptoms listed in Box 28-3.

Initial management of facial fractures should be directed toward the immobilization of fractured segments, early antibiotic therapy for open fractures, and pain control.[12] Definitive treatment should then be performed by a qualified specialist.

---

**BOX 28-2**

### Signs and Symptoms of Maxillary or Midface Fractures

(Patients may present with any or all of the following.)
1. Altered occlusion
2. Numbness in the infraorbital nerve distribution
3. Double vision
4. Periorbital ecchymosis (bruising)
5. Facial asymmetry or edema
6. Limited mandibular opening
7. Subcutaneous emphysema (skin cracking upon palpation)
8. Nasal hemorrhage
9. Ecchymosis of the palatal or buccal mucosa
10. Mobility or crepitus upon manipulation of the maxilla

---

### Odontogenic Infections

Infections of odontogenic origin are common in child and adolescent patients. Classic signs and symptoms of infection include redness, pain, swelling, and local and systemic temperature increases. Because of wider marrow spaces in the child, an odontogenic infection can rapidly spread through the bone, possibly resulting in damage to the erupting teeth. Most odontogenic infections in the child are not serious and can be easily managed with pulp therapy or removal of the involved tooth. There are serious complications that uncommonly arise from an odontogenic infection, including cavernous sinus thrombosis, brain abscess, airway obstruction, and mediastinal spread of infection. Signs and symptoms of a more serious infection include an elevated systemic temperature (102°F to 104°F), difficulty in swallowing, difficulty in breathing, nausea, fatigue, and sweating. The child with an odontogenic infection may become dehydrated as a result of his or her refusal to take fluids because of oral pain.

Management of odontogenic infections is directed at providing adequate drainage of the infection. This can be accomplished in minor infections by way of a pulpectomy or extraction. Management of more serious odontogenic infections is best accomplished by way of surgical incision and drainage.[13] It is often necessary to identify the causative organism or organisms in

## BOX 28-3

### Signs and Symptoms of Mandibular Fractures

(Patients may present with any or all of the following.)
1. Mandibular hemorrhage
2. Numbness in the mental or inferior alveolar nerve distribution
3. Altered occlusion
4. Ecchymosis or abrasion of the chin

5. Ecchymosis of the floor of the mouth or buccal mucosa
6. Periauricular pain
7. Mandibular deviation on opening
8. Mobility or crepitus upon manipulation of the mandible

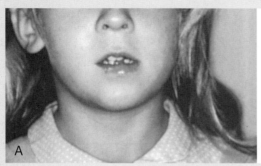
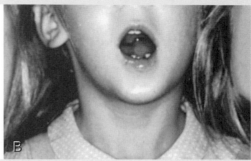

**A,** This child suffered a fracture of her left condyle. Note the deviation of the mandible to the left. **B,** The deviation of the mandible toward the side of the condylar fracture is more evident upon opening.

order to prescribe the most appropriate antibiotic. Because most oral infections are mixed infections (aerobic and anaerobic), penicillin remains the antibiotic of choice for initial therapy.

## REFERENCES

1. Allen KD, Kotil D, Larzelere RE et al: Comparison of a computerized anesthesia device with a traditional syringe in preschool children. *Pediatr Dent* 24(4):315-320, 2002.
2. Benham NR: The cephalometric position of the mandibular foramen with age. *J Dent Child* 43:233, 1976.
3. Bennett CR: *Monheim's Local Anesthesia and Pain Control in Dental Practice,* 7th ed. St Louis, Mosby, 1984, p 68.
4. Brannstrom M, Lindskog S, Nordenvall KJ: Enamel hypoplasia in permanent teeth induced by periodontal ligament anesthesia of primary teeth. *JADA* 109:735, 1984.
5. Brownbill JW, Walker PO, Bourcy BD, Keenan KM: Comparison of inferior dental nerve block injections in child patients using 30-gauge and 25-gauge short needles. *Anesth Prog* 34:215-219, 1987.
6. Fifield CA: Surgery and orthodontic treatment for unerupted teeth. *JADA* 113:590, 1986.
7. Gibilisco JA: *Oral Radiographic Diagnosis.* Philadelphia, Saunders, 1985, p 224.
8. Hersh EV, Helpin ML, Evans OB: Local anesthetic mortality: report of case. *J Dent Child* 58:489-491, 1991.
9. Kruger G: *Textbook of Oral and Maxillofacial Surgery,* 6th ed. St Louis, Mosby, 1984, p 52.
10. Malamed SF: The periodontal ligament (PDL) injection: an alternative to inferior alveolar nerve block. *Oral Surg* 53:117, 1982.
11. Malamed SF: *Handbook of Local Anesthesia,* 5th ed. St Louis, Mosby, 2004.
12. Rowe N, Williams J: *Maxillofacial Injuries.* Edinburgh, Churchill Livingstone, 1985, p 538.
13. Sanders B: *Pediatric Oral and Maxillofacial Surgery.* St Louis, Mosby, 1979.
14. Shojaei, AR, Haas DA: Local anesthetic cartridges and latex allergy: a literature review. *J Can Dent Assoc* 68(10):622-626, 2002.
15. teDuits E, Goepferd S, Donly K et al: The effectiveness of electronic dental anesthesia in children. *Pediatr Dent* 15(3):191-196, 1993.
16. United States Pharmacopeia: *Dispensing Information for the Health Care Professional,* 17th ed. Rockville, Md, United States Pharmacopeial Convention, 1997.

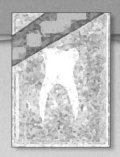

# PART 4

# THE TRANSITIONAL YEARS: SIX TO TWELVE YEARS

The dentist who follows a child from age 6 to age 12 will see many changes in the child. The physical changes will be dramatic, and those that have to do with facial form, occlusion, the advent of the permanent teeth, and the aesthetic appearance of these permanent teeth are the professional responsibility of the dentist. He or she must supervise the exfoliation of the 20 primary teeth in the 6-year-old and supervise through the next 6 years the eruption of the 28 permanent teeth that are found in most 12-year-olds. The dentist must provide answers to parents concerned about the appearance of their child, intercept those developing malocclusions that are within his or her treatment talents, and when appropriate, refer those malocclusions that need specialist care.

The dentist who can deliver the child from age 6 to adolescence with no amount or just a modest amount of hard tissue disease, no remarkable soft tissue diseases, allegiance to prevention and developed home care habits, and harmonious dentofacial relationships has indeed mastered the ultimate obligations in treating this age group.

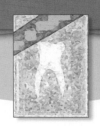

# CHAPTER 29
## The Dynamics of Change

## PHYSICAL CHANGES

### Body

*Jimmy R. Pinkham*

The average 6-year-old in the United States is approximately 3 feet, 10 inches tall and weighs about 48 pounds. By the time the child reaches age 12, he or she will be about 5 feet tall and will weigh about 85 pounds. This represents, from age 6 to age 12, an approximately 5% to 6% height increase per year and a weight adjustment of about 10% per year.[1]

By age 6, the child's overall body proportions are fairly close to what they will be in adulthood. The most remarkable proportional change in the body during these years results from the lengthening of the child's limbs.

During the years between the ages of 6 and 12, boys as a group are generally slightly taller than girls until around age 10. From age 10 to around age 15, girls are slightly taller than boys. From a weight standpoint, boys are slightly heavier than girls until around age 11, when girls overtake boys in weight for a brief time. The reasons why boys eventually become taller than girls are considered in the discussion of the body's physical changes in the later section on adolescence (Chapter 36).

Other growth and developmental changes that are noteworthy during these years are further increases in blood pressure, continuing decreases in the pulse rate, increased mineralization of the skeleton, and increases in muscular tissue. In addition, the lymphatic tissues reach a peak in development during these years to the point where they exceed the amounts found in adults.

## REFERENCE

1. Watson EN, Lowrey GH: *Growth and Development of Children*, 5th ed. Chicago, Year Book, 1967.

### Craniofacial Changes

*Jerry Walker*

The years from ages 6 through 12 represent a continuous progression of the growth in the head and neck noted in the 3- to 6-year-old. In a comparison of the differential growth rates of the craniofacial components from ages 5 to 10 (approximately the age range of interest here), neural and cranial growth are found to be almost entirely complete (Fig. 29-1). During this same age span, the jaws ($A = 2$ and $B = 3$ of Fig. 29-1) grow at a faster rate than the cranium. Despite this faster rate, considerable general growth is experienced after age 10.

Using the Bolton standards for illustrative purposes, nasal projection and increased mandibular prominence are demonstrated (Fig. 29-2). The nasal cartilage and mandibular condyle continue to grow by endochondral bone formation for some time, although the female mandibular growth spurt is most likely completed, and the male's is yet to come. Growth modification can therefore be performed in this age group. Changes in cranial base length caused by endochondral bone formation at the sphenooccipital synchondrosis cease in early adolescence, but some appositional changes continue to occur at the basion and nasion. Vertically, there is a continued lowering of the palatal vault with sutural growth and apposition on the oral side of the palate and resorption on the nasal side as the intramembranous process of bone formation continues.

In the transverse plane, there is continued growth at the maxillary suture and appositional widening of the dentoalveolar ridge with eruption of the permanent teeth (Fig. 29-3). This is especially noticeable with the canines and premolars. Widening of the anterior arch accompanies lateral incisor eruption.

Growth Increments

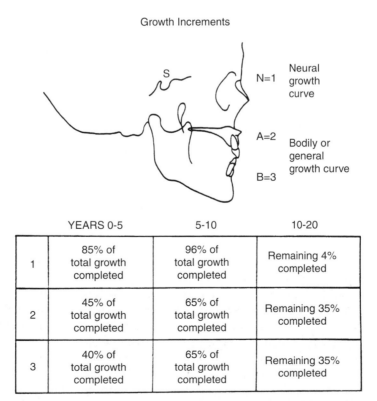

| | YEARS 0-5 | 5-10 | 10-20 |
|---|---|---|---|
| 1 | 85% of total growth completed | 96% of total growth completed | Remaining 4% completed |
| 2 | 45% of total growth completed | 65% of total growth completed | Remaining 35% completed |
| 3 | 40% of total growth completed | 65% of total growth completed | Remaining 35% completed |

**Figure 29-1**    Differential growth center rates of craniofacial components. (From Behrents RG: *Growth in the Aging Craniofacial Skeleton.* Center for Human Growth and Development. Ann Arbor, University of Michigan, 1985.)

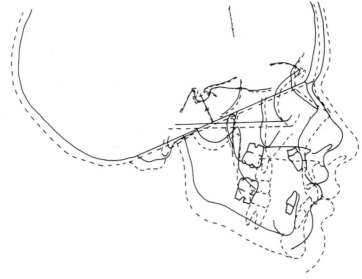

**Figure 29-2**   This anterior cranial base superimposition of the Bolton Standard for 6- and 12-year-olds (*solid line* and *dashed line,* respectively) demonstrates the magnitude of anteroposterior and vertical skeletal growth during this period as well as the soft tissue change. (Redrawn from Broadbent BH Sr, Broadbent BH Jr, Golden WH: *Bolton Standards of Developmental Growth.* St Louis, Mosby, 1975.)

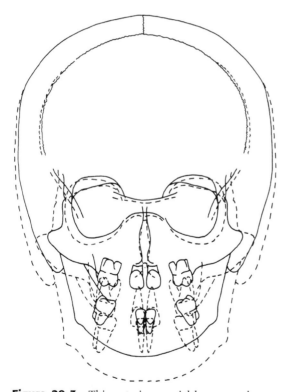

**Figure 29-3**   This anterior cranial base superimposition of the Bolton Standard for 6- and 12-year-olds (*solid line* and *dashed line,* respectively) demonstrates the magnitude of transverse and vertical skeletal growth during this period. (Redrawn from Broadbent BH Sr, Broadbent BH Jr, Golden WH: *Bolton Standards of Developmental Growth.* St Louis, Mosby, 1975.)

By the end of these transitional years, the complete permanent dentition with the exception of the third molars has erupted (Fig. 29-4). Most of the residual space resulting from either idiopathic spacing or leeway spacing has closed by this time. Further eruption and drift occur in response to continued growth.

## REFERENCE

1. Broadbent BH Sr, Broadbent BH Jr, Golden WH: *Bolton Standards of Developmental Growth.* St Louis, Mosby, 1975.

### Dental Changes

*Clemons A. Full*

Early during this period of time, many children experience the eruption of all four first permanent molars and the exfoliation of the mandibular and maxillary primary central and lateral incisors with a subsequent eruption of permanent incisors between the ages of 6 and 7 years (see Table 12-4). The maxillary permanent lateral incisors may erupt later than age 7 in some children.

With the exception of the third molars, all of the permanent teeth usually have erupted by the end of the twelfth year. Except for the third molars, the enamel of all of the permanent teeth

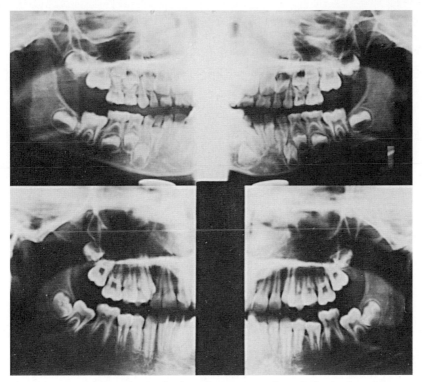

**Figure 29-4**    These two panoramic radiographs show the transition from the beginning of the permanent dentition to its completion with the exception of the third molars.

is complete by age 8. In the mandibular arch and following the first permanent molars and central incisors, the teeth erupt in immediate succession, that is, centrals, laterals, cuspids, first and second premolars, and second permanent molars from 6 to 7 years through 11 to 13 years of age. The same sequence takes place in the maxillary arch except for the maxillary cuspid, which usually erupts after the bicuspids or premolars and at about the same time as or before the eruption of the second permanent molars (Fig. 29-5).

The mandibular central incisor roots are complete by age 9. The roots of the four first permanent molars, the maxillary central incisors, and the mandibular lateral incisors are usually com-

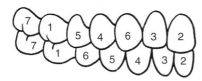

**Figure 29-5**    Desirable eruption sequence for the permanent teeth. (From McDonald RE, Avery DR, Dean JA: *Dentistry for the Child and Adolescent,* 8th ed. St Louis, Mosby, 2004.)

plete by age 10. The roots of the maxillary lateral incisors are complete by age 11.

Because the position of the dental lamina of the permanent teeth is located to the lingual of all of the primary teeth (except for the dental lamina coming off the second primary for the three permanent molars), the anterior teeth develop in their vault or crypt lingual to and near the apex of the primary incisors. When the roots begin to form on the permanent teeth, they start to migrate to the oral cavity. Generally, they follow a pattern such that they come across the primary root, resorbing it and erupting slightly labial to the location sustained by the primary tooth (Fig. 29-6). Therefore the permanent teeth are usually always angulated more buccally compared with their primary predecessors (Fig. 29-7). The developing bicuspids develop between the roots of the primary molars and continue to erupt in a slightly mesial position. The permanent molars develop from one dental lamina and, like the bicuspids or premolars, erupt in or at a mesial inclination or angle.

Compared with the primary incisors, the permanent incisors are larger and develop in a more restricted area.[1] Their growth, although perpet-

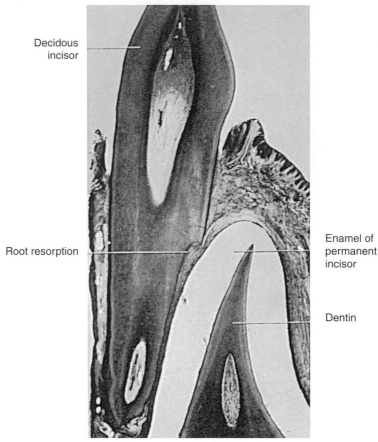

Decidous incisor

Root resorption

Enamel of permanent incisor

Dentin

**Figure 29-6**    Resorption of root of primary incisor owing to pressure of erupting successor. (From Bhaskar SN, editor: *Orban's Oral Histology and Embryology*, 11ᵗʰ ed. St Louis, Mosby, 1990.)

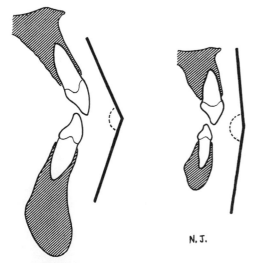

N. J.

**Figure 29-7**    Angulation of permanent and primary incisors. (From Moyers RE: *Handbook of Orthodontics*, 3ʳᵈ ed. Chicago, Year Book, 1973.)

ual, occurs at a much slower rate during their eruption than the primary incisors. The inclinations of the eruptive paths of the permanent incisors account for their flared appearance. Also, it is natural to find diastemas between the incisors, particularly in the maxilla. The permanent canine in the maxillary arch is usually the last permanent tooth to erupt mesial to the first permanent molar. As the permanent canine begins to erupt, its mesial component of force is often adequate to straighten the incisors and close the diastemas. This period of development has been called the "ugly duckling stage" (Fig. 29-8).[1]

## REFERENCE

1.  Finn SB: *Clinical Pedodontics*, 4ᵗʰ ed. Philadelphia, Saunders, 1973.

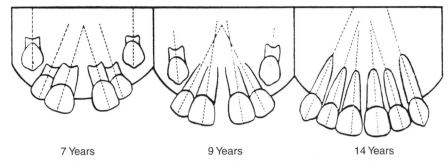

7 Years                    9 Years                    14 Years

**Figure 29-8**   The "ugly duckling" stage. (From Finn SB: *Clinical Pedodontics,* 4th ed. Philadelphia, Saunders, 1973; after Broadbent BH: *Angle Orthodont* 1:183-208, 1937.)

## COGNITIVE CHANGES

*Jimmy R. Pinkham*

A book could easily be written describing the incredible cognitive acquisitions, adjustments, and sophisticated changes occurring in a child from age 6 to age 12. Mental capacity alone grows extensively. For example, by age 12 a child can outline on paper or mentally recall the travels of Marco Polo. However, at age 6 the concept of a man from ancient Italy traveling to China would not be remarkable and probably would be mentally unretainable.

In 1968, White concluded that between the ages of 5 and 7 years a reorganization of the central nervous system may take place that accounts for a dramatically increased ability to remain diligent at a task or attentive to a problem.[1] Unquestionably, the attention span of the child older than 7 years is substantially greater than that of the child younger than 5 years.

The school-aged years of 6 to 12 are when a child becomes literate. Before age 6 few children can do much more than print their names. After age 12 most children have accomplished an appropriate approach to grammar and syntax and have the ability to produce increasingly sophisticated oral and written communications. In some parts of the world it is not uncommon for a child to be fluent in a second language by age 12.

According to Piaget, the ages between 6 and 12 roughly approximate the third major developmental stage of cognition, that is, the phase of concrete operations. Piaget proposed the following four major periods of intellectual development:

1. *Sensorimotor:* birth to 18 months
2. *Preoperational:* 18 months to 7 years
3. *Concrete operations:* 7 to 12 years
4. *Formal operations:* 12 years and onward

So far this book has presented a study of the child through the sensorimotor and preoperational stages. In the concrete operations stage, Piaget described numerous sophisticated changes in the child's mental abilities. For instance, the 5-year-old may be able to walk "two blocks down, one block right to the second white house" to get to his or her aunt's residence, but the same 5-year-old could not draw this route on a piece of paper. However, by age 7 or 8, the child could portray the route on a self-drawn map. In other words, mental representations of actions become a part of the cognitive abilities of the child during these years. For the dentist who instructs children in the process of tooth decay, it may be helpful in designing his or her preventive presentation to understand the differences in mental representation ability between preschoolers and school-aged children. Obviously, two different presentations are needed.

During the years from 6 to 12 (7 to 12, according to Piaget), children acquire the ability to understand the constancies between length, mass, number, and weight despite external differences. Relativity also emerges in the child's evaluation system. To the 4-year-old, the word "dark" means black. The 10-year-old can talk about a "dark" green car. In summary, the child between the ages of 6 to 12 grows up cognitively. By the age of 12 years, his or her mind and mental prowess have matured, and he or she is capable of assimilating real as well as theoretical or abstract information.

## REFERENCE

1. White SH: Changes in learning processes in the late preschool years. Presented at a meeting of the American Education Association, Chicago, 1968.

## EMOTIONAL CHANGES

*Jimmy R. Pinkham*

The years from 6 to 12 are years of matriculation toward the acceptance by the child of societal norms of behavior. Crying, tantrums, and other rages will, in normal children, be relinquished as possible modes of expression of frustration. Whereas the preschooler needs and perhaps demands immediate rewards and satisfaction, the child in the transitional years masters the emotional ability to delay gratification. This awareness of delay is reinforced by the child's schooling, and increasingly the child is guided toward the appropriate investment of his or her time in worthwhile activities. Homework, household chores, caring for pets, delivering newspapers, scouting, team sports, and piano lessons are some of the behaviors expected of this age group, which were almost impossible during the preschool years.

Another emotional refinement that is developed from age 6 to 12 is the ability to utilize life's tasks in ways effective enough to stave off boredom. Previously, the preschooler immersed his mind in an activity until all his energy and attention were spent. Then, at the point of burnout, he looked to his parents or other attendants to find something else for him to do. Between ages 6 and 12, however, the need for adults to direct the child's attention rapidly recedes, and by age 12 a child usually has a ledger of wants and desires, a sense of the time that should be spent in their pursuit, and an ability to set priorities for which wants and desires should come first or last.

In this age range, body image starts to become an emotional feature of the child's life. Unquestionably, for the majority of children the importance of body image becomes most dramatic during adolescence, but its emergence certainly occurs during these years. Whereas the 6-year-old usually couldn't care less about having ketchup on his face or mud on his pants, the 12-year-old may agonize over a blemish or over wearing clothes that are not stylish. In summary, body appearance becomes a subject of emotional awareness and emphasis during these years. Unquestionably, this has dental ramifications. The mottled enamel of the 6-year-old may have disturbed only the parents. The child was indifferent. By age 12, this condition may account for a lack of smiling, social withdrawal, and a feeling of forlornness by the child. Teasing may exacerbate the problem.

Although there certainly are exceptions, the majority of children from age 6 to 12 find overall emotional satisfaction only when they are accepted socially by their peers. Lack of acceptance, outright ostracism, and teasing can certainly be very damaging emotionally. During these years, with the help of parents, teachers, role models, and other significant individuals, it is important for the child to become emotionally resilient. The abilities to handle and recover from humiliation, frustration, loss, and disappointment should at least begin to emerge during these years. If they do not, then adolescence presents a real danger.

## SOCIAL CHANGES

*Jimmy R. Pinkham*

The years between ages 6 and 12 are often called middle childhood. These years are clearly more complicated socially than the earlier years because of school, the increasing importance of peers, and the enormous expansion of the child's social environment. These years see the child intensifying his or her focus on and pursuance of existing motives while minimizing or eliminating others.

School is extremely important for this age group and represents an extrafamilial world that may reinforce social responses learned at home, provide new ones, and even discourage others. Whether the teacher is encountered earlier in preschool or now for the first time at school, he or she is likely to be the first significant, day-by-day, authoritative adult known outside the child's immediate family. Also, as opposed to baby sitters and relatives, the teacher is encountered by the child in an environment in which the teacher has control. In 1964, Franco concluded that a child's feelings about her or his first teacher correlate closely with the child's feelings about her or his mother.[1]

Perhaps surprisingly, most children anticipate school positively and remain enthusiastic about their experiences there. It has also been noted that children's self-importance, self-control, and ability to be independent (e.g., getting one's own cereal for breakfast) increase quickly during the first few months of school.[2] These findings are less true for children from disadvantaged homes.

Also, unfortunately, enthusiasm for school and teachers tends to decline in later years, and this decline appears to be more significant in children from disadvantaged homes than in those from more affluent social classes. It has been suggested by some investigators that middle- and upper-middle-class parents may be better role models regarding school because their children see them reading, studying, and pursuing other intellectual activities.

Unquestionably, teachers have an important impact on the socialization of a child. Space is far too limited in this text to discuss how different teacher attributes affect pupils, but certainly the characteristics of fairness and consistency, the capacity to maintain order without being overly authoritative, and the ability to praise effectively are appreciated by children and have very positive social effects.

The peer group that a child joins also can be a powerful socializing force. Sometimes the values of the peer group are antithetical to those of the teacher and parents. This presents a conflict for the child in that he or she may risk reprimand from authoritative adults or ridicule or rejection from his or her peers if he or she conforms to one or the other's expectations. It is important for parents to understand these conflicts and how socially influential peer pressure can be for children in this age group. It is also important to note that the child who eagerly accepts a peer value that disappoints her or his parents may in fact be doing so to gain the feelings of acceptance and nurturing that were not provided sufficiently at home.

One last factor marks the middle childhood years. This is the advent of increasingly stronger, more stable, and more meaningful friendships. Generally, friendships are made with children of the same sex. Friends at this age level as a rule also share similar socioeconomic status, intelligence, maturity, and interests.

## REFERENCES

1. Franco D: The child's perception of "the teacher" as compared to his perception of "the mother." *Dissert Abstr* 24:3414-3415, 1964.
2. Stendler CB, Young N: Impact of first grade entrance upon the socialization of the child: changes after eight months of school. *Child Dev* 22:113-122, 1951.

## EPIDEMIOLOGY AND MECHANISMS OF DENTAL DISEASE

*Steven M. Adair*

Dental caries is the most common chronic disease of childhood. Even though caries prevalence declined substantially in the latter part of the twentieth century, it still affects a majority of U.S. school-aged children and is five times more common than asthma.[24] This section will review the epidemiology of caries during the period of the transitional dentition, as well as dietary factors related to caries.

### Epidemiology of Caries in the Transitional Dentition

Comprehensive data on the caries experience of U.S. school children were compiled by the Epidemiology and Oral Disease Prevention Program of the National Institute of Dental Research (NIDR)[6] in a nationwide study conducted in 1986–1987. More than 39,000 children, ages 5 to 17, were examined using visual-tactile criteria.

Figure 29-9 shows the mean number of decayed, missing, and filled permanent tooth surfaces (DMFS) for children by age and sex. The mean DMFS for 5-year-olds, who as a group have few erupted permanent teeth, was 0.07. For 8-year-olds, who would generally have permanent first molars and all permanent incisors erupted, the mean DMFS was about 10 times higher (0.71). By age 13, near the end of the transitional dentition, the mean DMFS was 3.76. These increases reflect the effects of time on an increasing number of permanent tooth surfaces available for decay as children progress through the transitional dentition years. Girls had slightly higher DMFS scores than boys.

More recent data from the National Health and Nutrition Examination Survey (NHANES III)[17] indicate that 58.6% of children and adolescents ages 5 to 17 years have experienced dental caries.

During the period of the transitional dentition, primary teeth may become carious as well. The 1986–1987 survey determined the number of decayed and filled primary tooth surfaces (DFS) for children ages 5 to 9 years to be 3.91. This is a 26% decline in primary tooth decay from the

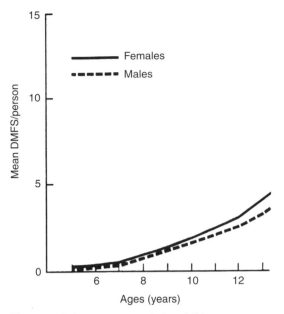

**Figure 29-9** Mean DMFS for children ages 5 to 13 years in the United States by age and sex. (Redrawn from *Oral Health of United States Children*, Epidemiology and Oral Disease Prevention Program, National Institute of Dental Research, 1989).

previous large-scale epidemiologic study carried out by the NIDR in 1979–1980.[14]

In general, the 1986–1987 survey found that the DMFS of whites was slightly lower than that of nonwhites, and the DMFS of urban children was slightly lower than that of children from rural areas. The explanation for this latter difference is the higher percentage of urban children who were exposed to optimally fluoridated public water supplies.

The disparity of permanent tooth dental caries experience by family income level was demonstrated in the NHANES III study. As shown in Table 29-1, the percentage of children with decayed and filled permanent teeth decreased with increasing family income. Similarly, the DMFT of children ages 6 to 14 years generally declined with increasing income level (Table 29-1).[25]

*Comparisons*
The degree to which the prevalence of caries has declined in this country can best be appreciated by comparison with similar surveys. The most complete surveys for comparison are those conducted by the National Center for Health Statistics (NCHS) in 1963–1965[15] and 1971–1974,[16] and by NIDR in 1979–1980,[14] as illustrated in Table 29-2.[2] Data for the NCHS studies were collected on subjects ages 6 to 11. Consequently the same age groups have been selected from the NIDR studies as well. The diagnostic criteria used were practically identical in all studies. As illustrated, the mean DMFT for children in the transitional dentition had declined by 50% since 1963–1965, and by 58% since the 1971–1974 NCHS study.

A similar comparison of the can be made for the percentage of caries-free 6- to 11-year-old children from each study. As illustrated in Table 29-3, that percentage increased markedly between 1963–1965 and 1986–1987.[2]

## TABLE 29-1

**Percentage of Children Ages 6 to 14 Years with Decayed and Filled Permanent Teeth by Family Income Level**

| INCOME LEVEL (% OF FPL) | PERCENTAGE WITH AT LEAST ONE DECAYED PRIMARY TOOTH (SE) | PERCENTAGE WITH AT LEAST ONE FILLED PRIMARY TOOTH (SE) | DMFT (CI) |
|---|---|---|---|
| 0–100 | 19.5 (2.1) | 25.3 (2.6) | 1.08 (0.88–1.28) |
| 101–200 | 14.3 (2.1) | 28.6 (2.7) | 1.13 (0.93–1.33) |
| 201–300 | 8.7 (1.4) | 29.9 (3.0) | 1.02 (0.82–1.22) |
| ≥301 | 3.4 (0.9) | 30.2 (3.2) | 0.89 (0.69–1.09) |
| Total sample | 11.3 (0.9) | 28.7 (1.7) | 1.03 (0.83–1.23) |

Data from Vargas CM, Crall JJ, Schneider DA: Sociodemographic distribution of pediatric dental caries: NHANES III, 1988–1994. *JADA* 129:1229, 1998.
*FPL,* Federal poverty level; *SE,* standard error of the percentage; *CI,* 95% confidence interval.

## TABLE 29-2

### Mean DMFT of 6- to 11-Year-Old Children in Four National Caries Surveys, 1963–1987

| NCHS 1963–65 | NCHS 1971–74 | NIDR 1979–80 | NIDR 1986–87 |
|---|---|---|---|
| 1.4 | 1.7 | 1.1 | 0.71 |

Modified from Brunelle JA, Carlos JP: *J Dent Res* 61(special issue):1346-1351, 1982.
NCHS, National Center for Health Statistics; NIDR, National Institute of Dental Research.

*Basis for Caries Reductions*

Caries results from the interaction of specific microflora with fermentable carbohydrate on a susceptible tooth surface (see Chapter 12 [section "Epidemiology and Mechanisms of Dental Disease"]). There is no evidence to suggest that mutans streptococci have become less pathogenic or less prevalent in the population, although it has been proposed that the increased use of antibiotics may have some effect on the oral microflora. Similarly, there is no evidence that per capita consumption of sugars has changed significantly during the intervening decades. While per capita consumption of sucrose has declined somewhat since the mid-1970s, it has been replaced with fructose and other sugars that are also cariogenic. It is unlikely, therefore, that there has been any discernible change in the disease process itself.

The best explanation for the reduction in caries prevalence is the increased exposure to fluoride in its various forms, such as fluoridated

## TABLE 29-3

### Percentage of Caries-Free 6- to 11-Year-Old Children in Four National Caries Surveys, 1963–1987

| NCHS 1963–65 | NCHS 1971–74 | NIDR 1979–80 | NIDR 1986–87 |
|---|---|---|---|
| 51.1 | 43.6 | 56.7 | 74.3 |

Modified from Brunelle JA, Carlos JP: *J Dent Res* 61(special issue):1346-1351, 1982.
NCHS, National Center for Health Statistics; NIDR, National Institute of Dental Research.

community water, fluoride-containing dentifrices, and self-administered fluoride supplements. Evidence for this view is supported by the fact that the major caries reductions have occurred on proximal surfaces. These smooth surfaces benefit most from fluoride's protective effects (see Chapter 17 [section "Epidemiology and Mechanisms of Dental Disease"]).

In the United States, the population exposed to optimally fluoridated water supplies doubled from 40 million to 80 million during the 1960s, and has risen at a lower rate since that time. Many of the children examined in 1979–1980 and in 1986–1987 benefited from lifetime exposure to optimally fluoridated water. Further evidence for this hypothesis can be found by comparing the DMFS scores of children from rural areas and urban areas. A higher proportion of children from cities have been exposed to artificially fluoridated water supplies, and this is reflected in the lower caries prevalence among these children. However, the increase in the numbers of school children from fluoride-deficient areas who participated in school fluoride mouth-rinse programs and other caries prevention programs has led to reductions in the prevalence of caries in these communities as well.

Other miscellaneous factors may also have contributed to the reduction in caries prevalence. These include an increase in the distribution to fluoride-deficient areas of foods and beverages prepared with fluoridated water, known as the "halo effect." A general improvement in education and socioeconomic status may also lead to a more health-conscious population with concomitant changes in dietary patterns. It is also possible that other, as-yet-unclear factors contributing to increased human life span may have some influence on oral health, just as it is possible that improved oral health can contribute to increased longevity.

Dental caries continues to be a common health problem among children. Dental disease has been referred to as "the silent epidemic."[24] The progress made in recent decades is significant and encouraging, but further substantial reductions in caries prevalence will require redoubled effort. Increases in the use of self-applied fluoride, whether by fluoride-containing dentifrices, high-fluoride prescription gels, or dietary fluoride supplements, should continue to be beneficial. Maximizing the use of pit and fissure sealants could greatly reduce the proportion of the caries that is minimally affected by fluoride.

## Dietary Factors and Dental Caries

As mentioned in Chapter 12, sugars (sucrose, fructose, glucose, and others) are one of the major etiologic factors in dental caries. Sucrose has been labeled the "arch criminal of dental caries,"[18] but in fact animal studies have shown other sugars, notably glucose and fructose, to be as cariogenic as sucrose.[11,20] This poses potential difficulties in making dietary recommendations, since many fruits and vegetables contain substantial amounts of natural sugars.[1]

### Sucrose

Speculation has centered on the role of sucrose in caries formation once scientific study of the disease began. One of the first controlled studies to document sucrose as an etiologic factor was the Vipeholm study.[9] In this study, 436 inmates in a mental institution near Lund, Sweden were given sugar in various forms to supplement the relatively sugar-free institutional diets. The sugar was offered as sucrose in solution or in retentive forms, such as sweetened bread and toffee. The sucrose in solution and the bread were introduced with meals, whereas the other forms were given between meals. The study showed that an increase in sucrose intake was associated with an increase in caries activity. Furthermore, this caries activity decreased when the sucrose-rich foods were discontinued. The cariogenic potential of the sucrose was enhanced when it was given between meals and in a more retentive form (caramels and toffees). The time required for the sugar to clear the oral cavity was closely related to the caries activity. The study also pointed out that caries formation varied among individuals and that caries formation continued in some individuals even after a return to low-sucrose diets. The subjects who received only 30 g of sucrose per day, all at mealtimes, developed an average of 0.27 new carious lesions per year. Those who ingested 330 g of sucrose per day, 300 g of which was in solution, were only slightly worse off, with 0.43 new carious surfaces per year. However, subjects in the group that received 24 sticky toffees per day developed 4.02 new lesions per year. This group ingested 300 g of sucrose per day, but 40% of it was eaten between meals. Although there were flaws in the design of this study, the magnitude of the differ-

ences in caries development are impressive. The questions regarding the ethics of this type of study ensure that it will probably never be repeated.

Another study corroborating the role of sucrose was conducted with 3- to 14-year-olds who resided at Hopewood House in Bowral, New South Wales, Australia.[22,23] Almost all of these institutionalized children had lived there since infancy and were fed an almost pure vegetarian diet supplemented with milk and an occasional egg yolk. The vegetables were generally served raw, and refined carbohydrate was rigidly restricted. In spite of poor oral hygiene, the caries prevalence of the children was very low. Primary dentition involvement was almost nonexistent, while the caries prevalence of the permanent teeth was about one tenth that of the mean score for other Australian children. Almost one third of the children remained caries free throughout the 5-year study. Children who left Hopewood House at an older age experienced a significant increase in dental caries.

Though there are still some who question the primary role of sucrose and other sugars in the etiologic development of caries,[26] there is overwhelming evidence to demonstrate its relationship to caries as part of a multifactorial process.[4]

### Other Food Factors

The multiplicity of food factors requires that estimations of the relative cariogenicity of foods be approached with caution. These factors include carbohydrate-sucrose concentration, retentiveness, oral clearance rate, detergent quality, texture, effect of mixing foods, sequence of ingestion, frequency of ingestion, and pH of the food itself. For example, most fruits will depress plaque pH by virtue of their own low pH. This occurs even though the low pH of the food inhibits natural fermentation of its sugar content. Low-pH fruits can also demineralize enamel by the direct action of their acids. At the same time, low-pH fruits stimulate a flow of saliva that buffers plaque pH drops; other foods, such as vegetables, stimulate salivary flow through the chewing reflex. On balance, however, there is not a strong case for a caries-protective effect from fruits and vegetables.[1]

Another food factor that has received much attention is stickiness or retentiveness. This characteristic has often been equated with the oral clearance of the food, with the underlying assumption being that longer oral clearance times can prolong the period of plaque acid production. However, our concepts of food retention on teeth have been challenged in recent years by research that shows a poor correlation between foods judged to be "sticky" and the time required for oral clearance.[10] Caramels and candy bars, judged by a lay group to be among the stickiest foods, were found to clear the oral cavity rather quickly; potato chips and white bread, judged as relatively nonsticky foods, were among the last to clear the mouth. Foods high in starch content (breads, cereals, potato chips) were slower to clear the oral cavity, whereas those high in sucrose exhibited a rapid clearance from the mouth. It has also been shown that the presence of starch increases the acid production from sucrose[3] and may allow fermentation to take place under otherwise inhibiting concentrations of sugar. On the other hand, high levels of sugar appear to increase the solubility of starchy foods and hasten the clearance from the oral cavity. Clearly, no one cariogenicity test can account for all these factors, except possibly trials in humans. Even in human trials, individual variations exist in plaque composition and amount, salivary buffering capacity, and enamel resistance to dissolution with or without the ability to remineralize.

The frequency with which cariogenic foods are ingested has a strong relationship to the risk of caries development. More frequent contact with sugars at mealtime and frequent between-meal snacks result in prolonged or multiple pH challenges to the teeth, and possibly to longer oral clearance times. The net result is an increased likelihood of enamel demineralization that has been demonstrated in animal models.[8]

Certain food components and factors may have cariostatic or caries-inhibiting effects. Phosphates, principally sodium metaphosphate, have been shown to reduce caries in animal studies.[19] The effect is probably local, related to buffering capacity, a reduction of enamel solubility, and other bacterial and biochemical properties. Unfortunately, clinical trials with phosphate supplements in human diets have not proved as effective.[12] Other animal studies[7] have shown that foods high in fat, protein, fluoride, or calcium may protect against caries. Such foods include cheese, yogurt, bologna, chocolate, and peanuts. Fats may protect by coating the teeth and reducing the retention of sugar and even plaque by changing the enamel surface activity. Fats also may have toxic effects on oral bacteria and may

decrease sugar solubility. Protein elevates the urea level in saliva and increases the buffering capacity of the saliva. Protein may also have an enamel-coating effect. Protein and fat in combination may raise plaque pH after exposure to carbohydrate. Tannins and other components of cocoa have been shown to suppress caries activity. The addition of fluoride to dietary sucrose in concentrations as low as 2 ppm has also been found to significantly reduce decay in rats.[13] Similar studies in humans have yet to be undertaken.

It has been proposed that the fibrous quality of some foods, such as celery or apples, may have a detergent effect on the teeth.[5] Such foods may remove gross debris during mastication, but they are ineffective at plaque removal. By requiring vigorous chewing, these foods may stimulate salivary flow, which in turn buffers plaque acid and promotes remineralization of enamel.

*Dietary Counseling*

Many of these findings have challenged long-accepted notions that have formed the basis of dietary recommendations to reduce the caries activity in children. Is sugared cereal worse than plain breakfast cereal if, in fact, it is cleared from the oral cavity more rapidly? Are potato chips a viable alternative to candy as a snack food?

Stookey[21] has enumerated the attributes of the ideal snack as follows: (1) It should stimulate salivary flow by its physical form; (2) it should be minimally retentive; (3) it should be relatively high in protein and low in fat, have minimal fermentable carbohydrate, and have a moderate mineral content (especially calcium, phosphate, and fluoride); and (4) it should have a pH above 5.5 so as not to decrease oral pH, with a large acid buffering capacity and a low sodium content. Certain foods, such as raw vegetables, meet most or all of these requirements. Present-day food technology should make it possible to create snacks that are nutritious and noncariogenic, but this will not happen until the food industry finds a reliable cariogenicity test and the incentives to invest in such production.

In the meantime, we are left with the difficult task of attempting to alter the dietary habits of caries-susceptible patients. While such attempts often fail, the profession has an obligation to make dietary information available to them. Although it is neither feasible nor desirable to eliminate sugar completely from the diet, we can recommend that between-meal snacks be should acquire the skills and knowledge to conduct effective personal oral hygiene.

4. *Participation in health care decisions.* Classically, dentists are taught to see the school-aged child as a passive recipient of care. Unfortunately, the result may be poor compliance and a tendency for the child to consider the dentist rather than himself or herself as responsible for his or her own health.

## THE HISTORY

Elements of history taking and recording are discussed in Chapter 18. The parent remains the historian of choice, yet the older school-aged child can provide corroborative information. An important aspect of history taking in this group should be the involvement of the child, whose role initially may be that of listener but can evolve into that of participant. By adolescence, the child can provide accurate, valuable information. Some instances in which this involvement may have profound benefits for both health care provider and patient are (1) when antibiotic premedication for heart disease is required, (2) when there is a history of illness that accompanies a complicated medical history, or (3) when there is a history of a positive reaction to the hepatitis antigen. The payoff for imparting this knowledge to the young patient through a good physician-patient relationship may not be evident until the child seeks care as an adolescent. A health history form should address issues similar to those applicable to the younger child but with different expectations. The differences in patient history for children in this age group in general include the following:

1. *Medical intervention has usually occurred.* Most children have a physician and may have experienced an emergency visit or some invasive procedure. School enrollment has required a physical examination and other treatment for the majority of children.

2. *A health history has evolved.* The coagulation and immunologic systems have been tested, and a developmental profile is available. Most childhood-onset disorders manifest themselves at some time during this period, but some have not been noted. Therefore, symptoms remain an important aspect of history taking.

3. *A dental history should be evolving,* and caries experiences and prevention, care delivery, and dental development should be established. Children usually have undergone a dental visit as part of school enrollment.

4. *The history should capture those children early on the curve of health experiences.* We would be naïve to presume that children are not exposed to different environmental, social, and other issues than a generation ago. The history form, unfortunately, should address substance use and pregnancy.

## THE EXAMINATION

As in younger children, the dental examination includes a behavioral assessment; general appraisal; and head and neck, facial, intraoral, and radiographic examinations.

### Behavioral Assessment

Another advantage for the dentist is the child's emergence into a period when few children experience behavioral problems that cannot be resolved with a simple tell-show-do method. Even early in this period, most children can be reasoned with to accept dental treatment. The child who resists attempts at careful and compassionate explanations of care may be suffering from a more significant emotional or psychological problem. Significant behavior problems in the presence of normal intelligence signal a serious deviation from normal. The diagnostic process for behavioral problems is clearer in this age group because so few children resist care. The dentist's diagnostic approach should include ruling out major behavioral problems by a history and general appraisal. The next step is to "chair-test" the child, using the dentist's proven techniques of managing children. The technique used may be tell-show-do, positive reinforcement, voice control, or some other method that has worked consistently in the past. Remember that consent should be obtained from the parent if the behavior management technique used is not one that a reasonable parent would expect.[10] If behavioral intervention fails, the dentist should consider further evaluation or referral. Some causes of extreme behavior problems in this age group include substance abuse, physical or sexual abuse, family problems, or a minor learning disability.

## General Appraisal

The school-aged population provides a wide range of physical and emotional profiles, yet the general appraisal should be easier from several standpoints. First, the school-aged child should have developed gross motor skills, and any variations from normal should be obvious. For example, the toddler may be active but still clumsy. The school-aged child, even at the early end of this age group, can play with skill. Speech development should also well exceed that of the preschooler, as should the child's emotional and intellectual status. This adaptation is really a manifestation of development of the brain and is one reason why schooling begins at this age.

One advantage available to the dentist who treats children in this age group is the host of health professionals with whom he or she can work if problems are noted. School placement often has identified problem areas, and the appropriate therapy usually has been initiated. These professionals can assist in clarifying findings made during the dental visit. Box 30-1 lists some characteristics of the school-aged child that are important in the diagnostic process.

## Head and Neck Examination

The head and neck examination should be completed in a manner similar to that outlined in Chapter 18.

## Facial Examination

Facial examination of the 6- to 12-year-old child is a systematic examination of the face in three planes of space. It is essentially the same as the facial examination described in Chapter 18, and the reader should review that information if

---

### BOX 30-1

### Selected Developmental Characteristics of the 6- to 12-Year-Old Child

**Intellectual Development**
Demonstrates school readiness early in this period
    Should be able to read and write in this period
    Becomes capable of logical thought

**Psychological Development**
Acquires a sense of accomplishment for tasks
    Learns responsibility for actions
    Develops a sense of right and wrong
    Looks outside the home for standards or values

**Physical Development**
Refinement of motor skills occurs as central nervous system develops
    Spine straightens to improve posture
    Sinuses enlarge
    Lymphoid system reaches high point of development

**Physiologic Development**

| | 6-Year-Old | 9-Year-Old | 12-Year-Old |
|---|---|---|---|
| *Height* | Boys = 121 cm<br>Girls = 119 cm<br>(Growth rate is approximately 6 cm/yr in this period.) | Boys = 140 cm<br>Girls = 137 cm | Boys = 154 cm<br>Girls = 157 cm |
| *Weight (75th percentile)* | Boys = 24 kg<br>Girls = 23 kg<br>(Growth rate is approximately 3 to 3.5 kg/yr in this period.) | Boys = 33 kg<br>Girls = 32 kg | Boys = 44 kg<br>Girls = 45 kg |
| *Pulse (average for age)* | 100/min | 90/min | 85–90/min |
| *Respiration (50th percentile)* | 23/min | 20/min | 18/min |
| *Blood pressure (average for age)* | 105/60 mm Hg | 110/65 mm Hg | 115.65 mm Hg |

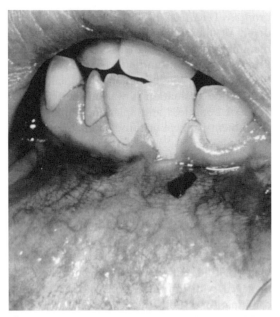

**Figure 30-4**  This labial gingival cleft is caused by a lack of attached gingival tissue, an abnormally high (coronal) muscle attachment, an anterior crossbite, less than ideal gingival health, or a combination of these factors.

must be repositioned prior to or after orthodontic treatment because they pull on attached marginal tissue and compromise gingival health or prevent space closure.

3. *Identification of problem areas, such as mandibular and maxillary anterior teeth.* Calculus accumulation, inflammation secondary to anterior crowding, poor cleaning, and eruptive gingivitis are examples of localized problems that require specialized attention.

Numerous gingival indices exist to assess inflammation.[29] The gingival index (GI)[17] can be adapted for pediatric use. The GI uses the following scoring system: 0 = normal gingiva; 1 = mild inflammation: slight change in color, slight edema, no bleeding on probing; 2 = moderate inflammation: redness, edema, and glazing, or bleeding on probing; 3 = severe inflammation: marked redness and edema, tendency toward spontaneous bleeding, ulceration.

In the private-practice setting, it may be easier to modify an existing index, using key teeth to provide baseline readings and progress. These readings can be recorded on the examination form adjacent to the data for the teeth being examined. Routine performance of full-mouth probing is not warranted.

**Oral hygiene evaluation.**  The assessment of clinical needs and patient skills in oral hygiene is a part of the examination process. The history should reveal a pattern of personal care, and the clinical examination should document the effectiveness of care and address problem areas in the oral cavity. A patient's brushing skills and dexterity in flossing can be judged at chairside and are generally directly correlated with classically difficult-to-clean areas such as plaque accumulation on teeth opposite to the side on which the brush is held, buccally placed canine teeth, and lingual surfaces. This information should be used to formulate an individual hygiene strategy. If orthodontic treatment is being considered, oral hygiene instructions should be given before orthodontic treatment is started and should be consistently reinforced during the treatment.

*Occlusal Evaluation*

The occlusal evaluation is organized around a systematic approach to alignment and the anteroposterior, transverse, and vertical planes of space.[26]

**Alignment.**  The intraoral occlusal examination in the mixed dentition begins with an assessment of arch form and alignment characteristics. An ideal arch should be symmetric in the anteroposterior and transverse dimensions. Minor asymmetry may exist but is usually confined to the anterior region if there is inadequate space for eruption of the permanent incisors. Significant asymmetry is rare, and is usually indicative of skeletal asymmetry or some type of oral habit or crossbite that has displaced the teeth and alveolus. Arch form is described as being either U or V shaped. Alignment problems are usually the result of a true arch length deficiency or a transitional arch length deficiency due to the size of the erupting permanent teeth. These are most common in the anterior portions of the arch but can occur anywhere. The type of alignment problem should be noted during the examination. The teeth can be tipped, bodily positioned, or rotated in their aberrant location. These types of positioning errors have definite implications for the type of treatment that can be recommended.

**Tooth number.**  After the form and symmetry of each arch have been characterized, it is imperative to count the number of permanent and primary teeth. A clinical examination and appropriate radiographs allow the practitioner to determine which teeth are present, developing, or missing. Disturbances in the initiation and proliferation stage of tooth development may lead to an abnormal number of teeth. Teeth that do not form are referred to as congenitally missing (Fig. 30-5). The most common missing teeth in the permanent dentition, with the exception of the maxillary and mandibular third molars, are the maxillary lateral incisor and the mandibular second premolar.[32,20] In general, the most distal tooth in a class of teeth is most liable to be congenitally missing. Some have looked at whether there is a genetic component to missing and impacted teeth. It is reported that patients with palatally impacted canines exhibit a higher incidence of missing permanent teeth than the general population and that several generations in the family will exhibit the same palatal impaction[25] (Fig. 30-6).

Supernumerary teeth are teeth added to the normal complement of teeth. These teeth are most often found in the maxillary midline region and are called mesiodens (Fig. 30-7). Supernumerary teeth are also frequently found distal to the maxillary molars and in the mandibular premolar regions.[33]

Although not a tooth in the strictest sense, the odontoma is discussed in this section on tooth number. The odontoma is a benign mixed tumor of enamel and dentin that is diagnosed radiographically. Two types of odontomas are identified. Odontomas that resemble teeth are called compound odontomas; those that are irregularly shaped are labeled complex odontomas. Both types may interfere with normal tooth eruption and are usually treated by surgical removal before eruption problems arise but late enough to avoid

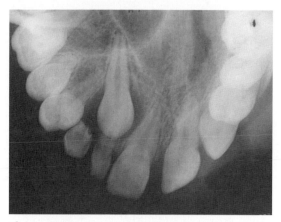

**Figure 30-6** The occurrence of multiple anomalies of tooth position, number, and shape linked by genetics is demonstrated in this patient with a mesially positioned maxillary right canine, a maxillary right peg lateral, and congenitally missing maxillary left lateral incisor.

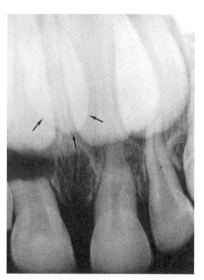

**Figure 30-7** A midline supernumerary tooth, or mesiodens, is situated between the unerupted maxillary central incisors. Arrows indicate the position of the mesiodens, which can cause disturbances in eruption and adjacent tooth formation.

surgical trauma to adjacent developing teeth (Fig. 30-8).

**Tooth structure.** Disturbances in the morphodifferentiation and histodifferentiation stages of tooth development result in alterations of tooth size and shape. Each arch should be examined for generalized large (macrodontia) or small (microdontia) teeth and for localized tooth size discrepancies. Generalized large or small teeth usually can be aligned so that there is a

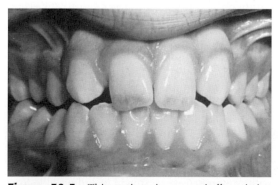

**Figure 30-5** This patient is congenitally missing both maxillary lateral incisors. The most common missing teeth in the permanent dentition, besides the third molars, are the maxillary lateral incisor and the mandibular second premolar.

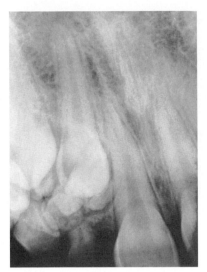

**Figure 30-8**    An odontoma is impeding the eruption of the maxillary right lateral incisor and canine. The odontoma should be surgically removed before eruption problems arise but late enough to avoid surgical trauma to the adjacent developing teeth. (Courtesy Dr. Phillip R. Parker.)

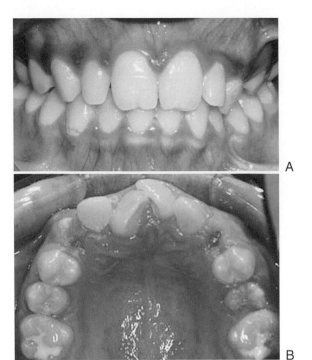

**Figure 30-9**    **A,** This maxillary right lateral incisor is smaller than normal; such a tooth is often called a peg lateral owing to its mesiodistal tapered form. Localized tooth size problems of this type make it difficult to establish good dental relationships. **B,** The maxillary right central incisor shown here in a lingual position is at least 2 mm larger than normal. Isolated teeth such as these often require mesiodistal interproximal reduction to fit harmoniously in a final occlusion.

compatible occlusal relationship if the teeth in both arches are equally affected. However, localized tooth size problems make it difficult to establish good dental relationships. Again, the most distal tooth in the dental class is the one most often affected. Undersized maxillary lateral incisors and mandibular second premolars are the most common isolated problems in tooth size (Fig. 30-9, *A*). Sometimes complex orthodontic and restorative treatment is necessary to achieve a harmonious occlusal relationship and satisfy aesthetic requirements when local tooth size problems exist. This type of treatment usually amounts to distributing space between the teeth so that when the teeth are restored to normal size and contour, they fit in a good occlusal relationship with good anterior aesthetics. Other times, treatment may mean reducing the mesiodistal dimension of oversized crowns through interproximal reduction (Fig. 30-9, *B*).

Teeth with abnormal crown and root morphologic characteristics may create occlusal problems. Careful clinical and radiographic examination is necessary to diagnose these problems. If the abnormality involves the crown (maxillary peg lateral or talon cusp), either the crown should be recontoured by addition of restorative material to increase its size or the talon cusp should be reduced in size by selective equilibration to elimi-

nate occlusal interference. Both conditions usually require tooth movement prior to definitive restorative care to obtain an aesthetically pleasing and functional result. Root structure abnormalities such as significant dilaceration may make orthodontic movement of teeth difficult (Fig. 30-10). Often the portion of the root apical to the irregularity is resorbed or remodeled during tooth movement. If a tooth with root abnormalities is scheduled for extraction, it may be prudent to refer the patient to a specialist because the abnormality will certainly complicate the extraction. Finally, fused or geminated teeth can pose difficulties due to their size. Often this situation requires tooth removal and prosthetic replacement. In some cases the teeth can be managed with comprehensive treatment including endodontics, surgery, orthodontics, and restorative care.[4,37]

**Tooth position.**    The position of erupted and unerupted permanent teeth in this age group should be noted and compared with the normal

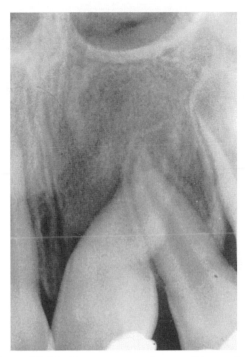

**Figure 30-10** Root structure abnormalities, such as this dilacerated maxillary left central incisor, make orthodontic movement of teeth very difficult. A dilaceration of this magnitude makes the root more susceptible to apical resorption and complicates the final positioning of the crown and root.

sequence and time of eruption. Minor asymmetry in dental eruption is normal, and there is little cause for concern if less than 6 months difference in eruption exists between contralateral sides of the mouth. Four tooth positioning problems are associated with the mixed dentition: ectopic eruption, transposition, impaction, and primary failure of eruption and the midline diastema. Interestingly, there appears to be a genetic component to some of these tooth position problems. Several studies have shown a genetic link between missing teeth, tooth anomalies, and altered eruption paths.[1,21,22,23] There seems to be clustering of these problems. For example, a missing maxillary lateral incisor is often associated with an altered canine eruption pattern. If one of these conditions is identified, the clinician should examine the patient for these other related problems.

*Ectopic eruption* describes a path of eruption that causes root resorption of a portion or all of the adjacent primary tooth. Ectopic eruption is most often associated with the permanent maxillary first molar, mandibular lateral incisor, and maxillary canine.[9,16,24] In ectopic eruption of the permanent first molar, a portion of the erupting

first molar resorbs the distal root of the primary second molar and is inhibited from erupting by the distal portion of the primary molar (Fig. 30-11). In many cases, the permanent molar spontaneously "jumps" or moves distally and erupts into the correct position. In other cases, the permanent molar lodges under the primary molar crown and no longer erupts. Usually, no pain or discomfort is associated with ectopic eruption unless a communication develops between the oral cavity and the pulpal tissue of the primary molar, causing an abscess. Permanent molar ectopic eruption is often detected during clinical examination and confirmed with routine bitewing radiographs.

The prevalence of permanent first molar ectopic eruption is reported to be 3% to 4%.[15] Several possible causes of ectopic molar eruption have been proposed as follows: (1) the maxillary teeth are larger than normal, (2) the maxilla is smaller than normal, (3) the maxilla is positioned further posteriorly than normal in relation to the cranial base, or (4) the angulation of the erupting maxillary permanent first molar is abnormal.[2,28]

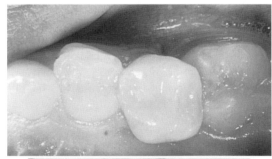

A

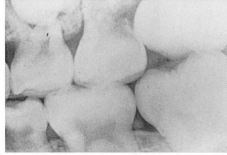

B

**Figure 30-11** In ectopic eruption, the permanent first molar resorbs a portion of the distal root of the primary second molar. **A,** In this case, the permanent first molar has lodged under the primary second molar crown. In other cases, the permanent molar spontaneously "jumps" or moves distally and erupts into the normal position. **B,** The distal resorption of the primary molar root is evident on this radiograph.

Although ectopic molar eruption may occur in the mandibular arch, it is more common in the maxilla. Ectopic eruption of the permanent lateral incisor is most common in the mandibular arch. The erupting incisor resorbs all or a portion of the primary canine root because the path of eruption is abnormal, there is transitional crowding from the primary to the permanent dentition, or there is a true arch length deficiency. The diagnosis is generally signaled by premature primary canine exfoliation, often accompanied by a midline shift to the side of the ectopic eruption or impeded eruption of the lateral incisor, or it is discovered on an occlusal radiograph (Fig. 30-12). The third common type of ectopic eruption occurs with maxillary permanent canine eruption and associated resorption of the permanent lateral incisor (Fig. 30-13). Studies have shown that if canines erupt from a more medial position in the dental arch and with a slightly more mesial horizontal path of eruption (an average of 10 degrees), there is a greater risk of lateral incisor resorption. It is recommended to remove the primary canine to promote more ideal canine eruption if the canine cusp in periapical, occlusal, or panoramic films is positioned medially to the midline of the lateral incisor.[5,6] A related phenomenon is *lingual eruption* of the permanent incisors, predominantly the mandibular incisors (Fig. 30-14). The prevalence of lingually erupting mandibular incisors is about 10%.[9] The cause of ectopic and lingually erupting incisors is not well established. One explanation suggests that ectopic and lingual eruption of the incisors results

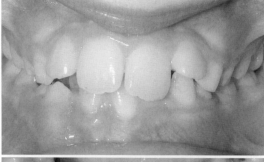

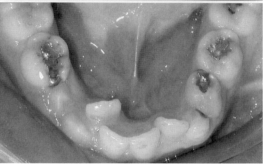

**Figure 30-12** When a primary canine is lost due to ectopic eruption of a permanent lateral incisor, the midline often shifts to the side of the lost primary canine. **A,** It is apparent from this view that the mandibular midline has shifted to the patient's right. **B,** The permanent right lateral incisor is now blocked to the lingual as a consequence of the mandibular midline shift.

from an abnormal pattern of resorption. Alternatively, it has been suggested that lingual eruption is a variation of the normal eruption pattern because the lower incisor tooth buds form lingual to the primary incisors and may not migrate facially.

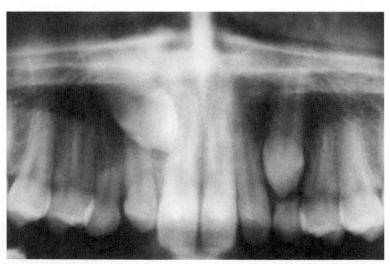

**Figure 30-13** The maxillary right canine has erupted into the lateral incisor space and resorbed a portion of the root. This type of resorption is more common than believed, but often not to this extent.

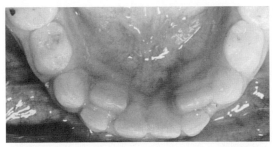

**Figure 30-14** Ectopic eruption of the permanent lateral incisors is most common in the mandibular arch. In this example, the mandibular lateral incisors erupted lingual to their ideal position and the primary laterals are still present. In some cases, the lateral incisors erupt into a more normal position but cause premature exfoliation of the primary canine.

*Transposition* occurs when there is "a positional interchange of two adjacent teeth, especially their roots or the development or eruption of a tooth in a position occupied normally by a nonadjacent tooth."[23] Usually transpositions are observed later in the transitional dentition years. The early-stage transposition is uncommon but is the type of transposition observed in the early mixed-dentition years (Fig. 30-15). This usually is a transposition of the mandibular lateral incisor and canine.[22] The lateral incisor will show distal tipping, resorption of the primary canine (and sometimes the primary first molar), and rotation as it migrates. Other transpositions that are observed later in the transitional years are likely to be the mature mandibular lateral and canine, and

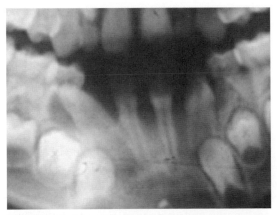

**Figure 30-15** Early-stage transposition of the mandibular lateral incisors and the canines. Note that the permanent mandibular right lateral incisor has resorbed the primary canine and the primary first molar is about to be lost. If intercepted early, true transposition will not occur.

the more prevalent transpositions of the maxillary canine and first premolar and maxillary canine and lateral incisor.[23]

*Tooth impaction* is diagnosed during the clinical examination or from appropriate radiographs. Overretained primary teeth, supernumerary teeth, severe crowding, or a failure in the eruption mechanism cause impaction of the anterior teeth (Fig. 30-16, *A*). The permanent tooth usually erupts if the overretained primary tooth or supernumerary tooth is removed. If the tooth is impacted as a result of crowding, it is necessary to provide space either orthodontically or by extraction to allow eruption. Generally, the last tooth to erupt in an arch or quadrant is impacted because all of the space is previously spoken for. This mechanism or the aberrant eruption direction usually is the cause of impaction of the maxillary canine. The maxillary canine is most often the last tooth to erupt into the arch. It also erupts or travels the longest distance to take its place in the arch. These two factors combine to make the maxillary canine the most common impacted tooth in the maxillary arch and indeed the mouth (Fig. 30-16, *B*). Posterior tooth impaction is normally the result of inadequate arch length. Inadequate arch length is caused by a tooth–jaw size discrepancy or space loss as a result of premature primary tooth loss. If the arch length problem is generalized, either permanent teeth should be removed or the arch should be expanded to allow eruption of all the permanent teeth. Limited, localized crowding due to space loss can be treated by orthodontically regaining the lost space.

*Primary failure of eruption* is an unusual eruption problem that affects the posterior teeth. It is diagnosed when a tooth fails to erupt despite the presence of adequate space and the absence of overlying hard tissue that prevents eruption. Furthermore, all teeth distal to the affected tooth also fail to erupt. The cause of primary failure of eruption is unknown but appears to have a genetic component.[27,30]

A small, maxillary *midline diastema* in the early mixed dentition is normal. Typically it is caused by the position of the unerupted lateral incisors or canines (Fig. 30-17). The unerupted teeth are positioned superior and distal to the roots of the central incisors and direct the central incisor roots toward the midline and the crowns toward the distal (Fig. 30-18). As the lateral incisors or canines erupt, the incisors upright themselves

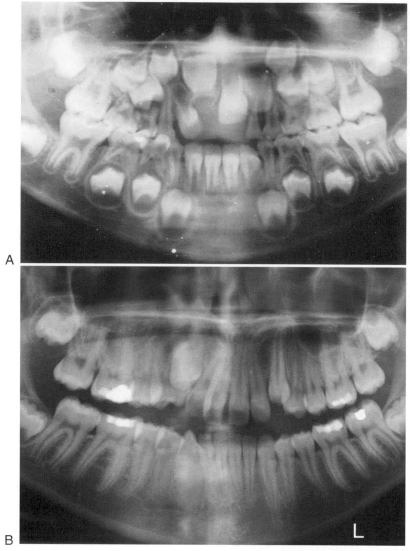

**Figure 30-16**   In the transitional years, tooth impaction in the anterior region is usually caused by overretained primary teeth, supernumerary teeth, or severe crowding. In a few cases, a failure in the eruption mechanism is responsible for the delayed eruption. **A,** In this case, the maxillary right central incisor is completely inverted and is directed toward the nasal cavity. **B,** The ultimate sequela of a lack of space is illustrated by this impacted maxillary right canine even though the orientation of the tooth is correct. Note that the maxillary left canine will successfully erupt.

slowly and the midline space begins to close. Treatment to close a diastema is usually delayed until the permanent canines are fully erupted unless the space available for eruption of the lateral incisors is severely limited. If the diastema is larger than 3 mm, the cause may be a mesiodens (see Fig. 30-7), a localized tooth size problem, or abnormal incisor positioning. A mesiodens is usually discovered on radiographic examination, and its removal normally allows the diastema to close. A size mismatch between the upper and lower teeth may result in a diastema. Normally,

the maxillary incisor crowns are small or excessively tapered, although the mandibular teeth may be too large in relation to the maxillary teeth. If large spaces are present, a combination of tooth movement and anterior restorations is required to correct the size discrepancy. Abnormal incisor positioning and protrusion also may result in a midline diastema. The abnormal positioning may be due to past or present finger habits or to abnormal eruption. Its best treatment is to first eliminate the habit and then to retract the incisors orthodontically and consolidate space.

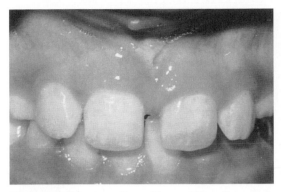

**Figure 30-17** A small maxillary midline diastema is normal in the mixed dentition. The diastema tends to close with the eruption of the permanent maxillary lateral incisors and canines.

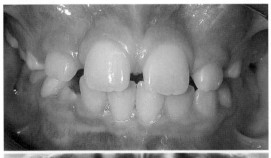

A

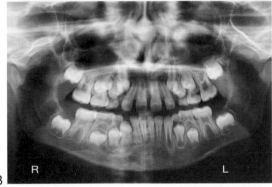

B

**Figure 30-18** **A,** The "ugly duckling" stage is evident when the crowns of the lateral incisor tip distally and open diastema between the anterior teeth. **B,** The permanent canines are pushing against the roots of the permanent lateral incisors.

**Anteroposterior dimension.** Permanent molar and canine relationships should be noted and compared with the anteroposterior skeletal relationships that were determined during the extraoral examination. Permanent molar and canine relationships are illustrated in Figure 30-19. Dental relationships generally reflect the underlying skeletal relationships, including asymmetry, although it is feasible to have different

dental and skeletal relationships if teeth are missing or have drifted. For example, a person with a class I skeletal relationship may have a class II molar relationship if there has been posterior space loss and the permanent maxillary first molar drifted forward into the space (Fig. 30-20).

If the permanent teeth are properly aligned in the alveolar bone at a normal angulation, overjet is a direct measurement of the relationship between the dental arches. Normal overjet is approximately 2 mm; therefore, the discrepancy between the arches can be calculated by subtracting 2 mm from the measured overjet. Incisor position is not always ideal, however, and estimates of dental arch discrepancies must be adjusted if both upper and lower anterior teeth are not protrusive or retrusive.

**Transverse relationship.** Dental midline and posterior crossbite evaluation is conducted in the same manner as described in Chapter 18. Usually, dental midline deviations are the result of simply moderate to severe crowding or ectopic eruption and tooth loss with a shift of the midline as teeth realign in the newly available space (see Fig. 30-12). Functional deviations of the mandible are identified by noting discrepancies between centric relation and centric occlusion (see Figs. 18-11 and 18-12). Posterior crossbites are determined to be either unilateral or bilateral. In the early mixed-dentition years, treatments for both skeletal and dental crossbites are essentially the same. As the child becomes older, it becomes more critical to identify whether a crossbite is due to skeletal or dental causes. However, management of posterior crossbite in the complete permanent dentition varies according to whether the crossbite is skeletal or dental in origin and the estimate of whether the midpalatal suture is bridged or closed.

**Vertical dimension.** The vertical dental examination is concerned with overbite and open-bite measurements and ankylosis. Normal overbite in this age group is approximately 2 mm. If there is a deviation from normal, the clinician should try to determine if the deviation is due to a dental or a skeletal problem. If the facial examination revealed a vertical skeletal problem, it is sometimes reflected in the dental relationships. Treatment of the malocclusion varies with the source of the problem.

Ankylosis of the primary teeth can present several problems because of the magnitude of vertical dentoalveolar growth. Dental eruption

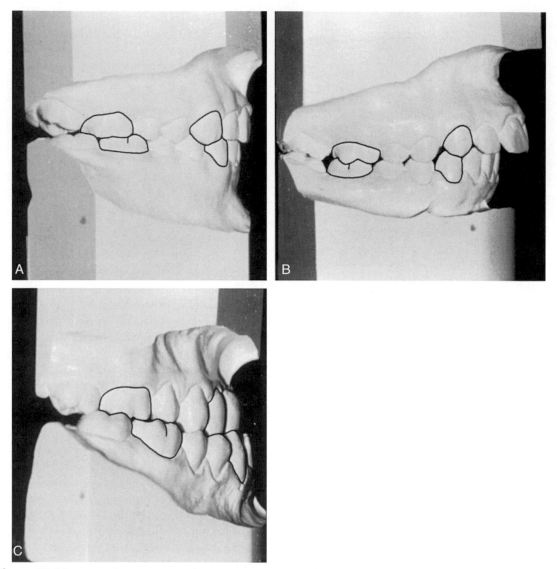

**Figure 30-19** **A,** In the permanent dentition, permanent molar and canine relationships are determined and compared with the anteroposterior skeletal relationships. To determine molar relationships, the position of the mesiobuccal cusp of the permanent maxillary first molar is related to the position of the facial groove of the permanent mandibular first molar. If the mesiobuccal cusp occludes in the facial groove, the molar relationship is called class I. The canine relationship is determined by the relationship of the maxillary canine to the embrasure between the mandibular canine and the first premolar (or primary first molar). If the maxillary canine occludes in the embrasure, the canine relationship is also called class I. **B,** If the mesiobuccal cusp of the permanent maxillary first molar occludes mesial to the mandibular facial groove, the molar relationship is called class II. The canine relationship is called class II if the maxillary canine occludes mesial to the mandibular canine–first premolar embrasure. **C,** If the mesiobuccal cusp of the permanent maxillary first molar occludes distal to the mandibular facial groove, the molar relationship is called class III. The canine relationship is class III if the maxillary canine occludes distal to the mandibular canine–first premolar embrasure.

and vertical growth of the alveolus may amount to as much as 10 mm from age 6 to age 12. Thus, ankylosis of a primary tooth at an early age may result in large marginal ridge discrepancies, tipping of adjacent teeth, and vertical bone loss. Most of these problems, with the exception of

space loss, resolve when the succedaneous tooth erupts. Ankylosed teeth and associated problems are discussed in Chapter 18, and the reader is referred to that chapter for a more detailed discussion. One aspect of ankylosed primary teeth that must be addressed differently is when the

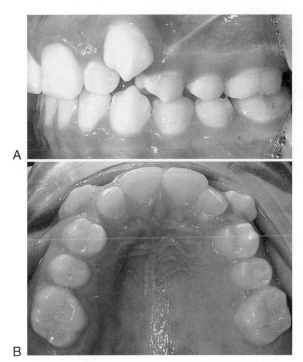

**Figure 30-20**   Space loss can cause dental relationships to not reflect skeletal relationships. **A,** This patient had maxillary posterior space loss with mesial drift so that the molars are class II and not reflective of the skeletal class I relationships. **B,** The space loss caused the permanent canines to be block to the facial.

primary tooth is ankylosed and the succedaneous tooth is missing. If the vertical occlusal step becomes exaggerated, and by definition the vertical bone level relative to adjacent teeth is exaggerated, intervention is indicated. This is the case because there is no permanent tooth to erupt and bring alveolar bone with it. If the primary tooth is allowed to remain, its eventual extraction will leave a bony defect adjacent to the remaining permanent teeth (Fig. 30-21). Timely removal of the primary tooth and further treatment will have to be considered. Loss of bone due to extraction of a primary tooth without a successor is more rapid and severe in the anterior than in the posterior areas of the mouth.

## SUPPLEMENTAL ORTHODONTIC DIAGNOSTIC TECHNIQUES

### Photographs

Among the most basic diagnostic records routinely obtained are facial and intraoral photographs. These images can be obtained with conventional photography and result in prints or transparencies (slides). Recently, digital imaging has become a feasible alternative to conventional photography. Digital imaging offers the advantage of immediate confirmation of an image and easy storage and copying. Usually three extraoral images of the face are obtained: a frontal face with lips relaxed, a frontal face with posed smile, and a lateral face with lips relaxed. Five intraoral images consisting of a frontal, right and left lateral, and maxillary and mandibular occlusal views are obtained. These images can be unified electronically in a montage for the patient's record and printed or stored (Fig. 30-22).

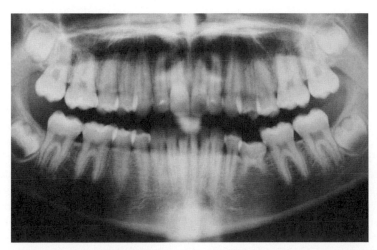

**Figure 30-21**   The ankylosed primary mandibular second molar demonstrates the alteration of bone level that can occur when ankylosed primary teeth without successors are maintained too long. Timely removal of the ankylosed tooth and treatment planning for orthodontic movement of the adjacent teeth or prosthetic replacement is critical.

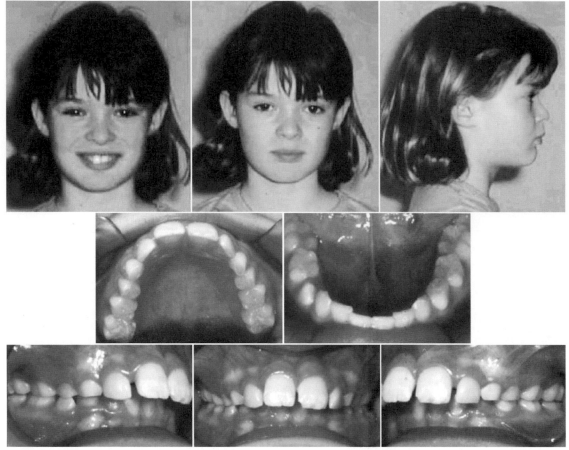

**Figure 30-22**   Digital images of pre- and posttreatment extra- and intraoral views of orthodontic patients can be stored electronically in the patient record or printed as a hard copy. This method circumvents the problems of losing images to either poor photographic technique or filing methods.

## Diagnostic Casts

Orthodontic treatment in the mixed dentition is more complex than treatment in the primary dentition. The clinician must consider the difference in size between the primary and permanent dentitions, the amount of space available for the permanent teeth, and the dental and skeletal status of the patient. This formidable job requires supplemental information to make accurate orthodontic diagnoses and to develop coherent treatment plans. Diagnostic study casts are an essential part of a thorough evaluation if problems are detected during the examination and definitive analysis or if treatment is required. These study casts can be conventional stone casts (see Fig. 18-15) or digital representations of stone casts. In the former case, the impressions are poured, separated, trimmed, and finished. In the latter case, the impression is disinfected and sent to a commercial laboratory where the impression

is poured and the resulting model scanned. A digital representation of the casts is transmitted to the practitioner via the Internet (Fig. 30-23). These digital images are less likely to be misplaced or broken and present no storage problems. They can also be manipulated to view all relationships for analysis (see Fig. 30-23). These digital images can be imported to the patient's record as static images for electronic archiving or printing (Fig. 30-24). The digital casts also can be analyzed and measured like conventional casts (Fig. 30-25). Findings recorded during the clinical examination are reviewed and confirmed using the casts. Alignment and tooth position characteristics should receive special attention because appliance design must be appropriate for each rotation and displacement.

After the diagnostic casts are studied, analyses should be performed to determine tooth size relationships and arch length adequacy using

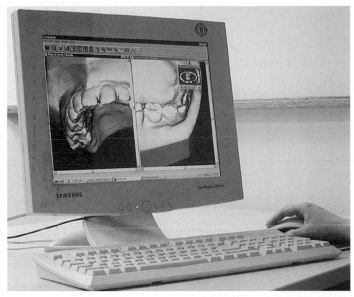

**Figure 30-23**  Digital casts can be displayed from the web or stored in image management software. The digital casts can be manipulated so that the casts can be separated or occluded and rotated or tipped to reveal all relationships. This prevents problems with loss and breakage of the casts and reduces the store space problems. (Courtesy OrthoCAD by Cadent, Inc.)

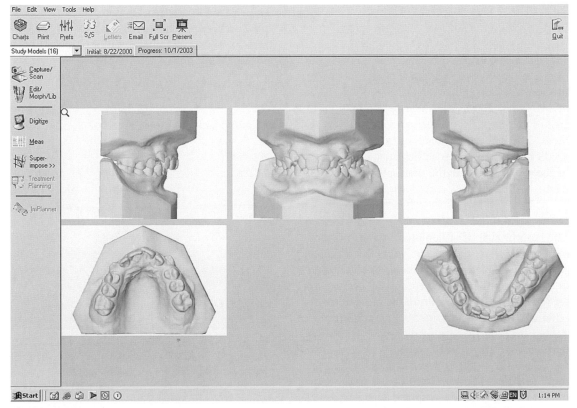

**Figure 30-24**  This screen capture demonstrates that the casts also can be printed or stored as static images. (Courtesy OrthoCAD by Cadent, Inc.)

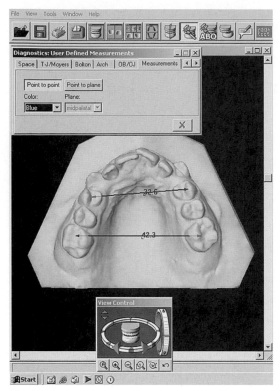

**Figure 30-25** The digital casts can also be measured electronically like conventional plaster casts so that arch dimensions can be evaluated. (Courtesy OrthoCAD by Cadent, Inc.)

either classical stone casts or digital images. The tooth size analysis attempts to compare the size of the teeth in one arch with the size of the teeth in the other. Tooth size must be compatible to ensure that teeth fit together correctly after treatment. The arch length analysis is an attempt to predict whether there is sufficient space available in the dental arch for the unerupted permanent teeth.

*Tooth Size Analysis*

The tooth size is calculated using Bolton's method.[3] Bolton selected 55 cases of excellent occlusion and measured the mesiodistal diameter of all teeth on the casts except for the permanent second and third molars. From the measurements obtained, Bolton determined that a certain ratio existed between the size of the upper and lower permanent teeth. A ratio could be determined for either the 6 anterior teeth or all 12 of the measured teeth. Little constructed a table based on the Bolton ratios to simplify tooth size determinations.[26] To use the table, the mesiodistal width of each permanent tooth is measured with

a needle-pointed divider or sharp Boley gauge (Fig. 30-26). The widths of the teeth are summed, and the intersection of the mandibular and maxillary totals is located on the table. The intersection gives the tooth size discrepancy in millimeters (Fig. 30-27). Because there is some error in measuring the casts and some error in the analysis itself, tooth size discrepancies of 1.5 mm or less are not considered significant. This analysis can be performed using the digital casts and the associated software (Fig. 30-28). Ultimately, when tooth-size problems are complex, diagnostic setups are required to determine which teeth should be positioned in specific orientations so that final diagnostic decisions can be made. Diagnostic setups are addressed in Chapter 37.

Several clinical situations contribute to tooth size discrepancy. Maxillary lateral incisors are commonly smaller than normal, resulting in a mandibular anterior tooth size excess (relatively speaking, the lower teeth are too large even though the problem is in the maxillary arch) (see Fig. 30-9, *A*). The size of the second premolar also varies highly. When significant tooth size discrepancies are discovered, the child is best referred to a specialist because simple tooth movement does not produce an aesthetically satisfactory result or good occlusion. Management of tooth size discrepancies often requires a combination of tooth movement and restorative dentistry.

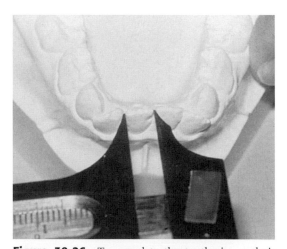

**Figure 30-26** To complete the tooth size analysis developed by Bolton, the mesiodistal width of each permanent tooth (except for second and third molars) is measured with a Boley gauge or a needle-pointed divider. The measurements are added together to provide totals for the six anterior teeth and for the overall arch.

## BOLTON ANALYSIS

### Maxillary Anterior Excess

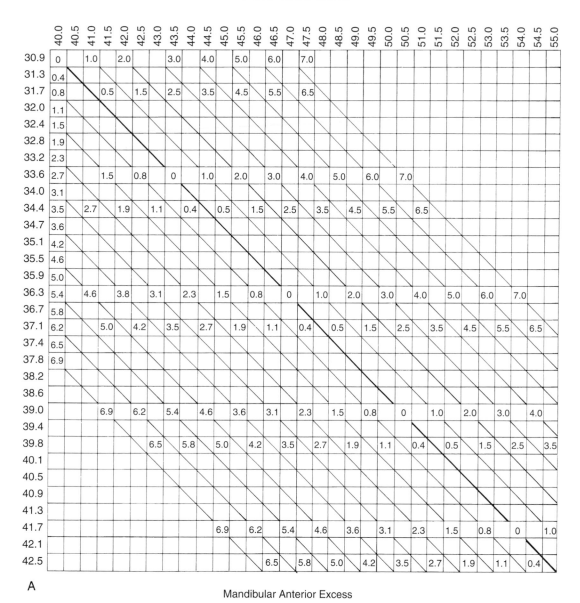

A

Mandibular Anterior Excess

**Figure 30-27**   To determine whether there is an anterior or overall tooth size discrepancy, the intersection of the maxillary and mandibular totals is located on the appropriate table. **A,** The width of the mandibular anterior teeth is indicated on the vertical axis, and the width of the maxillary anterior teeth is found on the horizontal axis. The intersection indicates whether a tooth size discrepancy exists and whether it is a maxillary or mandibular excess, and it indicates the size of the discrepancy in millimeters. (Courtesy Dr. Robert Little. From Proffit WR, Ackerman JL: Orthodontic diagnosis: the development of a problem list. In: Proffit WR et al, editors. Contemporary Orthodontics. St Louis, 1992, Mosby.)     *Continued*

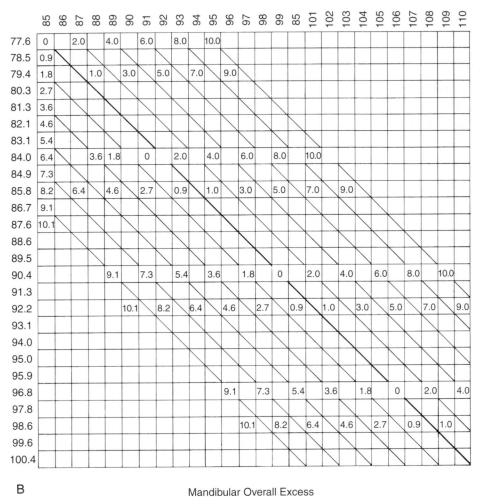

BOLTON ANALYSIS

Maxillary Overall Excess

**B**    Mandibular Overall Excess

**Figure 30-27—cont'd**    B, This table provides the same information for overall tooth size relationships.

*Space Analysis*

The space analysis is normally completed in the mixed dentition and is used to predict the amount of space available for the unerupted permanent teeth. A number of different methods of space analysis exist; however, all space analyses have two features in common. First, the permanent first molars and the mandibular incisors must be erupted to allow one to perform the analysis. Second, the mandibular incisors (sometimes in addition to other measurements) are used to predict the size of the unerupted canines and premolars. The following four assumptions are made in calculating a space analysis:

1. *All permanent teeth are developing normally.* Although this seems obvious, the analysis is meaningless if teeth are congenitally missing.

2. *There is a correlation between the size of the erupted mandibular incisors and the remaining succedaneous teeth.* The prediction of unerupted tooth size is more accurate if the correlation is strong.

3. *The prediction tables are most valid for a specific population.* The ethnic background of the patients used in most space analysis studies is northwestern European. If the patient is not of northwestern European descent, the analysis should be interpreted with some caution.

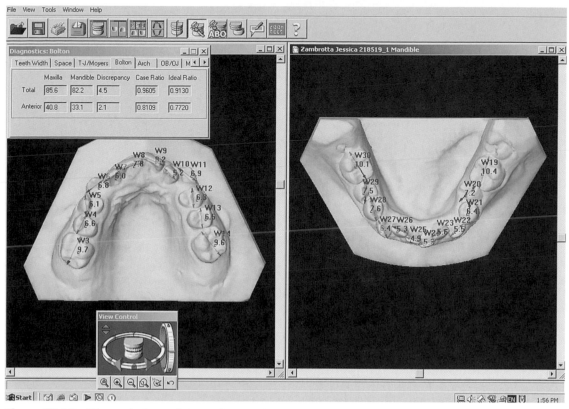

**Figure 30-28**   The tooth size analysis can be completed on conventional casts or electronically using digital casts. This screen capture shows that the teeth have been measured electronically using the cursor and mouse and then the analysis calculations performed by the software. (Courtesy OrthoCAD by Cadent, Inc.)

4. *Arch dimensions remain stable throughout growth.* This assumption is made to simplify the procedure, although it is recognized that the intercanine width, intermolar width, and arch length dimensions do change with age and eruption of teeth. Skeletal growth patterns may also affect arch dimension stability. Patients with class II mandibular deficiency tend to have proclined mandibular incisors to compensate for the deficiency, whereas those with class III deficiency tend to have more upright or retroclined mandibular incisors.

The most accurate space analysis currently available is a modification of the Hixon-Oldfather analysis.[34] This analysis uses lower incisor widths and the width of the unerupted premolars measured from radiographs to predict permanent tooth size. The Tanaka-Johnston analysis is most clinically useful because it requires no additional radiographs or tables to predict tooth size.[36] The first step in the Tanaka-Johnston analysis is to determine the available arch length. The distance

from the mesial of the permanent first molar to the mesial of the contralateral permanent first molar is measured by dividing the arch into several segments (Fig. 30-29, *A*). Each segment is measured over the contact points and incisal edges of the teeth. The segments are added together to provide an approximation of total arch length. The second step in the analysis is measurement of the width of the four mandibular incisors (Fig. 30-29, *B*). The widths of the four incisors are added together to determine the amount of room necessary for ideal alignment. The mesiodistal width of the unerupted mandibular canine and premolars in one quadrant is predicted by adding 10.5 mm to half the width of the four lower incisors (Fig. 30-29, *C*). The final step in the space analysis is to subtract the width of the lower incisors and two times the calculated premolar and canine width (both sides) from the total arch length approximation (Fig. 30-29, *D*). If the result is positive, there is more space available in the arch than is needed for the unerupted teeth. If the result is negative, the unerupted teeth

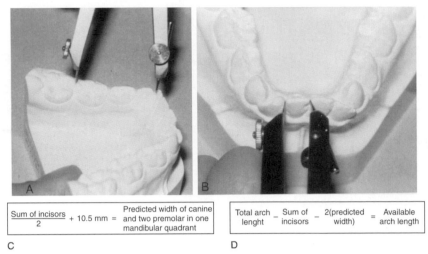

$$\frac{\text{Sum of incisors}}{2} + 10.5 \text{ mm} = \begin{array}{c}\text{Predicted width of canine}\\ \text{and two premolar in one}\\ \text{mandibular quadrant}\end{array}$$

C

$$\begin{array}{c}\text{Total arch}\\ \text{lenght}\end{array} - \begin{array}{c}\text{Sum of}\\ \text{incisors}\end{array} - \begin{array}{c}\text{2(predicted}\\ \text{width)}\end{array} = \begin{array}{c}\text{Available}\\ \text{arch length}\end{array}$$

D

**Figure 30-29 A,** The first step in the Tanaka-Johnston space is to determine available arch length. This is accomplished by dividing the arch into several segments and measuring each segment over the contact points and incisal edges of the teeth. **B,** The second step is to measure the width of the four mandibular incisors and add them together. **C,** The mesiodistal width of the unerupted canine and premolars in one quadrant is calculated by using the above formula. In the mandibular arch, 10.5 mm is used to determine the canine-premolar widths. In the maxillary arch, half the sum of the mandibular incisors is still used, but 11.0 mm is substituted for 10.5 mm because the unerupted permanent maxillary teeth are slightly larger. **D,** The final step in the analysis is to subtract the width of the four incisors and the predicted canine-premolar width from the total arch length. The remainder is the available arch length. If the remainder is positive, there is adequate space in the arch. If the remainder is negative, the permanent teeth require more room to erupt than is available in the arch.

require more space than is available to erupt in ideal alignment.

The maxillary space analysis is conducted in the same way. Maxillary arch length is measured, the width of the maxillary incisors is determined, and 11.0 mm is added to half the width of the four lower incisors to predict the size of the unerupted maxillary canine and premolars in one quadrant. The incisor width and the predicted canine-premolar width are subtracted from the total arch length to determine the amount of space available in the maxillary arch. This analysis also can be performed using the digital casts and the associated software (Fig. 30-30).

After the arch length predictions are made, the clinician should return to the cast and decide whether the results make sense. For example, if the arch appears to be crowded and the analysis predicts 5 mm of excess space, the analysis should be repeated or scrutinized for mistakes. Furthermore, the results should be considered in the context of the patient's soft tissue profile. The space analysis may indicate that the patient is moderately short of space, yet because he or she has very retrusive lips and incisors, the treatment of choice would be to expand the arch by moving

the incisors facially to provide better lip support (Fig. 30-31). Conversely, an analysis may predict that there is no crowding, yet extractions are considered necessary because the patient has very protrusive teeth and lips (Fig. 30-32). Dental protrusion and dental crowding are actually manifestations of the same problem. Whether the arch is crowded or the incisors are protrusive depends on the interaction between the pressure of the resting tongue and the circumoral musculature.

Two factors must be considered when using the Tanaka-Johnston analysis. It tends to overpredict slightly the width of the unerupted teeth. This makes the extent of crowding appear more severe than it actually is. In addition, if the patient is not of northwestern European background, it is difficult to know whether the prediction is over- or understated. An alternative method for determining available space is to measure arch length and incisor width as noted previously and then obtain periapical radiographs of the canines and premolars. The mesiodistal widths of the unerupted teeth are measured on the periapical films and then corrected for magnification by comparing the width of erupted teeth on the films with the actual width of these teeth on the

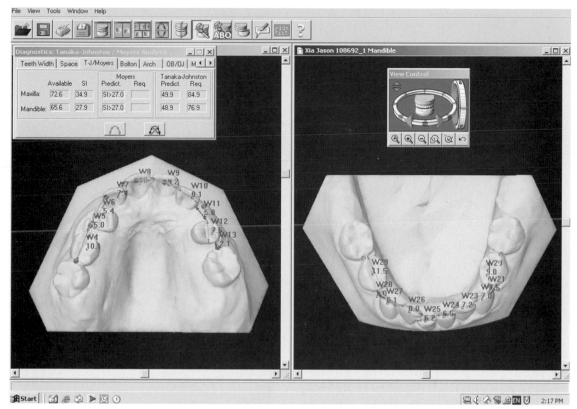

**Figure 30-30** The software packages that support the digital casts provide for several methods of space analysis. Again, using the tooth dimensions measured from the casts, the analyses are calculated. The accuracy of the result is contingent on careful management of the cursor for tooth measurement and how the arch dimensions are defined by the arch form, which is shown here as the overlying arc on each arch. (Courtesy OrthoCAD by Cadent, Inc.)

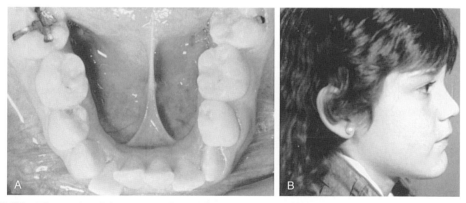

**Figure 30-31** The results of the space analysis (**A**) are considered in the context of the patient's soft tissue profile. In this example, the space analysis indicates that the arch length is short. The profile analysis (**B**), however, indicates that the patient cannot tolerate further loss of lip support. It is more prudent to expand the arch in this case to provide additional space than to extract teeth.

cast. With this technique, an individual space analysis can be performed for every patient. The disadvantages of this technique are that the patient is exposed to more radiation and undistorted radiographs of the canines are difficult to obtain.

## Analysis of Cephalometric Head Films

The facial profile analysis should be used by the clinician to gather basic information about the spatial relationships of the teeth and jaws. If the clinician identifies significant anteroposterior

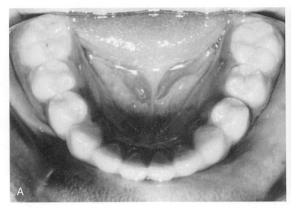

**Figure 30-32**    In this example, the space analysis (**A**) indicates that there is no shortage of arch length. The profile analysis (**B**), however, indicates that the patient has extremely protrusive lips and incisors. It is more prudent to extract teeth and retract the incisors and lips in this case. This figure illustrates the fact that dental crowding and dental protrusion are actually manifestations of the same problem.

or vertical discrepancies, the patient should be evaluated by a specialist. At that time, a lateral cephalometric radiograph may be used to obtain a more precise assessment of the problem. Analysis of lateral cephalometric head films is an additional diagnostic aid used to determine the relationship between the skeletal and dental structures. The cephalometric head film is normally ordered when significant skeletal discrepancies exist and comprehensive orthodontic treatment is being considered. The cephalometric analysis is an adjunct to the facial profile analysis. It provides confirmation of the clinical examination and possibly more specific information about the contribution of each skeletal and dental component to the malocclusion, and therefore must be viewed carefully.[8]

A large number of cephalometric analyses exist; however, the common goal of all analyses is to determine the size and position of the skeletal structures and the position of the teeth. The first step in the cephalometric analysis is to obtain a diagnostic head film. For the radiograph to be diagnostic, the head must be positioned in a cephalostat in a natural, relaxed posture (Fig. 30-33). In other words, the patient's head should not be tipped up or down or to one side or the other because this alters the perceived relationship of the skeletal structures and makes interpretation of the landmarks more difficult, even to the point of leading one to suspect skeletal

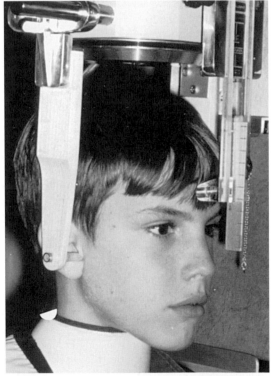

**Figure 30-33**    The first step in the cephalometric analysis is to obtain a diagnostic head film. After the patient has been appropriately draped with lead aprons, the head is placed in the cephalostat in a natural, relaxed position. Natural head position is produced by having the patient look at the distant horizon.

asymmetry. A mandibular deficiency may not be apparent if the patient's head is tipped upward. Natural head position is produced by having the patient look at the distant horizon. The teeth should be together and the lips relaxed when the film is exposed.

After the head film is made, the radiograph should be screened for pathologic findings. Traditionally, if no pathologic findings were found, landmarks were located on a piece of matte acetate paper placed over the film, the structures traced, and relationships measured (Fig. 30-34). These linear angular and proportional measurements made from the tracing provided the basis for the analysis. Nowadays landmarks can be located on a scanned or digital radiographic image using a mouse and desktop computing software (Fig. 30-35). The software generates linear and angular measurements, and a graphic image of the face constructed from the digitized landmarks provides the basis for the cephalometric analysis (Fig. 30-36). These same programs can be used to project treatment goals.

The analysis, regardless of how the measurements and comparisons are obtained, should evaluate the position of the maxilla and mandible in relation to that of the cranial base and the relationship of the maxilla and mandible to one another. Analysis also should evaluate the position of the teeth in each jaw and the relationship of the upper teeth to the lower teeth. Vertical relationships between total, upper, and lower facial heights of the anterior face should be determined. Finally, the analysis should evaluate the soft tissue profile and the position of the lips in relation to the teeth, nose, and chin. A cephalometric analysis requires two reference lines to orient the position of the teeth and jaws. Historically, the Frankfort horizontal plane has been used as the horizontal reference line because it was thought to be parallel to the true horizontal plane when the patient was looking at a distant point. The Frankfort horizontal plane connects the upper rim of the external auditory meatus (porion) with the inferior border of the orbital rim (orbitale) (Fig. 30-37). Although the Frankfort horizontal plane is not always parallel to the true horizontal plane, it is still the most widely used horizontal reference line. The vertical reference line can be either a true perpendicular (to the horizon) through the nasion (the bony bridge of the nose) or a line perpendicular to the Frankfort plane through the nasion. The position and size of the maxilla and mandible are evaluated by comparing A point (maxilla) and pogonion (mandible), the most anterior points on these

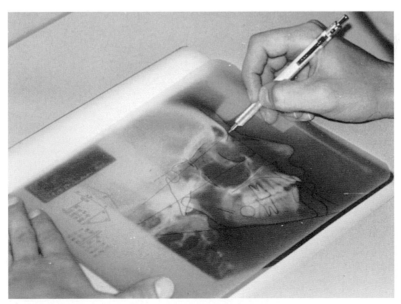

**Figure 30-34** After the head film has been screened for pathologic findings, a piece of matte acetate paper is placed over the film, the anatomic structures are traced, and landmarks are identified. Linear and angular measurements can be made manually from this tracing by using a protractor and ruler. These measurements provide the basis for the cephalometric analysis.

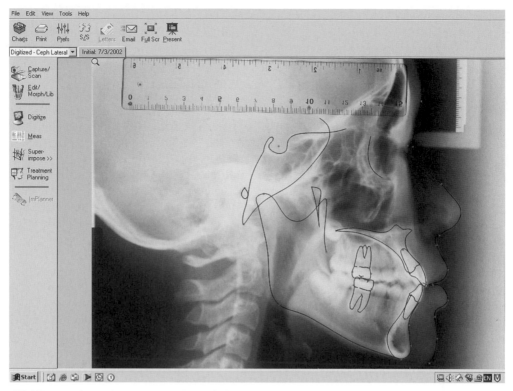

**Figure 30-35**   An alternative to tracing the cephalometric radiograph by hand is to digitize the critical points and have the measurements performed electronically by the software package (Dolphin). It is no longer necessary to have a separate digitizer for this purpose. This procedure can be performed with a personal computer and mouse using a digital radiographic image. The computer will provide various representations of traced landmarks and anatomy as well as lines and planes.

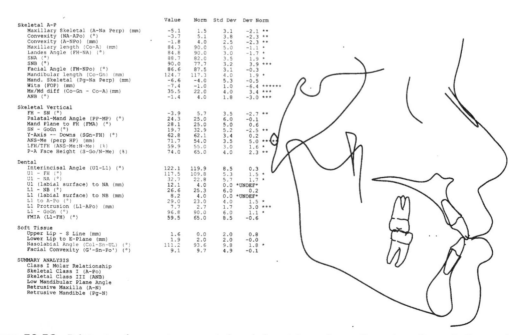

| | Value | Norm | Std Dev | Dev Norm |
|---|---|---|---|---|
| **Skeletal A-P** | | | | |
| Maxillary Skeletal (A-Na Perp) (mm) | -5.1 | 1.5 | 3.1 | -2.1 ** |
| Convexity (NA-APo) (°) | -3.7 | 5.1 | 3.8 | -2.3 ** |
| Convexity (A-NPo) (mm) | -1.8 | 4.0 | 2.5 | -2.3 ** |
| Maxillary length (Co-A) (mm) | 84.3 | 90.0 | 5.0 | -1.1 * |
| Landes Angle (FH-NA) (°) | 84.8 | 90.0 | 3.0 | -1.7 * |
| SNA (°) | 88.7 | 82.0 | 3.5 | 1.9 * |
| SNB (°) | 90.0 | 77.7 | 3.2 | 3.9 *** |
| Facial Angle (FH-NPo) (°) | 86.6 | 87.5 | 3.1 | -0.3 |
| Mandibular length (Co-Gn) (mm) | 124.7 | 117.3 | 4.0 | 1.9 * |
| Mand. Skeletal (Pg-Na Perp) (mm) | -6.6 | -4.0 | 5.3 | -0.5 |
| Wits (FOP) (mm) | -7.4 | -1.0 | 1.0 | -6.4 ****** |
| Mx/Md diff (Co-Gn - Co-A) (mm) | 35.5 | 22.0 | 4.0 | 3.4 *** |
| ANB (°) | -1.4 | 4.0 | 1.8 | -3.0 *** |
| **Skeletal Vertical** | | | | |
| FH - SN (°) | -3.9 | 5.7 | 3.5 | -2.7 ** |
| Palatal-Mand Angle (PP-MP) (°) | 24.3 | 25.0 | 6.0 | -0.1 |
| Mand Plane to FH (FMA) (°) | 28.1 | 25.0 | 5.0 | 0.6 |
| SN - GoGn (°) | 19.7 | 32.9 | 5.2 | -2.5 ** |
| Y-Axis -- Downs (SGn-FH) (°) | 62.8 | 62.1 | 3.4 | 0.2 |
| ANS-Me (perp HP) (mm) | 71.7 | 54.0 | 3.5 | 5.0 ** |
| LFH/TFH (ANS-Me:N-Me) (%) | 59.9 | 55.0 | 3.0 | 1.6 * |
| P-A Face Height (S-Go/N-Me) (%) | 74.0 | 65.0 | 4.0 | 2.3 ** |
| **Dental** | | | | |
| Interincisal Angle (U1-L1) (°) | 122.1 | 119.9 | 8.5 | 0.3 |
| U1 - FH (°) | 117.5 | 109.8 | 5.3 | 1.5 * |
| U1 - NA (°) | 32.7 | 22.8 | 5.7 | 1.7 * |
| U1 (labial surface) to NA (mm) | 12.1 | 4.0 | 0.0 | *UNDEF* |
| L1 - NB (°) | 26.6 | 25.3 | 6.0 | 0.2 |
| L1 (labial surface) to NB (mm) | 8.2 | 4.0 | 0.0 | *UNDEF* |
| L1 to A-Po (°) | 29.0 | 23.0 | 4.0 | 1.5 * |
| L1 Protrusion (L1-APo) (mm) | 7.7 | 2.7 | 1.7 | 3.0 *** |
| L1 - GoGn (°) | 96.8 | 90.0 | 6.0 | 1.1 * |
| FMIA (L1-FH) (°) | 59.5 | 65.0 | 8.5 | -0.6 |
| **Soft Tissue** | | | | |
| Upper Lip - S Line (mm) | 1.6 | 0.0 | 2.0 | 0.8 |
| Lower Lip to E-Plane (mm) | 1.9 | 2.0 | 2.0 | -0.0 |
| Nasolabial Angle (Col-Sn-UL) (°) | 111.2 | 93.6 | 9.8 | 1.8 * |
| Facial Convexity (G'-Sn-Po') (°) | 9.1 | 9.7 | 4.9 | -0.1 |

**SUMMARY ANALYSIS**
    Class I Molar Relationship
    Skeletal Class I (A-Po)
    Skeletal Class III (ANB)
    Low Mandibular Plane Angle
    Retrusive Maxilla (A-N)
    Retrusive Mandible (Pg-N)

**Figure 30-36**   Printouts of computer-generated cephalometric analyses often take a form similar to the ones illustrated here (Dolphin). The resulting measurements can even be combined with a graphic image of the face. The content either can be customized by altering the anatomic landmarks and measurements to provide those most useful to the individual clinician or multiple analyses are available in the package.

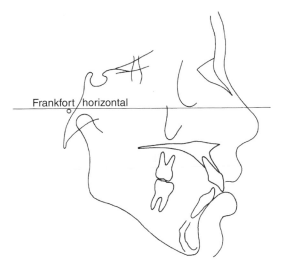

**Figure 30-37** Cephalometric analysis requires two reference lines to orient the position of the head and teeth. Historically, the Frankfort horizontal plane has been used as the reference line because it is felt to be parallel to the true horizontal when the patient is looking at the horizon. The Frankfort horizontal plane is constructed by connecting the upper rim of the external auditory meatus (porion) with the inferior border of the orbital rim (orbitale). The vertical reference line is either a true perpendicular to the nasion, the bony bridge of the nose, or a line perpendicular to the Frankfort plane through the nasion.

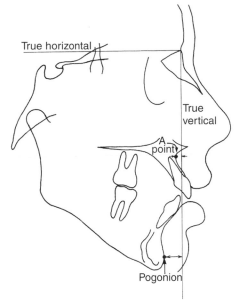

**Figure 30-38** The position and size of the maxilla and mandible are evaluated by comparing the A point (maxilla) and pogonion (mandible) with a vertical reference line. In a well-positioned maxilla, the A point is located 1 to 2 mm behind the vertical reference line. The pogonion is normally 5 mm behind the vertical line in a properly positioned mandible.

structures, to the vertical reference line. Normal maxillary position and size should place A point 1 to 2 mm behind the vertical line (Fig. 30-38).

The pogonion is normally 5 mm behind the vertical plane with a well-positioned mandible in a preadolescent patient.[19]

Angular and linear measurements can be used to compare the position of the maxilla with that of the mandible. The angle formed by connecting A and B points with the nasion has traditionally been used to describe the position of the two jaws (Fig. 30-39). In normally related jaws, the angle is between 2 and 5 degrees. Larger positive values suggest a class II relationship, whereas negative values indicate class III tendencies. The difference between the size of the lower and upper jaws, as determined from the Harvold measurements, can also be used to relate the jaws.[11]

Vertical facial proportions can be measured in two ways. The most direct method of determining vertical proportions is to measure total, upper, and lower anterior facial heights and to construct facial height ratios or compare linear

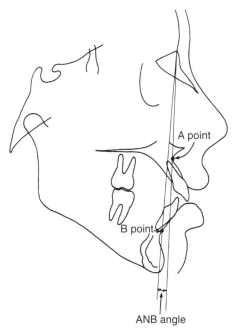

**Figure 30-39** The relative positions of the maxilla and mandible are also compared by using an angular measurement. In normally related jaws, the angle formed by connecting A and B points with nasion is between 2 and 5 degrees. Larger positive values suggest a class II relationship, whereas negative values indicate a class III tendency.

measurements with age-appropriate norms.[11,12] Total facial height is normally measured from nasion to menton. The division between the upper and lower facial heights is made at the anterior nasal spine (Fig. 30-40). The upper facial height should compose approximately 45% of the total facial height in a well-proportioned face.[38] Vertical facial height can be indirectly determined from the mandibular plane angle (the angle between the mandibular plane and the Frankfort horizontal plane). A long-faced person tends to have a large mandibular plane angle, whereas a short-faced person has a smaller mandibular plane angle (Fig. 30-41). Maxillary and mandibular dental position is evaluated by measuring overjet, overbite, and the axial and bodily position of the incisors. Overjet and overbite are simple measurements taken from the facial surfaces and incisal edges of the incisors, respectively (Fig. 30-42). The axial and bodily position of the maxillary incisor is determined relative to the nasion–A point line; the mandibular incisor position is related to the nasion–B point line. Axial inclination is determined from the angle

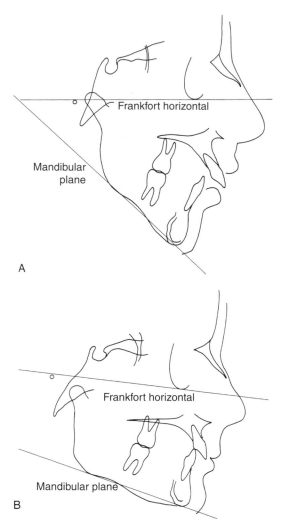

**A**

**B**

**Figure 30-41** **A,** Vertical facial height is determined indirectly from the mandibular plane angle (the angle between the mandibular plane and the Frankfort horizontal plane). This angle is usually approximately 24 degrees. A large mandibular plane angle is normally indicative of a long lower facial height. **B,** Conversely, a small mandibular plane angle is indicative of a short lower facial height.

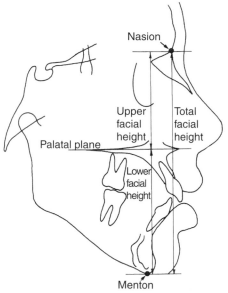

**Figure 30-40** Vertical facial proportions are determined by measuring total, upper, and lower facial heights. Total facial height is normally measured from the nasion to the menton. The division between upper and lower facial height is made at the palatal plane (a line connecting the anterior and posterior nasal spines). The measurements are used to construct facial height relations or are compared with age-appropriate norms.

formed by the intersection of the long axis of the incisor with the appropriate nasion–A point or nasion–B point lines. Bodily position is a measure of linear distance from the facial surface of the incisor to the reference line[35] (Fig. 30-43).

A number of soft tissue analyses exist to describe the facial profile. The major problem with soft tissue analysis is that the head film is a static representation of a dynamic object. Lip position may be different on the head film depending on whether the patient was in a relaxed

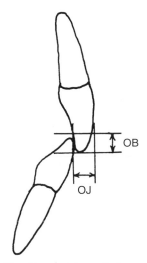

**Figure 30-42** The position of the maxillary and mandibular incisors and indirectly the entire dentition is evaluated by measuring the overjet and overbite. Overjet (OJ) is a horizontal measure of the distance between the most anterior points on the facial surfaces of the maxillary and mandibular central incisors. Overbite (OB) is a vertical measure of the overlap between the incisal edges of the maxillary and mandibular incisors.

posture (as recommended) or was straining to put the lips together when the film was made. This makes clinical assessment of the profile all the more important. Nevertheless, lip position is usually compared with the nose and chin. The Ricketts E line, which is convenient to use, is a line connecting the tip of the nose with the anterior contour of the chin (Fig. 30-44). In the permanent dentition, the upper lip is normally 1 mm behind the line and the lower lip is on the line or slightly behind it.[31]

It is important to realize that the numbers derived as norms serve as references and not as the diagnosis itself. Certain measurements may suggest a discrepancy, and this should be verified by the clinical examination. The clinician also should remember that hard and soft tissue analyses vary according to the ethnic background of the patient. Appropriate analyses and standards should be used. Serial cephalometric radiographs obtained prior to treatment, before and during treatment, or before and after treatment are often useful for evaluating growth, treatment progress, or treatment result, respectively.

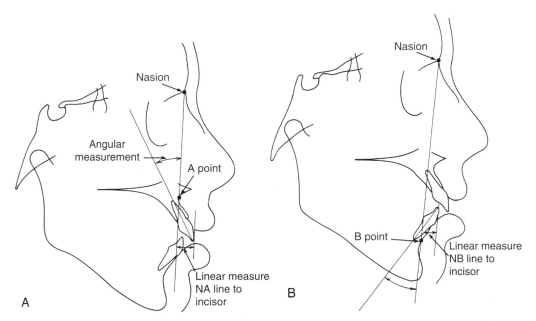

**Figure 30-43** **A,** The axial and bodily positions of the maxillary incisor are determined by making angular and linear measurements. Axial position is determined by drawing an angle formed by the intersection of the long axis of the incisor with the nasion–A point line. A large angle (more than approximately 22 degrees) suggests that the incisor is axially protrusive; a small angle suggests that the incisor is upright. The bodily position of the incisor is determined by measuring the linear distance between the facial surface of the incisor and the nasion–A point line. On the average, this distance is 4 mm. A large measurement suggests that the incisor is positioned too far anteriorly, whereas a small or negative measurement indicates that the incisor is positioned too far posteriorly in relation to the maxilla. **B,** The position of the mandibular incisor is similarly evaluated, although the nasion–B point line is used as a reference line. For these measurements, the average inclination is 25 degrees and the average linear distance is 4 mm.

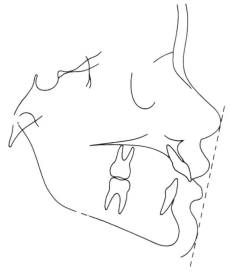

**Figure 30-44** The Ricketts E line is a convenient reference line used to assess the position of the lips in relation to the nose and chin. In the permanent dentition, the upper lip is normally 1 mm behind a line connecting the tip of the nose to the anterior contour of the chin. The lower lip is usually on or slightly behind this line.

Serial cephalometric head films can be superimposed on each other to illustrate changes in jaw and tooth positions. The observed changes are a combination of tooth movement and growth, and it is difficult to differentiate one from the other. To superimpose head films, one must locate an area in the head that is relatively unchanged over the time period in question, that is, an area that is not affected by growth or treatment from which change can be determined. Traditionally, three superimpositions are made with each pair of serial cephalometric radiographs when growth and treatment changes are being evaluated.

The first superimposition illustrates overall changes in the face. The comparison is made by superimposing the structures of the anterior cranial base or along the sella-nasion line registering at the sella. The amount and direction of change in the soft tissue profile and position of the jaws are readily apparent (Fig. 30-45, *A*). To demonstrate the amount and direction of dental change, structures of the maxilla and mandible are superimposed to eliminate all skeletal change from the evaluation (Fig. 30-45, *B, C*). In the maxilla, the pterygomaxillary fissure and zygomatic process are superimposed to find the best fit. In the mandible, the inner surface of the mandibular symphysis, the outline of the mandibu-

lar canal, and the unerupted third molar crypts are superimposed.

### Radiographic Evaluation

Transition into the mixed dentition requires modification of the basic pediatric survey. Some considerations for radiographs of children in this period are the following:

1. *Identification of missing teeth, supernumerary teeth, and the developmental status of permanent anteriors and premolars require greater periapical coverage on films.* The permanent second premolars are usually evident on radiographs at age 4, but they may not be apparent until age 8.

2. *Potential eruption problems may be diagnosed from the radiographs by study of the unerupted teeth.* Ectopic eruption of permanent first molars has been discussed and is diagnosed from routine bitewing radiographs. Ectopic eruption of incisors and canine impaction, which are other maxillary eruption problems, are often diagnosed from panoramic radiographs but can be erroneously evaluated in this manner if only a panoramic radiograph is used[13,18] (Fig. 30-46).

Labial or palatal positioning of the canine is best determined using the panoramic radiograph in conjunction with an occlusal radiograph, especially if the canines cannot be palpated on the facial aspect of the alveolus at approximately 9 to 10 years of age. The occlusal radiograph will provide a better estimate of the position of the canine to the lateral incisor. Also, by using the occlusal radiograph and the panoramic radiograph together, the image shift due to the change in beam position from the few degrees from the horizontal plane on which the panoramic radiograph is taken to the approximately 60 degrees of the occlusal radiograph provides the basis for the vertical parallax method that has proved reliable (Fig. 30-47).[14]

This is similar to the lateral beam shift method using two periapical radiographs. In that method the image of the canine on the two films shifts as the angulation of the central x-ray beam changes. If the image of the canine moves in the same direction (relative to the other teeth or reference structure) as the central x-ray beam from the first film to the second, the canine is positioned lingual or palatal to the other teeth. If the image moves in the opposite direction to the beam from the first film to the second, the canine is located buccal to

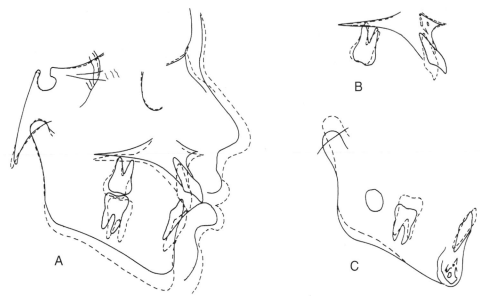

**Figure 30-45** **A,** Serial cephalometric head films are superimposed to illustrate changes in jaw and tooth positions during growth and orthodontic treatment. To assess overall change, a stable area within the head that is not influenced by growth or treatment is located. These overall changes in the face are illustrated by superimposing them on structures of the anterior cranial base. In this case, the solid line represents the patient before orthodontic treatment was initiated. The second or dashed line represents the patient after treatment was completed. During treatment, the maxilla moved slightly forward and downward. The horizontal position of the mandible remained virtually unchanged. However, the mandible did move vertically. The position of the lips improved during the treatment period as well. **B,** To illustrate the amount and direction of dental change, structures in the maxilla and mandible are superimposed. In this case, the maxillary superimposition, based on a best fit of palatal morphologic appearance, shows that the incisor and molar were both tipped distally. In addition, there was a change in the vertical position of the incisor. The change in incisor and molar position contributed to an improvement in molar relationships and overjet reduction. **C,** The mandibular superimposition, made by overlaying the inner aspect of the mandibular symphysis, the canal of the inferior alveolar nerve, and the unerupted third molar crypt, shows that both the incisor and molar erupted vertically.

the teeth. In the vertical parallax method, the same interpretation is made only with a change in vertical position. This technique may also be used to locate supernumerary teeth or other abnormal structures.

3. *Small palate size, especially early in the school-age period, prevents or complicates maxillary periapical radiography via a long-cone film-stabilizing apparatus.*

4. *Greater anteroposterior length in the posterior occlusion requires more bitewing coverage.*

In the early mixed-dentition period, a radiograph should be taken to expose supernumerary or missing teeth in the anterior maxilla. All tooth-bearing areas should be surveyed during the early mixed-dentition years. This survey could consist of a panoramic radiograph and posterior bitewing films. The panoramic radiograph offers the advantage of showing the temporomandibular

joint (TMJ). Definitive TMJ films are indicated when there are clinical signs of dysfunction or a history of TMJ abnormalities. A traditional intraoral film survey in this age group is composed of appropriate anterior occlusal views, at least one periapical view in each posterior quadrant, and posterior bitewing views (Fig. 30-48). The number of films should be dictated by the size of the tooth-bearing areas, the adequacy of tissue coverage by the size of films tolerated, and the needs of the child. A 12-film survey (four posterior periapical, six anterior periapical, and two posterior bitewing films) should suffice even for the older school-aged child if it is performed well.

Radiographic techniques used in children, especially the youngest in this age group, may include modifications. The anterior area requires placement of the film positioner deeper in the palate to obtain proper orientation. Two alternatives are to use the prong end of the Snap-a-Ray

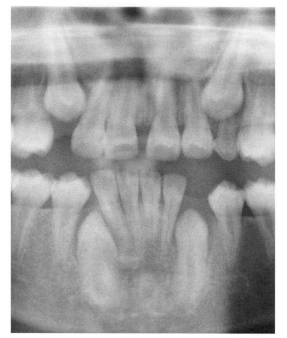

A

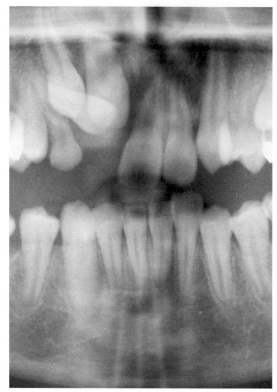

A

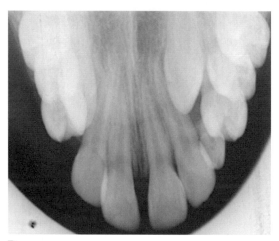

B

**Figure 30-46** Often images of unerupted canines and lateral incisors are distorted on panoramic radiographs and can be better visualized on occlusal radiographs. **A,** The panoramic radiograph shows little overlap of the maxillary left canine and lateral incisor. **B,** The occlusal radiograph shows considerable overlap of the same canine and lateral incisor.

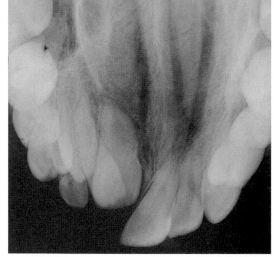

B

**Figure 30-47** Using a panoramic and occlusal radiograph appears to be a productive way to localize unerupted teeth. The panoramic radiograph is usually already available as a part of routine pretreatment records, so only the additional occlusal image is required. Applying the vertical parallax rules to this (**A**) panoramic and (**B**) occlusal radiograph that is taken at a higher angle, it is apparent that as the tube head moves up, the lateral incisor moves vertically relative to both the central incisor and the canine, indicating that it is located lingual to both these teeth.

device (Rinn Corporation, Elgin, Ill.) with a bisecting-angle technique or to use a film with cotton rolls attached (Fig. 30-49). The long-cone technique for posterior teeth is the same as that used in adults with two modifications to help improve the product. Figure 30-50 demonstrates the use of increased vertical angulation to pick

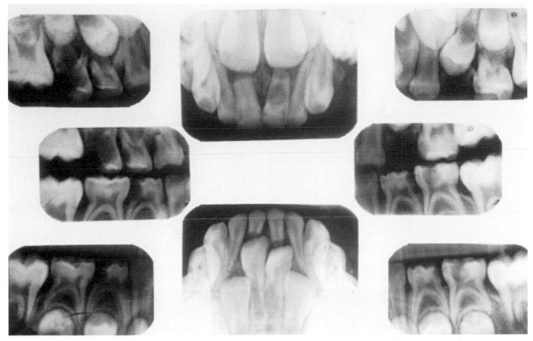

**Figure 30-48** An appropriate radiographic examination in this age group consists of anterior occlusal radiographs, at least one periapical film in each posterior quadrant, and posterior bitewing radiographs. The number of films should be dictated by the size of the tooth-bearing areas, the adequacy of tissue coverage by the size of the films, and the needs of the child.

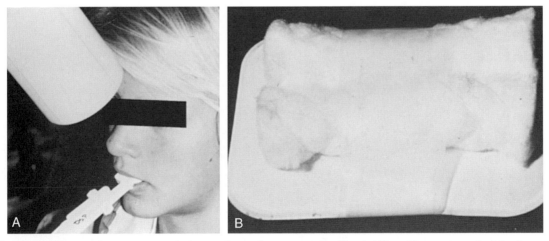

**Figure 30-49** **A,** The Snap-a-Ray device can be used as an anterior film stabilizer. The prong end of the Snap-a-Ray is used to hold a film in place by the child. A bisecting-angle technique is used. **B,** Alternatively, cotton rolls can be used to stabilize the film. Taping two or three cotton rolls can help fill the space in the palate and stabilize an anterior film. Care must be taken not to bend the film. Bisecting-angle technique is used.

up the developing teeth. Figure 30-51 shows the placement of cotton rolls on the bite block to facilitate positioning in small mouths or when teeth needed for stabilization are absent. A Styrofoam bite block may be used to obtain anterior films with a bisecting-angle technique (Fig. 30-52). The bitewing technique used in this age group is essentially the same as that used in the preschooler. It may take more skill to open contacts by careful positioning of the beam. Larger films may be preferable because they cover more area in each exposure.

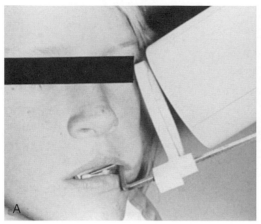
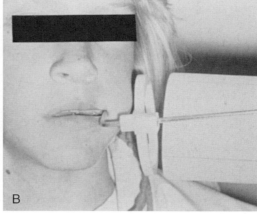

**Figure 30-50** Increasing the vertical angulation of posterior periapical films will provide more coverage of periapical tissue. This helps the radiographs to include developing premolar roots in this age group.

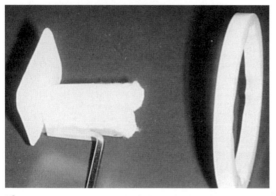

**Figure 30-51** Several cotton rolls will help to hold the film holder in place when palate depth is insufficient or teeth are missing. Rolls can be taped both above and below the holder's bite block.

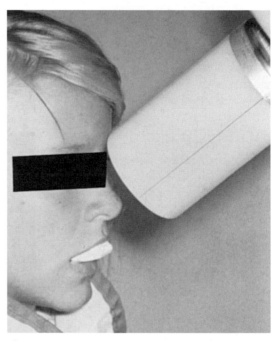

**Figure 30-52** A Styrofoam bite block can be used to aid in film positioning. Most plastic holders can be cut down to fit the child with transitional dentition better.

Selection criteria also apply to this age group. Justification of a full-mouth survey of some type is based on the need to identify dental developmental problems and pathologic processes. The number of films made should reflect the adequacy of composite exposure provided by individual views. This translates to making as few films as necessary to reveal tissue areas. In the age range of 6 to 12 years, a variety of combinations of films is possible. No single set of projections is considered best.

## Determining Growth Status

In order to make changes in skeletal relationships, children must be growing. When they are increasing in stature, their faces are also growing. Most girls grow steadily and rapidly during the 6- to 12-year period, and the majority achieve their peak growth and begin to slow down. Commonly, boys enter their somatic and facial growth spurts later than girls and show accelerated statural and facial growth near the end of this period and later. The most common critical determination regarding growth is 0 whether girls have completed their growth or are growing so slowly that facial growth modification cannot be successful. The methods to make this assessment are discussed in Chapter 37.

## TREATMENT PLANNING FOR NONORTHODONTIC PROBLEMS

The planning of care for this age group usually centers on orthodontic considerations, although many patients require additional treatment. Some elements of treatment planning that may have to be addressed but are only peripherally related to orthodontics include the following:

1. *Management of primary caries.* Within this age period, many primary teeth normally exfoliate. A decision to extract a tooth or restore it must be made with its remaining lifespan in mind as well as the length of time that the child will be without a replacement. Prosthetic replacement for a short time may not be indicated if adequate functional surfaces are available elsewhere and space maintenance is not indicated.

2. *Management of pathosis.* Some forms of oral pathosis, such as supernumerary teeth, odontomas, or missing teeth, are given definitive management in this period owing to the child's increased ability to cooperate and the impending effects of the problem.

3. *Prevention of dental disease.* The choice of sealants is also made during this period, as are decisions about how to manage incipient interproximal lesions of permanent teeth. Topical fluoride regimens may be considered if the caries pattern changes for the worse.

4. *Health issues.* Children with disabilities or serious illnesses are in a transitional time. The child with cancer, orofacial clefting, cerebral palsy, or a host of other conditions may need special consideration in regard to such issues as lifespan, realistic functional requirements, retention of teeth for growth purposes, and the role of the appearance of teeth in social acceptance. Decisions regarding these issues are often complex, and input from parents, the child, and other professionals is helpful in decision making. The dentist's role is to provide information about the need for care, the benefits anticipated, the alternatives to care (including no treatment), and the burden of maintenance of care. These special patients may tax the dentist's skills in planning care, and they may require careful and frequent observation rather than treatment.

Regardless of the specific situation, dental and periodontal diseases are addressed first and stabilized. Restorative care is rendered next, and more definitive prosthodontic or orthodontic treatment is completed last.

## REFERENCES

1. Baccetti T: Tooth anomalies associated with failure of eruption of first and second permanent molars. *Am J Orthod Dentofacial Orthop* 118:608-610, 2000.
2. Bjerklin K, Kurol J: Ectopic eruption of the maxillary first permanent molar: etiologic factors. *Am J Orthod Dentofacial Orthop* 84:147-155, 1983.
3. Bolton WA: Disharmony in tooth size and its relation to the analysis and treatment of malocclusion. *Am J Orthod Dentofacial Orthop* 28:113-130, 1958.
4. Braun A, Appel T, Frentzen M: Endodontic and surgical treatment of a geminated maxillary incisor. *Int Endod J* 36:380-386, 2003.
5. Ericson S, Kurol J: Early treatment of palatally erupting maxillary canines by extraction of the primary canines. *Eur J Orthod* 10:283-295, 1988.
6. Ericson S, Kurol J: Resorption of maxillary lateral incisors caused by ectopic eruption of the canines. A clinical and radiographic analysis of predisposing factors. *Am J Orthod Dentofacial Orthop* 94(6):503-513, 1988.
7. Fields HW, Proffit WR, Nixon WL et al: Facial pattern differences in long-faced children and adults. *Am J Orthod Dentofacial Orthop* 85:217-223, 1984.
8. Fields HW, Sinclair PM: Dentofacial growth and development. *J Dent Child* 57:46-55, 1990.
9. Gellin ME, Haley JV: Managing cases of overretention of mandibular primary incisors when their permanent successors erupt lingually. *J Dent Child* 49:118-122,1982.
10. Hagan PP, Hagan JP, Fields HW et al: The legal status of informed consent for behavior management technique in pediatric dentistry. *Pediatr Dent* 6:204-208, 1984.
11. Harvold EP: *The Activator in Orthodontics.* St Louis, Mosby, 1974.
12. Isaacson JR, Isaacson RJ, Speidel TM et al: Extreme variation in vertical facial growth and associated variation in skeletal and dental relations. *Am J Orthod Dentofacial Orthop* 41:219-229, 1971.
13. Jacobs SG: Localization of the unerupted maxillary canine: how to and when to. *Am J Orthod Dentofacial Orthop* 115(3):314-322, 1999.
14. Jacobs SG: Radiographic localization of unerupted teeth: further findings about the vertical tube shift method and other localization techniques. *Am J Orthod Dentofacial Orthop* 118(4):439-447, 2000.

15. Kimmel NA, Gellin ME, Bohannan HA et al: Ectopic eruption of maxillary first permanent molars in different areas of the United States. *J Dent Child* 49:294-299,1982.

16. Kurol J, Bjerklin K: Ectopic eruption of maxillary first permanent molars: a review. *J Dent Child* 53(3):209-214, 1986.

17. Loe N, Silness J: Periodontal disease in pregnancy: 1. Prevalence and severity. *Acta Odont Scand* 21:553, 1963.

18. Mason C, Papadakou P, Roberts GJ: The radiographic localization of impacted maxillary canines: a comparison of methods. *Eur J Orthod* 23(1):25-34, 2001.

19. McNamara JA Jr: A method of cephalometric analysis. In: McNamara JA, Ribbens KA, Howe RP, editors. *Clinical Alteration of the Growing Face.* Monograph 12, Craniofacial Growth Series. Ann Arbor, University of Michigan, Center for Human Growth and Development, 1983, pp 81-105.

20. Nordgarden H, Jensen JL, Storhaug K: Reported prevalence of congenitally missing teeth in two Norwegian counties. *Community Dent Health* 19(4):258-261, 2002.

21. Peck S, Peck L, Kataja M: Concomitant occurrence of canine malposition and tooth agenesis: evidence of orofacial genetic fields. *Am J Orthod Dentofacial Orthop* 122:657-660, 2002.

22. Peck S, Peck L, Kataja M: Mandibular lateral incisor-canine transposition, concomitant dental anomalies, and genetic control. *Angle Orthod* 68:455-466, 1998

23. Peck S, Peck L: Classification of maxillary tooth transpositions. *Am J Orthod Dentofacial Orthop* 107:505-517, 1995.

24. Portela MB, Sanchez AL, Gleiser R: Bilateral distal ectopic eruption of the permanent mandibular central incisors: a case report. *Quintessence Int* 34(2):131-134, 2003.

25. Pirinen S, Arte S, Apajalahti S: Palatal displacement

of canine is genetic and related to congenital absence of teeth. *J Dent Res* 75(10):1742-1746, 1996.

26. Proffit WR, Fields HW: *Contemporary Orthodontics,* 3rd ed. St Louis, Mosby–Year Book, 2000.

27. Proffit WR, Vig KWL: Primary failure of eruption: a possible cause of posterior open-bite. *Am J Orthod Dentofacial Orthop* 80:173-190, 1981.

28. Pulver F: The etiology and prevalence of ectopic eruption of the maxillary first permanent molar. *J Dent Child* 35:138-146, 1968.

29. Ramfjord SP: The periodontal index. *J Periodontol* 38:610, 1967.

30. Rasmussen P, Kotsaki A: Inherited primary failure of eruption in the primary dentition: report of five cases. *J Dent Child* 64(1):43-47, 1997.

31. Ricketts RM: Perspectives in the clinical application of cephalometrics. *Angle Orthod* 51:115-150, 1981.

32. Rolling S, Paulson S: Oligodontia in Danish schoolchildren. *Acta Odontol Scand* 59(2):111-112, 2001.

33. Neville B, Damm, DD, Allen CM, Bouquot J: *Oral and Maxillofacial Pathology,* 2nd ed. Philadelphia, Saunders, 2002.

34. Staley RN, O'Gorman TW, Hoag JF et al: Prediction of the widths of unerupted canines and premolars. *JADA* 108:185-190, 1984.

35. Steiner CC: The use of cephalometrics as an aid to planning and assessing orthodontic treatment. *Am J Orthod Dentofacial Orthop* 46:721-735, 1960.

36. Tanaka MM, Johnston LE: The prediction of the size of unerupted canines and premolars in a contemporary orthodontic population. *JADA* 88:798-801, 1974.

37. Velasco LF, de Araujo FB, Ferreira ES, Velasco LE: Esthetic and functional treatment of a fused permanent tooth: a case report. *Quintessence Int* 28(10):677-680, 1997.

38. Wylie WL, Johnson EL. Rapid evaluation of facial dysplasia in the vertical plane. *Angle Orthod* 22:165-182, 1952.

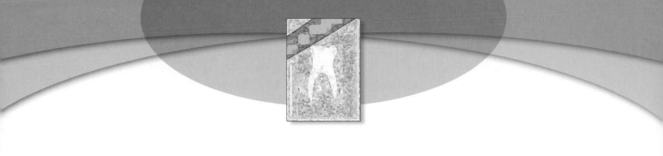

# CHAPTER 31

## Prevention of Dental Disease

*Arthur Nowak and James J. Crall*

The patient between 6 and 12 years of age presents an interesting professional challenge for the dentist. At the beginning of this period, the dentist is dealing with a patient who continues to depend on the parents but is now thrust into a new environment—school—for approximately 8 hours a day. By the end of this period, the dentist is dealing with a patient who has gained partial independence from his or her parents and is nearly ready for junior high school and, in the case of the female patient, approaching womanhood.

In addition, all through this period a number of oral-facial changes are taking place. Most of the primary teeth will be replaced with permanent teeth during this period. The alignment and occlusion of the teeth are developing, and the "adult face" is emerging. What "I" look like becomes important, as does the opinions of others, especially peers.

Diet and dietary practices are severely challenged by the educational environment and social pressures both during the day and after school hours. Requirements vary from year to year in this period. As the growth pattern of the patient changes from slow progressive physical growth early in the period to substantial physical growth at the end of the period, the requirements of the child must stay in tune. These dietary requirements depend not only on growth and development but on the level of physical and mental activity engaged in by the child. Snacking becomes a common practice during this period. With vending machines easily available, convenience stores on many street corners, and the influence of commercial media always pervasive, children are constantly prompted to think about food and eating.

Many changes in manual dexterity take place during this period. Although continuing gross motor development prevails, this is the period when fine motor skill begins to mature. Luckily so, because during this period the child is challenging the parents for independence, especially in areas of personal hygiene, clothes selection, and dietary choices. Conflicts emerge between the parents' desires and the child's wishes. It is a time when parents must have a strong daily influence on all types of activity, including oral care. With eruption of the permanent teeth, topical fluoride needs take on added importance. Periodic assessments and input by the dentist is important so that the child receives the optimal protection available.

## FLUORIDE ADMINISTRATION

The period from 6 to 12 years is extremely important with regard to fluoride administration for three major reasons: (1) the crowns of many permanent teeth continue to form during this period; (2) the posterior permanent teeth erupt and are at greater risk for developing caries until the process of "posteruptive maturation" has occurred; and (3) the child becomes increasingly responsible for the maintenance of his or her oral health. The optimal use of all forms of fluoride should be employed to provide protection during this first phase of carious attack on those teeth that will constitute the permanent dentition.

### Systemic Fluorides

Studies suggest that a substantial portion of the anticaries protection provided by water fluoridation in humans occurs during the preeruptive period.[5,16] Additional studies in laboratory animals have reported that daily doses of fluoride administered via gastric intubation during the period of tooth formation reduced the incidence of caries in these teeth after eruption.[8] Because systemically acquired fluoride may be deposited and redistributed in developing teeth during the mineralization phase as well as during the subsequent period prior to eruption, current recommendations call for systemic fluoride sup-

plements for all children residing in areas where the water is fluoride deficient until they reach the age of 16. This protocol should help to ensure maximum protection for the posterior teeth, which are more vulnerable to carious attack. Supplemental fluoride dosages remain constant for children between the ages of 6 and 16.

### Topical Fluorides

During the period from 6 to 12 years of age, the child should become increasingly responsible for the maintenance of his or her dentition. Many forms of topical fluoride are appropriate for children in this age group, including fluoride toothpastes, fluoride mouth rinses, and concentrated fluoride preparations for professional and home application.

Accumulating evidence continues to support the effectiveness and importance of frequent application of agents that contain relatively low concentrations of fluoride. The two principal forms of these agents in the United States are fluoride toothpastes and fluoride mouth rinses.

#### Fluoride Toothpastes

The daily use of a fluoride-containing dentifrice should form the foundation of the child's preventive dental activities. Although many toothpastes include fluoride in their formulations, products that have obtained approval by the Council on Dental Therapeutics of the American Dental Association (ADA) should be recommended. Formulations of toothpastes that have not obtained ADA approval may impede the release of fluoride from these products, thereby compromising their effectiveness.[4] Currently approved fluoride toothpastes contain sodium fluoride (NaF) or sodium monofluorophosphate (MFP) as active ingredients. In the United States, the maximal allowable concentration of fluoride in toothpastes that have not received New Drug Approval from the Food and Drug Administration is 1100 parts per million (ppm).[17] Parents should be advised that some over-the-counter products contain higher fluoride concentrations (e.g., 1500 ppm).

#### Fluoride Mouth Rinses

The use of fluoride mouth rinses has increased considerably as a result of increased use in the home as well as in school-based mouth rinsing programs. The most popular preparations contain neutral NaF, although stannous fluoride and acidulated phosphate fluoride rinses also are available. Several fluoride mouth rinses, including many 0.05% NaF products, are available on an over-the-counter (nonprescription) basis.

Numerous clinical trials conducted in the 1960s and 1970s reported caries reductions in the 20% and 40% range among children in non-fluoridated areas who rinsed either weekly with a 0.2% NaF rinse or daily with a 0.05% NaF product.[4] More recent studies, conducted since the overall decline in dental caries in children became evident, have reported that (1) the expected benefits from fluoride rinsing in terms of the actual number of tooth surfaces saved from becoming carious are generally less than previously reported and (2) rinsing appears to have a greater effect in older children (10 years of age).[4] Nevertheless, the observation that fluoride rinsing provides greater protection to erupting teeth during the time when rinses are being applied provides a rationale for their use in the 6- to 12-year age group.

Rinses are particularly indicated for persons deemed to be at high risk for caries. Included in this category are those who lack the motivation or manual dexterity necessary to carry out effective oral hygiene procedures, patients who wear orthodontic appliances or prostheses that may complicate the process of plaque removal, and patients who have medical conditions that place them at increased risk. Examples of persons in the last group are patients undergoing head and neck radiation therapy, which may compromise their salivary flow, and patients who are required to take frequent doses of liquid or chewable medications that have a high sugar content.

### Concentrated Agents for Professional Application or Home Use

Applications of more concentrated forms of fluoride should be considered for persons who are at elevated risk for dental caries, including those who cannot or do not make optimal use of the high-frequency, low-concentration forms of fluoride therapy. Generally, this implies semiannual applications of concentrated fluoride gels or forms in the dental office. Fluoride varnish applications have also been suggested for high-risk patients (see Chapter 14).

Several fluoride gels and solutions, including combinations of acidulated phosphate fluoride and stannous fluoride, are available for home use.

Practitioners should be aware that some of these products contain concentrations of fluoride that are similar to those found in fluoride toothpastes or over-the-counter rinses, and in most cases they have not undergone clinical testing. Some of these low-concentration products have also been advocated for professional application, but they are unlikely to be effective when used infrequently.[6] Therefore, the advantage of these less concentrated products over commercially available fluoride toothpastes and mouth rinses is questionable. More concentrated fluoride gels (0.5% APF) have been shown to be effective in reducing the incidence of caries and may be useful in high-risk patients with rampant caries.

## HOME CARE

With school activities now emerging as a major influence in the daily schedule of the child, routine personal hygiene must be scheduled. The development of a routine ideally has been reinforced with the routines established during the preschool period. Unfortunately, it is not only the school activity that fills the daily schedule. Music lessons, sports activities, dance and voice lessons, homework, religious instruction, daily chores, babysitting, and Internet surfing all begin to influence the daily schedule and the time remaining for personal hygiene.

Although brushing after all meals is ideal, such a schedule is probably unrealistic. A compromise should be worked out. An appropriate recommendation would be for a thorough brushing of the teeth with fluoride toothpaste and massaging of the gingiva before bed with additional brushing at the start of each day.[4] Brushing after lunch in school is impractical because most children do not remember to bring their toothbrush and they are more interested in physical activity after lunch. Swishing vigorously with water after lunch helps to dislodge any large particles of food remaining and neutralize any acid that may be present. Brushing after the dinner meal if eaten at home also should be encouraged.

Parents should remain active in supervising mouth care during this period. Interference from TV, radio, and computer games cannot be tolerated. A firm stand with appropriate discipline if required is recommended to develop and maintain this important hygiene practice.

Periodic inspection of the mouth by the parent is indeed appropriate. Because fine motor activity is further developing during this period, parental assistance is required to remove all plaque, especially on the buccal surfaces of the posterior maxillary molars and the lingual surfaces of the mandibular posterior molars. Brushes of the appropriate size and contour should be selected to meet the child's needs.[11] With increasing oral dimensions and numbers of teeth, larger brushes should be considered. Soft nylon bristled brushes are recommended over other varieties.

Although mechanical toothbrushes have been available for some time, there has recently been a dramatic increase in their development and promotion. All types, shapes, head size variations, rotations, and vibrations (oscillating and ultrasonic powered) are now available. Some are modified and promoted for children, others only for adults. Some studies show dramatic improvements in plaque removal and gingival health; others report results that are not so impressive.[7,12] The novelty of the device may increase children's compliance with daily brushing. One has to consider the initial cost and the cost of brush head replacements when recommending a mechanical brush. Supervision by a caregiver is required for younger children. For patients with special health care needs, especially those with limited motor activity, a discussion as to the benefits is indicated with the caregiver.

With the increased size and independence of the child, the bathroom becomes the ideal location for cleaning. The previously recommended supine position to increase visibility and stability is no longer appropriate. A well-lit bathroom with a wall mirror or hand mirror greatly aids the cleaning process.

Use of disclosing tablets or solutions helps the child and parent to evaluate the thoroughness of the cleaning. At least weekly, the teeth should be disclosed, and with the parent's supervision, the child's mouth should be inspected. Areas of disclosed plaque should be noted with instructions on modification of technique so that it will be removed daily.

With the exfoliation of primary teeth and the eruption of permanent teeth, the mouth may be sore, causing the child to hesitate to do a thorough cleaning. Generally, with the "loosening" of a primary tooth, the gingiva will be tender and even swollen. Careful wiping of this area with the brush should maintain the health of the tissues.

As the permanent teeth erupt, the alignment may be irregular, and the gingival tissue may lose its "knife edge" anatomy with the tooth. Instead, a ledge of gingival tissue may emerge that allows plaque to accumulate (Fig. 31-1). Careful manipulation of the brush is necessary until the gingival contour assumes a smooth margin with the tooth. In mouths with a developing discrepancy between arch length and tooth size, the malalignment of the teeth causes retention of food and plaque. Until corrected, additional manipulation of the brush by both child and parent may be necessary.

Toward the end of this period the child may have developed enough fine motor activity to be able to learn the process of flossing. Like any other motor activity, this skill must be learned and practiced frequently. Parents can be helpful in assisting the child. Inappropriate use of the floss by "snapping" it into the interproximal surfaces can injure the gingiva. Once passed through the contact, the floss must be carefully manipulated along one surface of the tooth and then the opposite surface, making sure that it reaches the area just under the gingival crevice. One of the many commercially available floss holders may greatly assist in the process.

Children with developmental disabilities may require partial or total assistance in oral care, depending on their mental and physical capabilities. If a parent must help with or be totally responsible for mouth care, a mouth prop may be helpful (Fig. 31-2). With good head stability and mouth propping, the cleaning process is enhanced. With severely disabled children, more than one person may be necessary. Stabilization and proper positioning may be necessary, and if so, the bathroom may be an inappropriate loca-

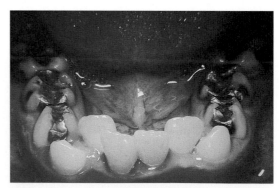

**Figure 31-1**    Early mixed dentition. Note crowding of teeth and ledge of gingiva.

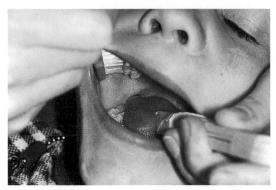

**Figure 31-2** A tongue blade mouth prop can be used to facilitate mouth care in a child with a disability.

tion. Use of the bedroom or other living area with available floor space, beds, or couches allows the child to be placed in a supine position and stabilized. In these situations the use of a dentifrice further complicates the process because of the foaming and the need to expectorate.

Last, as the child extends his or her social activities, overnight, weekend, or extended periods away from home occur. As they "pack their bags," toothbrushes, dentifrices, and floss will probably be thought of last, if at all. Again, parents must be responsible for making sure that the appropriate tools are available; whether they will be used is another question.

## DIET

Although children are introduced to a new variety of foods during the preschool years, it is during this period, the primary grades, that the real challenge to well-established dietary habits begins. Again, exposure to a full day in school with frequent treats and school lunches, either from home or purchased at school, vending machines,[1] and a multitude of after-school activities, usually associated with food, all influence the child's

---

## Toothbrush Innovations
*M. Catherine Skotowski, RDH, MS*

Billions of dollars is spent on oral health care products each year. The toothbrush is the most commonly used oral health care product for removing plaque and delivering toothpaste to the teeth. Until recent years, toothbrushes designed for children varied only slightly from those designed for adults, primarily by size, colors, and designs *on* the toothbrush. Now, however, a consumer can stroll down any oral health care aisle of a grocery store, pharmacy, or department store and find several types of toothbrushes in many shapes and sizes, designed specifically for children. Toothbrush handles have been ergonomically designed for better grip control and the varying levels of a child's manual dexterity development. Toothbrush bristles are usually soft but are often arranged in various heights to optimize plaque removal on all sides of the teeth. While some manufacturers have added longer bristles at the tip of the brush head to facilitate plaque removal on the distal surfaces of the most posterior teeth, others have extended bristle lengths at the outer portions of the brush head to aid in cleansing buccal and lingual surfaces. Bristles can be multicolored merely for appearances; however, in one manufacturer's case, a small section of colored bristles have been added to "indicate" when it is time to replace the toothbrush.

One of the most noticeable advances to the toothbrush market is the advent of power toothbrushes designed specifically for children. Although power toothbrushes were first introduced in the 1960s, it has only been in the last 10 years or so that manufacturers have targeted the children's power toothbrush market. Smaller brush heads, the use of brighter colors, popular cartoon characters, and built-in timers (some with musical tunes) are some of the features designed to make power brushes more appealing to children and adolescents. Some of the power toothbrushes have rechargeable stands that require electricity whereas others on the less expensive end are battery operated. In terms of plaque removal, power toothbrushes appear to be as effective if not better than manual toothbrushes.

The novelty toothbrushes, both manual and power, may provide some extra motivation for those who use them because they are unique, fun to use, and possibly more appealing. The ultimate desired outcome of their use is improved oral hygiene efforts on the part of children and adolescents (the wish of many dedicated oral health professionals).

dietary habits. In addition, the child is heavily influenced by the commercial media, especially television. The effect of food choices and purchases has been carefully studied, and although advocacy organizations have attempted to influence the number of commercials related to food shown during the daytime hours, it remains common for the school-aged child to be exposed to many enticements during a period of TV or radio entertainment. If children accompany parents to the market (a practice not encouraged), the purchases they request are frequently related to television and radio commercials.

Although some dramatic changes have occurred recently in food selection and dietary practices, we know that a large percentage of a family's meals are eaten on the run or in fast food restaurants, seldom with the entire family present, and too often in front of the television set. Per capita consumption of sweeteners is around 152.4 pounds annually,[15] although there has been a substantial decrease in the use of ordinary refined table sugar. Annual per capita consumption of soft drinks has increased since the early 1970s from 22.7 gallons to 55.7 gallons in 2000. Forty-three percent of the sweeteners used are refined sugar from sugarcane and beets; 57% are from corn sweeteners. High daily rates of consumption and between-meal intake of sugars remain a risk factor for children susceptible to proximal caries even though caries development is now declining in the United States.[3] Nevertheless, caries rates have been dramatically reduced during the last 15 years even as dramatic changes have been taking place in our dietary practices. Can we as dentists make any further impact on the way children eat and what they eat?

For children with a severe caries problem, the dentist must evaluate all etiologic factors, including diet and dietary practices. As noted earlier, the dietary history, whether a 24-hour recall or a 5-day history, is recommended. Once received, the dentist or a designated staff person reviews the history with the parent, paying particular attention to the number of exposures to carbohydrates per day and when they were eaten, whether during meals, after meals, or between meals. Every exposure to a food containing a refined carbohydrate, especially one that adheres to the teeth and dissolves slowly, produces acid in and around the plaque. If a pattern emerges, it should be defined and recommendations for substitute foods or modifications of a dietary practice provided. Identifying particular areas of concern and providing specific recommendations will be accepted more readily by both parent and child than sweeping changes of the entire diet. A series of small changes, successfully made over a period of time, eventually leads to a better diet for dental health.

A favorite activity of many school-aged children is gum chewing. Although frowned on by school officials and parents, it does in fact have an anticaries effect. Studies have reported an increase in salivary flow and mechanical pumping of saliva to the interproximal sites. This results in a neutralization of interproximal acids. These studies have used both sugarless and sugar-containing gums. All studies agree on the beneficial effects of sugarless gums; but a difference of opinion exists on the effect of sugar-containing gums.[2,9,10] Xylitol-containing gums continue to show decreased *Streptococcus mutans* levels in saliva and plaque when used on a routine basis. Reduction in caries incidences are reported in all age groups and when used by mothers may decrease the transmission of *S. mutans* from mother to child.[13]

As we learn more about the cariogenic potential of foods, foods that are "safe for teeth" will be identified and marketed. In the meantime, it is unrealistic to recommend to a parent of a 6- or 7-year-old child to cut out all candy and baked goods. It is better to advise them of possible substitutes, such as a chocolate candy instead of a caramel, or that intake of candy and baked goods should take place only after meals have been eaten rather than before or between meals. Children can learn appropriate eating habits, but the habits must be realistic, and the parents must be enthusiastic about the change.[14] Regarding meals at school, the parent must work with school authorities to provide wholesome and nutritious meals that also have eye appeal for the child. In addition, parents should work with specific teachers to encourage use of appropriate snacks and party foods for special occasions.

The diets of children with developmental disabilities may be modified for a number of reasons. To increase caloric requirements, supplements are frequently added to routine foods. Unfortunately, these supplements are frequently refined carbohydrates, which increase the risk of acid production. Foods may be altered, minced, pureed, or mashed to assist the child in swallowing and to meet the need for less chewing. Because of these modifications, retention of food in the mouth is enhanced and oral clearance decreased. Because of chewing and swallowing difficulties, fresh fruits and vegetables are withheld from the diet. Substitutes include pastries, canned fruits, puddings, and gelatin desserts, all with a high percentage of refined carbohydrates. The dentist and his or her staff must be aware of these modifications and be realistic in providing dietary recommendations to parents of children with developmental disabilities.

## REFERENCES

1. American Academy of Pediatric Dentistry: Policy on beverage vending machines in schools. *Pediatr Dent* 25:30, 2003.
2. Beiswanger BB, Elias A, Crawford JL et al: The effects of sugarless chewing gum use after meals on dental caries. *J Dent Res* 75 (Special Edition): 1003, 1996.
3. Burt BA, Eklund SA, Morgan KJ et al: The effects of sugar intake and frequency of ingestion on dental caries increment in a three-year longitudinal study. *J Dent Res* 67:1422-1429, 1988.
4. Centers for Disease Control and Prevention: Recommendations for using fluoride to prevent and control dental caries in the United States. *MMWR Morb Mortal Wkly Rep* 50 (RR-14):26, 2001.
5. Clarkson BH: Fluoride: biological implications and dietary supplementation. In: Pinkham JR, editor. *Pediatric Dental Care: An Update for the 90's*. Evansville, Ind., Bristol-Myers Squibb, 1991, pp 23-24.
6. Crall JJ, Bjerga JM: Fluoride uptake and retention following combined applications of APF and stannous fluoride in vitro. *Pediatr Dent* 6:226-229, 1984.
7. Grossman E, Proskin H: A comparison of the efficacy and safety of an electric and manual children's toothbrush. *JADA* 128:469-474, 1997.
8. Hunt CE, Navia JM: Pre-eruptive effects of Mo, B, Sr, and F on dental caries in the rat. *Arch Oral Biol* 20:497-501, 1975.
9. Jensen ME: Responses of interproximal plaque pH to snack foods and effect of chewing sorbitol-containing gum. *JADA* 113:262-266, 1986.
10. Jensen ME, Wefel JS: Human plaque pH responses to meals and the effects of chewing gum. *Br Dent J* 167:204-208, 1989.
11. Nowak AJ, Skotowski MC, Widmer R et al: A practice based evaluation of a range of children's manual toothbrushes: safety and acceptance. *Compendium* 23 (suppl 2):17-24, 2002.
12. Nowak AJ, Skotowski MC, Cugini M et al: A practice based study of a children's power toothbrush: efficacy and acceptance. *Compendium* 23 (suppl 2):25-32, 2002.
13. Peldyak J, Makinen KK: Xylitol for caries presentation. *J Dent Hyg* 76:276-285, 2002.
14. Singleton JC, Achterberg L, Shannon B: Role of food and nutrition in the health perceptions of young children. *J Am Diet Assoc* 92:67-70, 1992.
15. US Bureau of the Census: *Statistical Abstract of the United States: 2000*, 120th ed. Washington, DC, The Bureau, 2000.
16. van Eck AAMJ, Groenveld A, Backer Dirks O: Pre- and posteruptive caries reduction by water fluoridation. *Caries Res* 19(Abstr 28):163, 1985.
17. Whall C: Personal communications. American Dental Association Council on Dental Therapeutics, 1992.

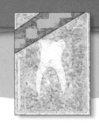

# CHAPTER 32

# Pit and Fissure Sealants and Conservative Adhesive Restorations: Scientific and Clinical Rationale

*John Hicks and Catherine M. Flaitz*

Increasingly, the attention of the dental profession has been directed toward prevention of dental caries in pits and fissures. For a number of decades, the prime area of concern has been related to reducing the incidence and prevalence of caries occurring in smooth surfaces. The most recent national surveys during the past several decades on caries incidence and prevalence in pediatric and adolescent groups have shown dramatic reductions in dental caries, especially with respect to smooth surface lesions.* This significant change in the caries status of children and adolescents has been attributed to a number of factors.[45-48,73,95,101] First, this generation of children may have benefited from the optimal use of both systemic and topical fluorides. Second, parents have become increasingly aware of the importance and need for both preventive and restorative dental care for their young children.

---

Thus parents bring their children to the dentist at an earlier age when perhaps only preventive measures or minimal restorative procedures are indicated. In addition, the dentist is provided an opportunity to educate both parents and children about the preventive practices available to minimize the caries experience for the child and adolescent. Third, group dental insurance, managed care, and government-funded programs that include expanded preventive and restorative dental care for young children are now common. The availability of such programs has removed some of the financial burden for children's dental care from the family. Fourth, the increase in dental manpower and availability has allowed easy access to technologically advanced dental care in both urban and rural communities. Finally, the interest of the dental profession in preventive dentistry has increased as the beneficial effects of preventive regimens on dental disease have become evident and both scientific and clinical bases for these regimens have been demonstrated.

Despite the dramatic improvement in the caries status of children, dental caries represents the most common childhood disease in the United States.[182] It is five times more common than asthma and seven times more common than allergic rhinitis (hay fever) in the 5- to 17-year-old population. By age 17 years, more than 75% of late adolescents have experienced caries, and slightly less than 10% have lost at least one permanent tooth to the ravages of caries. About 20% of 2- to 4-year-olds have had restorations placed or teeth extracted due to caries, with an additional 16% having untreated dental caries. Across all age groups, about one third of individuals have untreated dental caries. The sequelae of dental caries continue into adulthood, with more than 95% of adults experiencing caries and more than 25% being edentulous.

Particularly troublesome is the fact that 80% of the dental caries in the permanent dentition of 5- to 17-year-olds occurs in 25% of children.[10,17-20,49,210,242] Children in lower socioeconomic groups and of either Mexican-American or African-American descent have significantly greater caries prevalence than their higher income or non-Hispanic white counterparts. In these high-risk children, untreated caries is found in at least one third of primary teeth, which may be associated with pain, eating discomfort and difficulty, and underweight.

## EPIDEMIOLOGY OF PIT AND FISSURE CARIES

Tooth surfaces with pits and fissures are particularly vulnerable to caries development. With the permanent dentition, caries involving the occlusal surfaces account for almost 60% of the total caries experience in children and adolescents, according to the 1986–1987 NIDR survey and the 1988–1994 NHANES III survey* (Table 32-1). Previously, in the 1974 NCHS survey, occlusal caries represented 49% of total caries.[71,95,101,175,176] The increased proportion of caries experience attributed to pit and fissure caries is most likely due to the decreasing prevalence of caries with interproximal surfaces. Between the 1974 and 1980 surveys, a 53% reduction in interproximal caries occurred. A further reduction of 50% in interproximal caries occurred between 1980 and 1987 for all children. Surprisingly, interproximal caries declined an additional 25% from 1987 to 1994.[1,17-20,133] When considering children residing in fluoridated communities, the prevalence of interproximal caries decreased by 75% from 1980 to 1987 and by 88% from 1974 to 1987.

In fluoride-deficient communities, the reduction in interproximal caries was 37% between 1980 and 1987[†] (see Table 32-1) and may reflect the influence of fluoridated toothpastes, fluoride rinses, school-based water fluoridation programs, and professionally applied topical fluoride. From the information provided by the 1987 NIDR study,[‡] interproximal caries were decreased by 60% in fluoridated communities, whereas buccal or lingual and occlusal caries were decreased by only 10% in these fluoridated communities. This discrepancy emphasizes the fact that enamel forming pits and fissures does not receive the same level of caries protection from fluoride as smooth surface enamel. This finding may also partially explain the fact that occlusal caries are responsible for almost 60% of the total caries experience, although occlusal surfaces account for only 12.5% of the total number of tooth surfaces exposed to cariogenic challenges. The reason for this increased susceptibility is the presence of pits and fissures on these surfaces. When caries occurring in pits and fissures on buccal and

---

*References 17,18,70,72,114,177,178,211,213.
†References 1,10,17-20,82,91,133,142,175-178.
‡References 17,18,70,72,114,131,177,178,202,213.

## TABLE 32-1

### Dental Caries in School Children by Surface Type

|  | OCCLUSAL (DMFS) | BUCCAL/LINGUAL (DMFS) | PROXIMAL (DMFS) |
|---|---|---|---|
| NCHS 1971-74 | 49% (3.5) | 27% (1.9) | 24% (1.7) |
| NIDR 1979-80 | 54% (2.6) | 29% (1.4) | 17% (0.8) |
| NIDR 1986-87 |  |  |  |
| *All children* | 58% (1.8) | 29% (0.9) | 13% (0.4) |
| *Fluoridated* | 60% (1.7) | 31% (0.9) | 9% (0.2) |
| *Nonfluoridated* | 56% (1.9) | 30% (1.0) | 14% (0.5) |
| NHANES III 1988-91 | 56% (1.9) | 32% (0.8) | 12% (0.3) |

### CARIES REDUCTION (compared with NCHS 1971-74)

|  | NIDR 1986-87 | NHANES III 1988-94 |
|---|---|---|
| Occlusal surfaces | 49% | 60% |
| Buccal/lingual | 53% | 58% |
| Proximal surfaces posterior teeth | 74% | 82% |

### PIT AND FISSURE SURFACE CARIES REDUCTION: NHANES III 1988-94 (compared with NIDR 1979-80)

*Maxilla*

| First molar | Occlusal | 27 |
|---|---|---|
| Second molar | Occlusal | 33 |

*Mandible*

| First molar | Occlusal | 28 |
|---|---|---|
| First molar | Buccal | 23 |
| Second molar | Occlusal | 32 |

### TRANSITION OF CARIES IN SCHOOL CHILDREN (Risk Ratio Compared with Control)

|  | SOUND TO CARIOUS LESION | | | INTACT TO CAVITATION | | |
|---|---|---|---|---|---|---|
|  | BUCCAL/LINGUAL | PROXIMAL | OCCLUSAL | BUCCAL/LINGUAL | PROXIMAL | OCCLUSAL |
| Control | 1.0 | 1.1 | 3.7 | 1.0 | 2.1 | 6.7 |
| Sugar-free gum | 0.9 | 1.1 | 3.6 | 0.9 | 1.7 | 7.3 |
| Fluoride dentifrice | 0.9 | 1.2 | 3.3 | 0.8 | 1.7 | 5.6 |

Compiled from references 1,10,17-20,82,91,133,141,175-178,213.

lingual surfaces are taken into consideration, pit and fissure caries account for more than 80% of the total caries experience in all children and adolescents.[1,11,17-20,133] In fluoridated communities, more than 90% of dental caries occur in occlusal and buccal-lingual surfaces and represent, almost exclusively, pit and fissure caries.[17-20,45-48,133,178,227] According to NHANES III,[1,17-20,133,211,213] 88% of caries are found in surfaces associated with pit and fissure caries in children and

adolescents. From 1987 to 1994, interproximal caries was reduced by 25% whereas pit and fissure caries decreased by 18%.

In contrast to the permanent dentition, interproximal caries are more common in the primary dentition (Table 32-2).[19,133,146,213,241] In regional and national surveys,[17-20,133,241] caries experience is distributed almost equally among occlusal (35% to 40%), buccal/lingual (26% to 29%), and proximal (35%) tooth surfaces. Water fluorida-

**TABLE 32-2**

**Prevalence and Distribution of Caries for Primary Teeth**

| | DECAYED FILLED SURFACES, PRIMARY TEETH | CARIES-FREE | CARIES DISTRIBUTION BY SURFACE | | |
| --- | --- | --- | --- | --- | --- |
| | | | OCCLUSAL | BUCCAL/ LINGUAL | PROXIMAL |
| **Head Start Program (1990)** | | | | | |
| Fluoride-deficient community | 7.44 | 30.4% | 35.3% | 25.0% | 39.5% |
| Fluoridated community | 4.80 | 36.1% | 41.0% | 26.3% | 32.7% |
| All children | 5.67 | 34.2% | 39.2% | 25.9% | 34.9% |
| **NHANES III (1988-1994)** | | | | | |
| 2- to 4-year-olds | 1.2 | 83.1% | 25.0% | 36.5% | 36.5% |
| 5- to 9-year-olds | 4.1 | 50.3% | 39.0% | 24.4% | 36.6% |
| 2- to 9-year-olds | 3.1 | 62.1% | 35.5% | 29.0% | 35.5% |

Compiled from references 19,133,146,213,241.

tion reduces interproximal caries in primary teeth by 45%. In contrast, the prevalence of occlusal caries in fluoridated communities is decreased by 23%, whereas that for buccal/lingual caries is reduced by 32%. Pit and fissure caries in occlusal and buccal/lingual surfaces of primary teeth probably accounts for the lessened caries-preventive effect of water fluoridation seen with these surfaces when compared with interproximal surfaces.

Pit and fissure caries represents a disease process that has an early onset. Approximately 20% of children between the ages of 2 and 4 years have experienced caries in the primary dentition. In this age group, caries in occlusal surfaces alone may account for up to 67% of lesions. With the permanent dentition, 65% of first molars in 12-year-old adolescents either have been restored or currently have occlusal caries. In fact, in elementary schoolchildren from a fluoridated community, 90% of all lesions in the first permanent molars have been found to be pit and fissure caries.[*]

Although previously the incidence of pit and fissure caries in occlusal surfaces was thought to be greatest during the first 4 years following eruption, longitudinal studies of caries development in occlusal surfaces of permanent molars

(Table 32-3) provide some interesting findings.[†] The annual incidence of caries development in sound occlusal and interproximal surfaces has been determined over an 8-year period.[243] The development of pit and fissure caries in sound occlusal surfaces occurred at a rate of 15% and 10% for ages 8 and 9 years, respectively. From ages 10 through 15 years, pit and fissure caries continued to occur in previously sound first permanent molars at a rate of 4.3% to 6.8% per year. In contrast, interproximal caries occurred at an annual rate of 0.3% to 2.4%. When sound first permanent molars were followed in children from ages 8 to 15 years, it was found that 47% of occlusal surfaces developed pit and fissure caries whereas only 10% of interproximal surfaces succumbed to caries during this same period. The mean annual incidence of caries development in previously sound first permanent molars was 5.9% for occlusal surfaces and 1.3% for interproximal surfaces.

A separate clinical study (see Table 32-3) evaluated occlusal caries development in young adults aged 17 to 22 years.[229,230] During the 40-month study period, one third of these young adults developed occlusal caries without radiographic evidence of interproximal lesions in their permanent molars and premolars. An additional 10% developed occlusal caries with radiographic evidence of interproximal lesions. In this group of individuals, it appears that sealant placement during late adolescence or early adulthood would

[*]References 1,14,17-20,45-48,81,82,91,133,146,227,241.
[†]References 27,28,51,52,141,229,230,243.

## TABLE 32-3

### Annual Attack Rate of Occlusal and Interproximal Caries Development in Sound Permanent First Molars

| AGE | OCCLUSAL SURFACES (CARIES INCIDENCE) | INTERPROXIMAL SURFACES (CARIES INCIDENCE) |
|---|---|---|
| **Annual Attack Rate in 8- to 15-Year-Olds** | | |
| 8-year-olds | 15.0% | 0.3% |
| 9-year-olds | 10.1% | 1.1% |
| 10-year-olds | 5.8% | 0.9% |
| 11-year-olds | 6.4% | 0.9% |
| 12-year-olds | 5.2% | 2.4% |
| 13-year-olds | 5.9% | 1.8% |
| 14-year-olds | 4.3% | 1.3% |
| 15-year-olds | 6.8% | 2.1% |
| | | |
| **Average Annual Attack Rate During 8 Years** | | |
| | 5.9% | 1.3% |
| | | |
| **Total Percentage with Caries after 8 Years** | | |
| | 47% | 10% |
| | | |
| **Prevalence of Occlusal Caries in Molars of Young Adults** | | |
| *Coast Guard cadets (age range, 17 to 23 years)* | | |
| All molars | 11.9% | -- |
| First molars | 9.9% | -- |
| Second molars | 14.0% | -- |
| *Young military recruits (mean age, 20.9 years)* | | |
| Permanent molars | 25.4% | -- |
| | | |
| **Prospective Occlusal Caries Prevalence** | | |
| *Scandinavia* | | |
| 15-year-olds | 50 | -- |
| 20-year-olds | 75 | -- |
| *The Netherlands* | | |
| 17-year-olds | 63 | -- |
| 23-year-olds | 79 | -- |

| **Prevalence of Occlusal Caries in USA** | NCHS 1971-74 | NHANES III 1988-1994 |
|---|---|---|
| 10-year-olds | 55 | 15 |
| 16-year-olds | 68 | 25 |

Compiled from references 27,28,52,53,141,229,230,243.

have prevented restoration of the occlusal surfaces in more than 75% of cases. The incidence of occlusal caries development without interproximal lesions was found to be 9.9% for first permanent molars 11 to 16 years after eruption, 14.0% for second permanent molars 5 to 10 years after eruption, and 0.8% for premolars 7 to 12 years after eruption.

Assessment of the need for dental sealant placement in United States Air Force, Marines, and Navy recruits and active-duty military service personnel has provided interesting findings.[27,28,52,141]

In young military recruits (mean age 20.9 years, age range 17 to 25 years; see Table 32-3), occlusal caries were identified in 25% of permanent molars. It was also noted that at least one first or second molar needed sealant placement in 47% of the recruits. In almost one third of these young adults, occlusal caries could have been prevented by sealant application. Although the majority of pit and fissure caries were previously thought to occur within 4 years following eruption, these epidemiologic studies emphasize that pit and fissure caries continue to occur throughout late adolescence and well into early adulthood. In fact, it was found that 30% of the 24- to 25-year-old military recruits would benefit from sealant placement. The question of whether to place a sealant over a fissured surface should not be based on how long ago a tooth erupted into the oral cavity but on the clinical impression of whether a sealant is necessary to prevent caries.

## MORPHOLOGY OF SURFACES WITH PITS AND FISSURES

The dental profession has known for some time that susceptibility to caries on tooth surfaces containing pits and fissures is related to the form and depth of these pits and fissures. Because of the interest in caries formation in pits and fissures, attempts have been made to provide an elaborate classification system for pits and fissures. However, for the sake of simplicity, two main types of pits and fissures (Fig. 32-1) are usually described: (1) shallow, wide V-shaped fissures that tend to be self-cleansing and somewhat caries resistant, and (2) deep, narrow I-shaped fissures that are quite constricted and may resemble a bottleneck in that the fissure may have an extremely narrow slit-like opening with a larger base as it extends toward the dentinoenamel junction. These caries-susceptible, I-shaped fissures may also have a number of different branches extending toward or into the underlying dentin. The typical fissure usually contains an organic plug composed of reduced enamel epithelium, microorganisms forming dental plaque, and oral debris. Examination of fissures, even with a low level of magnification, reveals the reason for the caries susceptibility of tooth surfaces with pits and fissures. The fissure provides a protected niche for plaque accumulation. The rapidity with which dental caries occurs in pits and fissures is most likely related to the fact that the depth of the fissure is in close proximity to the dentinoenamel junction and the underlying dentin, which is highly susceptible to caries.[66,96,97,179,205]

The morphology of occlusal surfaces varies from one tooth to the next and from individual to individual. However, in general, the "typical" premolar (Fig. 32-2, A) has a prominent primary fissure with usually three or four pits. In the typical molar (Fig. 32-2, B), as many as 10 separate pits may be present in primary, secondary, and supplemental fissures. In addition, certain surface porosities that would not be noticed clinically

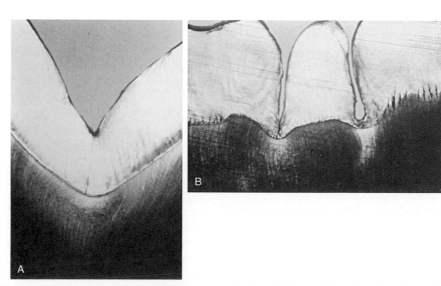

**Figure 32-1**  Histologic appearance of the main types of pits and fissures in occlusal surfaces (polarized light microscopy: water imbibition). **A,** Shallow, wide V-shaped fissure. **B,** Deep, narrow I-shaped fissure.

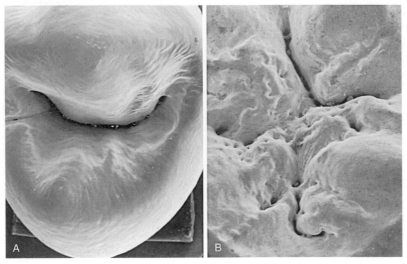

**Figure 32-2**   Surface morphologic appearance of caries-free premolar (**A**) and permanent molar (**B**) (scanning electron microscopy).

become apparent when the surface is examined microscopically.

## HISTOPATHOLOGY OF CARIES IN PITS AND FISSURES

At one time, caries formation in fissures was thought to begin at the base of the fissure, involving the deeper aspect of the underlying tooth structure before the walls and cuspal inclines of the fissure became involved in the caries process. This process was expected because the fissure extended into the tooth surface for a considerable depth. However, such is not the case. Rather, the inclines forming the walls of the fissures are affected first by the caries process. The first histologic evidence of lesion formation occurs at the orifice of the fissure and is usually represented by two independent bilateral lesions in the enamel composing the opposing cuspal inclines (Fig. 32-3, *A*). As the lesion progresses, the depths of the fissure walls become involved, and coalescence of the two independent lesions into a single, contiguous lesion occurs at the base of the fissure. The enamel at the base of the fissure is affected to a greater degree than that of the cuspal inclines, and the lesion spreads laterally along the enamel adjacent to the depth of the fissure and readily toward the dentinoenamel junction (Fig. 32-3, *B*). Once the caries process involves the dentin, the progress of the lesion is enhanced because caries susceptibility of dentin is increased compared with enamel. Eventually, cavitation of the fissure

occurs owing to loss of mineral and structural support from the adjacent affected enamel and dentin, resulting in a clinically detectable lesion. The unique process of caries formation in pits and fissures is due to the presence of an organic plug in the fissure. This organic plug acts as a buffer against the acid byproducts of plaque and provides a diffusion barrier, which results in a lessened acid attack at the fissural base during the initial phase of caries formation.[96,97]

Although systemic and topical fluoride use has been highly effective in prevention of caries on smooth surfaces, enamel surfaces with pits and fissures receive minimal caries protection from either systemic or topical fluoride agents. The reason why fluoride is less effective in preventing caries in fissured surfaces may be related to the total depth of enamel on smooth surfaces compared with that underlying the fissure.[96,97,217-219] On smooth surfaces, at least 1 mm of enamel is found superficial to the dentinoenamel junction. In contrast, the base of a fissure or pit may be relatively close to or lie within the dentin. When caries develop in a fissure, the underlying dentin becomes involved rapidly, resulting in a frank, clinically detectable lesion. When caries formation occurs in enamel on a smooth surface, a considerable amount of enamel must become involved before the dentin is involved. It is thought that 3 or 4 years may be required for dentinal involvement to occur. During this time period, remineralization of the smooth surface lesion following exposure to fluoride agents may occur, resulting in the arrest or reversal of the

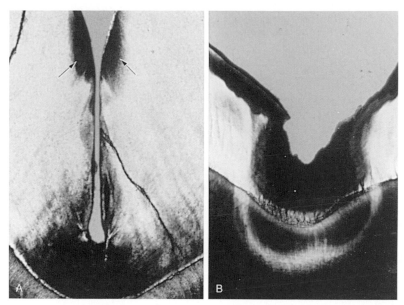

**Figure 32-3**   Histologic appearance of pit and fissure caries (polarized light microscopy: water imbibition). **A,** Caries formation *(arrows)* begins in the cuspal inclines just above the fissure orifice. The darkened appearance at the base of the fissure is due to the organic material present. **B,** The lesion progresses to the point at which the base of the fissure and underlying dentin become involved. With further progression, cavitation will occur, resulting in a clinically detectable lesion.

lesion. When pits and fissures are present on smooth surfaces (Fig. 32-4), the pattern of involvement is identical to that seen on occlusal surfaces, and progression of the lesion to a clinically detectable level appears to be related to the lessened thickness of the enamel present and the morphologic form of the pit or fissure.

## PREVENTION OF PIT AND FISSURE CARIES: HISTORICAL PERSPECTIVE AND PIT AND FISSURE SEALANT MATERIALS

During the 1920s, two different clinical techniques were introduced in an attempt to reduce the extent and severity of pit and fissure caries in occlusal and smooth surfaces.[13,123] In 1924, Thaddeus Hyatt[123] advocated prophylactic restoration. This procedure consisted of preparing a conservative class I cavity that included all pits and fissures at risk for caries development and then placing an amalgam restoration. The rationale for prophylactic restoration of an otherwise caries-free surface was that the procedure prevented further insult to the pulp from caries, decreased loss of tooth structure, and required less time for restoration when the tooth eventually succumbed to caries. A more conservative

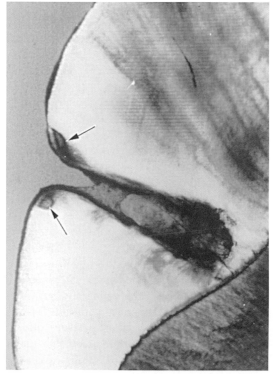

**Figure 32-4**   Histologic appearance of a pit in the buccal surface of a permanent molar tooth. Caries formation *(arrows)* is evident at the orifice of the fissure. An organic plug is present in the fissure. The base of the pit approaches the dentinoenamel junction (polarized light microscopy: water imbibition).

approach to prevention of pit and fissure caries was presented by Bodecker in 1929.[13] Initially, he advocated cleaning the fissure with an explorer and flowing a thin mix of oxyphosphate cement into the fissure in an attempt to "seal" the fissure. Later, he introduced an alternative method for caries prevention, the prophylactic odontotomy, which involved mechanical eradication of fissures in order to transform deep, retentive fissures into cleansable ones. These two techniques, prophylactic restoration and prophylactic odontotomy, were employed until the use of sealants became prevalent.

The development of pit and fissure sealants was based on the discovery that etching enamel with phosphoric acid increased the retention of resin restorative materials and improved marginal integrity considerably. The initial studies evaluating the effects of acid etching on enamel were performed by Buonocore in 1955.[21] The first sealant material that utilized the acid-etch technique was introduced in the mid-1960s and was a cyanoacrylate substance. Cyanoacrylates were not suitable as sealant materials owing to bacterial degradation of the material in the oral cavity over time. By the late 1960s, a number of different resin materials had been tested, and a viscous resin was found to be resistant to degradation and produced a tenacious bond with etched enamel. This resin was formed by reacting bisphenol A with glycidyl methacrylate, and this class of dimethacrylate resins has become known as BIS-GMA.[15]

BIS-GMA is a relatively large epoxy resin–like hybrid monomer in which epoxy groups are replaced by methacrylate groups.[22,92,168] BIS-GMA incorporates the rapid polymerization characteristic of methyl methacrylate with the minimal polymerization shrinkage property of epoxy resins. The vast majority of restorative resins are based on the BIS-GMA formulation. They differ from sealants in that restorative resin materials include filler particles such as quartz, glass, and porcelain to improve their strength, whereas the majority of sealants either are unfilled BIS-GMA or have relatively few filler particles added. However, some sealant products contain up to 50% filler particles intended to improve wear resistance.

BIS-GMA sealants differ in the ways in which the material is polymerized. Two methods of polymerization have been employed. Autopolymerization (chemically cured) systems involve mixing two liquids (a base resin and a catalyst resin). The material sets by an exothermic reaction, usually within 1 to 2 minutes. Photoactivated (visible light–cured) polymerization is currently the most popular method used for curing sealants. During the 1970s and early 1980s, ultraviolet light with a wavelength of 365 nm was used to initiate the setting reaction. However, due to the inconsistency of the wavelength from the ultraviolet light source and the potential for retinal damage with long-term exposure to ultraviolet light, this method of curing sealants was abandoned. In its place, photoactivation of sealant material with a visible–light source was introduced.

Photoactivated resins contain a diketone initiator such as camphoroquinone and a reducing agent such as a tertiary amine to initiate polymerization. This photoinitiator system is quite sensitive to light in the blue region of the visible light spectrum, with peak initiator activity centered around 480 nm. Use of visible light sources requires eye protection due to the intensity of the light created. The benefits of light-cured versus chemical-cured sealants are the following: (1) the sealant material sets in 10 to 20 seconds; (2) no mixing of resins is required, eliminating the incorporation of air bubbles that may occur with chemical-cured materials; (3) the viscosity of the sealant remains constant during infiltration of the etched enamel pores, and the sealant does not set until it is light activated. Laser curing of visible light–activated sealant and resin materials has been advocated.[12,103,134,193,259-261] In particular, the argon laser produces a visible blue-green light beam with a monochromatic wavelength similar to that used with visible light sources. The laser light beam also exhibits coherence and may be collimated and focused to a small spot size. The advantages of using a laser for initiating the setting reaction of sealants and restorative resins are (1) a further reduction in the setting time; (2) control over specific radiation energy, wavelength, and area of exposure; and (3) a decrease in the percentage of unpolymerized resin compared with conventional visible light curing. In addition, resin materials exposed to the laser have increased tensile and bond strengths,[133] and lased enamel along the sealant interface and forming the adjacent tooth surface has increased resistance to a cariogenic challenge.[103,259-261] The disadvantages of using a laser for curing resin materials are the cost of the instrument itself and the need for adequate training in laser operation and safety techniques. In the future, the laser may become more common in dental practices and may eventually replace visible light sources for polymerization of resin materials.

Opaque, tinted, colored, and clear sealant materials are commercially available. Opaque and tinted sealants have been advocated because of their ease of detection by the dentist, parents, and child, which allows monitoring of sealant retention.[45-48,204,222-227] Detection of a clear sealant requires tactile exploration of the sealed surface. A study has shown that the error rate among dentists in identifying the presence or absence of sealants is 1.4% for opaque sealants and 22.8% for clear sealants.[204] No apparent differences have been reported among opaque, tinted, or clear sealants for retention rates and caries prevention. Opaque sealants may not allow for caries detection under sealed pit and fissures using laser fluorescent devices. In addition to BIS-GMA sealants, conventional glass ionomer materials have also been used as pit and fissure sealants. Glass ionomers bond to both enamel and dentin by physicochemical mechanisms following polyacrylic acid conditioning.* The primary advantage of glass ionomers over conventional BIS-GMA sealants is the capability of glass ionomers to release fluoride. These materials are formed by reacting calcium aluminosilicate with polyacrylic acid in the presence of a fluoride flux. The ionomer powder is created by heating a variable mixture of silica, alumina, calcium fluoride as a flux, cryolite, sodium fluoride and/or aluminum phosphate to $1100°$ C to $1500°$ C. The liquid component is a copolymer of acrylic and itaconic acid or copolymers of maleic and tricarboxylic acids. The liquid component may be freeze dried and incorporated into the powder. In this situation, a dilute solution of water and tartaric acid as a chelating agent is used to activate the chemical acid-base setting reaction. The resulting material may contain as much as 19% fluoride by weight. This fluoride is readily exchangeable for hydroxyl and chloride ions from the adjacent enamel and dentin. Incorporation of the released fluoride into the adjacent enamel and dentin may enhance caries resistance, remineralize enamel caries and affected dentin, and alter the bacterial composition and metabolic byproducts of plaque.[92,102] The role of glass ionomer–containing "sealants" is currently being defined. Their potential for caries

reduction in pits and fissures seems to be high, although their long-term retention rate and wear resistance are questionable.

Hybrid materials composed of a variable mixture of glass ionomer and composite resin (resin-modified glass ionomers) have been advocated as possible pit and fissure sealants because of the improved physical characteristics over glass ionomers, relative ease of placement, adhesive compatibility with various dental substrates, and fluoride-releasing capability.* Such resin ionomers may be classified into resin-modified ionomers and ionomer-modified resins. The liquid components in both types are acidic monomers (hydroxyethyl methacrylate [HEMA], water, and polyacrylic acid analog with or without pendant methacrylic groups) that may copolymerize with dentin-bonding agents, unfilled bonding resins, or restorative composites and also react chemically via an ionomer type of acid-base reaction with glass fillers (fluoroaluminosilicate glass). The setting reaction is initiated by photoactivation of the resin component through methacrylate groups grafted onto the polyacrylic acid chain and methacrylate groups derived from HEMA. This is followed by an acid-base reaction between the filler and the matrix. Some materials also undergo chemical autocuring via generation of free radical methacrylates, which induce polymerization of the resin matrix polymer system and HEMA. Therefore it is possible that a resin may undergo dual curing or even tricuring with chemically cured and/or photoactivated resin curing in the presence of a chemical acid-base reaction characteristic for ionomers. These resin-modified ionomers still require a weak acid pretreatment of the tooth structure and visible light curing; however these materials are considered to be less technique sensitive than conventional glass ionomers. Ionomer-modified resins are also known as compomers and are composed of a glass filler with an anhydrous acid monomer matrix. The setting reaction between the glass filler and matrix occurs quite slowly while absorbing water after placement. Etching of dental substrates and placement of bonding primers may be necessary for long-term retention. Although the bond strength of compomers is higher than that for conventional glass ionomers, the occlusal wear resistance is considered to be low.

---

Selection of a specific sealant product depends on whether the practitioner prefers an opaque, tinted, colored, or clear sealant that is filled or unfilled and whether he or she prefers visible light curing or autopolymerization of the sealant material. The overall decision should be based on retention rates and caries incidences from longitudinal clinical trials. A number of sealant products (Table 32-4)[4,58] have met certain biologic, laboratory, and clinical guidelines established by the Council on Scientific Affairs of the American Dental Association (ADA, available at http:\\www.ada.org, 2004).[4] Sealant materials may receive a seal of acceptance from this testing agency. Periodically, updates on various dental materials, including sealants, are published by this ADA Council,[4] and these may serve as guides in selecting a sealant material.

During the mid-1990s, safety concerns were expressed regarding leaching of bisphenol A (BPA) and bisphenol A dimethacrylate (BPA-DMA) from sealants, and a possible estrogenic effect.[181] It is known that incomplete conversion of BPA during the setting reaction may allow release of this unreacted monomer into the oral environment. BPA and BPA-DMA possess estrogen-like effects in cultures of breast tumor cells, and this was the basis for the safety concerns

## TABLE 32-4
### Pit and Fissure Sealant Materials

| SEALANT MATERIAL | MANUFACTURER |
| --- | --- |
| **ADA Seal of Acceptance** | |
| Alpha-Dent Chemical Cure | Alpha-Dental Product Co. |
| Alpha-Dent Light Cure | Alpha-Dental Product Co. |
| Baritone L3 | Confi-Dental Products Co. |
| Helioseal F | Ivoclar-Vivadent, Inc. |
| Helioseal | Ivoclar-Vivadent, Inc. |
| Prisma Shield | Dentsply LD Caulk Division |
| Prisma Shield Compule Tips VLC Tinted Pit and Fissure Sealant | Dentsply LD Caulk Division |
| Prisma Shield VLC Filled Pit and Fissure Sealant | Dentsply LD Caulk Division |
| Seal-Rite | Pulpdent Corporation |
| Seal-Rite Low Viscosity | Pulpdent Corporation |
| | |
| **Other Sealants** | |
| Bisco Sealant (G-9200S) | Bisco Dental Products |
| Clinpro Sealant | 3M-ESPE |
| Copaliner | Harry J. Bosworth Company |
| Delton Plus | Dentsply Ash |
| EcuSeal | Zenith/DMG |
| Estiseal LC | Heraeus Kulzer Inc. |
| Fluroseal | Scientific Pharmaceuticals Inc. |
| FluorShield | Dentsply Caulk |
| FluRestore | DenMat Corporation |
| Guardian Seal | SDS-Kerr |
| Quikseal | Chameleon Dental Products |
| Team Sealant | Centrix |
| Teethmate-F | J Morita USA |
| Total-Seal Pit and Fissure Sealant | American Dental Hygienics |
| UltraSeal XT Plus Fissure Sealant | Ultradent Products Inc |

Compiled from references 4,58.

regarding sealants and composite resins. Sophisticated analysis of seven pit and fissure sealants with high-performance liquid chromatography, ultraviolet spectral analysis, and mass spectrography provide reassuring evidence regarding the safety of these materials.[174] BPA was below the level of detectability (less than 0.0001 μg BPA per mg of sealant tested) with all seven sealants. BPA-DMA was not detected in five of the seven sealants tested, with the remaining two having mean levels of 0.39 μg and 1.23 μg BPA-DMA per milligram of sealant tested. This laboratory investigation utilized 95% ethanol, which is a solvent for BPA and BPA-DMA, to extract leachable components. Additional studies using water have failed to demonstrate elution of BPA from sealants.[84] It appears that elution of possible estrogenic chemicals from sealants and composite resins does not necessitate the use of different sealant materials or restrict sealant usage in children or adults. Further clinical investigations[7,64,209] into salivary and serum levels of leachable chemicals from dental materials have shown that detectable levels of BPA are present in saliva shortly after placement (1 and 3 hours), but BPA is not detectable after 24 hours. More importantly, serum at all time intervals did not have detectable levels of BPA.[64] This implies that BPA may be released from a sealant into the oral cavity but that it is not systemically absorbed. No adverse health effects have been attributed to the leachable components in sealants or composite resins.[64,174]

## DIAGNOSIS OF PIT AND FISSURE CARIES

In 1968 at an ADA-sponsored conference on clinical testing of cariostatic agents,[196] the criteria for detection and diagnosis of pit and fissure lesions were defined as follows:

> Caries is present when the explorer catches or resists removal after insertion into a pit or fissure with moderate to firm pressure and when this is accompanied by one or more of the following signs of caries: (a) softness at the base of the area; (b) opacity or loss of normal translucency adjacent to the pit or fissure as evidence of undermining or demineralization; (c) softened enamel adjacent to the pit or fissure that can be scraped away with the explorer.

Although the incidence and prevalence of pit and fissure caries and the dental technology in dealing with this type of caries have changed dramatically since 1968, the dental profession is still using more or less the same criteria for diagnosis of pit and fissure caries. Diagnosis is based primarily on tactile evaluation with an explorer and visual assessment of the enamel appearance (visual-tactile inspection). Clinical examination is quite variable from one practitioner to another owing to the size and shape of the explorer tip, the force applied, and the judgment of the examiner.[120] In general, radiographic evaluation of occlusal surfaces has been found to be of minimal diagnostic value in detecting enamel caries and superficial dentinal caries.* Attempts to use fiberoptic transillumination to detect caries have been of value for interproximal surfaces but have failed to provide additional information about the caries status of occlusal surfaces.[203] Light-induced and infrared laser fluorescence devices for pit and fissure caries diagnosis has demonstrated promise over the past several years.†

There have been advocates for eliminating the explorer in evaluation of pit and fissure caries for fear of damaging the enamel lining pits and fissures, resulting in caries development and more rapid progression when enamel caries is present, and because it is felt that probing is unreliable in caries detection.[228,265] Clinical and laboratory studies have indicated that there is no difference in diagnostic accuracy when dentists use either visual-tactile or visual inspection alone. Perhaps this has more to do with the fact that reliability or reproducibility in diagnosis of pit and fissure caries is quite poor among dentists. In fact, it has been shown that with pit and fissure surfaces the correct diagnosis of caries occurs in only 42% of cases and only 20% to 48% of lesions histologically involving dentin are detected. However, it is more likely that dentists will treat carious teeth than restore sound teeth (sensitivity 62% and specificity 84%). Currently, there are a number of techniques to aid the dentist in diagnosis of pit and fissure caries. These include conventional, xeroradiographic, and digital radiography; fiberoptic transillumination; infrared laser and light-induced fluorescence; caries-detecting dye penetration; ultrasonic imaging; and electrical resistance.‡

---

*References 8,9,50,147,148,152,154,191,192,232,237.
†References 3,6,57,144,147,194,233,237.
‡References 5,144,152,188,214,228,232,237,262,265.

A promising ancillary diagnostic device introduced during the 1980s was the electronic caries detector, which was touted to be superior to the explorer because of its increased sensitivity, specificity, and consistency in pit and fissure caries diagnosis.* In laboratory studies comparing the clinical, radiographic, and histologic appearances of occlusal caries, the electronic caries detector was found to correlate well with the extent of histologic involvement of occlusal surfaces by caries. Electronic caries detection was found to have a high sensitivity (0.70 to 1.00) and high specificity (0.71 to 0.96) when compared with histologic extent of pit and fissure caries. In comparison, conventional bitewing radiography had a sensitivity of 0.62 and a specificity of 0.77. However, because of the expense of the instrument and the paucity of clinical studies, the electronic caries detector has not been readily accepted as a diagnostic instrument.

Quantitative laser fluorescence was introduced during the 1990s and has become commercially available as an instrument for detecting caries and following the clinical progress of enamel caries.† This device measures and quantifies the fluorescence of surface enamel that is induced after laser irradiation. Fluorescence differences between sound enamel and enamel caries occur due to a relationship between mineral loss and radiance of the fluorescence. Laser fluorescence has been stated to be best suited for shallow enamel caries on accessible smooth surfaces. A specific chairside laser fluorescence device for assessment of occlusal caries has been developed using fiber optics and a 655-nm diode laser light source. Changes in fluorescence attributed to demineralization are assigned a numeric value, compared with adjacent sound enamel. This device requires a clean surface because plaque, calcific deposits, and discoloration may give false or misleading values. Numeric values between 5 and 25 are considered to indicate enamel lesions, whereas values of 25 to 34 represent early dentinal caries, and values greater than 35 are considered to be advanced lesions in the dentin. These values may change with more current models and future models of this device. The sensitivity and specificity are similar to that for electronic caries monitors introduced in the 1980s, which were based on measurement of the electrical conductance. The highest sensitivity and specificity with laser fluorescence has been with dentinal caries, with lower sensitivity and specificity for enamel caries.

At this time, diagnosis of pit and fissure caries is based on visual assessment using a mouth mirror and adequate lighting, and tactile evaluation of the pits and fissures with a sharp explorer. Other ancillary devices may prove to be useful adjuncts but do not substitute for a thorough clinical examination of pit and fissure surfaces for caries detection and diagnosis.[6,130] The most important elements in diagnosis of and treatment planning for pit and fissure caries are clinical judgment and experience.

## PIT AND FISSURE TREATMENT ALTERNATIVES

With pits and fissures, a number of treatment options may be considered by the dental practitioner: (1) observation only; (2) sealant placement; (3) conservative adhesive restoration; (4) conservative restoration (glass ionomer-resin conservative restoration, glass ionomer conservative restoration, or sealant-amalgam conservative restoration); (5) amalgam, glass ionomer, glass ionomer–resin, or posterior composite restoration. The diagnostic criteria and recommended treatments are presented in Table 32-5.

Indications for sealant placement (Tables 32-5 and 32-6)* include the following: (1) deep, retentive pits and fissures, which may cause wedging or catching of an explorer; (2) stained pits and fissures with minimal appearance of decalcification or opacification; (3) pit and fissure caries or restoration of pits and fissures in other primary or permanent teeth; (4) no radiographic or clinical evidence of interproximal caries in need of restoration on teeth to be sealed; (5) use of other preventive treatment, such as systemic or topical fluoride therapy, to inhibit interproximal caries formation; (6) possibility of adequate isolation from salivary contamination. As noted previously, the development of pit and fissure caries in permanent molars may occur up to 16 years after eruption. Therefore, if a sealant appears to be indicated clinically for a premolar or first or second permanent molar in an older

---

*References 5,8,9,50,125,147,152,199,244,263.
†References 5,6,57,147,148,194,232,237.

*References 45,46,124,208,214,228,248,249.

adolescent or adult, a sealant should be placed to avoid caries development. In the past, the philosophy applied to pit and fissures was "drill and fill." With the present state of knowledge and technology in dentistry, the current philosophy should be "seal and heal."

Contraindications (see Tables 32-5 and 32-6)* for sealant placement are the following: (1) well-coalesced, self-cleaning pits and fissures; (2) radiographic or clinical evidence of interproximal caries in need of restoration; (3) presence of many interproximal lesions or restorations and no preventive treatment to inhibit interproximal caries formation; (4) tooth partially erupted and no possibility of adequate isolation from salivary

*References 45,46,124,208,214,228,248,249.

## TABLE 32-5
### Protocol for Pit and Fissure Treatment Alternatives

| DIAGNOSIS | TREATMENT |
| --- | --- |
| Caries-free surface: no explorer wedging* | No treatment |
| No explorer wedging*<br>Well-coalesced, self-cleansing shallow pits and fissures or no identifiable pits and fissures | Observation only and re-evaluation at 6-month recall examinations |
| Caries-free surface: no explorer wedging | No treatment |
| No explorer wedging<br>Stained pits and fissures | Observation only and re-evaluation at 6-month recall examinations |
| Caries-free surface: no explorer wedging | Sealant placement |
| No explorer wedging<br>Stained or minimal decalcified or opacified appearance of pits and fissures<br>No radiographic or clinical evidence of interproximal caries | Adequate isolation from saliva: place sealant<br>Adequate isolation not possible: allow further eruption and place sealant within 1 to 3 months.<br>Use hydrophilic bonding agent before sealant placement. Then close follow-up for possible sealant reapplication. |
| Caries-free surface: explorer wedging* | Sealant placement |
| Explorer wedging due to pit and fissure anatomy<br>Stained or decalcified appearance of pits and fissures<br>No radiographic or clinical evidence of interproximal caries | Adequate isolation from saliva: place sealant<br>Adequate isolation not possible: place sealant in accessible fissures and seal remaining fissures after further eruption (within 1 to 3 months); or remove overlying tissue and place sealant; or allow further eruption, and place sealant within 1 to 3 months.<br>Place sealant. |
| Incipient caries: minimal involvement | Conservative adhesive restoration placement<br>*(Restoration of isolated pits and fissures)* |
| Explorer catch[†] due to incipient or minimal caries involving limited areas of pits and fissures | Sealant/modified sealant (sealant alone; sealant and filled resin) |
| Decalcified appearance of pits and fissures indicative of incipient or minimal caries<br>Involvement of adjacent pit and fissure enamel with possible minimal involvement of underlying enamel and dentin<br>No or minimal undermining of isolated pits and fissures<br>No radiographic or clinical evidence of interproximal caries<br>Possible radiographic evidence of occlusal caries | Sandwich conservative resin/compomer restoration (glass ionomer liner, filled resin and sealant)<br>Glass ionomer conservative restoration (glass ionomer liner, glass ionomer restorative material and sealant)<br>Sealant-amalgam conservative restoration (amalgam in isolated pits and fissures without extension for prevention and sealant)<br>Glass ionomer-resin/compomer conservative restoration |

*Continued*

## TABLE 32-5

### Protocol for Pit and Fissure Treatment Alternatives—cont'd

| DIAGNOSIS | TREATMENT |
| --- | --- |
| Carious surface: obvious clinical caries | Restoration |
| Explorer catch with obvious clinical caries | Posterior resin/compomer restoration |
| Loss of enamel lining the pits and fissures | Amalgam restoration |
| Demineralized appearance of pits and fissures | Glass ionomer restoration |
| Generalized involvement of pits and fissures by caries with undermining of enamel | Glass ionomer-resin/compomer restoration |
| | Glass ionomer-posterior resin/compomer restoration |
| Probable radiographic evidence of occlusal caries | |
| No radiographic or clinical evidence of interproximal caries | |

* Explorer wedging: Wedging of a sharp explorer in pits of fissures on a clean, dry surface with the following characteristics: (1) pit or fissure is probed vertically; (2) explorer engages a fissure with no clinical or radiographic evidence of caries; (3) action may or may not be reproducible; (4) explorer penetrates into enamel only; and (5) probing by explorer may elicit slight discomfort.

†Explorer catch: An obvious catch of a sharp explorer in pits and fissures on a clean, dry surface with the following characteristics: (1) pit or fissure is probed vertically; (2) explorer engages a fissure with clinical evidence of incipient enamel or dentinal caries; (3) action is definitely reproducible; (4) explorer engages pit or fissure such that the explorer's weight is supported with minimal stabilization by the operator; (5) explorer penetrates both enamel and dentin; (6) pit or fissure may or may not have radiographic evidence of caries; and (7) explorer possibly elicits slight discomfort or pain on probing.

contamination. The presence of an operculum over the distal marginal ridge is associated with loss of sealant material and a reapplication rate of 54%.[35] Retreatment has been shown to be necessary in 26% of cases when gingival tissue is at the same height as the distal marginal ridge.[35] Sealant placement could be delayed if adequate isolation and tissue retraction is not possible. If the surface is at immediate risk for caries development, surgical removal of the operculum may be necessary to provide for adequate isolation. Another alternative is to use a hydrophilic bonding agent layer prior to placement of the sealant material.[45-48] In areas with saliva and water contamination, hydrophilic bonding agent has been shown to improve retention and provide significant caries reduction. Close follow-up for loss of sealant material is necessary in these difficult clinical situations. The contraindications are relative and should be taken into consideration when pits and fissures are being evaluated for sealant placement. However, if the clinical impression of whether or not to seal an occlusal surface is questionable, it is more appropriate to err toward sealant placement than toward observation of the surface and development of caries over a period of time.

In 1994 and 2002, consensus workshops were held to establish general guidelines for sealant use in individual patients as well as for community-based sealant programs.* A summary of the recommendations from these workshops is presented in Table 32-6.

A well-accepted clinical procedure used for restoring isolated pits and fissures and simultaneously preventing caries in the remaining unaffected pits and fissures was originally designated the "preventive resin restoration" and uses the acid-etch technique. This restorative technique has been renamed "conservative adhesive resin restoration," due to confusion of the original term with pit and fissure sealants. This innovative technique was introduced by Simonsen in 1978 as an alternative to either sealing questionable pits and fissures or restoring the entire surface with a conventional restorative material.* The technique involves widening the pits and fissures (enameloplasty) and removing only the enamel or dentin affected by caries. Depending on the extent of tooth structure removal, either an unfilled or a filled resin is used to "restore" the resulting conservative cavity. Typically, a composite resin is placed in the areas of dentin exposure after appli-

**TABLE 32-6**

## Guidelines from Workshop on Sealant Use

### PLACE SEALANTS
1. Questionable enamel caries in pit and fissures, but caries-free proximal surfaces
2. Enamel caries in pit and fissures, but caries-free proximal surfaces
3. Enamel caries and proximal caries not involving pit and fissures
4. Caries-free pit and fissures
    (a) Pit and fissure surface morphology at risk for caries
    (b) Patient's current and prior caries pattern (pit and fissure caries [≥1 lesion per year] or caries-free pattern in primary and/or permanent dentition)
    (c) Eruption status of teeth adequate for sealant placement
    (d) Patient's/parent's perception and desire for sealant placement
5. Medical history with factors associated with increased caries incidence or xerostomic medications
6. Routine dental care with active preventive dentistry program
7. Community-based sealant program
    (a) Identify population at moderate and high risk for caries
    (b) Individual caries-risk assessment
    (c) Sealant placement in pits and fissures of at risk teeth using above criteria

### DO NOT PLACE SEALANTS
1. Dentinal caries (consider preventive restoration, conventional restoration)
2. Proximal caries or restoration involves pit and fissures
3. Teeth cannot be isolated adequately (delay sealant until isolation possible)
4. Life expectancy of primary tooth is limited
5. Patient's risk pattern (caries-free or extensive caries pattern in primary and/or permanent dentition)
6. Pit and fissure morphology not at caries risk (monitor for change in caries risk)
7. Sporadic dental care and lack of preventive dentistry practices (instigate routine dental care and preventive practice)

### Recommendations from Pediatric Restorative Dentistry Consensus Conference 2002
1. Sealant effectiveness increased with placement by trained dental personnel using good technique, appropriate follow-up and resealing as necessary.
2. Sealant benefit increased with placement on surfaces judged to be at high risk or with existing incipient caries.
3. Risk assessment performed by experienced clinician based upon tooth morphology, prior caries history, prior fluoride history and current oral hygiene.
4. Caries risk exists in permanent and primary teeth with pits and fissures at any age.
5. Sealant placement employing careful cleaning of pits and fissures without appreciable removal of enamel or minimal enameloplasty.
6. Low viscosity, hydrophilic bonding layer enhances long-term sealant retention and effectiveness, especially in difficult to isolate situations.
7. Dental professionals remain alert to new preventive methods, technology and materials effective against pit and fissure caries.

Compiled from references 45,46,124,208,214,228,229,248,265.

cation of an appropriate base. Sealant material is placed over the remaining intact pits and fissures, as well as over the restored pits and fissures. It must be emphasized that only isolated pits and fissures with caries of clinical significance are prepared, and intact pits and fissures without clinical evidence of caries are not included in the preparations. Also, removal of additional tooth structure to aid retention is not necessary.

Recently, additional types of conservative adhesive restorations have been introduced to deal with more extensive caries in isolated pits and fissures that require restoration of the prepared cavities with dental materials of greater strength.* These techniques include (1) the glass

---

*References 47,93,94,117-119,121,122,220,221.

ionomer–resin/compomer conservative restoration; (2) the glass ionomer conservative restoration; and (3) the sealant-amalgam conservative restoration. These unconventional restorations adhere to the principle of conservation of tooth structure. With the glass ionomer–resin/compomer and the glass ionomer conservative restorations, no attempt is made to remove additional tooth structure for retention. Instead, these restorations rely on mechanical and physicochemical bonding of the materials to the tooth structure. With the glass ionomer–resin/compomer conservative restoration, a glass ionomer restorative material is placed in the deeper aspect of the prepared cavity, filling the lower third to half of the cavity and replacing the dentin that has been removed. A posterior composite resin or compomer material fills the remaining superficial portion of the cavity preparation, and sealant material is placed over the restoration, as well as over the remaining intact pits and fissures. In the glass ionomer conservative restoration, the dentinal cavity floor is covered with a glass ionomer lining material, and the remaining cavity is filled with a conventional glass ionomer, a glass ionomer–silver (cermet) restorative material, or a glass-ionomer modified resin. Again, the conservative restoration and remaining intact pits and fissures are coated with a sealant material. Finally, the sealant-amalgam conservative restoration attempts to preserve the maximal amount of tooth structure. However, the ultraconservative preparation of carious pits and fissures requires the dentist to pay some attention to retention form to allow placement of the amalgam material. There are some amalgam-bonding agents that are available, and these allow for reduction in leakage along the cavosurface, while releasing fluoride. Depending on the practitioner's preference, a glass ionomer lining material may be placed over the dentinal cavity floor. Amalgam restores the majority of the cavity preparation. Sealant material is placed over the ultraconservative amalgam restoration and the remaining intact pits and fissures. As is evident, these innovative techniques all share a common goal, namely, conservation of tooth structure with removal of only carious enamel and dentin. The original introduction of this technique almost three decades ago by Simonsen* has lead to recent advancement of a philosophy of minimally invasive dentistry. The goal of minimally invasive dentistry is to conserve healthy tooth structure by incorporating the dental science of detecting, diagnosing, intercepting, and managing dental caries on a microscopic level.[173,180,256,263] More recently, the World Health Organization (WHO) endorsed a minimal-intervention technique for management of dental caries in developing countries lacking dental personnel, equipment, and facilities.* It is estimated that more than 90% of dental caries in Africa go without treatment because restorative care is not available to the majority of Africans. Carious teeth will be left untreated and eventually be extracted because of pain, pulpal involvement, and jaw infections. In less economically developed countries, the predominant oral care procedure is extraction. Many of the citizens of these countries suffer from pit and fissure caries that over time become very extensive and result in pulpal involvement and eventual tooth loss. A minimal-intervention technique referred to as atraumatic restorative treatment (ART) has been touted by the WHO for controlling dental caries in disadvantaged countries. ART involves (1) isolation of the tooth with cotton rolls; (2) cleansing the tooth surface with water-moistened cotton pellets, followed by drying with cotton pellets; (3) widening the cavitated tooth surface with a dental hatchet by rotating the instrument backwards and forwards; (4) removing frank caries using a circular scraping motion with an excavator; (5) removing undermined, unsupported enamel with a dental hatchet and washing with lukewarm water; (6) placing calcium hydroxide paste over limited areas of very deep cavities; (7) cleansing the tooth surface with a wet cotton pellet; (8) applying dentinal conditioner to the cavity and tooth surface followed by cotton pellet washing and drying; (9) inserting glass ionomer and slightly overfilling; (10) applying pressure to entire occlusal surface using a petroleum jelly–coated gloved finger; (11) removing excess material if necessary; and (12) instructing the patient not to eat for at least 1 hour. The major advantages of the ART technique are that no anesthesia is required, no mechanical or electrical devices are needed, and the restorations may be applied by dental personnel or others trained in the procedure. This technique has undergone several years of clinical trials with impressive results. The WHO has established an electronic network for information regarding ART.[110]

---

*References 59-63,68,110-114,126,145,190,266,267.

The final treatment alternative is restoration of the entire occlusal surface with removal of all pits and fissures that are at risk for caries development. This treatment is reserved for surfaces that have generalized involvement of all pits and fissures and appear to be undermined clinically. These surfaces most likely have radiographic evidence of dentinal involvement without interproximal lesions. The choice of restorative material includes posterior composite resins, compomers, resin-modified glass ionomers, glass ionomer–silver (cermet), and amalgams. As with conservative adhesive restorations, a variety of clinical techniques incorporating the beneficial effects of different restorative materials are employed in restoring surfaces with pit and fissure caries.

## RETENTION AND CARIES PREVENTION WITH SEALANTS, CONSERVATIVE RESTORATIONS, AND ATRAUMATIC RESTORATIVE TREATMENT: CLINICAL TRIALS

### Pit and Fissure Sealants

Numerous clinical trials, ranging in length from 6 months to 20 years, have been carried out to assess retention rates, caries incidence, and the effectiveness of sealants in preventing pit and fissure caries (Fig. 32-5, A). In the majority of clinical studies, a single application of sealant is provided, followed by periodic evaluations to determine the retention rate and caries incidence. Clinical sealant trials carried out over periods of up to two decades have been reviewed* (Table 32-7). The complete retention rate varied from 92% after 1 year to 28% after 15 years with a single sealant application. Caries incidence increased from 4% after 1 year to 14% after 3 years. Seven years following a single sealant placement, caries incidence had increased to 31%. The 10-year results from two separate trials were encouraging, with a complete retention rate of 53% and a caries incidence of 22%.[207,223-227] Even 15 years after the initial sealant application, the caries incidence was found to be 31%, and the complete retention rate was 28%.[226,228] The effectiveness of a single application of sealant material in preventing caries ranged from 83% after 1 year to 53% after 15 years. A recent clinical study performed in a pediatric dentistry practice reported an 87%

*References 36,45-48,65,203,204,222-227,249,253-255,257.

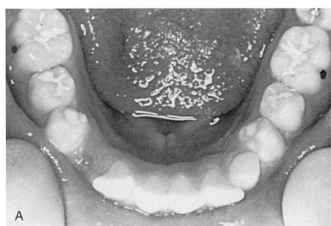

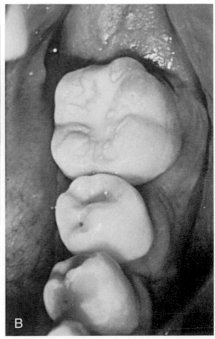

**Figure 32-5** Clinical appearance of fissure sealants and a conservative adhesive restoration. **A,** These sealants have been retained for 6 years with the permanent first molars and for 2 years with the premolar teeth. They are protecting the teeth from occlusal caries formation. **B,** After 5 years, this conservative adhesive restoration is still present and is responsible for the occlusal surface of the first molar remaining caries free.

## TABLE 32-7

### Retention and Effectiveness of Pit and Fissure Sealants in First Permanent Molar Teeth

| LENGTH OF TIME SINCE APPLICATION | COMPLETE RETENTION (MEDIAN) | CARIES RATE (MEDIAN) | EFFECTIVENESS OF SEALANTS (MEDIAN) |
|---|---|---|---|
| 1 year | 92% | 4% | 83% |
| 2 years | 85% | 7% | 81% |
| 3 years | 71% | 14% | 69% |
| 5 years | 67% | 26% | 55% |
| 6-7 years* | NA | NA | 41% Boys 38% Girls |
| 7 years | 66% | 31% | 55% |
| 10 years[†] | 53% | 22% | 68% |
| 10 years[‡] | 87% | 7% | NA |
| 15 years[§] | 28% | 31% | 53% |
| 15 years[¶] | 65% | 5% | |
| 20 years[#] | 65% | 13% | NA |

| PRIMARY MOLARS | COMPLETE RETENTION (MEAN) | CARIES |
|---|---|---|
| 2.8 years[#] | 76% | 9.8% |

*Represents single study.
[†]Represents results from two separate 10-year sealant studies.
[‡]Represents results from a single 10-year sealant study in a private pediatric dentistry practice.
[§]Represents a single 15-year sealant study.
[¶]Represents a single 20-year sealant study with sealant reapplication to first molars with deficient sealant when sealant was applied to second molars.
[#]Represents single study in 3-4 year-olds.
Compiled from references 35,36,45-48,51,65,116,204,205,222-227,249,257.

cumulative sealant survival probability over a 10-year period.[51] This result is quite impressive considering that the study population consisted of 810 children with 3194 sealants placed in permanent first molars. Of particular interest was the finding that risk for sealant failure was increased by threefold with dentists (n=4) and twofold with dental assistants (n=10) compared wtih dental hygienists (n=3). Sealant failure was greatest among the 10 dental assistants and ranged from 0 to 23%. Mean survival time for sealants placed by dentists and assistants was about 3.5 years, while that for hygienists was 7.7 years. Additional factors that were associated with significantly reduced sealant failure included age >10 years, caries-free status (DMFT=0), and availability of optimal water fluoridation. There was a trend toward less sealant failure with patients who had cooperative behavior and received systemic fluoride supplementation due to suboptimal water fluoridation.

The caries protection provided to pits and fissures by a single application of sealant material is therefore quite remarkable, especially considering the limited wear resistance of this resin material. In addition, even though sealant material may be judged clinically to be partially or completely lost, it may be present within the depths of pits and fissures and may provide protection against caries development.

Reapplication of sealants to pits and fissures that have lost their sealant provides an even greater degree of caries reduction than that reported by most single-application sealant trials. Clinical studies allowing reapplication of sealant material following sealant loss have shown that retention rates ranging from 88% to 96% at each annual evaluation may be achieved.[26,233,234] Over periods of up to 7 years it was found that 56% of sealed tooth surfaces required no retreatments, 28% required one reapplication, 8% required two reapplications, and only 8% required three reapplications. The anticipated annual reapplication rate is approximately 8%, with the highest rate of reapplication occurring 6 months following initial sealant application. The annual loss of sealant from 5% to 10% of teeth and need for sealant reapplication are consistent with others' findings.[45-48,227] The 5- to 7-year-old age group required the greatest number of sealant reapplications.[35] No doubt this high rate was due to the difficulty of isolating partially erupted first permanent molars from salivary contamination. With the current recommendation of bonding agent use with pits and fissures that are difficult to isolate from oral fluid contamination, the degree of sealant loss should become reduced over time.[37,45-48] When an operculum covered the distal marginal ridge, 54% of the sealed teeth required retreatment. Slightly less than one fourth required retreatment if the gingival tissue was at the same height as the distal marginal ridge.[35] If the gingiva was below the distal marginal ridge, no retreatments were required. Of interest was the fact that this type of sealant reapplication protocol was found to be 100% effective in preventing caries within pits and fissures. In a dental practice that maintains an active recall system for sealant evaluation and that advocates reapplication of sealant as necessary, a high degree of caries prevention may be anticipated.

A 20-year clinical trial[257] commencing in 1977 has shown exceptional results using a sealant placement and reapplication regimen (see Table 32-7). After 15 years, complete retention was found in 65% and partial retention was noted in 30%. Caries in or restoration of the pit and fissures had occurred in only 5% of teeth. At the 20-year follow-up, complete (65%) and partial (22%) retention were similar to that observed at the 15-year examination. Remarkably, some two decades after initial sealant placement, only 13% of the sealed surfaces had experienced caries or had been restored.

The effectiveness of sealants placed by dental students in a pediatric dentistry clinic[249] has been assessed and provides some interesting findings. A total of 7838 permanent molars had sealants placed and were followed for up to 7.9 years. Complete or partial retention not requiring sealant application was seen in 78.6% of molars. Reapplication of sealant was necessary in 13.2%. A conservative resin or one-surface composite restoration was placed in 6.4%. Caries requiring a one-surface or two-surface amalgam occurred in

1.0% and 0.8% of cases, respectively. Two thirds of sealant reapplications occurred in children younger than 8 years. This probably reflects the eruption status of the teeth at the time of sealant placement.

Although fewer sealant studies have been completed with primary teeth, caries incidence and retention rates are similar to those for permanent teeth.[45-48,88,222,245-247] Retention rates have been reported to be 95% and 93% after 1 and 3 years, respectively. During these time periods, none of the sealed primary molar surfaces developed caries. A recent clinical study compared retention rates in primary and permanent molars 36 months after placement of a fluoride-releasing sealant.[245-247] Complete retention was 95% for primary teeth and 96% for permanent teeth, whereas partial retention was 3% for primary teeth and 3% for permanent teeth. Less than 2% of the fluoride-releasing sealants were lost during the 36-month period. It is important to assess sealant placement on primary teeth in young children. A study of sealant placement on primary molars in 3- to 4-year-olds found a complete retention rate of 76% after a mean period of 2.8 years. Caries was found in less than 10% of the sealed teeth.[116] Several clinical studies (Table 32-8) have investigated the use of conventional glass ionomers, glass ionomer–silver cermets, and resin-modified glass ionomers as pit and fissure sealants.* Conventional glass ionomers used as pit and fissure sealants have a relatively low complete and partial retention rate when compared with resin-based pit and fissure sealants. Although conventional glass ionomers were assessed as completely lost in almost 50% of sealed teeth, only 5% of sealed teeth developed caries after 2 years. Two factors may account for the caries protection afforded by glass ionomers.[92] First, glass ionomer materials release a significant amount of fluoride. The released fluoride may become incorporated into the adjacent enamel forming the pits and fissures, providing increased caries resistance. Second, replica impression studies of surfaces that have experienced complete loss of their glass ionomer sealants have shown glass ionomer material within the depths of the pits and fissures in 93% of cases. These retained glass ionomer sealants may still provide an effective barrier against caries development. Both glass ionomer–

---

*References 54,111,153,156,183,187,189,235,236,240.

## TABLE 32-8

### Glass Ionomers As Pit and Fissure Sealants: Retention and Caries Preventive Effects

**Single-Application Glass Ionomer Materials as Pit and Fissure Sealants**

| Glass Ionomer | 12 MO | 24 MO |
|---|---|---|
| Complete retention | 20% | 26% |
| Partial loss | 70% | 26% |
| Complete loss | 10% | 48% |
| Caries development | 0% | 5% |

| Glass Ionomer (China) | 3 MO | 12 MO | 24 MO | 36 MO |
|---|---|---|---|---|
| Complete retention | 86% | 74% | 61% | 54% |
| Partial loss | 11% | 15% | 16% | 18% |
| Complete loss | 3% | 10% | 23% | 28% |
| Caries development | 0% | 0% | 0% | 2% |

| Glass Ionomer–Silver Cermet | 6 MO | 12 MO | 24 MO |
|---|---|---|---|
| Complete retention | 93% | 81% | 83% |
| Partial loss | 3% | 13% | 12% |
| Complete loss | 4% | 6% | 6% |
| Caries development | 0% | 0% | 0% |

| Resin-Modified Glass Ionomer | 6 MO | 12 MO |
|---|---|---|
| Complete retention | 78% | 51% |
| Partial loss | 22% | 49% |
| Caries development | 0% | 5% |

**Reapplication of Glass Ionomer As Pit and Fissure Sealants**

| | 6 MO | 12 MO | 24 MO | 36 MO |
|---|---|---|---|---|
| Complete retention | 37% | 41% | 51% | 53% |
| Partial loss | 46% | 28% | 20% | 17% |
| Complete loss | 17% | 31% | 29% | 30% |
| Caries reduction (compared with age-matched controls) | — | 76% | 70% | 67% |
| No reapplications required | — | 50% | 17% | 10% |

Compiled from references 54,111,153,156,183,187,189,235,236,240.

silver cermet and resin-modified glass ionomer sealants have improved retention rates when compared with conventional materials. Over a 2-year period, almost 95% of glass ionomer–silver sealants were retained, whereas all resin-modified glass ionomer sealants were retained over a 1-year period. Caries developed in 5% of teeth sealed with a resin-modified glass ionomer. In contrast, no caries developed in the pit and fissures protected by glass ionomer–silver cermets. With a reapplication protocol for conventional glass ionomer sealants, a considerable reduction in caries may be achieved. When compared with age- and gender-matched controls, pit and fissure caries was reduced by 76% after 1 year and by 67% after 3 years. Similar to conventional resin pit and fissure sealants, the highest percentage of reapplications occurred within 1 year of glass ionomer placement. By year 3 of the clinical trial, only 10% of sealed teeth required reapplication of the glass ionomer sealant. It is anticipated that if a reapplication protocol is used and resin-modified or glass ionomer–silver sealants are placed instead of conventional glass ionomer materials, the replacement rate would probably decrease while a high degree of caries protection would be provided. However, with the current success rate of resin-based sealants and the ability to incorporate releasable fluoride into these sealants, glass ionomer–based sealants have become less appealing for dental practitioners in developed countries.[45-48,227] Glass ionomer–based materials may be of greater benefit in developing countries, where the benefits of fluoride may overshadow the retention of the material and where clinical follow-up and reapplication of a traditional resin may not be possible.

## Conservative Adhesive Resin Restoration

Since the introduction of conservative adhesive resin restorations (see Fig. 32-5, *B*) in 1978, the retention rate of conservative adhesive resins and caries incidence have been investigated in both longitudinal and cross-sectional studies (Table 32-9). The results of a representative longitudinal trial indicated complete retention rates similar to those recorded for pit and fissure sealants.[47,117-119,121,122] However, the caries incidence was considerably reduced in comparison with pit and fissure sealants during the first 6.5 years of the study. Only 11% of surfaces with conservative resins had developed caries 78 months after placement. In comparison, caries incidence for surfaces with sealants was 31% after 84 months. Nine years after placement, almost 80% of the conservative resins were completely or partially retained. The caries incidence was 24% by year 9 and was similar to that for sealants that had been in place for 10 years. These findings are quite remarkable when one realizes that the clinical protocol allowed only for a one-time placement of the conservative resin material, followed by monitoring for restoration retention and caries development over the next 9 years. If periodic repair of the adhesive resin material had occurred, one can imagine that the caries incidence would have been reduced considerably with a concomitant increase in retention rate. The results from a cross-sectional study evaluated conservative resin restorations placed by dental students over a period of 3 to 65 months.[251] A relatively high retention rate was noted, with slightly more than 1% of restorations being completely lost. Considering the fact that the conservative resins had been in place for a mean period of 15 months, the caries incidence was at least comparable to that for pit and fissure sealants. In these longitudinal trials, it appears that conservative adhesive resin restorations may provide a retention rate and caries-protective effect similar to that associated with pit and fissure sealants.

The assessment of conservative resins placed by dental students in a pediatric dentistry clinic provides further support for the utility of this technique in simultaneous caries restoration and

---

**TABLE 32-9**

**Conservative Adhesive Restorations: Retention Rates and Caries Incidence/Prevalence**

| LENGTH OF TIME SINCE PLACEMENT | RETENTION | | | CARIES |
|---|---|---|---|---|
| | COMPLETE | PARTIAL | LOST | INCIDENCE/ PREVALENCE |
| **Longitudinal Conservative Adhesive Resin Restoration Study** | | | | |
| 3 years | 84.5% | 14.7% | 0.8% | 3.6% |
| 4 years | 77.2% | 18.8% | 4.0% | 6.9% |
| 5 years | 72.1% | 21.2% | 6.7% | 6.7% |
| 6.5 years | 65.4% | 19.2% | 15.4% | 10.6% |
| 9 years | 54.4% | 25.3% | 20.3% | 24.0% |
| **Cross-Sectional Conservative Adhesive Resin Restoration Studies** | | | | |
| 1.3 years (mean) (range = 0.3-5.5 years) | 81.7% | 11.9% | 1.2% | 5.2% |

Compiled from references 47,117-119,121,122,250,251.

prevention.[250] More than 5000 preventive resin restorations were followed for up to 6.5 years. No additional treatment was required in 83.2%, whereas 6.2% required replacement of the pit and fissure sealant component and another 1.5% were retreated with a conservative adhesive resin restoration. Slightly less than 7% required a one-surface restoration, with most of these being composite resin restorations (81%). Two or more surface restorations were placed in 3.6% of the teeth. It was observed that the most common reason for treatment intervention was either the loss of sealant material or failure to place sealant into the distal pits of maxillary molars and buccal pits of mandibular molars. Interproximal caries occurred in 3.6% of all teeth with conservative resins, whereas caries developed around conservative resin restorations in 8% of cases. Of the 10.6% of teeth restored, one third possessed intact conservative resin restorations but developed interproximal caries.

The conservative adhesive resin restoration is an acceptable alternative to restoration of an entire occlusal surface when only isolated pits and fissures with caries are present.[47] Currently, clinical trials involving glass ionomer preventive restorations are in progress but of limited duration. Because of the ability of glass ionomer materials to release considerable amounts of fluoride combined with the caries-preventive effects of the sealant material, results similar to those reported for conservative adhesive resin restorations are anticipated.

## Conservative Restorations (Minimal-Intervention Dentistry)

Relatively few clinical studies have evaluated conservative restoration of isolated pit and fissure caries followed by sealant placement over the restored areas and remaining intact pits and fissures.[157-165] The 10-year results from a clinical trial of sealant-amalgam and sealant-composite restorations on paired molars and premolars have now been reported (Table 32-10).[157-165] Isolated pits and fissures with clinical and radiographic evidence of superficial dentinal caries were prepared for either conservative composite or amalgam restorations. With the sealant-composite restorations, no attempt was made to remove undermined demineralized enamel or affected dentin. With the sealant-amalgam restorations, a conservative preparation was performed with complete removal of caries and attention to retention form. During the 10-year study period, complete and partial retention of the sealant material was comparable in both the sealant-composite and sealant-amalgam restorations. Complete and partial retention rates ranged from 88% to 97% with sealant-amalgam restorations and from 76% to 95% with sealant-composite restorations. Complete loss of sealant material occurred more often with sealant-composite restorations, with 10% of restorations lost 6 years after initial placement and a dramatic increase in lost restorations by year 10. Cumulative failures after 10 years amounted to 22% for sealant-composite restorations and only 6% for sealant-amalgam restorations. Despite the higher number of failures in the composite group, caries occurred in only 1% of cases after 2 years. By year 10, an additional 1% had developed caries during the remaining period of the study in the composite resin group. The results from this longitudinal paired trial demonstrate quite convincingly the ability of sealant-composite and sealant-amalgam conservative restorations to provide a caries-protective effect for pits and fissures while conserving tooth structure, using minimal invasive dental techniques. In addition, the isolation of dentinal caries from the oral environment by the sealant-composite materials allowed arrest of these lesions, with no radiographic evidence of advancement in any case noted during the entire study period.

## Atraumatic Restorative Treatment

Field trials of ART (Table 32-11) have been performed in developing countries such as Thailand, Tanzania, Zimbabwe, Syria, Kuwait, and rural areas of China using a minimal-intervention technique for caries control.* In Thailand, extensive data are available regarding this WHO-endorsed tooth-saving technique. When compared with one-surface amalgams, ARTs are not retained to the same extent. Considering the lack of technology, personnel, and physical facilities and equipment necessary to place amalgam restorations in these underdeveloped rural country settings, ART is the only viable option, except for extraction when caries becomes extensive.

---

*References  59-63,68,110-113,145,151,167,190,235,236, 266,267.

**TABLE 32-10**

**Sealant-Amalgam and Sealant-Composite Conservative Restorations: Comparison of Sealant Retention, Caries Development, and Restoration Failure**

| LENGTH OF TIME SINCE PLACEMENT | SEALANT RETENTION | | | CARIES INCIDENCE | RESTORATION FAILURE (CUMULATIVE) |
|---|---|---|---|---|---|
| | COMPLETE | PARTIAL | LOST | | |
| **Sealant-Amalgam Conservative Restorations** | | | | | |
| 1 year | 68% | 28% | 4% | 0% | 2% |
| 2 years | 52% | 45% | 3% | 0% | 2% |
| 3 years | 46% | 51% | 3% | 2% | 3% |
| 4 years | 48% | 47% | 5% | 0% | 3% |
| 5 years | 43% | 54% | 3% | 0% | 3% |
| 6 years | 41% | 53% | 6% | 0% | 6% |
| 9 years | 23% | 71% | 6% | 0% | 6% |
| 10 years | 27% | 61% | 12% | 0% | 6% |
| **Sealant-Composite Conservative Restorations** | | | | | |
| 1 year | 74% | 21% | 5% | 0% | 1% |
| 2 years | 57% | 34% | 9% | 1% | 1% |
| 3 years | 59% | 32% | 9% | 0% | 8% |
| 4 years | 55% | 47% | 8% | 0% | 8% |
| 5 years | 50% | 40% | 10% | 0% | 9% |
| 6 years | 55% | 35% | 10% | 0% | 12% |
| 9 years | 28% | 48% | 24% | 1% | 16% |
| 10 years | 20% | 69% | 11% | 0% | 22% |

Compiled from references 157-165.

ARTs placed in occlusal surfaces of children by dentists have a slightly reduced retention rate than ARTs placed in nonocclusal surfaces of adults by dental nurses. Primary teeth and restoration of two or more tooth surfaces have much higher loss rates than one-surface restorations and permanent teeth restored with ARTs. During the 3-year clinical field trial in Thailand, 71% of ARTs were retained for up to 3 years. The Zimbabwe clinical trials also included placement and assessment of glass ionomer sealants. Over a 2-year period, less than 4% of sealed teeth developed caries despite the fact that the retention rate was less than 60%. A 6-year study in Tanzania found that almost 70% of class I ARTs in permanent teeth were retained, and this was similar to that for amalgam restorations. Both primary and permanent teeth with glass ionomer sealants had similar retention rates after 1 year. Glass ionomer sealants are retained in up to 70% of teeth, with a caries rate of only 4%. These findings from economically less developed countries, with limited resources and dental manpower, are very encouraging and emphasize the importance of using relatively simple, low-technology procedures to improve the dental health and overall quality of life for less advantaged populations. Even in developed countries, a technique such as ART, incorporating the use of modern dental equipment, may provide a rapid means for controlling rampant caries, provide a means for fluoride delivery via fluoridated glass ionomer materials, and alleviate dental pain in the moderately to severely caries-affected child. This interim ART method may then be followed by appropriate restorative care in a timely fashion.

## Longevity of Amalgam Restorations in Children

The longevity of sealants and conservative restorations compares favorably with the longevity of conventional amalgam restorations placed in children.[92,252,253] The median survival for

## TABLE 32-11

### Atraumatic Restorative Treatment and Glass Ionomer Sealants in Caries Management in Developing Countries: Retention Rates

| Thailand | 1 YEAR | 2 YEARS | 3 YEARS |
|---|---|---|---|
| Alloy restoration (one surface restorations) | 98% | 94% | 85% |
| Atraumatic restorative treatment (one surface restorations) | 93% | 83% | 71% |
| Children | 92% | 80% | 67% |
| Adults | 93% | 86% | 77% |
| Occlusal | 91% | 80% | 62% |
| Non-occlusal | 95% | 88% | 85% |
| Dentist placed | 92% | 79% | 66% |
| Dental nurse placed | 93% | 85% | 73% |
| *Primary teeth* | | | |
| One surface | 79% | | |
| ≥ Two surfaces | 55% | | |
| *Permanent teeth* | | | |
| One surface | 93% | | |
| ≥ Two surfaces | 67% | | |

| Zimbabwe | | 2 YEARS | 3 YEARS |
|---|---|---|---|
| Atraumatic restorative treatment (one surface restorations) | | 89% | 88% |

| *Glass ionomer sealants* | 1 YEAR | 2 YEARS | 3 YEARS |
|---|---|---|---|
| Primary teeth | 73% | — | — |
| Permanent teeth | 78% | 73% | 50% |
| Caries present | — | 1% | 4% |

| China | | | |
|---|---|---|---|
| *Permanent teeth* | 1 YEAR | | 3 YEARS |
| Small class I | 99% | | 92% |
| Large class I | 90% | | 77% |

| *Primary teeth* | 1 YEAR | 2.5 YEARS |
|---|---|---|
| Class I | 91% | 79% |
| Class II | 75% | 51% |
| Class V | 79% | 70% |

| *Glass ionomer sealant* | | 3 YEARS |
|---|---|---|
| Permanent teeth | | 70% |

| Kuwait | | |
|---|---|---|
| *Primary teeth* | 8 MONTHS | 22 MONTHS |
| *Atraumatic restoration* | | |
| Class I | 98% | 93% |
| Class II | 100% | 84% |
| Class V | 100% | 90% |

## TABLE 32-11

**Atraumatic Restorative Treatment and Glass Ionomer Sealants in Caries Management in Developing Countries: Retention Rates—cont'd**

**Kuwait—cont'd**

| Primary teeth | 8 MONTHS | 22 MONTHS |
|---|---|---|
| Amalgam restoration | | |
| Class I | 100% | 92% |
| Class II | 100% | 100% |

**Syria**

| Primary teeth | | 3 YEARS |
|---|---|---|
| Atraumatic class I | | 86% |
| Amalgam class I | | 80% |

**Tanzania**

| Permanent teeth | | 6 YEARS |
|---|---|---|
| Atraumatic class I | | 69% |
| Amalgam class I | | 74% |

Compiled from references 59-63,110-113,145,151,167,190,235,236,266,267.

amalgam restorations placed in first permanent molars ranged from 26 months for 6-year-olds to 8 years and 11 months for 12-year-olds. The overall median survival for amalgams placed in first molars of 5- to 15-year-old children was 71 months. The age of the child at the time of placement is a major factor in restoration longevity. The 5-year survival rate for occlusal amalgams is 30% in 5- to 7-year-olds, 43% in 7- to 9-year-olds, and 62% in 9- to 15-year-olds. Sealants, conservative restorations, and amalgam restorations appear to follow a similar course with respect to retention in children and adolescents. The major difference is that sealant and adhesive dental material placement are associated with conservative preventive techniques, whereas amalgam placement represents a restorative procedure in which considerable tooth structure loss occurs. In fact, it has been shown that conservative adhesive resin restoration results in significant conservation of tooth structure, with the restored portion occupying only 5% of the occlusal surface compared with 25% of the occlusal surface removed in order to place an amalgam restoration.[256] Perhaps even more importantly when defective amalgam replacement is necessary, the area of the cavity preparation is further increased by 38%, resulting in an even greater loss of tooth structure.[38]

## COMBINED EFFECT OF SEALANT AND FLUORIDE RINSING PROGRAMS

The combination of sealant and fluoride rinsing programs significantly reduces the incidence and prevalence of pit and fissure and smooth surface caries in schoolchildren from fluoride-deficient communities.* A longitudinal study compared the effect of fluoride rinsing alone with sealant placement combined with fluoride rinsing in caries-free second- and third-grade schoolchildren.[200,201] After a 2-year period, 78% of the children in the fluoride rinse group were caries free. In comparison, 96% of children receiving the benefits of both fluoride rinsing and sealant placement were caries free. The caries incidence in children in the fluoride rinse group was 13 times that noted in children in the combined fluoride-sealant group. Perhaps even more impressive is the effect of combined fluoride rinsing and sealant therapy in children living on the fluoride-deficient island of Guam.[231] Following a baseline survey of caries prevalence in schoolchildren in Guam (Table 32-12), a school-based fluoride rinsing program was initiated in 1976. Assessment

*References 24,25,33,45-48,115,170,171,200,201,212,227.

## TABLE 32-12

### Effect of Fluoride and Sealant Programs on Caries Prevalence in Fluoride-Deficient Communities

| | OCCLUSAL | BUCCAL/ LINGUAL | PROXIMAL | TOTAL |
|---|---|---|---|---|
| **Guam Preventive Dentistry Program** | | | | |
| Before fluoride rinse DMFS | 3.27 | 2.48 | 1.31 | 7.06 |
| Fluoride rinse DMFS (% reduction) | 3.04 (7%) | 1.72 (31%) | 0.51 (61%) | 5.27 (25%) |
| Sealant and fluoride rinse DMFS (% reduction) | 1.38 (54%) | 1.09 (37%) | 0.46 (10%) | 2.93 (44%) |
| Water fluoridation, sealant, and fluoride rinse DMFS (% reduction) | 0.92 (72%) | 0.72 (71%) | 0.28 (79%) | 1.92 (73%) |
| **Nelson County School Preventive Dentistry Program** | | | | |
| *7- to 11-year-olds* | | | | |
| School fluoride program DMFS | 0.88 | 0.56 | 0.06 | 1.50 |
| Fluoride and sealant DMFS (% reduction) | 0.19 (78%) | 0.26 (54%) | 0.04 (33%) | 0.49 (67%) |
| *14- to 17-year-olds* | | | | |
| School fluoride program DMFS | 3.71 | 1.78 | 0.73 | 6.22 |
| Fluoride and sealant DMFS (% reduction) | 2.43 (35%) | 1.32 (26%) | 0.33 (55%) | 4.07 (35%) |

Compiled from references 117,212,231.

of caries prevalence in 1984 indicated that fluoride rinsing had resulted in a 25% reduction in the mean incidence of decayed, missing, and filled tooth surfaces (DMFS). The effects were most prominent in the proximal (60% reduction) and buccal-lingual surfaces (31% reduction). As would be expected, fluoride rinsing had the least effect on the occlusal surfaces (7% reduction). In 1984 a sealant application program was initiated while the fluoride rinsing program was maintained. In 1986, 2 years after the sealant program had begun, caries prevalence on surfaces with pits and fissures decreased dramatically. During this 2-year period, a more than 50% reduction in caries occurred on the occlusal surfaces, and a 36% reduction occurred on the buccal-lingual surfaces. The proximal surfaces showed the least degree of change, with a slightly less than 10% decrease in caries prevalence. With the addition of sealant placement to the existing fluoride rinsing program, caries prevalence was reduced by 44%. In Guam, the total reduction in caries prevalence from 1976 until 1986 was slightly less than 60%, translating to more than four tooth surfaces per child being saved from caries involvement. In 1986, community water fluoridation (0.5 to 1.0 ppm)

reaching more than 90% of the island's population was successfully implemented. This allowed an evaluation in 1989 of the effect of adding water fluoridation to the ongoing fluoride rinse and sealant programs. Three years after water fluoridation, the use of three preventive regimens in concert provided an overall reduction of over 70% in the DMFS for all surfaces when compared with the 1976 baseline prior to fluoride rinsing. The introduction of water fluoridation resulted in an additional DMFS reduction of 35% over that for the combined fluoride rinsing and sealant program. Proximal surfaces experienced a 40% DMFS reduction, while occlusal surfaces had a 33% decrease in DMFS. Over the 13-year period since the initial introduction of fluoride rinsing, 5.1 tooth surfaces per child were saved from dental caries. Perhaps even more impressive is the fact that children from Guam in 1989 had a mean DMFS of 1.92 whereas U.S. children in 1991 had a mean DMFS of 2.50. This further emphasizes that with optimization and integration of various caries-preventive regimens, including sealants, further reductions in caries experience may be achieved.

Within the United States, a longitudinal study was performed to assess a preventive program in a fluoride-deficient community which initially instituted a weekly school-based fluoride rinsing regimen and later introduced school-based sealant application.[117,212] After an 11-year fluoride rinsing program, the overall prevalence of dental caries was lowered by 65%. Four years after implementing the sealant program (see Table 32-12), the DMFS had decreased by two thirds in 7- to 11-year-olds and by one third in 14- to 17-year-olds. The younger group had a 78% reduction in occlusal caries, whereas the older age group experienced a 35% reduction in occlusal caries. Buccal/lingual caries, which is considered to predominantly involve pits and fissures, decreased by 54% in the younger group and by 26% in the older group. Proximal caries had a lower percent reduction in 7- to 11-year-olds, whereas these surfaces had the greatest caries decrease in 14- to 17-year-olds. This probably reflects the fact that 14- to 17-year-olds are in a period when proximal surfaces may be more susceptible to caries development, and the caries-preventive effect of the fluoride rinsing program on smooth surfaces is becoming realized.

The combination of a weekly fluoride rinsing program with the application of pit and fissure sealants in children at high risk for dental caries in a nonfluoridated region of Australia has shown the synergistic effects of fluoride and sealants on caries reduction.[33,170,171] Compared with age-matched early adolescents who were not the beneficiaries of fluoride rinsing and sealant application, there was a 1.49% reduction in DMFS over a 3-year period. It was noted that 70% of the caries reduction occurred with pit and fissure tooth surfaces.

## CLINICAL TECHNIQUE: SEALANT APPLICATION AND CONSERVATIVE ADHESIVE RESTORATION PLACEMENT

### Sealant Application

#### Step 1: Isolate Tooth Surface from Salivary Contamination

Isolation of the tooth from salivary contamination should be carried out, ideally by using rubber dam isolation (Fig. 32-6). Cotton roll isolation with adequate suctioning to remove saliva from the operating field is also acceptable and is the preferred method of isolation for many practitioners.

#### Step 2: Cleanse Tooth Surface

Prophylaxis of the tooth surface to be sealed should be carried out, using a pumice slurry applied with a rubber cup or pointed bristle brush in a prophy angle. An alternative method is to clean the surface with an air-polishing device using an air-powder abrasive (sodium bicarbonate slurry) system.[78] Some practitioners simply use a toothbrush prophylaxis with toothpaste or pumice followed by copious water rinsing to prepare the pits and fissures.[248] Rinse the tooth surface thoroughly to remove the prophylactic paste or slurry and oral debris. Trace the pits and fissures with a sharp, fine-pointed explorer to remove any cleansing material lodged within the pits and fissures. If a sodium bicarbonate slurry has been used, it is necessary to neutralize the retained slurry with phosphoric acid for 5 to 10 seconds. Some practitioners recommend cleaning the surface with 3% hydrogen peroxide after using a prophylactic paste to remove additional debris from the fissure. Once the tooth surface has been thoroughly cleansed, rinse and air dry the surface.

#### Step 3: Acid-Etch Tooth Surface

Apply the etching agent to the tooth surface with a fine brush, a cotton pledget, or a minisponge using the manufacturer's recommended exposure time. Exposure time varies from 15 seconds for permanent teeth to 15 to 30 seconds for primary teeth[45-48,124,195,227] with additional etching time for fluorosed teeth. Gently rub the etchant applicator over the tooth surface, including 2 to 3 mm of the cuspal inclines and reaching into any buccal and lingual pits and grooves that are present. Periodically add fresh etching agent to the tooth surface. Care should be taken to avoid spillage of the etchant onto the interproximal surfaces. Interproximal etching may lead to gingival irritation or sealing of adjacent interproximal surfaces together. The sealant may be either a gel or a liquid agent. The advantage of the gel material is increased control over the areas to be etched and a decreased likelihood of spillage onto the interproximal surfaces.

#### Step 4: Rinse and Dry-Etched Tooth Surface

Rinse the etched tooth surface with an air-water spray for 30 seconds.[124] This will remove the etching agent and reaction products from the etched enamel surface. Dry the tooth surface for at least 15 seconds[124] with uncontaminated com-

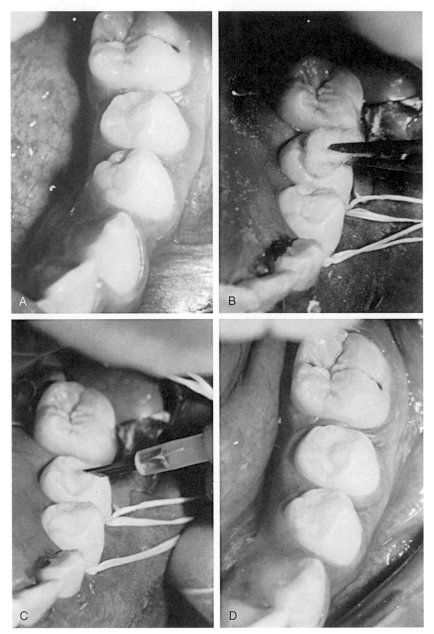

**Figure 32-6**   Sealant application. **A,** Sealant application to the occlusal surfaces of these premolar teeth is necessary because of the presence of deep retentive fissures. **B,** Following rubber dam isolation and pumice prophylaxis, phosphoric acid is applied to the teeth for 60 seconds, using a cotton pledget. The etched surface is then rinsed thoroughly and dried. **C,** An opaque sealant is applied with a fine brush. Polymerization of the sealant is completed with a visible light unit for 20 seconds. With chemically cured sealants, setting time varies from 1 to 2 minutes following mixing of the materials. **D,** Following removal of the rubber dam, the occlusion should be evaluated to determine if adjustment is necessary.

pressed air. If cotton roll isolation has been used, replace the cotton rolls at this time, making certain that salivary contamination of the etched enamel does not occur. The dried, etched enamel should have a frosted-white appearance. If the enamel does not have this appearance, repeat the etching step. If salivary contamination occurs at this stage, reisolate the tooth, rinse the entire tooth surface, dry thoroughly, and repeat the etching process. Avoid contact with the dry, etched enamel surface. If it is impossible to avoid salivary/water contamination, application of a hydrophilic bonding agent prior to sealant application may improve retention with teeth that cannot be isolated properly.[45-48,227,248,265]

### Step 5: Apply Sealant to Etched Tooth Surface

Apply the sealant material to the etched tooth surface and allow the material to flow into the pits and fissures. With mandibular teeth, apply the sealant at the distal aspect and allow it to flow mesially. With maxillary teeth, apply the sealant at the mesial aspect and allow it to flow distally. Allowing the sealant material to flow into the etched pits and fissures should prevent incorporation of air into the material and creation of voids. Add material as necessary to seal all pits and fissures. Using a fine brush, minisponge, or applicator provided by the manufacturer, carry a thin layer of sealant up the cuspal inclines to seal secondary and supplemental fissures, and flow the sealant material into buccal or lingual pits and grooves. With autopolymerizing sealants, working time varies from 1 to 2 minutes. With photo-activated sealants, the setting reaction is initiated by exposing the sealant to visible light and usually requires 10 to 20 seconds for complete setting. The manufacturer's recommended curing time should be considered a minimal exposure period, and the addition of 5 to 10 seconds of curing time to that recommended may allow for maximal polymerization. With light-cured sealants, penetration of the resin into the etched enamel may be increased by up to 300%, based on resin tag length, if curing is delayed for 10 seconds.[29] This delay in curing may be possible if isolation from salivary contamination is adequate.

### Step 6: Explore the Sealed Tooth Surface

Explore the entire tooth surface for pits and fissures that may not have been sealed and for voids in the material. If deficiencies are present, apply additional sealant material. Usually a sticky layer of apparently unreacted sealant will be present on the tooth surface. This is an air-inhibited layer of sealant that has not undergone polymerization. Remove the rubber dam or cotton rolls.

### Step 7: Evaluate the Occlusion of Sealed Tooth Surface

Evaluate the occlusion of the sealed tooth surface to determine whether excessive sealant material is present and must be removed. A small discrepancy in occlusal interference with an unfilled sealant is easily tolerated by the child because the sealant will abrade away, allowing proper inter-digitation. With filled sealant materials and in adult and adolescent age groups, occlusal adjustment should be completed to avoid discomfort due to excess material. Evaluate the interproximal regions for inadvertent sealant placement by performing tactile examination with an explorer and passing dental floss between the contact regions.

### Step 8: Periodically Reevaluate and Reapply Sealant as Necessary

During routine recall examination, it is necessary to reevaluate the sealed tooth surface for loss of material, exposure of voids in the material, and caries development. The need for reapplication of sealant material is usually highest during the first 6 months after placement. Should reapplication be necessary, the steps involved in reapplying sealant material to an existing sealant are identical to those used for initial placement.

## Placement of Conservative Adhesive Resin Restoration

A conservative adhesive resin restoration (Fig. 32-7) requires the same steps as those used for sealant placement except that caries are removed from isolated pits and fissures.

### Step 1: Isolate Tooth Surface from Salivary Contamination

Isolate tooth surfaces as described previously.

### Step 2: Remove Caries from Isolated Pits and Fissures

Remove caries from isolated pits and fissures using an inverted cone-shaped, round, or pear-shaped bur in a high-speed handpiece. The size of the bur and the resulting cavity preparation will be dictated by the amount of caries present. Caries should be removed making no attempt to incorporate retention into the preparation.

### Step 3: Cleanse Tooth Surface

Perform prophylaxis as previously described, followed by rinsing and drying.

### Step 4: Place Cavity Base or Lining Material

If dentin is exposed, a calcium hydroxide or glass ionomer base should be placed prior to acid etching.

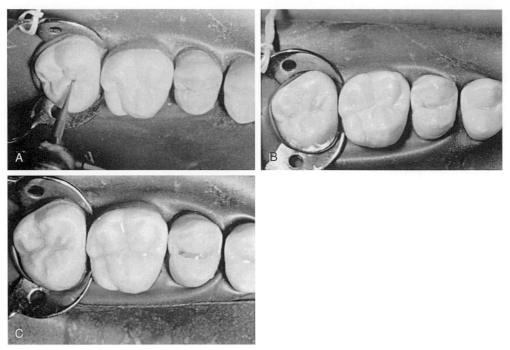

**Figure 32-7**    Conservative adhesive restoration placement. **A,** Following isolation with a rubber dam, pits and fissures with caries of clinical significance are removed with a round bur in a high-speed handpiece. **B,** Following minimal cavity preparation, a pumice prophylaxis is carried out. If dentin is exposed, a cavity base should be placed prior to etching the occlusal surface. **C,** After a conservative adhesive restoration has been completed, the occlusion should be evaluated to determine if adjustment is necessary.

### Step 5: Acid-Etch Tooth Surface

Etch, rinse, and dry tooth surface as previously described.

### Step 6: Place Resin and Sealant Material

Place a thin layer of resin bonding agent or dentinal bonding agent in the cavity preparation, followed by composite resin when the cavity extends into dentin. If the restorative material is chemically cured, allow time for complete setting reaction to occur. Expose light-cured material to the visible light source to initiate the setting reaction. If adequate isolation is present, allow resin to penetrate into etched tooth structure for 10 seconds before initiating light curing. Apply sealant material over the restored area and the adjacent intact etched pits and fissures. Carry the sealant material up the cuspal inclines for 2 to 3 mm and into the buccal-lingual grooves and pits. Initiate the sealant setting reaction.

### Step 7: Explore the Sealed and Restored Tooth Surface

Explore the sealed and restored surface as previously described. If necessary, apply additional sealant material. Remove rubber dam or cotton roll isolation.

### Step 8: Evaluate the Occlusion of Sealed and Restored Tooth Surface

Evaluate the occlusion of the sealed and restored tooth surface to determine whether excessive material is present and adjust as necessary. Evaluate the interproximal regions for inadvertent resin placement by tactile examination with an explorer and passage of dental floss between the contact regions.

### Step 9: Periodically Reevaluate the Conservative Adhesive Restoration, Repair and Reapply Sealant as Necessary

During routine recall examinations, it is necessary to reevaluate the sealed and restored tooth surface for loss of material and development of caries. Repair of the restored regions and reapplication of sealant material may be necessary periodically.

Although both techniques involved in sealant application and conservative adhesive resin restoration placement appear to be simple, a high failure rate may occur if the practitioner does not pay strict attention to the steps in the acid-etch technique. Of particular importance to the success of the acid-etch procedure is avoidance of salivary contamination of the enamel surface once the surface has been etched.

The remaining types of conservative restorations follow in general the same steps outlined for the conservative adhesive resin restoration. The major difference lies in the selection and substitution of different restorative materials. Each of the materials requires certain modifications in the restoration steps. (The reader is referred to Chapters 20 and 21 for details on glass ionomer, resin-modified glass ionomer, compomer, posterior composite, and amalgam restorative materials.)

## SCIENTIFIC BASIS FOR THE ACID-ETCH TECHNIQUE

The initial studies of acid etching of surface enamel used a solution of 85% phosphoric acid. Since the 1950s, a considerable number of laboratory and clinical studies have been performed to determine the appropriate acid type, acid concentration, and etching time that would yield optimal bonding characteristics with minimal loss of surface enamel. Phosphoric acid in the range of 35% to 40% with an application time of 15 to 60 seconds for permanent and primary teeth has been shown to produce adequate resin bonding while minimizing the loss of surface enamel.[40,45-48,198,216-219,227,239] No significant differences in sealant retention rates or caries incidence have been found with variations in the etching time for either primary or permanent teeth. The currently recommended etching times are 20 seconds for permanent teeth and 30 seconds for primary teeth.[124,248] The etching time should be extended for fluorosed teeth.

Acid etching of surface enamel has been shown to produce a certain degree of porosity.[216-219] In fact, sound enamel etched with phosphoric acid is affected at three levels microscopically (Fig. 32-8).

First, a narrow zone of enamel is removed by etching. In this manner, plaque and surface and subsurface organic pellicles are effectively dissolved. Fully reacted, inert mineral crystals in the surface enamel are also removed, resulting in a more reactive surface, an increased surface area, and a reduced surface tension that allows resin to wet the etched enamel more readily. This etched zone is approximately 10 mm in depth. The second zone is the qualitative porous zone, which is 20 mm in depth. Due to the relatively large porosities created by the etching process, this zone may be distinguished qualitatively from adjacent sound enamel using polarized light microscopy. The final zone is the quantitative porous zone; as its name implies, it has relatively small porosities created by the etching process that may be identified only by quantitative methods using polarized light microscopy. This zone extends into the enamel for an additional 20 mm. Following acid etching and creation of these various zones, sealant material is applied to the etched enamel, and the resin material penetrates into the porosities created. This provides a mechanical bond between the etched enamel and the resin material that may extend 40 mm or more into the underlying tooth structure.

Three characteristic etching patterns occur following exposure of sound enamel to phosphoric acid (Fig. 32-9). The type 1 etching pattern has lost the prism cores, but the prism peripheries remain. In the type 2 etching pattern, the prism peripheries are lost, and the prism cores appear to be relatively intact. Some regions of etched enamel show a generalized surface roughening and porosity with no exposure of prism cores or peripheries. This surface morphology is characteristic of the type 3 etching pattern. No specific etching pattern is preferentially created during the

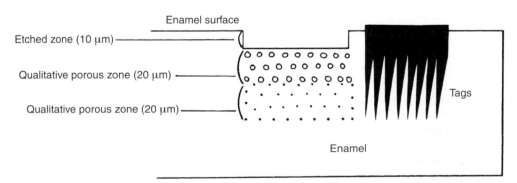

**Figure 32-8** Histologic zones created in sound enamel by the acid-etch technique. Resin penetrates into the porosities in etched sound enamel, forming retentive resin tags.

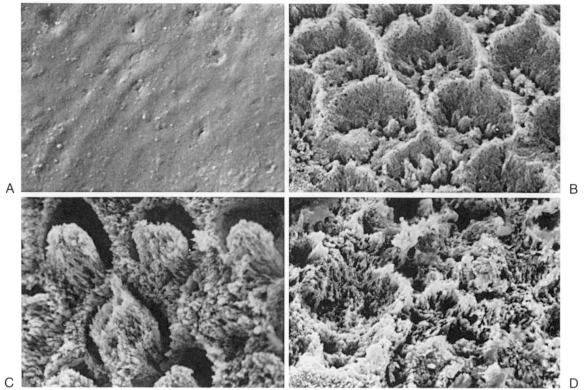

**Figure 32-9**    Effects of the acid-etch technique on surface morphology (scanning electron microscopy). **A,** The surface of sound enamel is relatively smooth, with occasional depressions representing terminations of enamel prisms. **B,** Type 1 etching pattern, with loss of prism cores following etching. **C,** Type 2 etching pattern, with loss of prism peripheries following etching. **D,** Type 3 etching pattern, with surface porosities but without a distinct prism morphologic appearance.

etching procedure, and the three types of etching pattern are often found adjacent to one another. The type of etching pattern has not been found to be related to increased or decreased sealant retention rates or caries incidence.[215-218]

## ENAMEL-RESIN INTERFACE

Following sealant application to an etched occlusal surface, the pits and fissures are occluded with resin material (Fig. 32-10 A, B). The surface morphology then changes from one in which plaque and oral debris can accumulate easily (see Fig. 32-2) to a self-cleansing surface with no readily apparent pits or fissures (Fig. 32-10, *A, B*). The interface between enamel and resin is intimate and shows no detectable microspaces between the resin and the adjacent etched enamel (Fig. 32-10, *B, C*).

Sealant materials do not simply bond to the enamel surface but actually penetrate into the microporosities created in the surface enamel

during the etching procedure (Fig. 32-10, *C, D*). Infiltration of the etched enamel results in formation of resin tags, which provide the mechanical means for sealant retention. Typically, resin tags penetrate etched enamel to a depth of 25 to 50 mm, with some tags terminating at depths of up to 100 mm.[216-219] As noted previously, resin tag length may be increased by allowing visible-light–cured resin to penetrate the etched enamel for 10 seconds or more prior to initiating the setting reaction.[29]

Resin tags serve a number of functions. They provide a mechanical means for retention of the sealant. The resin tags surround the enamel crystals and may provide resistance to demineralization by acid byproducts from plaque. BIS-GMA sealant materials are resistant to acid dissolution and provide protection against caries formation along the enamel-resin interface (Fig. 32-11). Finally, the enamel-resin interface creates a protective barrier against bacterial colonization of the sealed fissure and does not allow passage of nutriments into the fissure.[105-108]

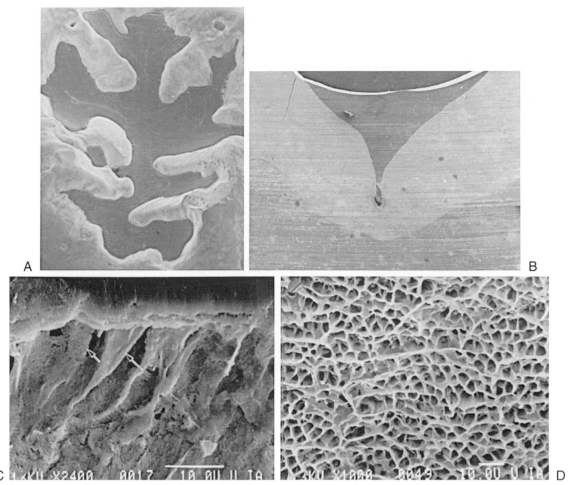

**Figure 32-10** The enamel-resin interface (scanning electron microscopy). **A,** Following sealant placement, the pits and fissures on this occlusal surface are protected from cariogenic challenges by the acid-resistant sealant. **B,** The interface between the enamel forming the fissure and the sealant appears to be an intimate one, with no apparent space between the etched enamel and sealant. **C,** Following partial demineralization of enamel that has been sealed, resin tags (arrows) may be seen in the etched enamel. **D,** Complete demineralization of enamel that has been sealed allows one to visualize the appearance of the acid-resistant resin tags.

Although the acid-etch technique produces an intimate, interdigitating interface between the etched enamel and the resin, microspaces are present between the cavosurface enamel and amalgam and glass ionomer materials used in restoration.[92-94,102] These microspaces may allow passage of acidic bacterial byproducts from plaque along the restoration-enamel interface and may result in secondary caries formation in the cavosurface enamel. With amalgam restorations, release of metallic ions, which may be bacteriostatic or bactericidal, into the microspace occurs. This may reduce bacterial colonization of the amalgam-enamel interface. In addition, certain amalgam materials produce corrosion-like products that may effectively seal the microspace over time. With glass ionomers, fluoride released into the microspace may become incorporated into the cavosurface enamel, providing increased caries resistance. In addition, the acidic nature of glass ionomers enhances the antimicrobial effects of fluoride on plaque. Clinical studies have shown that secondary caries is responsible for replacement of amalgams in over 70% of cases.[92,167,168] In limited clinical studies of glass ionomers used as sealants, massive clinical loss of material from pits and fissures occurs; however, only 1% of previously sealed surfaces developed caries.[156,183]

These clinical findings are consistent with laboratory studies[92-94,97-100,102,103,105-107] on artificial secondary caries formation around restorative materials (see Fig. 32-11). Typically, secondary

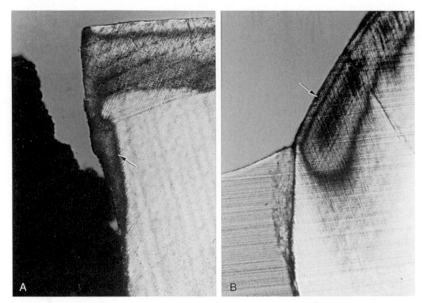

**Figure 32-11**   Caries-like lesion formation adjacent to amalgam and sealant materials (polarized light microscopy: water imbibition). **A,** Secondary caries formation (arrow) may be seen along the cavity wall of this amalgam restoration, indicating that microleakage between the restoration and cavity wall has occurred. Fracturing of the restoration occurred during preparation of the section for microscopic examination. **B,** The primary surface lesion (arrow) terminates at the point where bonding occurs between the etched enamel and sealant material. No secondary cavity wall lesion exists. Resin tags provide resistance against a cariogenic challenge at the enamel-resin interface.

caries-like lesions form along the amalgam-enamel interface in all cases. This reflects the ready access of acidic byproducts to the microspace between the amalgam and the cavosurface enamel. In contrast, artificial secondary lesions are found in up to 17% of cases when sealants or composite resins have been placed using the acid-etch technique. With glass ionomer materials, up to 7.5% of specimens develop artificial secondary caries. The difference in prevalence of secondary lesions between amalgams and sealants reflects the intimate interface created by the acid-etch technique during placement of the resin material. However, the differences noted between sealant and glass ionomer materials are related to the fluoride released from glass ionomers. This release results in incorporation of fluoride into the cavosurface enamel, thereby enhancing the resistance of the enamel to caries. The effect of glass ionomers on caries formation is also seen in the surface enamel adjacent to the restoration. In fact, primary surface lesions are reduced by 40% to 50% when the surface enamel is in close proximity to a glass ionomer restoration or a fluoride-releasing sealant.[92,97,98,100,102,106] The importance of protecting the cavosurface enamel and the enamel-dental material interface from secondary caries formation cannot be overemphasized.

## FLUORIDE-RELEASING SEALANTS

Initial attempts to incorporate fluoride into BIS-GMA sealants were disappointing. Typically, a relatively large amount of fluoride was released during the first 24 hours following sealant placement; however, fluoride levels returned to baseline within a 1-week period. The great majority of the fluoride incorporated into the sealant was trapped within inert sealant material and was unavailable for release. Loosely bound fluoride that was present on the surface of the sealant was responsible for the initial burst of fluoride released into the oral environment.[202] Instead of incorporating fluoride into an inert sealant material, ion-exchanging resins were developed.[197,238] These resins have a relatively high fluoride content and exchange fluorine ions from the sealant material for hydroxyl and chloride ions in the oral environment. In laboratory studies, fluoride levels of 5 to 10 ppm/day are released for periods of up to 2 years. Inhibition of caries formation and remineralization of enamel caries have been shown to occur in vitro and in vivo. A significant level of fluoride is taken up by the sealed enamel. Both superficial and deep enamel layers incorporate the released fluoride, with fluoride levels of 3500 ppm and 1700 ppm reported for enamel biopsy depths of 10 mm and 60 mm, respectively. In comparison, fluoride levels in contralateral control teeth were 650 ppm and 200 ppm for enamel biopsy depths of 10 and 60 mm, respectively. The potential benefits of these fluoride-exchanging resins in prevention and remineralization of both smooth surface and pit and fissure caries appear to be considerable.

Fluoride-releasing sealant material composed of modified urethane–BIS-GMA resin have become available for routine clinical use.* Laboratory and clinical studies have shown that a burst of fluoride release occurs during the first week following sealant placement, and a relatively constant release of low levels of fluoride follows for many months to years. In clinical trials, retention rates have been similar to those reported for conventional sealants, and caries incidence has been identical or slightly reduced compared with non–fluoride-containing sealants. The caries-protective effect of this fluoride-releasing sealant has also been assessed using an artificial caries system.[92,97,98,100,102] A reduction of approximately 60% of secondary caries formation occurs with use of the fluoride-releasing sealant compared with conventional sealant material. In addition, primary caries formation in surface enamel adjacent to the fluoride-releasing sealant shows about a 35% reduction in lesion depth, indicating an enhanced degree of caries resistance. Similar results are seen with permanent and primary teeth. The fluoride released from the sealant material apparently becomes incorporated into the adjacent enamel and provides an increased level of caries resistance. Currently, there are many pit and fissure sealants that contain and release fluoride into the oral environment. No differences have been noted in the handling characteristics of these materials, and they have identical retention rates to their non–fluoride-releasing sealant counterparts in both the primary and permanent dentition.

The effect of the amount of fluoride release to the local environment and the degree of demineralization has led to the development of experimental methods to improve the delivery of fluoride from fluoride-containing preventive and restorative materials.[67,76,77,92,104] It is possible

to increase the fluoride load within a resin-based material. This may result in substantial increases in fluoride released in the local environment and may reduce the effect of a cariogenic challenge.[76,77,92] Incorporation of organic fluorides in resin materials also enhances fluoride release while maintaining the physical properties of the resin material.[75,76,91] Organic fluorides that may be incorporated into polymer matrix of dental materials include: methacrylol fluoride–methyl methacrylate, acrylic amine–hydrogen fluoride salt, t-butylaminoethyl methacrylate hydrogen fluoride, morpholinoethyl methacrylate hydrogen fluoride, and tetrabutylammonium tetrafluoroborate. These organic fluorides are in the testing stage and show promising laboratory and clinical results.

## SALIVARY CONTAMINATION OF ETCHED ENAMEL

Perhaps the most common reason for sealant failure is a lack of care for proper isolation of etched enamel from contamination with saliva (Fig. 32-12). In the initial sealant studies, the effect of salivary contamination on the success of the acid-etch technique was not known. A high level of sealant loss and caries development most likely occurred because saliva had contaminated the etched enamel and prevented resin penetration into the porosities of the etched enamel.

Protection of the etched enamel from salivary contamination is considered the key to success

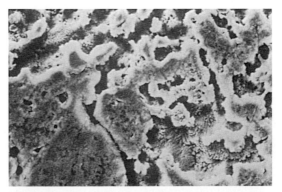

**Figure 32-12** Etched enamel that was exposed to saliva for only 10 seconds. A tenacious surface coating, which would interfere with resin bonding, is present, even though the surface was rinsed thoroughly following salivary contamination (scanning electron microscopy).

---

*References  31,45-48,66,97,98,100,128,135,172,227,245-248.

with the acid-etch technique. Rapid formation of a tenacious surface coating occurs over etched enamel surfaces exposed to saliva (see Fig. 32-12). These coatings form within a few seconds of salivary contamination and cannot be removed entirely by rinsing with an air-water spray unless the etched enamel has been exposed to saliva for 1 second or less. This means that if salivary contamination occurs, the tooth surface should be reisolated from saliva and then rinsed and dried thoroughly; repetition of the etching step in its entirety follows prior to placement of the resin.[219,248] As noted previously, the use of a hydrophilic bonding agent prior to sealant placement may improve sealant retention in areas that are difficult, if not impossible, to isolate from moisture contamination. Similar retention and caries protection have been reported with the use of a hydrophilic bonding agent in conjunction with sealants.[37,45-48,90,227]

In general, two methods of isolation from salivary contamination are used: the rubber dam and cotton roll isolation.[39] Approximately two thirds of practitioners prefer to use cotton roll isolation during placement of sealants, and the remainder prefer rubber dam isolation. Retention rates for sealants placed using the rubber dam or cotton roll have recently been compared. In one study in which a single-application protocol was used, retention rates were 96% for rubber dam isolation and 88% for cotton roll isolation 2 years after placement of the sealant.[39] A separate 3-year study in which a sealant reapplication protocol was used showed no difference in retention rates between the two isolation methods.[234] When sealant reapplication was used, the average retention rate at each 6-month recall period was 95% for cotton roll isolation compared with 94% for rubber dam isolation. If the need for sealant reapplication had been classified as sealant loss, the retention rates would have been 65% for cotton roll isolation and 62% for rubber dam isolation after 3 years. Using the reapplication protocol, 68% of sealed surfaces required no reapplication, 25% required one reapplication, 5% required two reapplications, and 1% required three reapplications. During the 3-year study period, no carious lesions developed.

A potential source of contamination of etched enamel is the air-water syringe. It is possible for oil or water to contaminate the air line. If contamination occurs, a thin film of oil or water may be deposited on the etched surface, which would interfere with resin penetration into the etched enamel. Periodically, the air line should be evaluated for contamination by blowing air onto a mirror surface. If oil or water droplets form on the mirror surface, contamination of the air line has occurred, and filtration to remove these contaminants is necessary.

## SEALING OVER CARIES

Because caries may be present histologically for a considerable time before it is detected clinically and radiographically, it is possible that sealant placed over a clinically caries-free surface may result in sealing over enamel caries and cariogenic organisms within pits and fissures. This has caused a great deal of concern among practitioners and has resulted in limited use of sealants since they were introduced. It should be reassuring to the practitioner that the acid-etching procedure itself eliminates 75% of the viable microorganisms from pits and fissures. Clinical studies in which sealants were placed over intact pits and fissures with radiographic evidence of dentinal lesions showed that after a 2-week period, only 4.5% of microorganisms were viable. Two years following sealant placement, a reduction of 99.9% of viable microorganisms was found. Of the remaining viable microorganisms, less than 3% were of an acidogenic variety associated with caries formation. Sealant placement effectively creates an impermeable barrier that isolates the remaining viable organisms from their source of nutriments and prevents colonization of the sealed fissure by other oral microorganisms.*

Of clinical significance is the radiographic appearance of sealed surfaces with caries. Following sealant placement, the dentinal lesions are arrested, and some studies report reversal of these lesions in up to 89% of cases. In longitudinal studies it has been shown that although dentinal lesions in matched control teeth progressed an average depth of 640 mm, dentinal lesions present beneath the contralateral sealed teeth were arrested and advanced no further. This finding is convincing because each pair of control and sealed molars was exposed to the same intraoral cariogenic environment. On removal of the sealant and bacterial sampling of the underlying

---

*References 45-48,69,76,85-88,129,157-165,227.

dentin, the superficial affected dentin was noted to be dry, leathery, and somewhat powdery. The more deeply situated dentin had become sclerotic with a glassine appearance, which was indicative of reparative dentin formation.[85-88,157-165]

Retention rates of sealants placed over carious and sound tooth surfaces have been found to be similar. After a 2-year period, complete retention was 64% and 65% for sealed carious and sound molars, respectively. Partial retention of sealant material was present in 35% of carious molars and 34% of sound molars.[85-88] Similar results were obtained for sealant-composite preventive restorations in which dentinal caries remained sealed beneath the resin material.[157-165] At the end of this 6-year clinical trial, complete or partial retention was present in 90% of cases, with caries occurring in only 1% of cases. These findings are not surprising because previous laboratory studies showed identical etching patterns for both sound enamel and enamel caries.[107,108] It has also been shown that if the sealant appears to be lost clinically from an etched surface, resin tags remain embedded in the enamel and provide protection against a cariogenic challenge.[69,107,108] The placement of an unfilled resin over caries-like lesions has been shown to protect against caries progression.[69]

These results obtained from sealing over caries involving enamel and dentin emphasize the fact that if sealants are applied properly and are monitored periodically, caries arrest beneath a sealant can be expected. If clinically undetectable dentinal involvement has occurred, sealing over the lesion may allow odontoblasts to effect biological repair of the affected dentin.

## SEALANT UTILIZATION

Since the introduction of commercially available sealant products in the early 1970s, dental practitioners have been somewhat hesitant to incorporate sealants into their practices. The initial ADA sealant utilization survey in 1974 found that only 38% of general dentists were placing sealants.[71] The reasons given for the poor acceptance of sealants were concern about the effectiveness of sealants in preventing caries, the possibility of sealing over caries, and the longevity of sealants. A follow-up survey by the ADA in 1982 showed a modest increase in the proportion of practitioners placing sealants.[70] Almost 60% of

general dentists had accepted sealants as a preventive procedure and provided this service for their pediatric patients. Because of the overwhelming laboratory and clinical results attesting to the caries-preventive capabilities and retention rates of sealants, one would have expected an even higher level of acceptance. However, this lack of acceptance can be explained in part by the fact that 41% of surveyed dentists believed that amalgam restorations were very effective in preventing pit and fissure caries in children whereas only 10% believed that sealants were very effective in preventing caries. The reasons given for limiting sealant usage included concerns about sealing over caries, lack of reimbursement by third party providers, and a preference for restoration of pits and fissures.

During the late 1980s and the 1990s, it became apparent that sealants had been incorporated into the preventive regimens of almost all general and pediatric dentists. Both regional and national surveys (Table 32-13) have indicated that between 80% and 95% of general dentists use sealants in their practice to some extent.* This rapid adoption of sealants since the previous ADA survey is consistent with the finding that slightly more than 50% of dentists have been using sealants for 3 years or less.[42,43] In a limited 2001 survey,[210] general dentists indicated that they placed sealants very often or often (79%) in permanent teeth. There was only a small percentage who rarely or never placed sealants (6%), with the remainder indicating that they sometimes placed sealants. The majority (53%) indicated that they rarely or never used sealants with primary teeth. About 20% indicated that sealants were placed often or very often with primary teeth. The majority of general dentists also reported that they placed conservative adhesive resin restorations often or very often (44%) or sometimes (21%).

Using a self-assessment method for determining sealant usage (see Table 32-13), a regional survey found that 83% of general dentists and 96% of pediatric dentists used sealants.[23,100] Although 73% of pediatric dentists indicated that they used sealants routinely, only 40% of general dentists claimed to be routine users of sealants. Perhaps more important, only 17% of general dentists and 4% of pediatric dentists did not place

---

*References  2,16,23,30,32,34,42-44,79,80,89,99,127,132, 140,169,184-186,195,206,210,214,215.

## TABLE 32-13

### Comparison of Sealant Usage by Colorado Pediatric and General Dentists

| | PEDIATRIC DENTISTS | GENERAL DENTISTS |
|---|:---:|:---:|
| **Self-Assessment Category** | | |
| Routinely Use Sealants | 73% | 40% |
| Occasionally Use Sealants | 16% | 33% |
| Seldom Use Sealants | 7% | 10% |
| Do Not Use Sealants | 4% | 17% |
| **Sealant Utilization Category** | | |
| High Use (>20 sealants/wk) | 38% | 8% |
| Moderate Use (11-20 sealants/wk) | 27% | 12% |
| Low Use (1-10 sealants/wk) | 31% | 53% |
| Non-Use (0 sealants/wk) | 4% | 27% |
| **Percentage of Children in Private Practice Receiving Sealants** | | |
| 0% | 6% | 31% |
| 1-9% | 11% | 13% |
| 10-19% | 14% | 18% |
| 20-39% | 21% | 19% |
| 40-59% | 18% | 11% |
| 60-79% | 17% | 5% |
| 80-89% | 8% | 2% |
| 90-100% | 7% | 2% |
| **Average Percentage of Children in Private Practice Receiving Sealants** | 39% | 19% |
| **Delegation of Sealant Placement** | 61% | 53% |
| **Sealant Placed B** | | |
| Dentist | 50% | 40% |
| Dental hygienist | 9% | 51% |
| Dental assistant | 18% | 9% |
| Dental assistant or hygienist | 23% | — |

Compiled from references 23,99.

sealants. By grouping dentists into sealant usage categories based on the number of sealants placed per week, it can be seen that most general dentists (53%) are in the low-use category and the majority of pediatric dentists (65%) are in the moderate-use and high-use categories. These figures may reflect the relatively low proportion of children in general dentistry practices, resulting in less frequent applications of sealants during a specific time period. Still, pediatric dentists placed sealants in slightly less than 40% of their patients, whereas less than 20% of children in general dentistry practices have received sealants.[30,206] Almost 50% of general dentists reported placing sealants in less than 10% of their child patients. In contrast, 50% of pediatric dentists indicated that they placed sealants in more than 40% of their patients. Delegation of sealant placement is similar for pediatric and general dentists, with slightly over half delegating the responsibility for sealant placement to hygienists or assistants.[44,52,54] Pediatric dentists tend to delegate this responsibility more frequently to dental assistants, whereas general dentists delegate more frequently to dental hygienists. This probably reflects the fact that relatively few pediatric dentistry practices employ hygienists.

Incorporation of sealants into general practice is associated with the dentist's age and number of years in practice.[23,42,43,99,215] In fact, one survey found that 97% of dentists younger than 30 years provided sealants for their child patients. Among dentists in practice for 10 years or less, 90% used sealants, whereas among dentists with 30 or more years of practice approximately two thirds used sealants. In the latter group, slightly less than 50% used sealants either routinely or occasionally, whereas 78% of dentists with 10 years or less of practice experience claimed to use sealants routinely or occasionally.

Although incorporation of sealants into general practice has become more or less a standard of care, the proportion of children receiving the benefits of sealants is unexpectedly low (Table 32-14). In both regional and national surveys carried out between 1985 and 1994, the proportion of children who had had sealants placed ranged from 6% to 21%.[139,184-186,213,224] In a 1989 U.S. Public Health Service survey, a trend toward an increased prevalence of sealants was noted, with 17% of 8-year-olds and 13% of 14-year-olds having received sealants.[184-186]

The most recent NHANES III survey of sealant prevalence (see Table 32-14) indicates a continuing increase in sealant application by dentists.[213] Sealants are found in 18.5% of all children and adolescents. Slightly more than 25% of 14-year-olds have had sealants placed, whereas slightly more than 20% of 8-year-olds have received sealants. The highest sealant application rates are associated with children of white, non-Hispanic race. Overall, both Hispanics and blacks have sealants applied infrequently. The rate of sealant use in 18- to 24-year-olds is slightly greater than 5%. In contrast, individuals older than 25 years rarely have sealants present.

An exemplary, aggressive campaign for sealant placement in Ohio (see Table 32-14) has been waged in conjunction with state and local dental societies, a sealant product manufacturer, and federal agencies.[184-186] Sealant prevalence in second graders in one Ohio community increased from 7% to 24% between 1986 and 1992. Among third-grade students evaluated in 1992, sealants were found to be present in 35%. Perhaps even

## TABLE 32-14

### Prevalence of Sealants in U.S. Children, Adolescents, and Young Adults

| | INDIVIDUALS WITH SEALANTS |
|---|---|
| **Michigan Sealant Prevalence Study 1985-86** | |
| All age groups | 6.4% |
| **NIDR Sealant Prevalence Study 1986-87** | |
| All regions of US | 7.6% |
| **USPHS Sealant Prevalence Study 1987** | |
| 8-year-olds | 11% |
| 14-year-olds | 8% |
| **USPHS Sealant Prevalence Study 1989** | |
| 8-year-olds | 17% |
| 14-year-olds | 13% |
| **NHANES III 1988-91** | |
| *8-year-olds* | 20.9% |
| White | 26.6% |
| Hispanic | 9.9% |
| Black | 8.6% |
| *14-year-olds* | 28.2% |
| White | 35.7% |
| Hispanic | 10.9% |
| Black | 4.7% |
| *5- to 17-year-olds* | 18.5% |
| Males | 17.1% |
| Females | 19.9% |
| White | 21.7% |
| Hispanic | 7.0% |
| Black | 6.9% |
| *18- to 24-year-olds* | 5.5% |
| *25- to 34-year-olds* | 1.6% |
| *>35-year-olds* | 0.6% |
| **Tennessee: 1996-97** | |
| Low socioeconomic status | 11% |
| Moderate socioeconomic status | 18% |
| High socioeconomic status | 22% |
| **US Military Recruits: 1994** | 14.8% |

*Continued*

| **TABLE 32-14** | |
| :--- | :--- |
| **Prevalence of Sealants in U.S. Children, Adolescents, and Young Adults—cont'd** | |
| | INDIVIDUALS WITH SEALANTS |
| Active Duty US Military Personnel: 1994 | 6.8% |
| 2nd and 3rd Grader School Children: 1997 | 23% |
| 8th and 9th Grader School Children: 1997 | 20% |
| Low risk insured children: 1991-97 | |
| 5.5- to 8-year-olds | 8% |
| 11.5- to 14-year-olds | 5% |
| **Ohio Bureau of Dental Health Sealant Project 1986-1999** | |
| 1986    8-year-olds | 11% |
| 1992    8-year-olds | 26% |
| 1999    8-year-olds | 30% |
| 1999    8-year-olds | 34% |

| | SEALANT PROGRAM | NO SEALANT PROGRAM |
| :--- | :--- | :--- |
| | 57% | 28% |
| White | 62% | 30% |
| Black | 51% | 18% |
| Male | 57% | 28% |
| Female | 56% | 28% |
| Lunch program eligible | 54% | 29% |
| Lunch program ineligible | 65% | 34% |
| No insurance | 55% | 24% |
| Medicaid | 58% | 22% |
| Private insurance | 58% | 34% |

| **Upstate New York Targeted School-Based Program (2nd Graders): 2002** | |
| :--- | :--- |
| Caries-free children | 18-91% |
| Caries affected children | 47-88% |
| **US Indian Health Services Sealant Project 1990** | |
| 9-year-olds | 74% |

| **TABLE 32-14** | |
| :--- | :--- |
| **Prevalence of Sealants in U.S. Children, Adolescents, and Young Adults—cont'd** | |
| | INDIVIDUALS WITH SEALANTS |
| USPHS Oral Health Goal for 8- to 14-Year-Olds for the Year 2000 (goal not met) and 2010 | 50% |

Compiled from references 2,16,23,30,32,34,42-44,52, 53,79,80,89,127, 132,140,169,184-186,195,206,210,214,215.

more surprising was a program initiated by the Indian Health Service to provide sealants to at least 75% of 9-year-old American Indian children by 1990 to complement the preventive effects of water fluoridation.[184-186] In 1990, the Indian Health Service announced that 74% of 9-year-olds had received sealants. Also in 1990, the director of the U.S. Public Health Service established oral health goals for the next decade.[184-186] One of the 16 goals for the year 2000 is to achieve sealant protection of the pits and fissures of permanent molar teeth in at least 50% of U.S. schoolchildren between the ages of 8 and 14. Most decidedly, this goal was not met, and the United States surgeon general's "Healthy People 2010" goal for sealant placement in 8- to 14-year-olds remains at 50%. If past trends continue along the same path, it is unlikely that 50% of U.S. schoolchildren will have sealants in place by the year 2010.

With children who had sealants present, the number of permanent teeth with sealants and tooth type (Table 32-15) were analyzed in the NHANES III survey.[213] In the 5- to 11-year age group, four teeth had been sealed in 50% of children, whereas in the 12- to 17-year age group, 8 teeth had been sealed in 14%, 3 teeth in 21%, and 1 tooth in 13%. The number of permanent teeth sealed was quite variable with as many as 16 teeth sealed in 12- to 17-year-olds. The most frequently sealed tooth types were maxillary and mandibular first molars (10.5% to 15.6%), followed by maxillary and mandibular second molars (5.5% to 9.5%). Less than 3% of premolars had been sealed in 12- to 17-year-olds.

Even though remarkable increases are occurring in the number of children with sealants, there

## TABLE 32-15

### Sealant Placement: Number of Teeth Sealed and Tooth Type Sealed

| NUMBER OF PERMANENT TEETH SEALED | 5- TO 11-YEAR-OLDS | 12- TO 17-YEAR-OLDS |
|---|---|---|
| 1 tooth | 8.0% | 12.7% |
| 2 teeth | 18.3% | 8.8% |
| 3 teeth | 18.6% | 21.3% |
| 4 teeth | 50.5% | 8.8% |
| ≥ 5 teeth | 4.6% | — |
| 5 teeth | — | 8.9% |
| 6 teeth | — | 7.1% |
| 7 teeth | — | 5.2% |
| 8 teeth | — | 14.1% |
| 9 to12 teeth | — | 3.8% |
| 13 to16 teeth | — | 5.9% |

| PERMANENT TOOTH TYPE SEALED | 5- TO 11-YEAR-OLDS | 12- TO 17-YEAR-OLDS |
|---|---|---|
| **Maxillary** | | |
| First molar | 15.6% | 10.5% |
| Second molar | 5.5% | 8.0% |
| First premolar | 0.8% | 2.5% |
| Second premolar | 0.6% | 2.6% |
| **Mandibular** | | |
| First molar | 15.3% | 11.7% |
| Second molar | 5.6% | 9.5% |
| First premolar | 0.6% | 2.4% |
| Second premolar | 1.7% | 2.7% |

Compiled from reference 213.

still appears to be a significant discrepancy between the percentage of dentists using sealants in their practices and the proportion of children receiving sealants. Perhaps the most frequent reason cited for limiting sealant usage may help to explain why more children are not receiving the caries-protective benefit of sealants (Table 32-16). Although concerns about sealing over caries, sealant retention, and cost-effectiveness were cited, lack of reimbursement for sealant placement was the most frequently reported reason for limiting sealant usage.[99,213,227] In fact, dentists report that only 11% of their patients' insurance policies cover sealant placement.[30,206] In addition, lack of insurance coverage influenced the level of sealant use by slightly more than 50% of dentists. In one regional survey, approximately 15% of dentists did not place sealants in their patients

because insurance plans did not provide reimbursement for this procedure.[42,43] Without insurance coverage, parents are required to accept financial responsibility for sealant placement or decline this preventive procedure. Without sealant placement, susceptible tooth surfaces will most likely develop caries and require placement of a permanent restoration that will be covered by the patient's insurance program. The lack of insurance coverage for sealants and the reimbursement for restorative procedures may partially explain the lower than expected prevalence of sealants in children. However, when one examines the reasons for limiting sealant use by sealant nonusers and sealant users, the major concerns expressed by the nonusers are based on lack of confidence in sealants' effectiveness in preventing caries and being retained. With sealant

## TABLE 32-16

### Reasons for Limiting Use of Pit and Fissure Sealant by General Practitioners

|  | RANKING (1 = MOST FREQUENT) |
|---|:---:|
| Lack of insurance reimbursement | 1 |
| Concern with sealing over caries | 2 |
| Concern with sealant retention | 3 |
| Cost effectiveness of sealants low | 4 |
| **Sealant Nonusers** | |
| Concern regarding sealing in decay | 1 |
| Occlusal fillings preferred | 2 |
| Sealants do not last long | 3 |
| Patients not requesting sealants | 4 |
| Additional research necessary | 4 |
| Better materials needed | 4 |
| Insurance coverage lacking | 4 |
| **Sealant Users** | |
| Patients unwilling to pay for sealants | 1 |
| Insurance companies do not reimburse | 2 |
| Patients do not understand value of sealants | 3 |
| **Other Concerns (not ranked)** | |
| Difficulty in placing sealants | |
| Maintenance and repair required for effectiveness | |

Compiled from references 2,23,30,42,43,45-48,83,99,206, 213,215,227.

## TABLE 32-17

### Reasons for Limited Coverage of Sealants by Third-Party Payment Plans

| REASON | RANKING (1 = MOST FREQUENT) |
|---|:---:|
| Cost effectiveness of sealants low | 1 |
| Guidelines for sealant placement not defined | 2 |
| More clinical research necessary | 3 |
| Potential for inappropriate use and fees | 4 |
| Most insurers do not provide sealant coverage in policies | 5 |
| Sealants are temporary treatment | 6 |
| Policy premiums would increase | 7 |
| Employers exclude sealant coverage from dental plans | 7 |

Compiled from references 74,75.

(2) guidelines for sealant placement not defined; (3) more clinical research deemed necessary; and (4) potential for inappropriate usage and fees. It is quite obvious that these reasons for non-reimbursement are not well founded. Because the same third-party providers reimburse the patient for restoration placement, it seems logical to assume that sealant placement may provide additional savings for the insurance companies based on the cost to place and maintain sealants compared with that to place amalgam restorations. Of the insurance companies that do provide sealant coverage, approximately two thirds define certain clinical conditions for reimbursement. Some of these conditions are age limitations; restriction of sealant placement to permanent teeth, with some specifying first and second molars only; and caries-free status of teeth to be sealed. One insurance company required that only opaque sealants be used.[42]

Significant gains have been realized in sealant coverage by Medicaid programs. In 1985, less than 10% of Medicaid programs covered sealant reimbursement.[75] A 1991 ADA survey found that 58% of Medicaid programs covered sealant protection.[184] In 1992, it was reported that 92% of Medicaid programs provided reimbursement for sealant placement,[184] and by October 1994 all 50 states included sealants in their Medicaid programs.[214] With the oral health goal for the year

nonusers, the least common reasons cited for limiting sealant usage are related to insurance coverage issues. In contrast, sealant users appear to limit sealant usage in their practices when the parents are unwilling to pay for sealant placement, insurance does not reimburse for sealants, or the patients/parents do not understand the value of sealants in preventing caries.

Surveys of insurance companies that do not provide sealant coverage have been carried out to determine the reasons for lack of reimbursement.[74,75] The most frequently cited reasons for nonreimbursement (Table 32-17), in descending order, were (1) low cost-effectiveness of sealants;

2000 of sealant protection provided to 50% of schoolchildren, it is hoped that inclusion of sealants in comprehensive dental insurance plans will become common among third-party and managed care providers.

## SEALANT USE AND PRACTICES AMONG PEDIATRIC DENTISTS

A survey of a large proportion of U.S. pediatric dentists and pediatric dentistry departments in dental schools was conducted to assess the sealant use and practices in pediatric dentistry (Table 32-18).[195] The survey included almost 900 pediatric dentists in six states representing different regions of the United States. As expected, all pediatric dentists place sealants. However, caries risk assessment, criteria for placement, and application techniques varied somewhat. The majority of dentists place sealants based on the perceived susceptibility of the pits and fissures to caries in children with all levels of caries risk. Permanent molars are more commonly sealed than primary molars and premolars. The only criterion for not placing a sealant was clinically obvious caries. The majority of dentists depend on visual and tactile examination for caries detection. The minority use rubber dam isolation for isolation of the tooth during sealant placement, and most use cotton rolls and dry angles. A number of different surface-cleansing techniques are employed, with the explorer and pumice paste being the most popular. Almost 90% perform surface preparation with burs or air abrasion. Acid etching, rinsing, and drying times conform to the standards suggested by manufacturers and prior workshops on sealant techniques. Both opaque and fluoride-releasing sealants are used relatively frequently, whereas flowable composites and dentin-bonding agents are used less frequently. Polymerization is primarily with a visible light source. Autopolymerized sealants are rarely used (3%) in these pediatric dental practices. Evaluation of the sealant immediately following placement is done with a displacement test to assess for defects and for occlusal interferences. Clinical assessment of sealant success was estimated to be about 80% for retention with caries in only 6% over a 3-year period. Reapplication of sealants is estimated at 5% to 8% per year, which is within that expected from prior clinical trials. When reapplication is necessary, the policy varies

with most dentists charging a fee after 1 year (57%). If the sealant fails and caries develops, one third of dentists charge a reduced fee for the subsequent restoration whereas about 60% assess the entire fee. Some of the issues not addressed were the parties responsible for payment, parents' willingness to pay for sealants when not covered by insurance, the fee schedule for sealants, the percentage of children receiving sealants, and delegation of sealant placement.

## PARENTAL AND PHYSICIAN KNOWLEDGE AND ATTITUDES ABOUT SEALANTS

Education of parents and physicians regarding the importance of caries prevention is of considerable importance in improving the dental health of infants and young children. With the majority of dentists claiming to use sealants in their practices, expansion of the knowledge base and attitudes of parents and physicians may be required to advance the acceptance of this preventive technique. Certain parental factors (Table 32-19) are associated with acceptance of sealants for their children.* Some of the parental factors associated with sealant acceptance as a preventive measure include (1) education beyond high school; (2) female parent decision maker; (3) recommendation by dentist or dental staff; and (4) regular dental care for children. Although a number of parents have heard about sealants from friends or the popular press, recommendations by the dentist and his staff are most important. Dental coverage for sealants is more commonly associated with sealant placement. The parental knowledge of preventive and restorative dental care may also give the dentist a sense of the parents' knowledge base and the need for education in caries prevention. While most parents understand the importance of professional prophylaxis, restoring carious teeth and decreasing sucrose intake, a large percentage (44% to 66%) are not certain of the effect of sealants on caries prevention. Many times pediatric and general dentists are dependent on the knowledge base and attitude of pediatricians and family practice physicians for referral of infants and young children in need of preventive and restorative care.[16] More than two thirds of physicians are not familiar with sealants

---

*References 16,79,80,109,127,150,211

## TABLE 32-18
### Sealant Survey of U.S. Pediatric Dentists

**Criteria for Sealant Placement**

*Caries Risk Status*

| | |
|---|---|
| All caries risk categories | 75% |
| Low caries risk only | 6% |
| High caries risk only | 19% |

*Patient Behavior*

| | |
|---|---|
| Cooperative only | 62% |
| Cooperative and non-cooperative | 38% |

*Tooth Type*

| | |
|---|---|
| Permanent molars | 100% |
| Premolars | 58% |
| Primary molars | 42% |

*Tooth Eruption Status*

| | |
|---|---|
| Complete eruption only | 77% |
| Complete or partial eruption | 23% |

*Post-Eruption Period*

| | |
|---|---|
| Less than 3 years only | 44% |
| Any post-eruption tooth age | 56% |

*Pit and Fissure Caries Status*

| | |
|---|---|
| Caries-free only | 31% |
| Caries questionable | 48% |
| Incipient caries | 21% |
| Obvious caries | 0% |

*Caries Detection Technique*

| | |
|---|---|
| Visual and tactile | 100% |
| Radiographic | 55% |
| Transillumination | 5% |

**Sealant Placement Practice**

| | |
|---|---|
| Antisialagogue | 15% |

*Saliva Isolation*

| | |
|---|---|
| Cotton roll/dry angle | 89% |
| Saliva ejector | 54% |
| Rubber dam | 33% |

*Surface Cleansing*

| | |
|---|---|
| Explorer | 54% |
| Pumice paste | 45% |
| Rotary cup | 15% |
| Toothbrush | 13% |
| No cleansing | 11% |
| Hydrogen peroxide | 5% |
| Air abrasion | 2% |

## TABLE 32-18
### Sealant Survey of U.S. Pediatric Dentists—cont'd

*Surface Preparation*

| | |
|---|---|
| High-speed bur | 53% |
| Low-speed bur | 16% |
| Air abrasion | 18% |
| No preparation | 13% |

*Acid-Etching Time (mean)*

| | |
|---|---|
| Primary teeth | 29 seconds |
| Permanent teeth | 23 seconds |
| Post acid-etch rinsing time (mean) | 14 seconds |
| Post rinse drying time (mean) | 11 seconds |

*Sealant Material*

| | |
|---|---|
| Transparent sealant | 20% |
| Opaque sealant | 45% |
| Fluoride-releasing sealant | 40% |
| Flowable composite | 26% |
| Dentin bonding agent | 16% |

*Sealant Polymerization*

| | |
|---|---|
| Visible light polymerization | 94% |
| Autopolymerization (chemical) | 3% |
| Laser polymerization | 3% |

*Evaluation After Placement*
*Explorer*

| | |
|---|---|
| Forceful (displacement test) | 47% |
| Gentle (defect evaluation) | 44% |
| Visual inspection only | 10% |
| Occlusion interference | 40% |

| CLINICAL ASSESSMENT OF SUCCESS | 1 YEAR | 3 YEARS |
|---|---|---|
| Retention | 89% | 78% |
| Caries on sealed surface | 3% | 6% |
| Sealant requires reapplications | 8% | 16% |

**Sealant Reapplication Policy**

| | |
|---|---|
| No fee | 37% |
| Fee only after 1 year | 16% |
| Fee only after 2 years | 16% |
| Fee only after 3 years | 25% |
| Failed recall examinations | 4% |
| Fee always charged | 2% |

**Restoration Policy**

| | |
|---|---|
| Entire fee for restoration | 59% |
| Reduced fee for restoration | 33% |
| No fee for restoration | 8% |

Compiled from reference 195.

## TABLE 32-19
### Parental and Physician Knowledge and Attitude Toward Sealants

**Parental Factors Associated with Acceptance of Sealant Placement**

Education beyond high school, especially college educated

Caucasian race

Female parent decision-maker

Prior knowledge of sealants

Recommendation by dentist or dental staff

Regular dental care for children

Dental insurance coverage

Middle and upper socioeconomic group

**Parental Rating of Preventive and Restorative Dental Care**

|  | IMPORTANT | NOT IMPORTANT | NOT SURE |
|---|---|---|---|
| Professional cleaning | 76% | 10% | 13% |
| Filling decayed teeth | 88% | 3% | 10% |
| Decrease sugar intake | 88% | 7% | 5% |
| *Sealant placement* | 45% | 6% | 49% |
| Sealants prevent decay | 53% | 2% | 46% |
| Fluoride and sealants may prevent most caries | 53% | 3% | 44% |
| Sealants important for permanent teeth | 43% | 5% | 52% |
| Sealants protect for > 1 year | 31% | 3% | 66% |

**Physicians Knowledge Base Regarding Sealants**

| | |
|---|---|
| Not very familiar with sealants | 69% |
| Unsure which type of teeth to recommend for sealants | 64% |
| Sealants protect against caries | 35% |
| Benefit of combining sealants and fluoride | 32% |
| Acceptable to place sealant over incipient caries | 3% |

Compiled from references 16,79,80,109,127,150,211.

(see Table 32-19) and are unsure about which type of teeth benefit from sealant placement.[16] Only one third of physicians realize that sealants alone or in combination with fluoride protect against caries formation. It is quite obvious that the dental profession needs to develop educational material directed to parents and physicians regarding the role of sealants in a complete prevention program. With an expanded knowledge base and improved attitudes about sealants, parents' and physicians' requests for evaluation of children for sealant placement may result in an increase in the use of sealants in the pediatric and adolescent population.

## COST-EFFECTIVENESS OF SEALANTS

Although it has become apparent that sealants provide significant caries protection for pits and fissures, the use of sealants has been limited in the past owing to questions about their cost-effectiveness. In a regional survey of sealant use during 1987, the mean professional fee for sealant placement per tooth surface was $9.05.[42] In comparison, a national survey completed in 1988 found that mean costs for sealant placement were $13.50 and for amalgam placement were $26.50.[30] The average cost per child for sealant application and reapplication was determined to be $28.78 per year.[42] These fees are based on those reported by private practitioners. Cost analysis in 2000 placed the estimated sealant fee at $27 and a one-surface amalgam restoration fee at $73.77.[83]

An extensive study of dental insurance claims for sealants and one-surface posterior restorations placed in 1.35 million children across the United States over a 39-month period provided a means to calculate the cost ratio of sealant versus a one-surface restoration placement.[136,137] Of interest was the difference between the range of fees for sealant placement from $11.63 to $38.91 and those for one-surface restoration from $28.48 to $76.69. The mean cost of a sealant was $17.80, contrasted with $41.00 for a one-surface restoration. By applying a sealant to an at-risk surface, a cost reduction of 57% could be realized. Appropriate placement of a sealant would provide a significant initial savings for governmental health care agencies, third-party payors, and parents. Some additional maintenance expenses may be incurred secondary to sealant loss and caries development over time. It has been suggested that the cost of placing sealants may be reduced by as much as 80% if sealants are placed by dental auxiliaries either in the dental office or in a school-based public dentistry facility.[166]

The total expense incurred with sealant placement must be compared with the cost of restoration of the teeth should sealants not be placed and caries eventually develop. Over a 10-year period, it was found that the cost of restoring unsealed surfaces was 1.64 times the cost of a single application of sealant.[223-227] Using a sealant maintenance program that includes the cost of initial sealant placement, sealant reapplication, and restoration placement when sealants fail, the total expenditure for this type of program would be 25% less than that for restoration of unsealed surfaces when caries developed. Perhaps more important is the fact that even with a single application of sealant material, 4.7 and 4.1 tooth surfaces per child are "saved" from caries over a 10- and 15-year period, respectively.[223-227] When comparing the cost of a preventive program including sealants with the expense of restoration placement, one must also consider the intangible value of maintaining caries-free tooth surfaces and promoting a low incidence of dental caries in our child and adolescent population.

Studies of the cost-effectiveness of school-based sealant programs have shown a considerable savings.[33,170,171,258] The cost savings ranged from $42 per tooth surface in a dental clinic environment to $65 per tooth surface with a school-based program. These cost savings did not take into account additional hidden costs, such as time taken from work by parents, transportation time, lost school time, and waiting room time when sealants were placed in a dental clinic.

A survey of sealant placement in 5- to 7-year-old Medicaid children has shown a threefold reduction in claims for restorative services compared to children who did not have any sealants placed.[34] Over the 7-year period that Medicaid claims were reviewed, it was found that there was a 30% increase in cost for providing restorative care for children that had not had sealants placed compared with those with sealants. Children who did not receive sealants had a 3.3-fold increase in the number of claims for one-surface posterior amalgam or resin restorations. The cost savings in this pediatric Medicaid population was independent of race, gender, or age of the child.

Cost-effectiveness of sealants may be enhanced by (1) training auxiliaries to place sealants as allowed by local state laws; (2) using sealants with the highest retention rates and lowest caries rates based on evidence-based clinical studies; (3) sealant application in children, adolescents, and adults with low risk for interproximal caries; (4) combination with other caries-preventive agents, such as fluoride rinses, chlorhexidine rinses/toothpastes, fluoride varnishes, xylitol or casein phosphopeptide-amorphous calcium phosphate–containing chewing gum; and (5) sealant polymerization with an argon laser.[104,109]

## SUMMARY

Pit and fissure caries represent approximately 90% of the total caries experience in childhood and adolescence. The development of pit and fissure caries occurs not only in 6- to 14-year-old children but also in adolescents and young adults. With the introduction of sealants, a clinical approach to prevention of caries in pit and fissures became available. Laboratory studies and clinical trials have provided overwhelming evidence supporting the capacity of this resin material to resist caries development. With innovative applications of the acid-etch technique, tooth surfaces with isolated involvement of pits and fissures may also benefit from the conservation of tooth structure afforded by conservative adhesive resin restorations. It also appears that both fluoride-releasing sealant and glass ionomer–based materials act as fluoride reservoirs for adjacent enamel and dentin, provide enhanced caries resistance for sound enamel, and perhaps remineralize enamel and dentinal caries.

During the past two decades, increased acceptance of sealants as a preventive regimen has occurred, with 80% to 95% of dentists using sealants in their practice. It is hoped that sealants will be adopted as a standard of care for prevention of pit and fissure caries. However, the goal for Healthy People 2000 that called for placement of sealants in 50% of children between 8 to 14 years of age was not met. This goal has now been included as one of the objectives for Healthy People 2010. Although the percentage of children receiving sealants has increased over the past decade, certain factors still limit sealant utilization. The primary concern limiting sealant utilization is still lack of third-party reimbursement for this procedure. To make significant gains in caries reduction in the child, adolescent, and adult populations in the near future, it is necessary for the dental profession to educate and inform the general public, parents, physicians, underwriters of dental care plans, and funding agencies about the cost-effectiveness and caries-preventive benefits of sealants and preventive restorations. With widespread use of the acid-etch technique, it may be possible to provide the majority of children, adolescents, and adults with a caries-free dentition.

# REFERENCES

1. Adair SM: The role of sealants in caries prevention programs. *J Calif Dent Assoc* 31:221, 2003.
2. Albert DA: Sealant use in public and private insurance programs. *NY State Dent J* 65:30, 1999.
3. Alwas-Danowska HM, Plasschaert AJM, Suliborski S, Verdonschot EH: Reliability and validity of laser fluorescence measurements in occlusal caries diagnosis. *J Dent* 30:129, 2002.
4. American Dental Association, Council on Scientific Affairs: Available at www.ada.org/prof/prac/seal, 2004.
5. Angmar-Mansson B, ten Bosch JJ: Advances in methods for diagnosing coronal caries: a review. *Adv Dent Res* 7:70, 1993.
6. Anttonen V, Seppa L, Hausen H: Clinical study of the use of the laser fluorescence device DIAGNOdent for detection of occlusal caries in children. *Caries Res* 37:17, 2003.
7. Arenholt-Bindslev D, Breinholt V, Preiss A, Schmalz G: Time-related bisphenol-A content and estrogenic activity in saliva samples collected in relation to placement of fissure sealants. *Clin Oral Invest* 3:120, 1999.
8. Ashley P: Diagnosis of occlusal caries in primary teeth. *Int J Pediatr Dent* 10:166, 2000.
9. Ashley PF, Blinkhorn AS, Davies RM: Occlusal caries diagnosis: an in vitro histological validation of the electronic caries monitor (ECM) and other methods. *J Dent* 26:83, 1998.
10. Baelum V, Machiulskiene V, Nyvad B et al: Application of survival analysis to carious lesion transitions in intervention trials. *Community Dent Oral Epidemiol* 31:252, 2003.
11. Bell RM, Klein SP, Bohannon HM et al: *Treatment Effects in the National Preventive Dentistry Demonstration Program.* Publication R-3072-RWS, Santa Monica, CA, Rand Corporation, 1984.
12. Blankenau RJ, Kelsey WP, Powell GL et al: Degree of composite resin polymerization with visible light and argon laser. *Am J Dent* 4:40, 1991.
13. Bodecker CF: The eradication of enamel fissures. *Dent Items Interest* 51:859, 1929.
14. Bohannon HM, Disney JA, Graves RC et al: Indications for sealant use in a community-based preventive dentistry program. *J Dent Educ* 48:45, 1984.
15. Bowen RL: Composite and sealant resins: past, present and future. *Pediatr Dent* 4:10, 1982.
16. Bowman PA, Zinner KL: 'Utah's parent, teacher and physician sealant awareness surveys. *J Dent Hyg* 68:279, 1994
17. Brown LJ: The impact of recent changes in the epidemiology of dental caries on guidelines for the use of dental sealants. *J Public Health Dent* 55:274, 1995.
18. Brown LJ, Kaste LM, Selwitz RH, Furman LJ: Dental caries and sealant usage in US children, 1988–91. Selected findings from the third national health and nutrition examination survey. *JADA* 127:335, 1996.
19. Brown LJ, Wall TP, Lazar V: Trends in total caries experience: permanent and primary teeth. *JADA* 131:223, 2000.
20. Brown LJ, Wall TP, Lazar V: Trends in untreated caries in primary teeth of children 2 to 10 years old. *JADA* 131:93, 2000
21. Buonocore MG: Simple method of increasing the adhesion of acrylic filling materials to enamel surfaces. *J Dent Res* 34:849, 1955.
22. Burgess J, Norling B, Summitt J: Resin ionomer restorative materials: the new generation. *J Esthet Dent* 6:207, 1994.
23. Call RL, Mann J, Hicks J: Attitudes of general practitioners towards fissure sealant use. *Clin Prev Dent* 10:9, 1988.
24. Centers for Disease Control and Prevention:

Community and other approaches to promote oral health and prevent oral disease. In: Oral Health in America: Report of the Surgeon General. Available at www.surgeongeneral.gov/library/oralhealth. Last accessed 2003.

25. Centers for Disease Control and Prevention: Preventing dental caries. Children's oral health. Oral Health 2000: Facts and Figures. Available at www.cdc.gov/oralhealth.factsheets. Last accessed 2003.

26. Charbeneau GT: Pit and fissure sealants. *J Dent* 32:315, 1982.

27. Chisick MC, Poindexter FR, York AK: Dental sealants: prevalence and need in US military recruits. *Mil Med* 163:386, 1998.

28. Chisick MC, Poindexter FR, York AK: The need for and prevalence of dental sealants in active duty US military personnel. *Mil Med* 163:155, 1998.

29. Chosak A, Eidelman E: Effect of time from application until exposure to light on the tag length of a visible light–polymerized sealant. *Dent Mater* 4:302, 1988.

30. Cohen L, LaBelle A, Romberg, E: The use of pit and fissure sealants in private practice: a national survey. *J Public Health Dent* 48:26, 1988.

31. Cooley RL, McCourt JW, Huddleston AM et al: Evaluation of a fluoride-containing sealant by SEM, microleakage and fluoride release. *Pediatr Dent* 12:38, 1990.

32. Corbin SB, Clark NL, McClendon BJ et al: Patterns of sealant delivery under variable third party requirements. *J Public Health Dent* 50:311, 1990.

33. Crowley SJ, Campain AC, Morgan MV: An economic evaluation of a publicly funded dental prevention program in regional and rural Victoria: an extrapolated analysis. *Community Dent Oral Epidemiol* 17:145, 2000.

34. Dasanyake AP, Li Y, Kirk K et al: Restorative cost savings related to dental sealants in Alabama Medicaid children. *Pediatr Dent* 25:572, 2003.

35. Dennison JB, Straffon LH, More FG: Evaluating tooth eruption on sealant efficacy. *JADA* 121:610, 1990.

36. Dennison JB, Straffon LH, Smith RC: Effectiveness of sealant treatment over five years in an insured population. *JADA* 131:597, 2000.

37. Duangthip D, Lussi A: Microleakage and penetration ability of resin sealant versus bonding system when applied following contamination. *Pediatr Dent* 25:505, 2003.

38. Elderton RJ: The cause of failure of restorations: a literature review. *J Dent* 4:257, 1976.

39. Eidelman E, Fuks A, Chosak A: The retention of fissure sealants: Rubber dam or cotton roll isolation in private practice. *J Dent Child* 50:259, 1983.

40. Eidelman E, Shapira J, Houpt M: The retention of fissure sealants using twenty-second etching time: three-year follow-up. *J Dent Child* 55:119, 1988.

41. Erickson RL, Glasspoole EA: Bonding to tooth structure: a comparison of glass-ionomer and composite-resin systems. *J Esthet Dent* 6:227, 1994.

42. Faine RC, Dennen T: A survey of private dental 'practitioners' utilization of dental sealants in Washington state. *J Dent Child* 53:337, 1986.

43. Faine RC, Isman R: The use of dental sealants in the Washington state medical assistance program: a second-year report. *J Dent Child* 56:450, 1989.

44. Farghaly MM, Lang WP, Woolfolk MW et al: Factors associated with fissure sealant delegation: 'dentists' characteristics and office staffing patterns. *J Public Health Dent* 53:246, 1993.

45. Feigal RJ: Current status of pit and fissure sealants: improving effectiveness of the preventive strategy. *J Pediatr Dental Care* 2003:9:10.

46. Feigal RJ: The use of pit and fissure sealants. *Pediatr Dent* 24:415, 2002.

47. Feigal RJ: Sealants and preventive restorations: review of effectiveness and clinical changes for improvement. *Pediatr Dent* 20:85, 1998.

48. Feigal RJ, Musherure P, Gillespie B et al: Improved sealant retention with bonding agents: a clinical study of two-bottle and single-bottle systems. *J Dent Res* 79:1850, 2000.

49. Felding JE, Mullen PD, Brownson RC et al: Promoting oral health: interventions for preventing dental caries, oral and pharyngeal cancers, and sports-related craniofacial injuries. *MMWR Morb Mortal Wkly Rep* 50(RR21):1, 2001.

50. Flaitz CM, Hicks MJ, Silverstone LM: Radiographic, histologic, and electronic comparison of occlusal caries: an in vitro study. *Pediatr Dent* 8:24, 1986.

51. Folke BD, Walton JL, Feigal RJ: Occlusal sealant success over ten years in a private practice: comparing longevity of sealants placed by dentists, hygienists, and assistants. *Pediatr Dent* 26:426, 2004.

52. Foreman FJ: Sealant prevalence and indication in a young military population. *JADA* 125:182, 1994.

53. Foreman FJ: Effects of delegation, state practice acts, and practice management techniques upon sealant utilization: a national survey of pediatric dentists. *J Dent Child* 60:193, 1993.

54. Forss H, Halme E: Retention of glass ionomer cement and a resin-based fissure sealant and effects on carious outcome after 7 years. *Community Dent Oral Epidemiol* 26:21, 1998.

55. Forsten L: Fluoride release of glass ionomers. *J Esthet Dent* 6:216, 1994.

56. Forsten L: Fluoride release and uptake by glass ionomers and related materials and its clinical effect. *Biomaterials* 19:503, 1998.

57. Francescut P, Lussi A: Correlation between fissure discoloration, DIAGNOdent measurements, and caries depth: an in vitro study. *Pediatr Dent* 35:564, 2003.

58. Freedman G, McLauglin G: Sealants buyer guide. *Dental Products Rep* 16:112, 1997.

59. Frencken JE, Pilot T, Songpaisan Y, Phantumvanit P: Atraumatic restorative treatment (ART): rationale, technique and development. *J Public Health Dent* 56:135, 1996.

60. Frencken JE, Makoni F, Sithole WD: ART restorations and glass ionomer sealants in Zimbabwe: survival after 3 years. *Community Dent Oral Epidemiol* 26:372, 1998.

61. Frencken JE, Makoni F, Sithole WD, Hackenitz E: Three-year survival of one-surface ART restorations and glass-ionomer sealants in a school oral health programme in Zimbabwe. *Caries Res* 32:119, 1998.

62. Frencken JE, Songpaisan Y, Phantumvanit P, Pilot T: An atraumatic restorative treatment (ART) technique: evaluation after one year. *Int Dent J* 44:460, 1994.

63. Frencken JE, 'van't Hof MA, van Amerongen WE, Holmgren CJ: Effectiveness of single-surface ART restorations in the permanent dentition: a meta-analysis. *J Dent Res* 83:120, 2004.

64. Fung EYK, Ewoldsen NO, St Germain HA, Marx D et al: Pharmacokinetics of bisphenol A released from a dental sealant. *JADA* 131:51, 2000.

65. Gale TJ, Hanes CM, Myers DR, Russell CM: Performance of sealants applied to first permanent molars in a dental school setting. *Pediatr Dent* 20:341, 1998.

66. Galil KA, Gwinnett AJ: Three-dimensional replicas of pits and fissures in human teeth: a scanning electron microscopic study. *Arch Oral Biol* 20:493, 1975.

67. Ganss C, Klimek J, Gleim A: One year clinical evaluation of the retention and quality of two fluoride releasing sealants. *Clin Oral Invest* 3:188, 1999.

68. Gao W, Peng D, Smales RJ, Kip KHK: Comparison of atraumatic restorative treatment and conventional restorative procedures in a hospital clinic: evaluation after 30 months. *Quintessence Int* 34:31, 2003.

69. Garcia-Godoy F, Summitt JB, Donly KJ: Caries progression of white spot lesions sealed with an unfilled resin. *J Clin Pediatr Dent* 21:141, 1997.

70. Gift HC, Frew RA: Sealants: changing patterns. *JADA* 112:391, 1986.

71. Gift HC, Frew RA, Hefferren J: Attitudes toward and use of pit and fissure sealants. *J Dent Child* 42:460, 1975.

72. Gift HC, Newman JF: Oral health activities of US children: results of a national health interview survey. *JADA* 123:96, 1992.

73. Gilchrist JA, Brumley DE, Blackford JU: Community socioeconomic status and 'children's dental health. *JADA* 132:216, 2001.

74. Glasrud PH: Insuring preventive dental care: are sealants included? *Am J Public Health* 75:285, 1985.

75. Glasrud PH, Frazier PJ, Horowitz AM: Insurance reimbursement for sealants in 1986: report of a survey. *J Dent Child* 54:81, 1987.

76. Glasspoole EA, Erickson RL, Davidson CL: Demineralization of enamel in relation to the fluoride release of materials. *Am J Dent* 14:8, 2001.

77. Glasspoole EA, Erickson RL, Davidson CL: Protective effects of resin impregnation on demineralization of enamel. *Am J Dent* 12:315, 1999.

78. Goldstein RE, Parkins FM: Using air-abrasive technology to diagnose and restore pit and fissure caries. *JADA* 126:761, 1995.

79. Gonzalez CD, Frazier PJ, Messer LB: Sealant use by general practitioners: a Minnesota survey. *J Dent Child* 58:38, 1991.

80. Gonzalez CD, Frazier PJ, LeMay W et al: Sealant status and factors associated with sealant presence among children in Milwaukee, WI. *J Dent Child* 62:335, 1995.

81. Graves RC, Burt BA: The pattern of the carious attack in children as a consideration in the use of fissure sealants. *J Prev Dent* 2:28, 1975.

82. Greenwall AL, Johnsen D, DiSantis TA et al: Longitudinal evaluation of caries pattern from the primary to the mixed dentition. *Pediatr Dent* 12:278, 1990.

83. Griffin SO, Griffin PM, Gooch PM, Barker LK: Comparing costs of three sealant delivery strategies. *J Dent Res* 81:641, 2002.

84. Hamid A, Hume WR: Release of estrogenic component bisphenol-A not detected from fissure sealants in vitro. *J Dent Res* 76:321,1997.

85. Handelman SL, Leverett DH, Espeland M et al: Clinical radiographic evaluation of sealed carious and sound tooth surfaces. *JADA* 113:751, 1986.

86. Handelman SL, Leverett DH, Espeland M et al: Retention of sealants over carious and sound tooth surfaces. *Community Dent Oral Epidemiol* 15:1, 1987.

87. Handelman SL, Washburn F, Wopperer P: Two-year report on the sealant effect on bacteria in dental caries. *J Dent Res* 93:967, 1976.

88. Hardison JR, Collier OR, Sprouse CW et al: Retention of pit and fissure sealant on primary molars of 3- and 4-year-old children after 1 year. *JADA* 114:613, 1987.

89. Hassall DC, Mellor AC: An investigation into sealant restoration usage in general dental practice in England. *Br Dent J* 13:388, 2001.

90. Hebling J, Feigal RJ: Use of one-bottle adhesive as an intermediate bonding layer to reduce sealant microleakage on saliva contaminated enamel. *Am J Dent* 13:187, 2000.

91. Hennon DK, Stookey GK, Muhler JC: Prevalence and distribution of dental caries in preschool children. *JADA* 79:1405, 1969.

92. Hicks J, Garcia-Godoy F, Donly K, Flaitz C:

Fluoride-releasing restorative materials and secondary caries. *Dent Clin North Am* 46:247, 2002.

93. Hicks MJ: Preventive resin restorations: etching patterns, resin tag morphology and the enamel-resin interface. *J Dent Child* 51:116, 1984.

94. Hicks MJ: Caries-like lesion formation around occlusal alloy and preventive resin restorations. *Pediatr Dent* 6:17, 1984.

95. Hicks MJ, Flaitz CM: The epidemiology of dental caries in pediatric and adolescent population: a review of past and current trends. *J Clin Pediatr Dent* 18:43, 1993.

96. Hicks MJ, Flaitz CM: Caries-like lesion formation in occlusal fissures: an in vitro study. *Quintessence Int* 17:405, 1986.

97. Hicks MJ, Flaitz CM: Occlusal caries formation in vitro: comparison of resin-modified glass ionomer with fluoride-releasing sealant. *J Clin Pediatr Dent* 24:309, 2000.

98. Hicks MJ, Flaitz CM: Caries formation in vitro around fluoride-releasing pit and fissure sealant in primary teeth. *J Dent Child* 65:161, 1998.

99. Hicks MJ, Flaitz CM, Call RL: Comparison of pit and fissure sealant utilization by pediatric and general dentists in Colorado. *J Pedod* 14:97, 1990.

100. Hicks MJ, Flaitz CM, Garcia-Godoy F: Fluoride-releasing sealant and caries-like enamel lesion formation in vitro. *J Clin Pediatr Dent* 24:215, 2000.

101. Hicks MJ, Flaitz CM, Silverstone LM: The current status of dental caries in the pediatric population. *J Pedod* 10:57, 1985.

102. Hicks MJ, Flaitz CM, Silverstone LM: Secondary caries formation in vitro around glass ionomer restorations. *Quintessence Int* 17:527, 1986.

103. Hicks MJ, Flaitz CM, Westerman GH et al: Caries-like lesion initiation and progression around laser-cured sealants. *Am J Dent* 6:176, 1993.

104. Hicks J, Garcia-Godoy F, Flaitz C: Biologic factors in dental caries: role of remineralization and fluoride in the dynamic process of demineralization and remineralization (part 3). *J Clin Pediatr Dent* 28:203, 2004.

105. Hicks MJ, Silverstone LM: Fissure sealants and dental enamel: a histological study of microleakage in vitro. *Caries Res* 16:353, 1982.

106. Hicks MJ, Silverstone LM: The effect of sealant application and sealant loss on caries-like lesion formation in vitro. *Pediatr Dent* 4:111, 1982.

107. Hicks MJ, Silverstone LM: Acid-etching of caries-like lesions of enamel: a scanning electron microscopic study. *Caries Res* 18:326, 1984.

108. Hicks MJ, Silverstone LM: Acid-etching of caries-like lesions of enamel: a polarized light microscopic study. *Caries Res* 18:315, 1984.

109. Holloway PJ, Clarkson JE: Cost/benefit of prevention in practice. *Int Dent J* 44:317, 1994.

110. Holmgren CJ: ART-ODONT: an electronic network for information concerning minimal intervention techniques for caries. *J Public Health Dent* 56:166, 1996.

111. Holmgren CJ, Lo ECM, Hu DY, Wan HC: ART restorations and sealants placed in Chinese school children: results after three years. *Community Dent Oral Epidemiol* 28:314, 2000.

112. Holmgren CJ, Pilot T: Preliminary research agenda for minimal intervention techniques for caries. *J Public Health Dent* 56:164, 1996.

113. Honkala E, Behbehani J, Ibricevic H et al: The atraumatic restorative treatment (ART) approach to restoring primary teeth in a standard dental clinic. *Int J Pediatr Dent* 13:172, 2003.

114. Horowitz AM: Introduction to the symposium on minimal intervention techniques for caries. *J Public Health Dent* 56:133, 1996.

115. Horowitz HS, Meyers RJ, Heifetz SB et al: Combined fluoride, school-based program in a fluoride-deficient area: results of an 11-year study. *JADA* 112:621, 1986.

116. Hotuman E, Rolling I, Poulsen S: Fissure sealants in a group of 3-4-year-old children. *Int J Pediatr Dent* 1998:8:159.

117. Houpt M, Eidelman E, Shey Z et al: Occlusal restoration using fissure sealant instead of "extension for prevention." *J Dent Child* 51:270, 1984.

118. Houpt M, Eidelman E, Shey Z et al: Occlusal composite restorations: 4-year results. *JADA* 110:351, 1985.

119. Houpt M, Eidelman E, Shey Z et al: The composite/sealant restoration. Five-year results. *J Prosthet Dent* 55:164, 1986.

120. Houpt M, Fuks A, Eidelman E: Measuring the stickiness of pits and fissures in enamel. *Clin Prev Dent* 7:28, 1985.

121. Houpt M, Fuks A, Eidelmann E: The preventive resin (composite resin/sealant) restoration: nine-year results. *Quintessence Int* 28:155, 1994.

122. Houpt M, Fuks A, Eidelman E et al: Composite/sealant restoration: 6-year results. *Pediatr Dent* 10:394, 1988.

123. Hyatt TP: Occlusal fissures: their frequency and danger. How shall they be treated? *Dent Items Interest* 46:493, 1924.

124. IADR Sealant Symposium. *J Dent Res* 70(special issue):266, 1991.

125. Ile YL, Verdonschot EH, Schaeken MJM, 'van't Hof MA: Electrical conductance of fissure enamel in recently erupted molar teeth as related to caries status. *Caries Res* 29:94, 1995.

126. Ismail AI: Reactor paper: minimal intervention techniques for dental caries. *J Public Health Dent* 56:155, 1996.

127. Ismail AI, Gagnon P: A longitudinal evaluation of fissure sealants applied in dental practices. *J Dent Res* 74:1583, 1995.

128. Jensen OE, Billings RJ, Featherstone JD: Clinical

olds: a 6 year longitudinal study. *Caries Res* 37:29, 2003.

192. Pooterman JHG, Weerheijm KL, Groen HG, Kalsbeek H: Clinical and radiographic judgment of occlusal caries in adolescents. *Eur J Oral Sci* 108:93,2000.

193. Powell GL, Kelsey WP, Blankenau RJ et al: The use of an argon laser for polymerization of composite resin. *J Esthet Dent* 1:34, 1989.

194. Pretty OA, Edgar WM, Higham SM: Detection of in vitro demineralization of primary teeth using quantitative light-induced fluorescence (QLF). *Int J Pediatr Dent* 12:158, 2002.

195. Primosch RE, Barr ES: Sealant use and placement techniques among pediatric dentists. *JADA* 132:1442, 2001.

196. Radike AW: Criteria for diagnosis of dental caries. In: *Proceedings of the Conference on the Clinical Testing of Cariostatic Agents.* Held October 14–16, 1968. Chicago, American Dental Association, 1972, pp 87-88.

197. Rawls HR, Zimmerman BF: Fluoride-exchanging resins for caries protection. *Caries Res* 17:32, 1983.

198. Redford DA, Clarkson BH, Jensen ME: The effect of different etching times on sealant bond strength, etch depth and pattern in primary teeth. *Pediatr Dent* 8:11, 1986.

199. Ricketts DNJ, Kidd EAM, Liepins PJ, Wilson RF: Histological validation of electrical resistance measurements in the diagnosis of occlusal caries. *Caries Res* 30:148, 1996.

200. Ripa LW, Leske GS, Forte F: The combined use of pit and fissure sealants and fluoride mouthrinsing in second and third grade children: one-year clinical results. *Pediatr Dent* 8:158, 1986.

201. Ripa LW, Leske GS, Forte F: The combined use of pit and fissure sealants and fluoride mouth rinsing in second and third grade children: final clinical results after two years. *Pediatr Dent* 9:118, 1987.

202. Roberts MW, Shern RJ, Kennedy JB: Evaluation of an autopolymerizing fissure sealant as a vehicle for slow release of fluoride. *Pediatr Dent* 6:145, 1984.

203. Rock WP: The diagnosis of early carious lesions: a review. *J Pediatr Dent* 3:1, 1987.

204. Rock WP, Potts AJC, Marchment MD et al: The visibility of clear and opaque fissure sealants. *Br Dent J* 167:395, 1989.

205. Rohr M, Makinson OF, Burrow MF: Pit and fissures: morphology. *J Dent Child* 58:97, 1991.

206. Romberg E, Cohen LA, LaBelle AD: A national survey of sealant usage by pediatric dentists. *J Dent Child* 55:257, 1988.

207. Romcke RG, Lewis DW, Maze BD et al: Retention and maintenance of fissure sealants over 10 years. *Can Dent J* 56:235, 1990.

208. Rozier RG: Reaction paper. The impact of recent changes in the epidemiology of dental caries on guidelines for the use of dental sealants: epidemiologic perspectives. *J Public Health Dent* 55:292, 1995.

209. Schmalz G, Preiss A, Arenholt-Bindslev D: Bisphenol-A content of resin monomers and related degradation products. *Clin Oral Invest* 3:114, 1999.

210. Seale NS, Casamassimo PS: Access to dental care for children in the United States: a survey of general practitioners. *JADA* 2003:134:1630.

211. Selwitz RH, Colley BJ, Rozier RG: Factors associated with parental acceptance of dental sealants. *J Public Health Dent* 52:137, 1992.

212. Selwitz RH, Nowjack-Raymer R, Driscoll WS et al: Evaluation after 4 years of the combined use of fluoride and dental sealants. *Community Dent Oral Epidemiol* 23:30, 1995.

213. Selwitz RH, Winn DM, Kingman A et al: The prevalence of dental sealants in the US population: findings from NHANES III, 1988–1991. *J Dent Res* 75(special issue):652, 1996.

214. Siegal M: Promotion and use of pit and fissure sealants: an introduction to the special issue. *J Public Health Dent* 55:259, 1995.

215. Siegal MD, Garcia IA, Kandray DP et al: The use of dental sealants by Ohio dentists. *J Public Health Dent* 56:12, 1996.

216. Silverstone LM: The current status of fissure sealants and priorities for future research. Part I. *Comp Cont Educ* 5:204, 1984.

217. Silverstone LM: The current status of fissure sealants and priorities for future research. Part II. *Comp Cont Educ* 5:299, 1984.

218. Silverstone LM: State of the art on sealant research and priorities for the further research. *J Dent Educ* 48:107, 1984.

219. Silverstone LM, Hicks MJ, Featherstone MJ: Oral fluid contamination of etched enamel surfaces: an SEM study. *JADA* 110:329, 1985.

220. Simonsen RJ: Preventive resin restorations (I). *Quintessence Int* 1:69, 1978.

221. Simonsen RJ: Preventive resin restorations (II). *Quintessence Int* 2:95, 1978.

222. Simonsen RJ: The clinical effectiveness of a colored pit and fissure sealant at 36 months. *JADA* 102:323, 1981.

223. Simonsen RJ: Retention and effectiveness of a single application of white sealant after 10 years. *JADA* 115:31, 1987.

224. Simonsen RJ: Cost-effectiveness of pit and fissure sealants at 10 years. *Quintessence Int* 20:75, 1989.

225. Simonsen RJ: Why not prevention? *Quintessence Int* 20:785, 1989.

226. Simonsen RJ: Retention and effectiveness of dental sealants after 15 years. *JADA* 122:34, 1991.

227. Simonsen RJ: Pit and fissure sealants: review of the literature. *Pediatr Dent* 24:393, 2002.

228. Soderholm K-J M: Reactor paper. The impact of recent changes in the epidemiology of dental caries on guidelines for the use of dental sealants: clinical perspectives. *J Public Health Dent* 55:302, 1995.

229. Stahl JW, Katz RV: Occlusal dental caries incidence in college students: Implications for sealants. *J Dent Res* 71(AADR Abstr):250, 1992.

230. Stahl JW, Katz RV: Occlusal dental caries incidence and implications for sealant program in a US college student population. *J Public Health Dent* 53:212, 1993.

231. Sterritt GR, Frew RA, Rozier RG et al: Evaluation of a school-based fluoride mouthrinsing and clinic-based sealant program on a non-fluoridated island. *Community Dent Oral Epidemiol* 18:288, 1994.

232. Stookey GK, Gonzalez-Cabezas C: Emerging methods of caries diagnosis. *J Dent Educ* 65:1001, 2001.

233. Straffon LH, Dennison JB: Clinical evaluation comparing sealant and amalgam after 7 years. Final report. *JADA* 117:751, 1988.

234. Straffon LH, Dennison JB, More FG: Three-year evaluation of sealant: effect of isolation on efficacy. *JADA* 110:714, 1985.

235. Taifur D, Frencken JE, Beiruti N' et al: Effectiveness of glass-ionomer (ART) and amalgam restorations in the deciduous dentition: results after 3 years. *Caries Res* 36:437, 2002.

236. Taifur D, Frencken JE, van't Hof MA et al: Effects of glass ionomer sealants in newly erupted first molars after 5 years: a pilot study. *Community Dent Oral Epidemiol* 31:314, 2003.

237. Tam LE, McComb D: Diagnosis of occlusal caries: Part 2. Recent diagnostic technologies. *J Can Dent Assoc* 67:459, 2001.

238. Tanaka M, Ono H, Kadoma Y et al: Incorporation into human enamel of fluoride slowly released from a sealant in vivo. *J Dent Res* 66:1591, 1987.

239. Tandon S, Kumari R, Udupa S: The effect of etch-time on the bond strength of a sealant and on the etch pattern in primary and permanent enamel: an evaluation. *J Dent Child* 56:186, 1989.

240. Torppa-Saarinen E, Seppa L: Short-term retention of glass-ionomer sealants. *Proc Finn Dent Soc* 86:83, 1990.

241. Traubman A, Silberman SL, Meydrech EF: Dental caries assessment of Mississippi Head Start Program children. *J Public Health Dent* 49:167, 1989.

242. Vargas CM, Crall JJ, Schneider DA: Socioeconomic distribution of pediatric dental caries: NHANES III, 1988–1994. *JADA* 129:1229, 1998.

243. Vehkalahti MM, Solavaara L, Rytomaa I: An eight-year follow-up of the occlusal surfaces of first permanent molars. *J Dent Res* 70:1064, 1991.

244. Verdonschot EH, Rondel P, Huysmans MC: Validity of electrical conductance measurements in evaluating the marginal integrity of sealant restorations. *Caries Res* 29:100, 1995.

245. Vrbic V: Retention of a fluoride-containing sealant on primary and permanent teeth 3 years after placement. *Quintessence Int 30:835, 1999.*

246. Vrbic V: Sealing of primary and permanent teeth with Helioseal F. *J Dent Res* 76(special issue):191 (Abstr 1421), 1997.

247. Vrbic V: Retention of a fluoride-containing sealant on primary and permanent teeth 3 years after placement. *Quintessence Int 30*:825, 1999.

248. Waggoner WF, Siegal M: Pit and fissure sealant application: updating the technique. *JADA* 127:351, 1996.

249. Walker JD, Floyd K, Jakobsen J: The effectiveness of sealants in pediatric patients. *J Dent Child* 63:268, 1996.

250. Walker, JD, Floyd K, Jakobsen J, Pinkham JR: The effectiveness of preventive resin restorations in pediatric patients. *J Dent Child* 63:338, 1996.

251. Walker JD, Jensen ME, Pinkham JR: A clinical review of preventive resin restorations. *J Dent Child* 57:257, 1990.

252. Walls AWG, Wallwork MA, Holland IS et al: The longevity of occlusal amalgam restorations in first permanent molars of child patients. *Br Dent J* 158:133, 1985.

253. Weintraub JA: The effectiveness of pit and fissure sealants. *J Public Health Dent* 49:317, 1989.

254. Weintraub JA: Pit and fissure sealants in high-caries-risk individuals. *J Dent Educ* 65:1084, 2001.

255. Weintraub JA, Stearns SC, Rozier RC, Huang CC: Treatment outcomes and costs of dental sealants among children enrolled in Medicaid. *Am J Public Health* 91:1877, 2001.

256. Wellbury RR, Walls AWG, Murray JJ et al: The management of occlusal caries in permanent molars. A 5-year clinical trial comparing minimal composite with an amalgam restoration. *Br Dent J* 169:361, 1990.

257. Wendt L-K, Koch G, Birkhed D: On the retention and effectiveness of fissure sealants in permanent molars after 15–20 years: a cohort study. *Community Dent Oral Epidemiol* 29:302, 2001.

258. Werner CW, Pereira AC, Eklund SA: Cost-effectiveness study of a school-based sealant program. *J Dent Child* 67:93, 2000.

259. Westerman GH, Ellis RW, Latta MA, Powell GL: An in vitro study of enamel surface microhardness following argon laser irradiation and acidulated phosphate fluoride treatment. *Pediatr Dent* 25:497, 2003.

260. Westerman G, Hicks J, Flaitz C: Argon laser curing of fluoride-releasing pit and fissure sealant: in vitro caries development. *J Dent Child* 67:385, 2000.

the pulp-dentin complex.[38] Therefore, all procedures performed in the dentin will have an effect on the pulp.

## Reactions to Caries and Operative Procedures

The molecular and cellular changes that take place during primary dentinogenesis are mimicked during the dentin-pulp reactions to injury. Several bioactive molecules, particularly the transforming growth factors of the beta family (TGF-β), sequestrated within the dentin matrix during primary dentinogenesis, may be released during processes leading to tissue dissolution, as in dental caries.[87] Therefore, dentin matrix should not be considered as an inert dental hard tissue but rather as a potential tissue store of a cocktail of bioactive molecules (particularly growth factors) waiting to be released, if appropriate tissue conditions prevail.[87]

Kuttler[53] proposed the concept of tertiary dentin formation, encompassing a wide range of responses, from the secretion of a regular, tubular dentin to a very dysplastic atubular dentin. These responses are the result of different cellular and molecular processes, and express reactions to a mild or strong stimulus. Thus, tertiary dentin has been classified as either reactionary or reparative dentin, the former being secreted by surviving postmitotic odontoblasts in response to a mild stimulus, while reparative dentin is secreted by a new generation of odontoblast-like cells differentiated after the death of the original postmitotic odontoblasts.[79] Reparative odontogenesis encompasses a complex sequence of biological events, involving progenitor cell recruitment and differentiation prior to matrix secretion at the site of the injury. In cases of pulp exposure, reparative dentinogenesis can give rise to a dentin bridge formation, restoring the dentin matrix continuum around the pulp.[19]

In addition to the caries process, various factors associated with cavity preparation and restoration can influence the tertiary dentin response. Thus, the method of cavity preparation, the size of the cavity, the residual dentin thickness (RDT), etching of the cavity, the type of restorative material, and the method of application have an effect on the type and quality of the tertiary dentin. Several studies have reported that the pulpal changes related to these various factors are more important than those related to the restorative materials themselves.[18,54,61,62] RDT is apparently the most significant factor determining the secretion of reactionary dentin. Maximal reactionary dentin was observed in a study where the RDT in the cavities was between 0.5 mm and 0.25 mm. The reduced reactionary dentin beneath cavities with an RDT less than 0.25 mm, described in the same study, appeared to be related to reduced odontoblastic survival.[62] In these deep cavities, little more than 50% of the odontoblasts survived, whereas in shallow cavities, odontoblastic survival was about 85% or greater, and despite the cutting of the odontoblastic process, the cells responded by secreting reactionary dentin. The same authors demonstrated that the choice of the restorative material influenced the secretion of reactionary dentin to a lesser extent than the RDT. Of the materials tested, calcium hydroxide had the greatest influence, followed by resin composite, resin-modified glass ionomer, and zinc oxide–eugenol (ZOE) paste.[62]

The condition of the pulp-dentin complex is the main determining factor in treatment planning. Pulp exposures in young permanent teeth can result from caries, from operative procedures, or from traumatic injury. In carious exposures, the pulp and the dentin are infected, whereas in accidental exposures during operative procedures only the dentin may be infected; the pulp may be vital and sometimes not even inflamed. In traumatic pulp exposures the dentin is not infected, and the pulp tissue may remain vital and not infected if treatment is performed immediately after the injury.

To make the most accurate diagnosis of the pulp condition, information must be obtained from several sources, including a detailed medical history, characteristics of the pain, and a thorough clinical and radiographic examination.

## CLINICAL PULPAL DIAGNOSIS

### Patient History

Belanger[4] refers to the importance of assessing the type of pain described by the child, whether it is spontaneous or is precipitated by a stimulus. Spontaneous pain occurs without any external stimulus and frequently indicates that the damage to the pulp is irreversible. Sensitivity to pressure may indicate that the pulpal damage has extended to the periodontal ligament causing extrusion of the tooth from the socket. However, it may also be the result of a much more innocuous situation such as a sealant placed in excess or a high restoration causing hyperocclusion.[4] Children often complain of "toothaches" during the eruption of the first permanent molars. In these cases the dentist should carefully ascertain whether the complaint is due to a pericoronitis or to biting on an operculum, rather than to pain resulting from a pulp condition. Food impaction can also mimic the symptoms of an irreversible pulp condition. In cases of trauma, both patient and parents should be asked about the timing and nature of the injury, and whether previous traumatic incidents have occurred.

## Clinical Examination

As for primary teeth, a careful extraoral and intraoral examination is very important for the detection of a pulpally involved tooth. Redness and swelling of the vestibulum, or teeth with extensive caries with draining sinus tracts, are definitely indicative of pulpal pathoses. Sensitivity to palpation in the vestibule may also be indicative of an acute apical pathologic process. Special attention should be paid to fractured restorations or those with marginal breakdown, as these may also be indicators of pulp involvement.[30]

Heat, cold, and an electric pulp tester are commonly used to test pulp vitality. In young permanent teeth, these tests should be carefully interpreted, as immature teeth may not react to stimulation due to the incomplete development of the innervation system. It is always advisable to compare the results with those of an antimere or with an uninvolved tooth.

Tooth mobility and sensitivity to percussion should also be tested, and compared with the antimeres or other unaffected teeth. Increased mobility in teeth with extensive caries is usually indicative of periodontal ligament involvement.

## Radiographic Examination

Radiography to detect the presence of pulpal and periapical pathoses should follow a careful clinical examination. The interpretation of radiographs of young, immature permanent teeth can be difficult, due to their normally large and open apex. Less experienced dentists treating these teeth should avoid confusing pathologic changes with normal anatomy. Thus, a treatment decision

should not be made based on a single radiograph, and one of the antimeres should be taken for comparison. Other pathologic changes such as internal resorption may occur in permanent teeth but are less common than in primary teeth.

Radiographs of each central incisor should be obtained separately from a distal angulation to prevent overlapping of the periodontal ligament of the central incisor over the lateral incisor. Performing radiography in this manner is mandatory in teeth after traumatic injuries. The degree of root development and apical closure of the affected tooth and the amount of dentin apposition along the canal should be compared with those of the contralateral tooth.

## Direct Pulp Evaluation

In some instances, during the clinical treatment, a final diagnosis can only be reached by direct evaluation of the pulp tissue. The quality (color) and the amount of bleeding from a direct exposure of the pulp tissue must be assessed; profuse bleeding or pus exudate indicates irreversible pulpitis. Based on these observations, the dentist may decide to confirm or change the treatment plan for that particular tooth.

In summary, a clinical pulpal diagnosis must be based on clinical and radiographic findings as well as on knowledge of pulpal reactions. However, it is impossible to determine the histopathologic status of the pulp based on clinical symptoms and tests. Therefore, the accepted clinical classifications refer to pulp disease (pulpitis) as reversible versus irreversible, or treatable versus nontreatable. These classifications indicate whether treatment will aim to conserve pulp vitality or, if the pulp condition is irreversible and nontreatable, whether the choice will be pulpectomy followed by root canal treatment. Teeth diagnosed with reversible or treatable pulpitis will be treated according to the estimated status of the pulp-dentin complex, with treatment ranging from indirect pulp treatment, to direct pulp capping, to partial or cervical pulpotomy, depending on the progress of the inflammatory process within the pulp and the degree of root development. Clinically, the difference between reversible and irreversible pulpitis is frequently determined on the basis of the duration and intensity of the pain sensation. Overshoot to cold stimuli or spontaneous pain will frequently lead to a diagnosis of irreversible or untreatable pulpitis, and these performing direct pulp capping after accidental exposures during cavity preparation or after exposures following excavation of deep caries. His recommendation is to perform direct pulp capping only in fresh traumatic exposures, before bacterial plaque has become established on the exposed pulp. Conversely, Horsted et al.[43] showed an 82% survival rate after 5 years when direct pulp capping with calcium hydroxide was done in asymptomatic teeth exhibiting small incisal or occlusal exposures. Consequently, when direct pulp capping is indicated, it should be performed immediately after the exposure to prevent contamination of the pulp and damage of the cells. Another factor influencing the outcome of this procedure is the size of the exposure: the smaller the diameter, the better the prognosis. Also the characteristic of the pulp capping material is of significant importance: it must be biocompatible, nonresorbable, capable of adhering to the dentin, capable of establishing and maintaining a good seal to prevent bacterial contamination, and capable of promoting pulp repair. Ideally the dentin bridge formed after direct pulp capping should be without tunnel defects that could allow the penetration of bacteria into the pulp at a later stage.[51]

Various materials have been suggested for direct pulp capping; at present, the use of calcium hydroxide is the most frequently recommended. When a paste of calcium hydroxide and water is placed on a pulp wound, it causes superficial liquefaction necrosis. The tissue close to the wound loses its architecture, and coagulation necrosis can be observed beneath it. The coagulated necrotic tissue becomes diffusely calcified, and a hard tissue bridge is subsequently formed.[73,74]

Today the beneficial effect of calcium hydroxide as a capping material is believed to be due to its initial low-grade irritation of the injured pulp, allowing a favorable tissue response followed by dentin bridge formation. Calcium ions are released from the capping material, forming anorganic precipitations that have been associated with the mechanism controlling cytologic and functional changes in the interacting pulpal cells.[85] The high pH and low solubility of calcium hydroxide prolongs its antibacterial effect. However, this material is water soluble and, under leaky restorations, might dissolve and be washed out, leaving an empty space under the filling material. Hard-setting calcium hydroxide cements can induce dentin bridge formation, but they do not provide an effective long-term seal against bacteria or their byproducts.

The use of dentin-bonding agents for direct pulp capping (hybridization) has been recommended by some investigators.[47,48,70] The rationale for this recommendation is that hybridization provides an effective, permanent seal against bacterial invasion, allowing healing to occur. Costa et al.,[16] in a review on pulp capping with dentin adhesive systems, reported that self-etching adhesive systems caused inflammatory reactions, delay in pulpal healing, and failure of dentin bridging in human pulps capped with bonding agents. They stated that vital pulp therapy using acidic agents and adhesive resins seems to be contraindicated. Even if a hard tissue barrier has been formed and no clinical symptoms are present, histologic examination can reveal severe pulpal inflammation or necrosis. As the hard tissue barrier is often incomplete and has tunnel defects, leakage under a filling will bring bacteria in direct contact with the pulp tissue.[19,67]

Recently, a mineral trioxide aggregate, ProRoot MTA (Dentsply, Tulsa Dental, Tulsa, Okla.), was introduced for direct pulp capping. MTA is a biocompatible material with an antibacterial effect similar to that of calcium hydroxide that provides a biologically active substrate for cell attachment. This feature makes this material effective in preventing microleakage and improving the treatment outcome. MTA stimulated pulp healing with dentin bridge formation and minimal inflammatory reaction in exposed pulps in monkeys.[69] Its dentinogenetic effect in short-term capping experiments was demonstrated in dogs.[27] Tziafas[88] demonstrated in dogs that after direct pulp capping the underlying pulp tissue was consistently normal, and only at a later stage was some hemorrhaging in the pulp core observed. After 2 weeks, the beginning of a hard tissue barrier was observed, and reparative dentinogenesis was observed after 3 weeks, associated with a firm fibrodentin matrix. This material seems to be very promising as a direct pulp capping material and was approved for use by the ADA. A preliminary study in human teeth reports better results with MTA than with calcium hydroxide.[1] Long-term clinical studies in humans are underway.

### Direct Pulp Capping Technique

The technique of direct pulp capping with MTA is presented in Figure 33-2. The tooth should be isolated with a rubber dam. After cavity

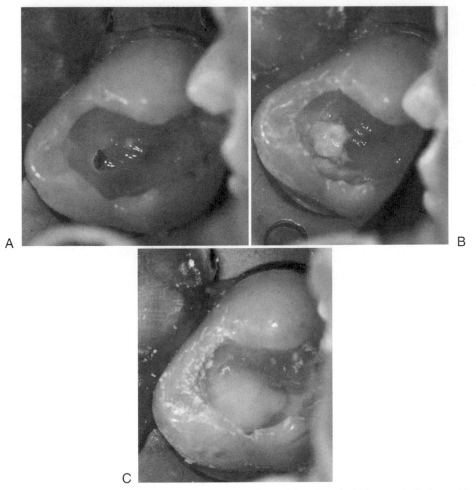

**Figure 33-2  A,** Carious exposure of a maxillary molar after rubber dam isolation and rinsing with sodium hypochlorite. **B,** The exposure site is capped with a mineral trioxide aggregate (MTA) paste. C, Glass ionomer cement (Vitrebond) placed over the MTA. The tooth was restored with a composite resin. (Courtesy Dr. D. Eidlitz.)

preparation with high speed under constant water spray and caries removal with slow speed, the cavity should be rinsed with diluted sodium hypochlorite, which disinfects the cavity and removes the blood clot, if present. If bleeding persists, application of pressure to the exposure site with a cotton pellet moistened with saline will stop it. If bleeding continues, direct pulp capping should not be performed and an alternative treatment should be considered. MTA should be prepared according to the manufacturer's instructions and placed using the carrier provided in the kit. The material should then be covered with a glass ionomer cement followed by a permanent restoration.

## Partial or Cervical Pulpotomy

Although use of direct pulp capping and pulpotomy in cariously exposed pulps in mature teeth

remains a controversial issue, these procedures are universally accepted in teeth with incomplete root formation. The pulpotomy procedure involves removing pulp tissue that has inflammatory or degenerative changes, leaving intact the remaining vital tissue, which is covered with a pulp-capping agent to promote healing at the amputation site.[14,31] The only difference between pulpotomy and pulp capping is that in pulpotomy additional tissue is removed from the exposed pulp. Traditionally, pulpotomy implied the removal of the entire coronal pulp up to the cervical area. Today the depth of tissue removal is based on clinical judgment: only tissue with profuse bleeding, judged to be inflamed or infected, should be removed, as the dressing should be placed on healthy tissue. Although many materials and drugs have been used as capping agents after pulpotomy, calcium hydroxide seems to be

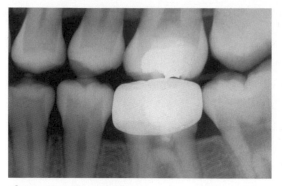

**Figure 33-3** Permanent molar with a carious exposure 2 years after treatment with a calcium hydroxide partial pulpotomy. Notice the dentin bridge. (Courtesy Dr. G. Holan.)

the treatment of choice to stimulate dentin bridge formation in young permanent teeth with exposed pulps[85] (Fig. 33-3). Trope et al.[84] demonstrated hard tissue formation in inflamed dog's teeth treated either with direct pulp capping or partial pulpotomy, both with calcium hydroxide. The authors emphasize that "the combination of a partial pulpotomy, calcium hydroxide and a bacterial-tight coronal restoration represent a viable technique for capping the inflamed pulp."

Recently, MTA has been successfully employed in pulpotomies in several human and animal studies.[23,42]

### Partial Pulpotomy or Cvek Technique

The tooth should be anesthetized and isolated with a rubber dam. If any loosening of the tooth has occurred, the rubber dam clamp must be applied to adjacent uninjured teeth. In traumatically exposed pulps, only tissue judged to be inflamed should be removed. Cvek has shown that, in exposures resulting from traumatic injuries, pulpal changes are characterized by a proliferative response, with inflammation extending only a few millimeters into the pulp.[21] When the hyperplastic tissue is removed, healthy pulp is found. Care should be taken to remove all the tissue coronal to the amputation site to prevent continuation of bleeding, contamination, and discoloration of the tooth. In teeth with carious exposure, it might be necessary to remove tissue to a greater depth in order to reach noninflamed pulp. Cutting of the tissue with an abrasive diamond bur, using high speed with water cooling, has been shown to be the least damaging to the underlying tissue.[36] Replacing the diamond

by a carbide #330 bur with high speed appeared to have similar results.[8] After pulp amputation, the preparation is thoroughly washed with saline and dried with cotton pellets.

Hemorrhage is controlled with cotton pellets slightly moistened with saline; the use of dry cotton pellets carries the risk of fibers being incorporated into the clot and causing hemorrhage during clot removal. Cox et al.[20] recommend the use of sodium hydrochloride (NaOCl) to control hemorrhage. They claim that this agent, in addition to promoting hemostasis, also kills bacteria. If hemorrhage persists, amputation should be performed at a more apical level, using a small endodontic spoon or a round diamond bur.[14] When this occurs in posterior teeth, it might be necessary to remove the tissue in the canal with reamers or files. Once hemorrhage has been controlled and the blood clot removed, a dressing of calcium hydroxide is gently placed over the amputation site. Care should be taken not to push the material into the pulp as it might cause inflammation, increasing the potential for failure of the procedure; on the other hand, if the pulpotomy is successful, such material in the pulp may create a tendency for calcific obliteration of the pulp. A creamy mix of zinc oxide and eugenol or other cement is flowed over the calcium hydroxide and allowed to set. When a composite is used, eugenol compounds must be avoided, as these cements interfere with the setting reactions of the composite. In these cases, a second layer of glass ionomer is placed. Unless a crown is necessary, amalgam is still the preferred material for posterior teeth, whereas aesthetic composite restorations are the treatment of choice for anterior teeth. Recently MTA has been utilized to replace the calcium hydroxide in pulpotomy procedures (Fig. 33-4).

### Cervical Pulpotomy

Pulpotomy in mature teeth is performed only when irreversible pulpitis is diagnosed, and it should be considered as an emergency treatment. In these teeth, root canal treatment will follow at the next appointment. In immature permanent teeth, pulpotomy is performed in molars to allow completion of root development; it may be regarded as an apexogenesis procedure. Pulpotomy is performed in teeth in which it is assumed that healthy pulp tissue, with a potential to produce a dentin bridge and complete the formation of the

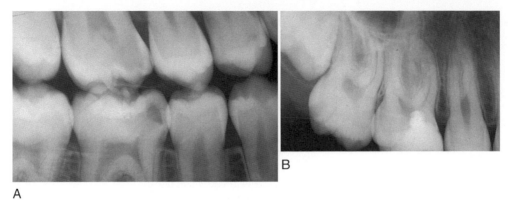

**Figure 33-4  A,** Maxillary molar with extensive caries treated with mineral trioxide aggregate deep partial pulpotomy. **B,** The same tooth 10 months later. No symptoms are present, and no pathologic process is evident in the radiograph. (Courtesy Dr. N. Jabarin.)

root, remains in the root canal. The technique for cervical pulpotomy in permanent teeth is similar to that for primary teeth, and the dressing material should maintain pulp vitality and function. Care should be taken to remove the blood clot prior to placement of a calcium hydroxide paste over the pulp stumps, as its presence may compromise the treatment outcome. It has been demonstrated that leaving the blood clot may result in the formation of dystrophic calcifications and internal resorption. A blood clot may also interfere with dentin bridge formation and serve as a substrate for bacteria in leaky restorations.[73] MTA seems to be an appropriate material for capping, with the main drawback being that it is impossible to remove from the canal after setting. Pulpotomy is frequently performed in teeth in which the histopathologic condition of the pulp stumps is not clear; often the symptoms continue and pulpectomy is needed. As MTA sets in about 4 hours and removing it to gain access to the root canal will be impossible, this material is not recommended for pulpotomies in these teeth. In the last few years, successful reports of pulpotomy using MTA in primary teeth have appeared in the literature.[23]

A dentin bridge may form under the calcium hydroxide dressing, indicating that the pulp tissue is normal with a dentinogenic potential, allowing further root development. Sometimes the calcium hydroxide dressing may form dystrophic calcifications, rendering the root canal difficult to negotiate if endodontic treatment becomes necessary. Clinical and radiographic follow-up of these teeth is essential to ensure that pulpal or periapical pathosis is not developing. It is of utmost impor-

tance to perform a permanent restoration as soon as possible to prevent bacterial leakage and ensure the success of the treatment.[41]

### Apexogenesis

Apexogenesis is done in immature teeth when part of the pulp tissue remains vital and uninflamed, as in carious exposures or in some trauma situations in which pulp exposure occurred and treatment was delayed. This procedure allows continuation of root formation apically to the calcium hydroxide. The root formed usually is irregular but nevertheless provides additional support for the tooth. Apexogenesis can be regarded as a very deep pulpotomy. Calcium hydroxide is placed over the vital pulp stump after hemostasis but before the formation of a blood clot (Fig. 33-5). It is difficult to determine the status of the pulp deep in the root canal or to predict the formation of a calcified barrier. Radiographic and clinical follow-up is mandatory, and if a barrier is not observed, apexification should follow.

## TREATMENT OF NONVITAL TEETH WITH EXPOSED PULPS: IMMATURE TEETH

### Apexification

Apexification is a method of treatment for immature permanent teeth in which root growth and development ceased due to pulp necrosis. Its purpose is to allow the formation of an apical barrier. Apexification is most often performed in incisors that lost vitality after a traumatic injury.

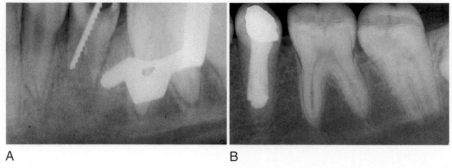

A          B

**Figure 33-5** **A,** Mandibular premolar with incomplete root development due to partial pulp necrosis. Apexogenesis with calcium hydroxide was instituted. **B,** Two years later apical closure was evident in the radiograph. Root canal treatment was completed using gutta-percha with a root canal sealant. (Courtesy Dr. E. Galon.)

It may also be indicated in nonvital immature teeth after carious exposures, and in certain anatomic variations such as dens invaginatus.

The apex in immature teeth may present in two variations: divergent and flaring apical foramen (blunderbuss apex) or parallel to convergent. In both forms conventional endodontic treatment cannot be performed, as it is difficult if not impossible to achieve an apical seal that will prevent extrusion of the filling materials.

This procedure may also be carried out in teeth with radiographic signs of rarifying osteitis. During apexification, healing of the bone will gradually be observed. Before deciding on this mode of treatment, a correct diagnosis should be determined based on clinical and radiographic assessment.

Medical and tooth history should be carefully documented. The teeth in both arches should be inspected for the presence of crown craze lines, fracture, or discoloration. Transillumination may reveal signs of pulp hemorrhage. Periodontal examination including pocket measurement should be done; a localized deep pocket may be pathognomonic of root fracture. If a sinus tract is observed, it should be traced using a gutta-percha point.

When a diagnosis of irreversible pulpitis, pulp necrosis, or acute or chronic apical periodontitis has been established, treatment should be planned. The most important consideration is whether the tooth can be restored to function and aesthetics. The apexification procedure can be done in young patients with short roots. However, because of the long duration of the treatment, patients' and parents' compliance is required. Apexification is a predictable procedure, and an apical barrier will be formed in 74% to 100% of cases.[75] The most common complication is cer-

vical crown or root fracture because the cervical portion of the tooth is very thin and may fracture easily.[22]

Apexification is traditionally performed using a calcium hydroxide dressing that disinfects the root canal and induces apical closure. The high pH and low solubility of calcium hydroxide keeps its antimicrobial effect for a long period.[28] Siqueira and Lopes discussed the mechanisms of its antimicrobial activity in detail.[76] Calcium hydroxide assists in the debridement of the root canal, as it increases the dissolution of necrotic tissue when used alone or in combination with sodium hypochlorite.[37] Apexification requires multiple visits and could take a year or more[52] to achieve a complete apical barrier that would allow root canal filling using gutta-percha and sealer. The time needed for apexification depends on the stage of root development and the status of the periapical tissue.

### Apexification Technique
Coronal access should be wide enough to include the pulp horns to prevent future contamination and discoloration. Gates-Glidden drills are used to remove the lingual eminence in the cervical portion of the root canal, facilitating instrumentation of all aspects of the canal. Debridement of the root canal, including irrigations with disinfecting solutions like 0.5% to 2.5% NaOCl or 0.2% chlorhexidine solution followed by sterile saline solution, should be done without pressure, verifying that the needle is loose inside the root canal. Minimal instrumentation is advised to prevent damage to the thin dentin walls. A calcium hydroxide dressing in a paste consistency can be then applied with a lentulo spiral mounted in a low-speed engine, with specially designed syringes

or with files followed by condensation with endodontic pluggers. If rotary instruments are used, care should be taken to prevent instrument breakage. The second appointment should be from 2 weeks to a month later. The aim of this visit is to complete the debridement and remove the tissue remnants denatured by the calcium hydroxide dressing that could not be removed mechanically in the first appointment. The length of the root canal should be determined radiographically, as electronic apex locators are not reliable in teeth with open apices.[45] At the second visit, a thick paste of calcium hydroxide will be packed in the root canal using endodontic pluggers.[59]

The tooth is monitored clinically and radiographically at 3-month intervals. When a calcified barrier can be seen in the radiograph, the tooth is reopened and biomechanically cleaned by NaOCl irrigation. The apical area should be examined using a file to the working length in order to determine the completeness of the apical barrier. If the barrier is incomplete and the patient feels the touch of the file, the apexification procedure is reestablished until a complete barrier is formed. The frequency with which the calcium hydroxide dressing should be changed is controversial. Some authors believe that frequent replacements can increase the speed of barrier detection but do not appear to affect its position.[50] Chosack et al.[15] demonstrated that changing the calcium hydroxide dressing did not enhance either the speed or the quality of the apical barrier in monkeys. Figure 33-6 shows an immature maxillary central incisor with a necrotic pulp and a sinus tract treated with calcium hydroxide apexification. The bone lesion healed, and the endodontic treatment was properly completed.

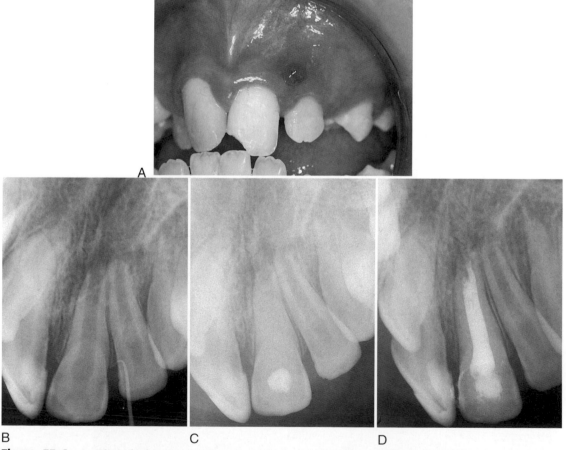

**Figure 33-6** **A,** Clinical photograph of a traumatized central incisor with pulp necrosis and a sinus tract. **B,** Radiograph of the same tooth showing an incompletely formed root, an open apex, and periapical bone destruction. **C,** Radiograph of the tooth filled with a calcium hydroxide paste to achieve apexification. **D,** Radiograph of the tooth after root canal treatment with gutta-percha and sealer. (Courtesy Dr. M. Solomonov.)

When a calcified barrier is formed coronal to the apex, it should not be perforated in order to fill the tooth to the apical end; the tissue forming the apical barrier should be regarded as healthy tissue. It has been reported that calcium hydroxide may significantly increase the risk of root fracture after long-term application. Therefore, in order to reduce this risk in immature teeth, it is advisable to minimize the time needed for apexification.[3]

Recently, it has been suggested that the process of apexification will be replaced by use of an MTA seal. MTA was introduced to function as the apical barrier, reducing the time needed for completion of the treatment and for restoration of the tooth. The treatment may be completed in just a few visits.[33]

After completion of the biomechanical cleaning of the root canal, MTA can be placed at the apical portion of the immature root and will act as an apical plug after setting. MTA cannot be removed from within the canal after it sets; retreatment, if necessary, can be done only by apical surgery. Therefore, complete debridement and disinfection of the root canal and of the dentin walls is mandatory. The MTA apical seal has a number of advantages: less patient compliance is required; the dentin will not lose its physical properties; and the material allows for earlier restoration of the tooth, thus minimizing the likelihood of root fracture.[3]

Placement of MTA at the apex is more complicated than the use of calcium hydroxide. After mixing according to the manufacturer's indications, the material is placed at the apical area, as determined by the radiograph, using special carriers or endodontic pluggers. The MTA is covered by a wet cotton pellet, and the tooth is sealed with a temporary filling (Fig. 33-7). After a few days, the root canal filling can be completed and the tooth can be restored with a composite resin and resin-reinforced fiberglass Luscent Anchors post (Dentatus, New York, N.Y.) (Fig. 33-8). It can also be done with the help of a Luminex post (Dentatus) to ensure the polymerization of the resin inside the canal.[40]

It was demonstrated that the resistance to fracture of immature teeth could be increased by using resin modified glass ionomer inside the root canal.[34]

## TREATMENT OF *NONVITAL* TEETH (EXPOSED AND NONEXPOSED PULPS): MATURE TEETH

### Root Canal Treatment in Young Mature Permanent Teeth

#### Special Considerations

Root canal treatment in mature teeth of children and adolescents is basically similar to that performed in adults. However, due to their wider canals and thinner dentin walls in comparison with those of adult patients, special precautions are needed, as described below:

#### Access

During opening of the access cavity with Gates-Glidden burs, care should be taken to remove only a minimal amount of dentin. Removing too much

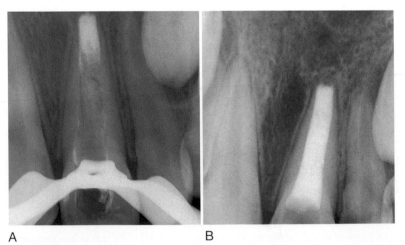

A                                    B

**Figure 33-7** **A,** Central incisor showing an apical seal with mineral trioxide aggregate (MTA). **B,** Root canal treatment completed with gutta-percha and sealer condensed against the MTA plug. (Courtesy Dr. T. Shimko.)

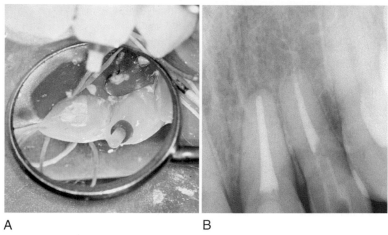

**Figure 33-8**  **A,** Root-treated central incisor reinforced with a Luscent post and composite resin to prevent fracture of the tooth. **B,** Control radiograph of the tooth reinforced with the Luscent post. (Courtesy Dr. R. Maor.)

dentin will weaken the tooth and may cause perforation, particularly on the furcation side.

### Instrumentation

The length of the root canal should be determined carefully using radiographs; an apex locator can also be used. Though the root canals are larger, they may be curved, so instrumentation should be done with precurved instruments in anticurvature filing motions. The use of nickel titanium (NiTi) rotary instruments will ease instrumentation.

### Irrigation

Irrigation during root canal treatment should be done only after making sure that the rubber dam is placed properly, and that leakage of fluids into the mouth cannot occur accidentally. The needle of the irrigation syringe is placed loosely in the root canal to avoid pushing the irrigation solution beyond the apex. Sodium hypochlorite is used in various concentrations (0.5% to 5.25%); low concentrations are preferable in young patients to prevent tissue damage in case of extrusion of the solution beyond the apical foramen. Chlorhexidine 0.2% to 0.5% can also serve as an irrigating solution and may be used in conjunction with 3% hydrogen peroxide.[39] However, it should not be used in combination with sodium hypochlorite, as dark sediments will form.

### Intracanal Dressing

When the initial diagnosis is chronic apical periodontitis, it is recommended that treatment be done in two sessions, with placement of an antiseptic dressing between visits. Calcium hydroxide paste is the preferred dressing material.[77,78] In recent experiments, a mixture of calcium hydroxide and 2% chlorhexidine gel proved to be more bactericidal than calcium hydroxide alone.[25,35] This combination is effective against *Enterococcus faecalis,* which is the microorganism most commonly isolated from failed endodontic treatments.[55,68] The placement of the dressing can be done using a lentulo spiral shorter than the length of the root canal, or using specially designed syringes or files.

### The Isthmus

The isthmus is a narrow connection between fused root canals that contains pulp tissue. Any root containing two canals has a high incidence of isthmuses,[83] and their number varies between 4.9% and 52%. The location is most frequently between midroot and the apex; partial isthmuses can be observed. An isthmus is formed when a root projection cannot close itself, and it will be larger in children where root formation is not fully complete. This web-like connection between root canals is part of the root canal system. It can function as a reservoir for bacteria and therefore should be cleaned and obturated during root canal treatment.[49]

### Obturation

The apex in young teeth is large, and adaptation of a master cone should be done carefully to avoid extrusion of filling materials that can easily occur during condensation. Obturation will require more accessory gutta-percha points; initial points should be placed such that they will not block access to the canal. Filling with warm gutta-percha or use of warm condensation techniques should be done cautiously to avoid overfilling.

# REFERENCES

1. Aeinehchi M, Eslami B, Ghanbariha M et al: Mineral trioxide aggregate (MTA) and calcium hydroxide as pulp-capping agents in human teeth: a preliminary report. *Int Endod J* 36:225, 2003.
2. American Academy of Pediatric Dentistry: Reference manual. Guideline for pulp therapy for primary and young permanent teeth. *Pediatr Dent* 24:86, 2002-2003.
3. Andreasen JO, Farik B, Munksgaard EC: Long-term calcium hydroxide as a root canal dressing may increase risk of root fracture. *Dent Traumatol* 18:134, 2002.
4. Belanger GK: Pulp therapy for young permanent teeth. In: Pinkham JR, editor. *Pediatric Dentistry: Infancy Through Adolescence.* Philadelphia, Saunders, 1999.
5. Bergenholtz G: Effect of bacterial products on inflammatory reactions in the dental pulp. *Scand J Dent Res* 85:122, 1977.
6. Bergenholtz G: Inflammatory response of the dental pulp to bacterial irritation. *J Endod* 7:100, 1981.
7. Bergenholtz G, Cox CF, Loesche WJ et al: Bacterial leakage around dental restorations: its effect on the dental pulp. *J Oral Pathol* 11:439,1982.
8. Bimstein E, Chen S, Fuks AB: Histologic evaluation of the effect of different cutting techniques on pulpotomized teeth. *Am J Dent* 2:151, 1989.
9. Bjorndal L, Larsen T, Thylstrup A: A clinical and microbiological study of deep carious lesions during stepwise excavation using long treatment intervals. *Caries Res* 31:411, 1997.
10. Bjorndal L, Thylstrup A: A practice-based study on stepwise excavation of deep carious lesions in permanent teeth: a 1-year follow-up study. *Community Dent Oral Epidemiol* 26:122, 1998.
11. Brannstrom M: Communication between the oral cavity and the dental pulp associated with restorative treatment. *Oper Dent* 9:57, 1984.
12. Browne RM, Tobias RS, Crombie IK et al: Bacterial microleakage and pulpal inflammation in experimental cavities. *Int Endod J* 16:147, 1983.
13. Camp JH: Pulp therapy for primary and young permanent teeth. *Dent Clin North Am* 28:651, 1984.
14. Camp JH: Pediatric endodontics: endodontic treatment for the primary and young permanent dentition. In: Cohen S, Burns RC, editors. *Pathways of the Pulp.* St Louis, Mosby, 2002.
15. Chosack A, Sela J, Cleaton-Jones P: A histological and quantitative histomorphometric study of apexification of nonvital permanent incisors of vervet monkeys after repeated root filling with a calcium hydroxide paste. *Endod Dent Traumatol* 13:211, 1997.
16. Costa CA, Hebling J, Hanks CT: Current status of pulp capping with dentin adhesive systems: a review. *Dent Mater* 16:188, 2000.
17. Cox CF, Keall CL, Keall HJ et al: Biocompatibility of surface-sealed dental materials against exposed pulps. *J Prosthet Dent* 57:1, 1987.
18. Cox CF, White KC, Ramus DL et al: Reparative dentin: factors affecting its deposition. *Quintessence Int* 23:257, 1992.
19. Cox CF, Subay RK, Ostro E et al: Tunnel defects in dentin bridges: their formation following direct pulp capping. *Oper Dent* 21:4, 1996.
20. Cox CF, Hafez AA, Akimoto N: Biocompatibility of primer, adhesive and resin composite systems on non-exposed and exposed pulps of non-human primate teeth. *Am J Dent* 11:S55, 1998.
21. Cvek M: A clinical report on partial pulpotomy and capping with calcium hydroxide in permanent incisors with complicated crown fracture. *J Endod* 4:232, 1978.
22. Cvek M: Prognosis of luxated non-vital maxillary incisors treated with calcium hydroxide and filled with gutta-percha. A retrospective clinical study. *Endod Dent Traumatol* 8:45, 1992.
23. Eidelman E, Holan G, Fuks AB: Mineral trioxide aggregate vs. formocresol in pulpotomized primary molars: a preliminary report. *Pediatr Dent* 23:15, 2001.
24. Ericson D, Zimmerman M, Raber H et al: Clinical evaluation of efficacy and safety of a new method for chemo-mechanical removal of caries: a multi-centre study. *Caries Res* 33:171, 1999.
25. Evans MD, Baumgartner JC, Khemaleelakul SU et al: Efficacy of calcium hydroxide: chlorhexidine paste as an intracanal medication in bovine dentin. *J Endod* 29:338, 2003.
26. Falster CA, Araujo FB, Straffon LH et al: Indirect pulp treatment: in vivo outcomes of an adhesive resin system vs calcium hydroxide for protection of the dentin-pulp complex. *Pediatr Dent* 24:241, 2002.
27. Faraco IM Jr, Holland R: Response of the pulp of dogs to capping with mineral trioxide aggregate or a calcium hydroxide cement. *Dent Traumatol* 17:163, 2001.
28. Fava LR, Saunders WP: Calcium hydroxide pastes: classification and clinical indications. *Int Endod J* 32:257, 1999.
29. Fitzgerald M, Heys RJ: A clinical and histological evaluation of conservative pulpal therapy in human teeth. *Oper Dent* 16:101, 1991.
30. Fuks AB: Pulp therapy for the primary dentition. In: Pinkham JR, editor. *Pediatric Dentistry,* 3rd ed. Philadelphia, Saunders, 1999.

31. Fuks AB: Pulp therapy for the primary and young permanent dentitions. *Dent Clin North Am* 44:571, 2000.

32. Fuks AB: Current concepts in vital primary pulp therapy. *Eur J Paediatr Dent* 3:115, 2002.

33. Giuliani V, Baccetti T, Pace R et al: The use of MTA in teeth with necrotic pulps and open apices. *Dent Traumatol* 18:217, 2002.

34. Goldberg F, Kaplan A, Roitman M et al: Reinforcing effect of a resin glass ionomer in the restoration of immature roots in vitro. *Dent Traumatol* 18:70, 2002.

35. Gomes BP, Souza SF, Ferraz CC et al: Effectiveness of 2% chlorhexidine gel and calcium hydroxide against *Enterococcus faecalis* in bovine root dentine in vitro. *Int Endod J* 36:267, 2003.

36. Granath LE, Hagman G: Experimental pulpotomy in human bicuspids with reference to cutting technique. *Acta Odontol Scand* 29:155, 1971.

37. Hasselgren G, Olsson B, Cvek M:. Effects of calcium hydroxide and sodium hypochlorite on the dissolution of necrotic porcine muscle tissue. *J Endod* 14:125, 1988.

38. Hasselgren G: Treatment of the exposed dentin-pulp complex. In: Orstavik D, Pitt Ford TR, editors. *Essential Endodontology.* London, Blackwell, 1998.

39. Heling I, Chandler NP: Antimicrobial effect of irrigant combinations within dentinal tubules. *Int Endod J* 31:8, 1998.

40. Heling I, Lustmann J, Hover R et al: Complications of apexification resulting from poor patient compliance: report of case. *J Dent Child* 66:415, 1999.

41. Heling I, Gorfil C, Slutzky H et al: Endodontic failure caused by inadequate restorative procedures: review and treatment recommendations. *J Prosthet Dent* 87:674, 2002.

42. Holland R, de Souza V, Murata SS et al: Healing process of dog dental pulp after pulpotomy and pulp covering with mineral trioxide aggregate or Portland cement. *Braz Dent J* 12:109, 2001.

43. Horsted P, Sandergaard B, Thylstrup A et al: A retrospective study of direct pulp capping with calcium hydroxide compounds. *Endod Dent Traumatol* 1:29, 1985.

44. Hu CC, Zhang C, Qian Q et al: Reparative dentin formation in rat molars after direct pulp capping with growth factors. *J Endod* 24:744, 1998.

45. Hulsmann M, Pieper K: Use of an electronic apex locator in the treatment of teeth with incomplete root formation. *Endod Dent Traumatol* 5:238,1989

46. Hutchins DW, Parker WA: Indirect pulp capping: clinical evaluation using polymethyl methacrylate reinforced zinc oxide-eugenol cement. *J Dent Child* 39:55, 1972.

47. Kashiwada T, Takagi M: New restoration and direct pulp capping systems using adhesive composite resin. *Bull Tokyo Med Dent Univ* 38:45, 1991.

48. Kanca J III: Replacement of a fractured incisor fragment over pulpal exposure: a case report. *Quintessence Int* 24:81,1993

49. Kim S, Pecora G, Rubinstein RA: The resected root surface and isthmus. In: *Color Atlas of Microsurgery in Endodontics.* Philadelphia, Saunders, 2001.

50. Kinirons MJ, Srinivasan V, Welbury RR et al: A study in two centres of variations in the time of apical barrier detection and barrier position in nonvital immature permanent incisors. *Int J Paediatr Dent* 11:447, 2001.

51. Kitasako Y, Murray PE, Tagami J et al: Histo-morphometric analysis of dentinal bridge formation and pulpal inflammation. *Quintessence Int* 33:600, 2002.

52. Kleier DJ, Barr ES: A study of endodontically apexified teeth. *Endod Dent Traumatol* 7:112, 1991.

53. Kuttler Y: Classification of dentin into primary, secondary and tertiary. *Oral Surg* 12:996, 1959.

54. Lee SJ, Walton RE, Osborne JW: Pulp response to bases and cavity depths. *Am J Dent* 5:64, 1992.

55. Love RM: *Enterococcus faecalis:* a mechanism for its role in endodontic failure. *Int Endod* 34:399, 2001.

56. Massler M, Pawlak J: The affected and infected pulp. *Oral Surg Oral Med Oral Pathol* 43:929, 1977.

57. McDonald RE, Avery DR: Treatment of deep caries, vital pulp exposure, and pulpless teeth. In: McDonald RE, Avery DR, editors. *Dentistry for the Child and Adolescent.* Philadelphia, Saunders, 1994.

58. Mertz-Fairhurst EJ, Adair SM, Sams DR et al: Cariostatic and ultraconservative sealed restorations: nine-year results among children and adults. *J Dent Child* 62:97, 1995.

59. Metzger Z, Solomonov M, Mass E: Calcium hydroxide retention in wide root canals with flaring apices. *Dent Traumatol* 17:86, 2001.

60. Mjor AI, Heyeraas KJ: Pulp-dentin and periodontal anatomy and physiology. In: Orstavik D, Pitt Ford TR, editors. *Essential Endodontology.* London, Blackwell, 1998.

61. Murray PE, About I, Lumley PJ et al: Postoperative pulpal and repair responses. *JADA* 131:321, 2000.

62. Murray PE, About I, Lumley PJ et al: Cavity remaining dentin thickness and pulpal activity. *Am J Dent* 15:41, 2002.

63. Nakamura Y, Hammarstrom L, Lundberg E et al: Enamel matrix derivative promotes reparative processes in the dental pulp. *Adv Dent Res* 15:105, 2001.

64. Nakamura Y, Hammarstrom L, Matsumoto K et al: The induction of reparative dentine by enamel proteins. *Int Endod J* 35:407, 2002.

65. Nakashima M: Induction of dentine in amputated pulp of dogs by recombinant human bone morphogenetic proteins-2 and -4 with collagen matrix. *Arch Oral Biol* 39:1085, 1994.

66. Nirschl RF, Avery DR: Evaluation of a new pulp

capping agent in indirect pulp therapy. *J Dent Child* 50:25, 1983.

67. Nyborg H: Healing processes in the pulp on capping. *Acta Odontol Scand* 32:61, 1955

68. Pinheiro ET, Gomes BP, Ferraz CC et al: Microorganisms from canals of root-filled teeth with periapical lesions. *Int Endod J* 36:1, 2003.

69. Pitt Ford TR, Torabinejad M, Abedi HR et al: Using mineral trioxide aggregate as a pulp-capping material. *JADA* 127:1491, 1996.

70. Prager M: Pulp capping with the total-etch technique. *Dent Econ* 84:78, 1994.

71. Rutherford RB, Wahle J, Tucker M et al: Induction of reparative dentine formation in monkeys by recombinant human osteogenic protein-1. *Arch Oral Biol* 38:571, 1993.

72. Rutherford RB, Spangberg L, Tucker M et al: The time-course of the induction of reparative dentine formation in monkeys by recombinant human osteogenic protein-1. *Arch Oral Biol* 39:833, 1994.

73. Schroder U: Effect of an extra-pulpal blood clot on healing following experimental pulpotomy and capping with calcium hydroxide. *Odontol Rev* 24:257, 1973.

74. Schroder U: A 2-year follow-up of primary molars, pulpotomized with a gentle technique and capped with calcium hydroxide. *Scand J Dent Res* 86:273, 1978.

75. Sheehy EC, Roberts GJ: Use of calcium hydroxide for apical barrier formation and healing in non-vital immature permanent teeth: a review. *Braz Dent J* 11:183, 1997.

76. Siqueira JF Jr, Lopes HP: Mechanisms of antimicrobial activity of calcium hydroxide: a critical review. *Int Endod J* 32:361, 1999.

77. Sjogren U, Figdor D, Spangberg L et al: The antimicrobial effect of calcium hydroxide as a short-term intracanal dressing. *Int Endod J* 24:119, 1991.

78. Sjogren U, Figdor D, Persson S et al: Influence of infection at the time of root filling on the outcome of endodontic treatment of teeth with apical periodontitis. *Int Endod J* 30:297, 1997.

79. Smith AJ: Dentin formation and repair. In: Hargreaves KM, Goodis HE, editors. *Seltzer and Bender's Dental Pulp II.* Carol Stream, IL, Quintessence, 2002.

80. Smith AJ, Smith G: Solubilization of TGFb1 by dentine conditioning agents. *J Dent Res* 77:1034 (Abstr 3224), 1998.

81. Stanley HR: Pulpal responses to ionomer cements: biological characteristics. *JADA* 120:25, 1990.

82. Straffon LH, Corpron RL, Bruner FW et al: Twenty-four-month clinical trial of visible-light-activated cavity liner in young permanent teeth. *J Dent Child* 58:124, 1991.

83. Teixeira FB, Sano CL, Gomes BP et al: A preliminary in vitro study of the incidence and position of the root canal isthmus in maxillary and mandibular first molars. *Int Endod J* 36:276, 2003.

84. Trope M, McDougal R, Levin L et al: Capping the inflamed pulp under different clinical conditions. *J Esthet Restor Dent* 14:349, 2002.

85. Tziafas D: Basic mechanisms of cytodifferentiation and dentinogenesis during dental pulp repair. *J Dev Biol* 39:281, 1995.

86. Tziafas D, Alvanou A, Papadimitriou S et al: Effects of recombinant basic fibroblast growth factor, insulin-like growth factor-II and transforming growth factor-beta 1 on dog dental pulp cells in vivo. *Arch Oral Biol* 43:431, 1998.

87. Tziafas D, Smith AJ, Lesot H: Designing new treatment strategies in vital pulp therapy. *J Dent* 28:77, 2000.

88. Tziafas D, Pantelidou O, Alvanou A et al: The dentinogenic effect of mineral trioxide aggregate (MTA) in short-term capping experiments. *Int Endod J* 35:245, 2002.

89. Warfvinge J, Dahlen G, Bergenholtz G: Dental pulp response to bacterial cell wall material. *J Dent Res* 64:1046, 1985.

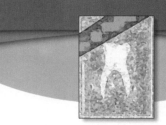

# CHAPTER 34

# Managing Traumatic Injuries in the Young Permanent Dentition

*Dennis J. McTigue*

Injuries to the primary dentition are discussed in Chapter 15. Also covered there are the following fundamental areas relevant to managing trauma in children of any age:

1. Classification of traumatic injuries to teeth
2. Medical and dental history
3. Clinical and radiographic examinations
4. Common reactions of teeth to trauma

This chapter deals with injuries to the young permanent dentition, but the reader is strongly advised to review the fundamental areas just noted in Chapter 15. Frequent reference will be made to them.

## ETIOLOGY AND EPIDEMIOLOGY OF TRAUMA IN THE YOUNG PERMANENT DENTITION

Falls during play account for most injuries to young permanent teeth. Children engaging in contact sports are at greatest risk for dental injury, though the use of mouth guards greatly reduces their frequency (see Chapter 40). In the teenage years, automobile accidents cause a significant number of dental injuries when occupants not wearing seat belts hit the steering wheel or dashboard. As noted in Chapter 15, children with seizure disorders also injure their permanent teeth more frequently. In contrast to the primary dentition, permanent teeth suffer crown fractures more frequently than luxation injuries. The lower

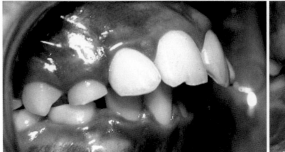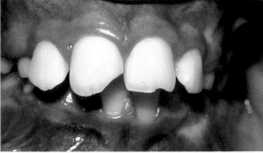

**Figure 34-1** **A,** Lateral view showing large horizontal overjet. **B,** Same patient with fractured central incisors. (From McTigue DJ: Management of orofacial trauma in children. Pediatr Ann 14:125, 1985.)

crown-to-root ratio and denser alveolar bone in the permanent dentition contribute to this phenomenon. Maxillary central incisors are again most commonly injured, and protruding incisors are at greatest risk[24] (Fig. 34-1).

## CLASSIFICATION OF INJURIES TO YOUNG PERMANENT TEETH

Classification of tooth fractures and luxation injuries is discussed in Chapter 15. Refer to Figure 15-1.

## HISTORY

The essential elements of the medical and dental history are discussed in Chapter 15. The use of a trauma assessment form to help organize the gathering of historical and clinical data is emphasized (see Fig. 15-8). The reader is reminded to determine the status of the child's tetanus prophylaxis and to consult the child's physician if there is any question about its adequacy.

Another issue worthy of review relates to the potential for injury to the central nervous system. Older children are likely to suffer harder blows at play, and thus the dentist should find out if the child lost consciousness or became disoriented or nauseated after the injury. Positive findings indicate immediate medical consultation. As noted in Chapter 15, significant head injuries can lead to symptoms many hours after the initial trauma, and parents should be cautioned to watch for the signs noted above for 24 hours, including waking the child every 2 to 3 hours throughout the night.[34]

## CLINICAL EXAMINATION

Refer to Chapter 15 for a thorough discussion of the clinical examination. An important difference between the primary and permanent dentition exists in respect to vitality testing. Whereas it is not routinely performed in the primary dentition, vitality testing can be a useful diagnostic aid in the permanent dentition. The dentist should be aware that pulp testing might not elicit reliable responses from erupting permanent teeth and from those with open apices. Furthermore, recently traumatized teeth may not respond to any vitality test for several months. Positive findings following a traumatic injury are thus more valuable for assessing pulp vitality than are negative responses.

Cold testing with agents like difluorodichloromethane or carbon dioxide snow yield the most reliable results,[38] although the thermal shock of the low temperature applied can cause infraction lines in the enamel.[3] Some clinicians prefer electrical vitality testing because it utilizes a stimulus that can be gradually increased and precisely recorded. Although carbon dioxide snow elicits more reliable results, laser Doppler flowmetry has potentially great clinical value as this technique directly measures blood flow and does not rely on sensory nerve response.[41] The technique is also painless and is reliable in teeth with immature apices.[29] However, modifications in this instrument's design and a significant reduction in its cost are necessary for it to achieve widespread use.

Principles of radiographic diagnosis for permanent teeth do not differ from those for primary teeth. A common error made by dentists in diagnosing traumatic injuries is to take an insufficient number of radiographs. Additional views taken from slightly different angles both vertically and horizontally can improve the accuracy of diagnosis to a significant degree.[2]

It is important to note the urgency of follow-up radiographs after injury. Reviewing radiographs at 1 month after injury will detect signs of pulpal necrosis and inflammatory resorption. At 2 months, replacement resorption can be detected.

## PATHOLOGIC SEQUELAE OF TRAUMATIZED TEETH

Refer to Chapter 15 for a discussion of the pathologic sequelae of traumatized teeth.

## TREATMENT OF TRAUMATIC INJURIES TO THE PERMANENT DENTITION

The dentist treating a traumatic injury follows essentially the same principles of gathering historical information and completing a clinical examination, regardless of the child's age. Furthermore, the pathologic sequelae of injuries to teeth are similar for both primary and permanent teeth. However, there are many significant differences in the way that injuries to permanent teeth are treated. As in the primary dentition, a complete diagnostic workup (described in Chapter 15) should precede all treatment. Even though a blow may cause little if any obvious injury to a permanent tooth, it may lead to pulp necrosis as a result of disruption of the neurovascular bundle at the apex of the tooth. Posttreatment evaluation is indicated for all traumatic injuries.

### Enamel Fractures

In some cases, minor enamel fractures can be smoothed with fine disks. Larger fractures should be restored using an acid-etch/composite resin technique (see Chapter 39).

### Enamel and Dentin Fractures

The primary issue in managing fractures that expose dentin is to prevent bacterial irritants from reaching the pulp. Standard care in the past called for covering exposed dentin with calcium hydroxide or glass ionomer cement to seal out oral flora. Recent research indicates that sealing exposed dentin with a bonding agent enables the unexposed pulp to form reparative dentin. Some clinicians are thus advocating simultaneous acid etching of dentin and enamel followed by dentin and enamel bonding without placement of calcium hydroxide or glass ionomer.[40] However, a recent review of pulp capping with dentin adhesive systems reported that these systems are not indicated owing to increased inflammatory reactions, delay in pulp healing, and failure of dentin bridge formation.[11] This author recommends covering the deepest portion of dentin fractures with glass ionomer cement, followed by a dentin-bonding agent (see Chapters 20 and 39). The tooth can then be restored with an acid-etch/composite resin technique (Fig. 34-2). If adequate time is not available to restore the tooth completely, an interim covering of resin material (a resin "patch") can temporize the tooth until a final restoration can be placed. Some dentists routinely place such a partial restoration to ensure an appropriate posttreatment evaluation when the patient returns for the final restoration. This is

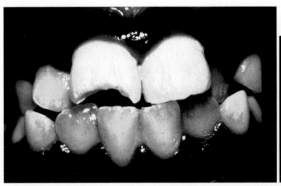
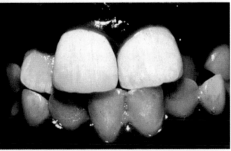

**Figure 34-2**   A fractured incisor (**A**) can quickly be restored using an acid-etch/composite resin technique (**B**).

a reasonable strategy provided that care is taken to assure an adequate seal.

## Fractures Involving the Pulp

Management of crown fractures that expose the pulp is particularly challenging (Fig. 34-3). Pertinent clinical findings that dictate treatment include the following:

1. Vitality of the exposed pulp
2. Time elapsed since the exposure
3. Degree of root maturation of the fractured tooth
4. Restorability of the fractured crown

The objective of treatment in managing these injuries is to preserve a vital pulp in the entire tooth (see Chapter 33). This allows for physiologic closure of the root apex in immature teeth. It is important to note that root end closure does not signal completion of root maturation. Progressive deposition of dentin normally continues in roots through adolescence, making them stronger and more resistant to traumatic insult. Maintaining a vital pulp in the tooth crown allows the clinician to monitor the tooth's vitality periodically.

It is not always possible to maintain vital tissue throughout the tooth. Three treatment alternatives are available, based on the clinical findings just noted:

1. Direct pulp cap
2. Pulpotomy
3. Pulpectomy

### Direct Pulp Cap

The direct pulp cap is only indicated in small exposures that can be treated within a few hours of the injury. The chances for pulp healing decrease if the tissue is inflamed, has formed a clot, or is contaminated with foreign materials.

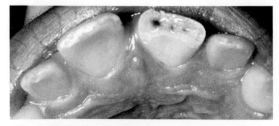

**Figure 34-3**   Crown fracture exposing the pulp.

The objective, then, is to preserve vital pulp tissue that is free of inflammation and physiologically walled off by a calcific barrier.

A rubber dam is applied, and the tooth is gently cleaned with water. Commercially available calcium hydroxide paste is applied directly to the pulp tissue and to surrounding dentin. It is essential that a restoration be placed that is capable of thoroughly sealing the exposure to prevent further contamination by oral bacteria. As in the management of dentin fractures, it is acceptable to use an acid-etch/composite resin system for an initial restoration. The calcific bridge stimulated by calcium hydroxide should be evident radiographically in 2 to 3 months.

In fractures exposing pulps of immature permanent teeth with incomplete root development, a direct cap is no longer the treatment of choice. Failure in these cases leads to total pulpal necrosis and a fragile, immature root with thin dentinal walls. Thus, the preferred treatment in pulp exposures of immature permanent teeth is pulpotomy.

### Pulpotomy

The objectives of the pulpotomy technique are to remove only the inflamed pulp tissue and to leave healthy tissue to enhance physiologic maturation of the root. As previously noted, this technique is favored for immature permanent teeth with exposed pulps. It is also indicated in large exposures or for pulps exposed for more than a few hours. Owing to its higher success rate, many clinicians have totally abandoned the direct pulp cap in favor of this technique.

It is difficult to determine clinically how far the inflamed pulp extends. The tooth shown in Figure 34-4 had been fractured for 4 days with a pulp exposure approximately 3 mm in diameter. The dentist elected to remove all tissue in the pulp chamber, with obvious success. Figure 34-4, *B* demonstrates complete maturation of the root, including apical closure and dentinal wall thickening as well as a calcific barrier at the amputation site. However, maintaining some pulp tissue in the crown allows the dentist to monitor the vitality of the tooth and thus is preferable when possible.

In 1978, Cvek noted that in most cases of pulps exposed for more than a few hours, the initial biological response is pulpal hyperplasia.[13] Inflammation in these cases rarely extends beyond 2 mm. In his study involving 60 teeth

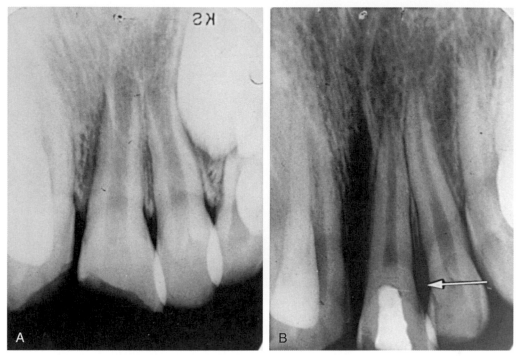

**Figure 34-4**  **A,** Crown fracture exposing the pulp in an immature permanent incisor. Note the open apex and thin dentinal walls in the root. **B,** A calcium hydroxide pulpotomy stimulated the formation of a calcific barrier *(arrow)* and enabled the root to mature.

with pulps exposed from 1 hour to 90 days, Cvek removed only 2 mm of the pulp and the surrounding dentin. He covered the pulp stumps with calcium hydroxide and reported a success rate of 96%.[13] The Fuks et al. 1993 report of long-term success confirms these findings and indicates that this conservative removal of tissue is the treatment of choice[19] (Fig. 34-5).

Rubber dam isolation to prevent contamination of the pulp with oral bacteria is essential. The inflamed pulp is gently removed to a level approximately 2 mm below the exposure site with a sterile diamond bur at high speed. Copious irrigation is mandatory to avoid pulp injury. The preparation should provide adequate space for the calcium hydroxide pulp dressing and a glass ionomer seal. Attaining a bacteria-tight coronal seal is essential for the success of this technique. The tooth can then be aesthetically restored with composite resin.

A relatively new material that is gaining favor as a pulp-capping agent is mineral trioxide aggregate (MTA).[32] It has been shown to perform well in pulpotomies casing dentinal bridge formation while maintaining normal pulpal histologic features.[31] See Chapter 33 for details on its use.

*Pulpectomy*

A pulpectomy involves complete pulp tissue removal from the crown and root and is indicated when no vital tissue remains. It is also indicated when root maturation is complete and the permanent restoration requires a post buildup. In the absence of inflammatory root resorption, treatment is to obturate the canal with gutta-percha. The reader is referred to standard endodontic textbooks for more information on this technique.

One of the greatest challenges facing the clinician is the treatment of a nonvital immature permanent tooth with an open apex. In this case, an apexification procedure is indicated wherein calcium hydroxide is carried to the root apex to contact vital tissues directly. The calcium hydroxide stimulates the formation of a cementoid barrier against which gutta-percha can subsequently be condensed. Even though a good apical seal can be achieved in this manner, no dentinal wall deposition will occur in the root, and it will remain thin and fragile (Fig. 34-6). These teeth are at increased risk for cervical crown or root fracture.[14] Refer to Chapter 33 for more detailed information regarding the apexification technique.

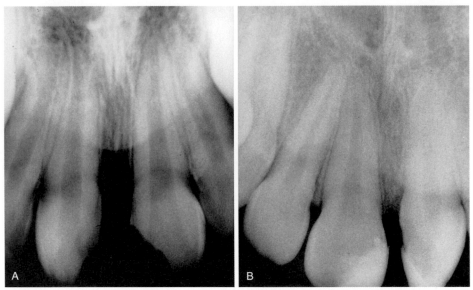

**Figure 34-5** **A,** Maxillary right permanent central incisor suffered crown fracture with pulp exposure. **B,** One-year postoperative radiograph of the same tooth successfully treated with a calcium hydroxide partial pulpotomy. Note completion of root development both apically and laterally.

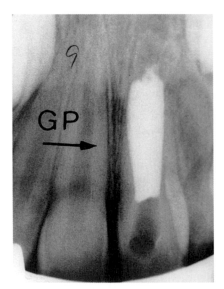

**Figure 34-6** An apexification procedure allowed this immature permanent tooth to be obturated successfully with gutta-percha *(GP).* The root, however, remains fragile and at increased risk of future trauma because no further dentinal wall apposition can occur.

An alternative to the apexification technique for managing devitalized immature incisors is the apical barrier technique.[21] This method employs the use of generic tricalcium phosphate (g-TCP) powder, which is condensed through the root canal to the apex. The material is mixed with saline to a wet sand–like consistency, inserted with an amalgam carrier, and condensed with amalgam or endodontic pluggers. Gutta-percha can then be packed against the g-TCP plugs during the same visit, significantly reducing the time and expense associated with the treatment of these teeth (Fig. 34-7). MTA is rapidly gaining favor for this technique as it is nonresorbable and has good marginal adaptability.[35]

Iwaya and others reported another interesting alternative to apexification of a necrotic immature tooth.[23] In an effort to promote physiologic maturation of the immature root in a premolar with a necrotic pulp, the authors cleansed the canal by copious irrigation and applied an antimicrobial paste. They did not mechanically cleanse the canal, were careful not to disrupt the tissue at the root apex, and left the canal unfilled. With this treatment they succeeded in removing the bacteria in the pulp canal and made it possible for the root to be revascularized by healthy apical pulp cells. The outcome was a physiologically mature root with thick dentinal walls. The effectiveness of this method will undoubtedly lead to its greater use in the future.

### Criteria for Success
Criteria to judge success of the techniques used to manage pulpal insult in fractured teeth include the following:

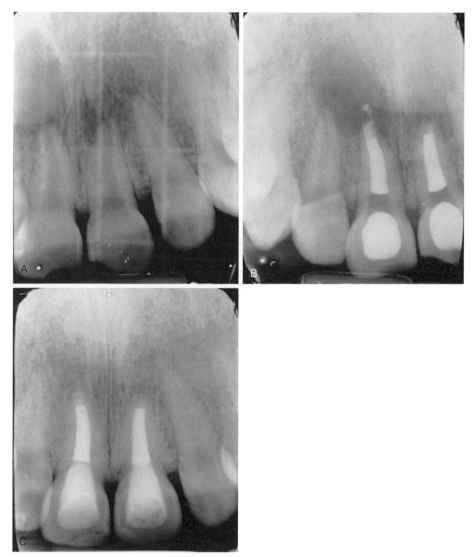

**Figure 34-7** Apexification using one visit, apical barrier technique. **A,** Preoperative view. **B,** Four-week postoperative view. **C,** 27-month postoperative view.

1. Completion of root development in immature teeth
2. Absence of clinical signs such as pain, mobility, or fistula
3. Absence of any radiographic signs of pathologic processes, such as periapical radiolucency of bone or root resorption

## Posterior Crown Fractures

Posterior crown fractures in the permanent dentition pose a restorative challenge for the clinician. These fractures usually occur secondary to hard blows to the underside of the chin, and vertical crown fractures may result (Fig. 34-8). Full cover-

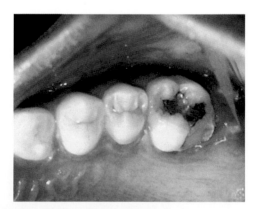

**Figure 34-8** A vertical crown fracture of the distolingual cusp *(arrow)* occurred secondary to a blow to the underside of this child's chin.

age with stainless steel or cast metal crowns is frequently the only alternative. The reader is reminded to watch for mandibular fractures and cervical spine injuries in these cases.[8]

## Root Fractures

The prognosis for root fractures is best when the fracture occurs in the apical one third of the root. The prognosis worsens progressively with fractures that occur more cervically on the root. Bender and Freedland reported that more than 75% of teeth with intraalveolar root fractures maintain their vitality.[7]

A tooth with a fractured root is usually mobile, and its coronal fragment is often displaced. Several baseline radiographs should be taken from various angulations to verify the extent of the fracture. Optimal results are obtained if the coronal fragment is repositioned as soon as possible.[17] The tooth position should be verified radiographically, and the pulp sensitivity should be tested. Accurate repositioning of the tooth enhances the likelihood of both hard tissue healing of the root fracture and pulp healing.[15] Immature teeth with incompletely formed root apices and positive pulp sensitivity at the time of injury are also significantly related to pulp healing and hard tissue repair of the fracture.

Tooth splinting techniques are detailed later in this chapter; however, recent findings have brought into question the recommendations for splinting root-fractured teeth. Former recommendations called for firm immobilization with a splint for several months.[3] Recent evidence indicates that root-fractured teeth may heal better if splinted for only 3 to 4 weeks with a functional splint that allows for some mobility of the teeth.[15] Further research is needed to resolve this question.

Root canal therapy should not be initiated until clinical and radiographic signs of necrosis or resorption are apparent. Even in those cases, treatment can often be limited to the coronal fragment because in most instances the apical fragments maintain their vitality.

## Managing Sequelae to Dental Trauma

In Chapter 15, common reactions of the teeth to trauma are described. Three of the most challenging sequelae include pulp canal obliteration, inflammatory resorption (both external and internal), and replacement resorption. These pathologic processes can occur following crown fractures or luxation injuries.

### Pulp Canal Obliteration

Pulp canal obliteration (PCO) is a degenerative pathologic process that ultimately leads to obliteration of the pulp canal (Figs. 34-9 and 34-10, *B*). F. Andreasen et al. have shown that its occurrence depends on the type of luxation injury sustained and the stage of root development.[1] Thus immature teeth with open apices suffering

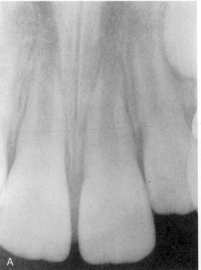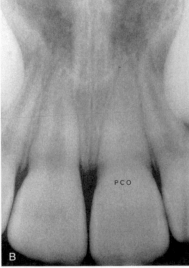

**Figure 34-9**  **A,** Ten-day postoperative view of immature maxillary left central incisor in 7-year-old child that had been extruded and repositioned. **B,** 16-month post-operative view demonstrating pulp canal obliteration (pco).

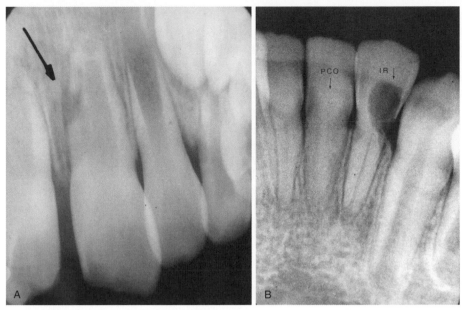

**Figure 34-10**    **A,** External inflammatory resorption *(arrow).* **B,** Internal inflammatory resorption *(ir)* of the lateral incisor; pulp canal obliteration *(pco)* of the permanent central incisor. (**B** from McTigue DJ: *Pediatr Ann* 14:125, 1985.)

moderate to severe injuries are likely to undergo PCO. It was noted previously that most primary teeth with PCO resorb normally, and thus treatment is usually not indicated. Controversy exists, however, regarding treatment of permanent teeth.

Some clinicians contend that as soon as PCO is diagnosed, a pulpectomy with gutta-percha should be performed. This treatment is advocated because of reports of later development of pulpal necrosis and periapical change. Furthermore, difficulty in completing routine endodontic procedures after pulp canals have calcified is noted. However, Andreasen counters that pulp necrosis is an uncommon sequelae of PCO, reportedly as low as 1%.[1] She also states that endodontic procedures can be successfully completed in a great majority of obliterated canals.[3] The dentist is advised, then, to closely monitor PCO in permanent teeth and to initiate endodontic procedures only when periapical changes are noted.

### Inflammatory Resorption

Inflammatory resorption can occur externally and/or internally (see Fig. 34-10). It commonly arises following luxation injuries when the periodontal ligament (PDL) is inflamed and the pulp is necrotic.[36] Odontoclastic activity can occur so rapidly that the teeth are destroyed in a matter of weeks.

Immediate management of inflammatory resorption is essential. As soon as this process is detected radiographically, the pulp tissue in the tooth is thoroughly extirpated. Copious irrigation with sodium hypochlorite assists in the dissolution of organic debris in the canal. In permanent teeth, calcium hydroxide is placed in the canal with a technique identical to that used to induce apexification (see Chapter 33). Here the objective is not to induce apical closure but to create an environment unfavorable for the resorptive process. It is theorized that calcium hydroxide has antiseptic properties because of its extreme alkalinity. This medicament apparently percolates through the dentinal tubules to the areas of resorption at the PDL and halts its progress.

Depending on the severity of the inflammatory resorption, calcium hydroxide may have to be retained in the tooth for 6 to 12 months. Repeated applications may be necessary if the resorption progresses. When radiographs confirm that the process is not continuing, gutta-percha is placed as the final filling material.

### Replacement Resorption (Ankylosis)

Replacement resorption occurs most commonly following severe luxation injuries like avulsions or intrusions in which PDL cells are destroyed. Alveolar bone directly contacts cementum on the involved tooth and becomes fused with it. Then as the bone undergoes its normal physiologic, osteoclastic, and osteoblastic activity, the root is resorbed or "replaced" with bone (Fig. 34-11). In young children with rapid bone turnover, roots are completely resorbed in 3 to 4 years. In adults, the process may take up to 10 years. Replacement resorption can be prevented by prompt and appropriate management of luxation injuries.

Recent reports indicate that replacement resorption may be delayed by treating the root surface with the enamel matrix protein Emdogain (Biora, Malmo, Sweden), which has been shown to stimulate regeneration of PDL following periodontal surgery in adults.[25] Short-term data indicate that a delay in ankylosis up to 1 year can occur,[16] but more research is needed to verify a longer term benefit.

## Treating Luxation Injuries in the Permanent Dentition

The reader is referred to Chapter 15 for the definition of the various types of luxation injuries. Luxation injuries damage the supporting structures of the teeth, that is, the PDL and alveolar bone. Additionally, in mature teeth with closed apices, the pulp frequently becomes necrotic. Pulp necrosis occurs less frequently when immature teeth with open apices are luxated but, as noted earlier, PCO is a common finding in these cases.

Vitality of the PDL is far more important than pulp vitality in determining the prognosis of luxated teeth. The primary objective of treatment in these injuries is to *maintain PDL vitality*.

### Concussion
Concussion injuries in permanent teeth must be followed closely. Although the prognosis is normally good, pulp necrosis and root resorption have been reported. Involved teeth can be carefully taken out of occlusion if the child complains of pain.

### Subluxation
Pulp necrosis occurs far more commonly in subluxated permanent teeth than in primary teeth. These teeth should be monitored closely with radiographs for at least 1 year, and root canal therapy should be instituted at the first sign of pathologic change. Immature teeth with open apices are less likely to undergo pulpal necrosis. Splinting of subluxated teeth should be avoided.

### Intrusive Luxation
The prognosis for intruded permanent teeth is not good. These teeth frequently undergo pulpal necrosis, root resorption, and alveolar bone loss.

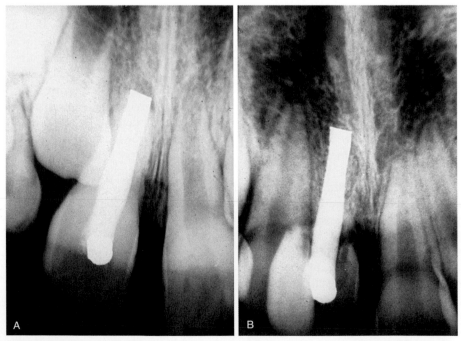

**Figure 34-11    A,** A permanent incisor that had been avulsed and stored dry for 3 hours was filled with gutta-percha prior to reimplantation. **B,** Three years later, replacement resorption has completely destroyed the root.

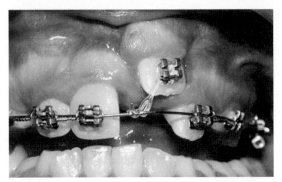

**Figure 34-12**  Orthodontic repositioning of intruded permanent incisor prevents replacement resorption (ankylosis) and alveolar bone loss.

The treatment of choice is to reposition the intruded teeth orthodontically, using light forces[33] (Fig. 34-12). The pulp should be extirpated within 2 weeks following the injury, and calcium hydroxide should be placed in the root canal using the same technique as described for apexification in Chapter 33. Radiographic monitoring of the tooth should occur for at least 1 year, and the calcium hydroxide in the canal should be replaced if signs of root resorption persist.

As opposed to the primary dentition, the author does not wait for the intruded permanent tooth to reerupt. Permanent teeth with closed apices reerupt very slowly, if at all, and are likely to undergo replacement resorption.[39] Those with open apices may reerupt but the process could take several months, in which time the root could be badly resorbed.

Current evidence indicates that immediate surgical repositioning is only indicated for intruded permanent teeth that are quite loose and freely mobile. Firmly intruded permanent teeth should not be surgically repositioned as this

may enhance both root resorption and alveolar bone loss.[3]

*Extrusion*
Extruded permanent teeth (Fig. 34-13, *A*) should be repositioned and splinted for 2 to 3 weeks. It normally takes the PDL fibers this period of time to reanastomose. Extruded permanent teeth with closed apices will undergo pulpal necrosis; therefore, root canal therapy should be initiated after the teeth are splinted. Extruded teeth with open apices have a chance to revascularize and maintain their vitality, so the decision to initiate therapy should be delayed until clinical or radiographic signs indicate necrosis.

*Lateral Luxation*
Alveolar bone fractures frequently occur in lateral luxation injuries and can complicate their management (Fig. 34-13, *B*). In the most severe cases, PDL and marginal bone loss occurs. Treatment is to reposition the teeth and alveolar fragments. A splint should then be applied for 3 to 8 weeks, depending on the degree of bone involvement. With good oral hygiene, alveolar bone regeneration can occur in children in approximately 8 weeks. The author's current protocol includes prescribing a 0.12% chlorhexidine mouth rinse. If the apices are closed, the pulps will likely become necrotic; therefore endodontic therapy should be instituted soon after the teeth are splinted. Again, teeth with open apices should be monitored until signs of necrosis are evident.

*Avulsion*
The prognosis for long-term retention of an avulsed permanent tooth worsens the longer that the tooth is out of its socket.[6] The primary

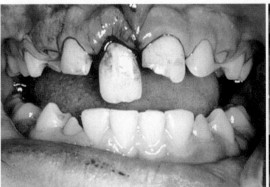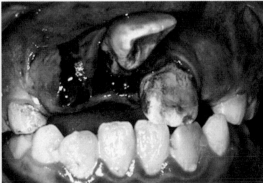

**Figure 34-13**  **A,** Extrusion injury of maxillary right central incisor and crown fracture of maxillary left central incisor. **B,** Laterally luxated tooth.

therapeutic concern is to maintain the vitality of PDL fibers, and the longer that they are out of the mouth, the worse the prognosis for their survival. *It is thus imperative that the avulsed tooth be immediately reimplanted by the first capable person,* whether that person is a parent, teacher, or sibling (Fig. 34-14).

Owing to a variety of circumstances, it is sometimes not possible to reimplant a tooth immediately. Research has shown that the best transport medium for avulsed teeth is cell culture media such as ViaSpan (DuPont, Wilmington, Del.) or Hanks balanced salt solution (HBSS).[22] ViaSpan is not readily available for clinical use but HBSS is commercially available as EMT Tooth Saver (Smart Practice, Phoenix, Ariz.). Use of HBSS significantly increases the likelihood of PDL cell survival for several hours.[26]

The best alternative storage medium if culture media is not available is milk.[9,12] It is readily available, relatively aseptic, and its osmolality is more favorable to maintaining the vitality of the PDL cells than is saline solution or tap water. Cool milk has been shown to maintain the ability of PDL precursor cells to reproduce for twice as long as room temperature milk.[27] While some studies have indicated that storing the tooth in the patient's mouth (saliva) may be favorable toward

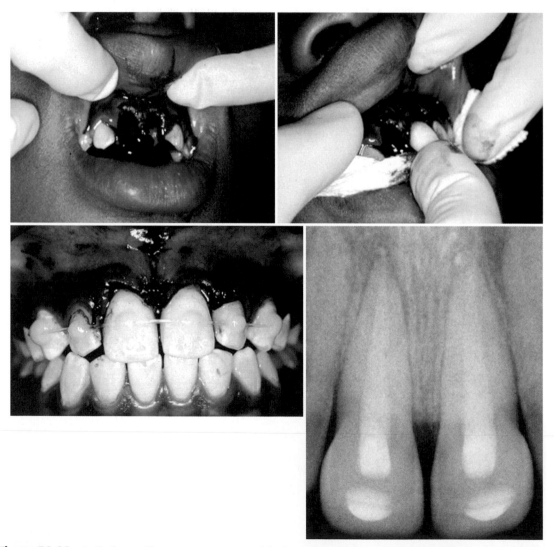

**Figure 34-14** **A,** Both maxillary permanent central incisors avulsed. **B,** Reimplanting avulsed teeth with finger pressure. **C,** Aesthetic, flexible splint fabricated using 50-pound test monofilament fishing line retained with composite resin. **D,** Calcium hydroxide pulpectomies completed to prevent inflammatory resorption. (Courtesy Dr. Jeff Hays.)

PDL survival, the danger of an alarmed child swallowing, aspirating or chewing on the tooth eliminates this option in the author's opinion. Water is not a good transport medium because it is a hypotonic solution and causes PDL cells to swell and rupture. Thus in these cases, with the tooth stored in milk, the patient should be taken to the dentist as soon as possible.

Because root resorption is so closely correlated with the extraoral period, the dentist should reimplant the tooth in its socket as soon as possible after the child arrives. Adequate evidence exists, however, to support the immediate placement of the avulsed tooth into HBSS while the patient is brought to the dental operatory and appropriate informed consent is being obtained from the parent.[37] Soaking the tooth may reduce ankylosis and help debride necrotic cells, foreign bodies, and bacteria.[28] The author's current protocol is again to prescribe an oral mouth rinse of 0.12% chlorhexidine used empirically to reduce the likelihood of bacterial invasion of the PDL space. Controversy exists regarding the benefit of systemic antibiotics for pulp or periodontal healing.[4,5] Given the evidence that systemic antibiotics can prevent bacterial invasion of the necrotic pulp,[20] Trope recommends a 1-week course of penicillin V for tooth avulsion patients.[38] Owing to tetracycline's antiresorptive properties,[30] doxycycline has been recommended for those patients older than 8 years and not susceptible to tetracycline staining.[18]

When immature teeth with open apices are avulsed, the ideal treatment objective is revascularization of the pulp in addition to maintenance of PDL health. This would enable physiologic maturation of the immature root, including apexogenesis and root wall thickening. The tooth should be splinted for approximately 1 week. Success in these cases has been reported; therefore dentists should await clinical or radiographic signs of necrosis prior to initiating root canal therapy. When the splint is removed, the dentist may note that the tooth is quite mobile. This mobility is preferable to long-term rigid splinting, as the latter has been correlated with an increased incidence of replacement resorption. The mobility of the tooth physiologically interrupts areas of incipient resorption/ankylosis on the PDL, allowing it to heal normally.

In mature teeth with closed apices, a splint that affords the tooth functional mobility should be applied for 7 to 10 days. The necrotic pulp should be extirpated and replaced with calcium hydroxide after 1 week to prevent the initiation of inflammatory root resorption (Fig. 34-14, *D*). Importantly, *root canal therapy should not be performed in the hand prior to reimplantation.* This extends the extraoral period and places the PDL at greater risk to injury as a result of the additional manipulation of the tooth. The calcium hydroxide can be removed and a gutta-percha pulpectomy performed after 1 month. In those cases where the pulp was not removed within 2 weeks of the reimplantation, or when inflammatory resorption is evident radiographically, the calcium hydroxide should be maintained in the tooth for a minimum of 3 months.

PDL cells on avulsed teeth that have been stored dry for more than 1 hour are necrotic, and these teeth will eventually ankylose and resorb. There is some evidence that the pace of this resorption can be reduced if these teeth are soaked in fluoride for approximately 20 minutes prior to reimplantation.[10] As noted earlier, Emdogain may be beneficial in delaying replacement resorption, and the International Association of Dental Traumatology recommends it use in these cases.[18]

In summary, the procedure for reimplantation of a mature tooth is as follows:

1. Hold the tooth by the crown to prevent damage to the PDL.
2. Gently rinse the tooth with tap water. No attempt should be made to scrub or sterilize the tooth.
3. Manually reimplant the tooth in the socket *as soon as possible.*
4. Apply a light, functional splint for 1 week.
5. Complete calcium hydroxide pulpectomy after 1 week and then remove splint.

### Splinting Technique

Various methods of splinting teeth have been advocated, but it is apparent that the ideal splint should possess the following characteristics. It should

1. Be passive and not cause trauma
2. Be flexible and allow functional movement of the tooth
3. Allow for vitality testing and endodontic access
4. Be easy to apply and remove

**BOX 34-1**

**Splinting Periods**

Avulsions: 1 to 2 weeks
Extrusions: 2 to 3 weeks
Lateral luxations with bone damage: 3 to 8 weeks
Root fractures: 3 to 4 weeks

Many splints can meet these criteria, and several good commercial products are available. To allow for flexibility, a light orthodontic arch wire or a 30- to 60-pound test monofilament fishing line can be used (Fig. 34-14, *C*). See Box 34-1 for a summary of splinting periods.

## SUMMARY

Advances in dental research have greatly improved the ability of dentists to ensure long-term retention of traumatized teeth in children. It is the dentist's responsibility to stay abreast of this new information and to be available to patients who need urgent treatment.

## REFERENCES

1. Andreasen FM: Pulp healing after luxation injuries and root fractures in the permanent dentition. *Endod Dent Traumatol* 5:111, 1989.
2. Andreasen FM, Andreasen JO: Diagnosis of luxation injuries: the importance of standardized clinical, radiographic and photographic techniques in clinical investigations. *Endod Dent Traumatol* 1:160, 1985.
3. Andreasen JO, Andreasen, FM: *Textbook and Color Atlas of Traumatic Injuries to the Teeth,* 3rd ed. Copenhagen, Munksgaard, 1994.
4. Andreasen J, Borum M, Jacobsen H, Andreasen F: Replantation of 400 avulsed permanent incisors. 2. Factors related to pulpal healing. *Endod Dent Traumatol* 11:59, 1995.
5. Andreasen J, Borum M, Jacobsen H, Andreasen F: Replantation of 400 avulsed permanent incisors. 3. Factors related to periodontal ligament healing. *Endod Dent Traumatol* 11:76, 1995.
6. Andreasen JO, Hjorting-Hansen E: Replantation of teeth. I. Radiographic and clinical studies of 110 human teeth replanted after accidental loss. *Acta Odont Scand* 24:263, 1966.
7. Bender IB, Freedland JB: Clinical considerations in the diagnosis and treatment of intra-alveolar root fractures. *JADA* 107:595, 1983.
8. Bertolami CN, Kaban LB: Chin trauma: a clue to associated mandibular and cervical spine injury. *Oral Surg* 53:122, 1982.
9. Blomlof L: Storage of human periodontal ligament cells in a combination of different media. *J Dent Res* 60:1904, 1981.
10. Coccia C: A clinical investigation of root resorption rates in reimplanted young permanent incisors: a five-year study. *J Endod* 6:413, 1980.
11. Costa CA, Hebling J, Hanks CT: Current status of pulp capping with dentin adhesive systems: a review. *Dent Mater* 16:188, 2000.
12. Courts FJ, Mueller WA, Tabeling HJ: Milk as an interim storage medium for avulsed teeth. *Pediatr Dent* 5:183, 1983.
13. Cvek M: A clinical report on partial pulpotomy and capping with calcium hydroxide in permanent incisors with complicated crown fracture. *J Endod* 4:232, 1978.
14. Cvek M: Prognosis of luxated non-vital maxillary incisors treated with calcium hydroxide and filled with gutta-percha. A retrospective clinical study. *Endod Dent Traumatol* 8:45, 1992.
15. Cvek M, Andreasen J, Borum M: Healing of 208 intra-alveolar root fractures in patients aged 7-17 years. *Dent Traumatol* 17: 53-62, 2001.
16. Filippi A, Pohl Y, von Arx T: Treatment of replacement resorption with Emdogain—a prospective clinical study. *Dent Traumatol* 18:138, 2002.
17. Flores M, Andreasen J, Bakland L et al: Guidelines for the evaluation and management of traumatic dental injuries. *Dent Traumatol* 17:97, 2001.
18. Flores M, Andreasen J, Bakland L et al: Guidelines for the evaluation and management of traumatic dental injuries. *Dent Traumatol* 17:193, 2001.
19. Fuks A, Gavra S, Chosack A: Long-term follow up of traumatized incisors treated by partial pulpotomy. *Pediatr Dent* 15:334, 1993.
20. Hammarstrom L, Pierce A, Blomlof L et al: Tooth avulsion and replantation: a review. *Endod Dent Traumatol* 2:1, 1986.
21. Harbert H: Generic tricalcium phosphate plugs: an adjunct in endodontics. *J Endod* 17:131, 1991.
22. Hiltz J, Trope M: Vitality of human lip fibroblasts in milk, Hanks balanced salt solution and Viaspan storage media. *Endod Dent Traumatol* 7:69, 1991.
23. Iwaya S, Ikawa M, Kubota M: Revascularization of an immature permanent tooth with apical periodontitis and sinus tract. *Dent Traumatol* 17:185, 2001.
24. Jarvinen S: Incisal overjet and traumatic injuries to upper permanent incisors: a retrospective study. *Acta Odontol Scand* 36:359, 1978.
25. Kenny D, Barrett E, Johnston D et al: Clinical management of avulsed permanent incisors using Emdogain: initial report of an investigation. *J Can Dent Assoc* 66:21, 2000.
26. Krasner P, Person P: Preserving avulsed teeth for replantation. *J Am Dent Assoc* 123:80, 1992.

27. Lekic P, Kenny D, Barrett E: The influence of storage conditions on the clonogenic capacity of periodontal ligament cells: implications for tooth replantation. *Int Endod J* 31:137, 1998.

28. Matsson L, Andreasen J, Cvek M, Granath L: Ankylosis of experimentally reimplanted teeth related to extra-alveolar period and storage environment. *Pediatr Dent* 4:327, 1982.

29. Mesaros S, Trope M: Revascularization of traumatized teeth assessed by laser Doppler flowmetry: case report. *Endod Dent Traumatol* 13:24, 1997.

30. Sae-Lim V, Wang C, Choi G et al: Effect of systemic tetracycline and amoxicillin on inflammatory root resorption of replanted dogs' teeth. *Endod Dent Traumatol* 14:216, 1998.

31. Salako, N, Joseph B, Ritwik P et al: Comparison of bioactive glass, mineral trioxide aggregate, ferric sulfate, and formocresol as pulpotomy agents in rat molar. *Dent Traumatol* 19:314, 2003.

32. Schmitt D, Lee J, Bogen G: Multifaceted use of ProRoot MTA root canal repair material. *Pediatr Dent* 23:326, 2001.

33. Spalding PM, Fields HW, Torney D et al: The changing role of endodontics and orthodontics in the management of traumatically intruded permanent incisors. *Pediatr Dent* 7:104, 1985.

34. Tecklenburg F, Wright M: Minor head trauma in the pediatric patient. *Pediatr Emerg Care* 7:40, 1991.

35. Torabinejad M, Watson T, Pitt Ford T: The sealing ability of a mineral trioxide aggregate as a root-end filling material. *J Endod* 19:591, 1993.

36. Tronstad L: Root resorption: etiology, terminology and clinical manifestations. *Endod Dent Traumatol* 4:241, 1988.

37. Trope M: Clinical management of the avulsed tooth. *Dent Clin North Am* 39:93, 1995.

38. Trope M: Clinical management of the avulsed tooth: present strategies and future directions. *Dent Traumatol* 18:1, 2002.

39. Turley PK, Joiner MW, Hellstrom S: The effect of orthodontic extrusion on traumatically intruded teeth. *Am J Orthod* 85:47, 1984.

40. White K, Cox C, Kanka J et al: Histologic pulpal response of acid etching vital dentin. *J Dent Res* 71:188, 1992.

41. Yanpiset K, Vongsavan N, Sigurdsson A, Trope M: Efficacy of laser Doppler flowmetry for the diagnosis of revascularization of reimplanted immature dog teeth. *Dent Traumatol* 17:63, 2001.

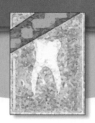

# CHAPTER 35

# Treatment Planning and Management of Orthodontic Problems

*John R. Christensen and Henry W. Fields, Jr.*

When considering treatment for problems during the mixed-dentition years, the precise problem and the goal of treatment must be clearly in mind. Few problems will receive definitive or complete treatment at this stage of development, although some simple and isolated dental problems may be resolved. As always, information regarding the patient's problems is gathered through an interview of the patient and the parents and a clinical examination. A list of orthodontic problems is generated from this database, and the problems are ranked in order from most to least severe.[42] Severity is determined by patient, functional, and aesthetic concerns. The clinician is specifically trained to identify functional and aesthetic problems but does not always consider the concerns of the parent and child. These concerns should be listened to carefully and often dictate treatment direction and treatment satisfaction outcomes. Many times the motivation for treatment can be elicited from these concerns. If the child patient desires to have treatment, cooperation will usually be good during treatment, and little parental support will be necessary. This is called internal motivation. External motivation, motivation supplied by the parent for treatment, will require continuous parental support to successfully complete treatment. If the chief complaint or reason for seeking treatment ranks low on the treatment priority list or will be addressed later in the treatment plan, an explanation should be provided to the child and parent to justify this situation.

After the problem list has been generated and each problem has been ranked in order of severity, possible solutions to each problem should be listed. The solution list should be comprehensive; that is, all reasonable solutions should be considered for each specific problem without regard for the other problems. After the solution list has been constructed, the clinician should look for similar solutions that are listed for more than one problem. In some cases, the best solution for one problem is the best solution for all problems, and the treatment plan is easily derived. Unfortunately, in most cases, a solution for one problem is not the solution for the others, and, worse, may actually magnify the second problem. Treatment planning is not entirely scientific, and clinical wisdom is needed to determine a plan in these cases.

## SKELETAL PROBLEMS

Orthodontic problems in the preadolescent patient are generally thought of as either dental or skeletal in origin. The complexity of these problems varies tremendously. Many dental problems are well within the treatment domain of the general practitioner. Skeletal problems, as diagnosed from the facial profile analysis and confirmed by supplemental means, are best managed by a specialist. However, the general practitioner should have an understanding of how skeletal discrepancies are treated.

Three basic alternatives for treating skeletal discrepancies exist: growth modification, camouflage, and orthognathic surgery. Growth modification is a means to change skeletal relationships by using the patient's remaining growth to alter the size or position of the jaws. Camouflage and orthognathic surgery usually are considered only in the nongrowing or adult patient. The camouflage type of orthodontic treatment is aimed at hiding a mild skeletal discrepancy by moving teeth situated on the jaws so that they fit together. The skeletal discrepancy still exists, but it is disguised by a normal occlusion and acceptable facial aesthetic appearance. Orthognathic surgery places the jaws and teeth in a normal or near-normal position through the use of surgical procedures and pre- and postsurgical orthodontic treatment.[43] For the mixed-dentition patient only growth modification or no treatment is a reasonable choice for skeletal intervention.

Growth modification during the early mixed-dentition years rests on several assumptions that are not as clear as many would presume. First, a child must be growing for the growth to be modi-

fied. Most normal children in the 6- to 12-year age group are actively growing, and their faces are also growing. Furthermore, clinicians have thought that it is easiest to correct skeletal problems if a child is undergoing maximal facial growth during treatment. Although the data to support this contention are not voluminous or clear,[19] clinicians have long sought to predict maximum somatic growth and maximal facial growth from other indicators. There appears to be wide variation in the amount of facial growth occurring at one time and an equally wide variation in the correlation of facial growth with overall body growth and other indicators that have been chosen.[10,41,48] Because of this state of inaccuracy, the clinician should use as many indicators as possible (personal growth history, skeletal growth maturation, and onset of menarche) to make an educated decision about whether the child is growing at an acceptable rate. Girls tend to enter the adolescent growth spurt as defined by obvious somatic growth at around 10 and boys at around 12.

The data are not totally clear that one must treat children when they are at a certain rate of facial growth to be successful, and experience has shown that most skeletal and dental problems can be managed a bit later in one phase during the transition from the mixed to permanent dentitions. For these reasons, a single stage of orthodontic treatment is most popular and adequately effective. This enables practitioners to successfully manage most problems and deal with a more mature patient who is both reasonably cooperative and compliant. Asynchrony between dental development and rapid facial growth may create a situation in which the patient may be ready for growth modification but not for orthodontic dental treatment, or vice versa. These patients must be handled individually by balancing the dental and skeletal interventions. Similarly, some patients have compelling problems that demand earlier treatment as described below.

The second assumption made when growth modification is undertaken is that the practitioner can accurately diagnose the source of the skeletal discrepancy and then design treatment that will apply the appropriate amount and direction of force to correct the discrepancy. Diagnosis is not an exact science and may be confusing even with the use of cephalometric measures,[15,24] and the discrepancy may be due to a number of small skeletal problems rather than to one easily identified discrepancy. It is important to remember that not all class II or class III mal-occlusions are created equal or have only one skeletal feature at fault. Force delivery to dental and skeletal structures also is inexact, and the clinical impression and treatment response may dictate alteration in the amount and direction of force applied to modify growth. Certainly orthodontic treatment for skeletal problems is not just a "see it" and "fix it" situation.

Third, growth modification is usually only one portion of a treatment plan. Most appliances used to modify growth—headgears and functional appliances, for example—are designed to alter skeletal structures rather than precisely move teeth. Although the appliances are capable of causing tooth movement, they are not as precise as fixed orthodontic appliances and usually are used prior to or in conjunction with fixed appliances. Therefore, most growth modification treatments are followed immediately or at a later time by traditional fixed orthodontic appliances to move the teeth into a final position.

There are several theories offered to explain how growth modification works to achieve the desired results. The first theory suggests that growth modification appliances change the absolute size of one or both jaws. For example, a class II skeletal profile may be treated by making a deficient mandible larger to fit a normal-sized maxilla or by limiting the size of an oversized maxilla. Clinical data show dramatic size changes, but there appears to be large variability in patient response to growth-modifying appliances, with moderate changes in various structures being the rule rather than the exception.

Alternatively, growth modification may work by accelerating the desired growth but not changing the ultimate size or shape of the jaw. A deficient mandible may not end up larger than it ultimately would have been, but it may achieve its final size sooner. This requires the clinician to make some final dentoalveolar changes or compensations to establish an ideal occlusion following growth modification. This type of growth modification response also shows large individual variability. There is support for this interpretation of growth modification based on recent randomized clinical trials that demonstrate little difference between an early- and a late-treatment group of patients with skeletal class II malocclusion.[50]

A third possibility is that growth modification may work by changing the spatial relationship of the two jaws. The ultimate size of the jaw and its rate of growth are not changed, but by modifying the orientation of the jaws to each other a more balanced profile may result. For example, a convex profile and an increased lower facial height could be made more proportional to each other if the vertical growth of the maxilla could be inhibited and the mandible allowed to rotate upward and forward. The profile would then become less convex and the vertical relations more ideal. Jaw reorientation would be successful in a concave class III patient with a short face if the mandible could be rotated downward and backward (more vertical) to create a more acceptable profile. Reorientation does not work well in class II short faces or class III long faces because correcting one problem (e.g., the vertical) makes the other problem (e.g., the anteroposterior) worse.

As you can see, growth modification is at best inexact. From the best available data, it appears that if a patient is growing, on average modest skeletal changes can be accomplished during the mixed-dentition years. These are reasonably comparable if attempted early or late in this period of development. It may be advisable to attempt these changes during the earlier mixed-dentition years if patients have aesthetic complaints or, in the case of class II patients, they are trauma prone. Otherwise, conventional late mixed-dentition treatment appears to be just as sensible.

## Growth Modification Applied to Anteroposterior Problems

Anteroposterior skeletal problems are class II and class III in nature. These descriptions are not very informative, however, because the source of the discrepancy may be the maxilla, the mandible, or a combination of the two. Therefore, the first step in patient evaluation is to identify the source of the problem and then design a treatment plan to resolve the problem. Although this approach appears to indicate that these problems are clearly identifiable and treatable with concise approaches, the previous discussion makes it clear that this is not the case. In many moderately severe cases of anteroposterior problems a number of approaches may work that rely more on patient compliance than clinical expertise.

### Class II Maxillary Protrusion
Class II maxillary protrusion is best managed by headgear therapy to restrict or redirect maxillary growth on the basis of retrospective studies and

randomized clinical trials.[4, 50] Headgear places a distal force on the maxillary dentition and the maxilla (Fig. 35-1). Theoretically, the relative movement of dental and skeletal structures depends on the amount and time of force application. In actual practice, it is probably not possible to move selectively only teeth or bones.[4] Generally, tooth movement is greater with higher forces, but skeletal change can successfully occur with either heavy or light forces. The best approach is probably to apply forces ranging from 12 to 16 ounces per side for 12 to 14 hours and then monitor the skeletal and dental changes and adjust accordingly. Certainly, the skeletal and dental response varies according to the type of headgear chosen and the resultant direction of force exerted by the headgear. The most common varieties, cervical and high pull, provide predominantly distal and occlusal and distal and apical forces, respectively. Traditionally, one avoids using a headgear that tends to extrude posterior teeth in a long-faced person or a person with limited overbite. On the other hand, a headgear that extrudes the molars is often useful in a patient with a short face and a deep bite.

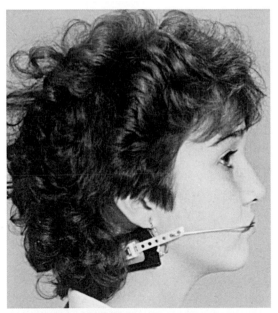

**Figure 35-1** The class II maxillary protrusive patient is best treated by headgear therapy to restrict or redirect maxillary growth. This patient is being treated with cervical headgear that places a distal and extrusive force on both maxillary skeletal and dental structures. The force is provided by a neck strap attached to the outer bows of the headgear.

Class II maxillary protrusion may also be managed with a removable functional appliance of the activator, bionator, or twin block type (Fig. 35-2). Although a functional appliance is primarily designed to stimulate mandibular growth, studies have indicated that it has some secondary effects of restricting forward maxillary skeletal and dental movement.[6,38,50] This happens because the mandible, which is postured forward, tends to return to a more distal position as a result of the distal muscle and soft tissue forces that are also transmitted through the appliance to the maxilla and the maxillary teeth. The maxillary teeth tend to tip lingually rather than to move bodily, and the mandibular teeth tip facially.

Another functional appliance is the Herbst appliance, which is a fixed appliance used to reposition the mandible forward. It is held in place with bands, stainless steel crowns, bonding, or a cemented cast framework (Fig. 35-3). A pin and tube apparatus forces the mandible forward and places constant force on the maxilla and maxillary and mandibular teeth as the mandible attempts to return to a normal and more distal posture. Maxillary teeth tend to move distally and mandibular anterior teeth move forward. This appliance has shown changes similar to those of functional appliances in randomized clinical trails.[38]

### Class II Mandibular Deficiency
The mandibular-deficient patient is usually treated with a removable or fixed functional appliance that positions the mandible forward in an attempt to stimulate or accelerate mandibular growth (see Fig. 35-2). Retrospective clinical studies have shown that these appliances can produce a small average increase in mandibular projection (2 to 4 mm/year).[34,44] This has been confirmed by randomized clinical trials.[23,50] Patient response varies greatly, and in many cases the increased growth does not totally correct the class II skeletal problem for several reasons. First, the amount of growth is not enough to overcome the discrepancy. Second, all the available growth would have to be directed to produce anteroposterior change. This is usually not the case because some dental eruption and vertical growth occurs. This interaction between anteroposterior and vertical dimensional changes decreases ultimate mandibular projection and class II correction because the mandible grows downward and forward and not straightforward. The rest of the anteroposterior

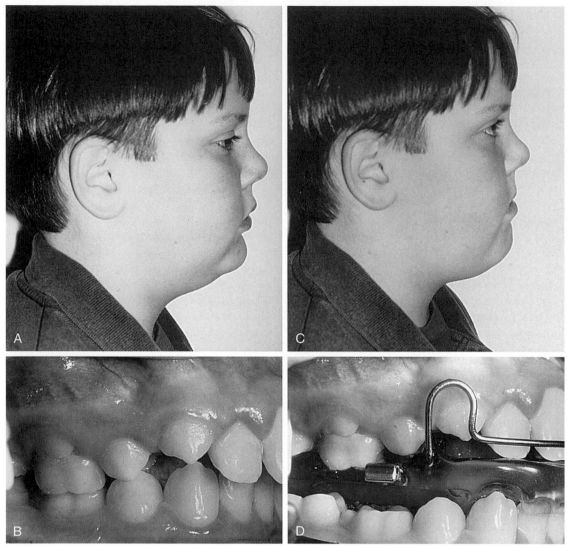

**Figure 35-2**    The class II mandibular deficient patient is usually treated with a functional appliance that positions the mandible forward in an attempt to stimulate, accelerate, or redirect mandibular growth. **A,** This patient has a class II mandibular deficient profile. **B,** The patient's molar and canine relationships reflect the skeletal class II relationship. **C,** The profile is immediately improved when the functional appliance is in place because the mandible is pushed forward into a class I relationship. **D,** Because functional appliances position the mandible forward using the upper and lower dental arches, there may be movement of the upper and lower teeth. Dental aspects of the malocclusion must be considered during treatment planning.

discrepancy is managed by restricting maxillary growth, tipping the maxillary teeth back, and tipping the mandibular teeth forward. Different appliances can be designed that exaggerate the secondary responses of maxillary restriction and dental movement if desired. The Herbst appliance, mentioned above, also has been used with mandibular-deficient patients. Some studies indicate that headgear treatment may cause an increase in mandibular growth.[3,23]

### Class III Maxillary Deficiency

True midface deficiency can be treated by using a reverse-pull headgear or facemask to exert anteriorly directed force on the maxilla (Fig. 35-4).[51] The facemask applies force to the maxilla through an appliance (either a removable splint or fixed appliance) attached to the teeth; tooth movement also occurs. Some clinicians also use the facemask in conjunction with maxillary expansion (either rapid or slow) in an effort to enhance the

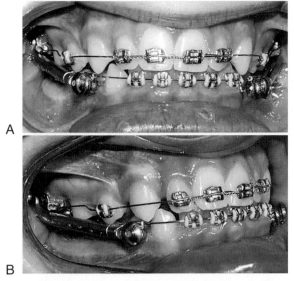

A

B

**Figure 35-3**  The Herbst appliance is a fixed appliance that uses a pin and tube apparatus to reposition the mandible into a more forward position. **A,** This class II patient demonstrates a near class I occlusion. **B,** Used in conjunction with fixed appliances, some of the dental effects can be more readily controlled.

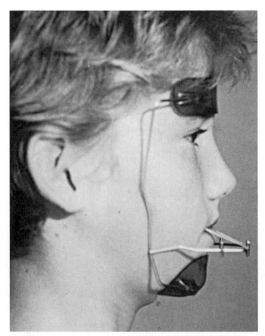

**Figure 35-4**  The class III maxillary deficient patient is treated by using a reverse pull headgear or facemask to exert anteriorly directed force on the maxilla. The force is provided by rubber bands extending from the facemask to intraoral hooks or wires.

transverse coordination of the arches or to facilitate anterior movement of the maxilla due to alteration of the bony interfaces with other skeletal structures. A comparison of clinical studies found that less maxillary incisor movement occurs when expansion accompanies protraction.[26] Timing of this treatment has been controversial. Some authors believe that the ideal time to attempt this treatment is soon after eruption of the permanent incisors, whereas others have waited a bit longer. Clearly, postpubertal treatment is not indicated for growth modification.[9] Data indicate that there is little anteroposterior difference in treatment effect whether treatment is applied early or late as long as the treatment is completed before 10 years of age.[2,26,35] Unfortunately, the longterm success of maxillary protraction is not clear. One fact appears to be emerging: mistaken diagnosis or treatment in patients whose class III malocclusion is the result of mandibular protrusion will usually fail.

Functional appliances designed to stimulate maxillary growth do not seem to be effective. The improvement in facial profile obtained by using these appliances in patients with very minor class III problems is usually the result of a downward and backward rotation of the mandible. The occlusion improves as a result of facial tipping of the maxillary incisors and lingual tipping of the lower incisors

### Class III Mandibular Protrusion

Class III mandibular protrusion has been historically managed with chin cup therapy (Fig. 35-5). The theory of chin cup therapy is to apply a distal and superior force through the chin that inhibits or redirects growth at the condyle. Again, studies in animals have shown some change in absolute mandibular size, but clinical application in humans routinely has been less successful.[45,46] The typical short-term treatment response to chin cup therapy is a distal rotation of the mandible and lingual tipping of the lower incisors. Therefore, chin cup therapy is well tolerated in patients with mild mandibular protrusion and short to normal vertical proportions. It is contraindicated, however, in a person with a long lower face because the anteroposterior correction would come at the expense of an increased vertical dimension. The long-term results of chin cup therapy indicate that although a transient positive change can occur, the long-term results are difficult to differentiate from those in untreated patients.[46]

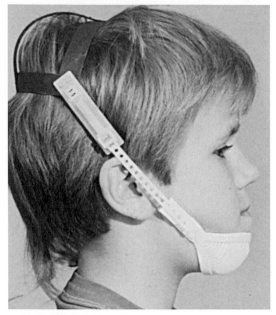

**Figure 35-5** The class III mandibular protrusive patient has historically been treated with chin cup therapy. The chin cup was designed to apply a distal and superior force through the chin to inhibit growth at the condyle. In clinical practice, this device has not proved to be routinely successful, although chin cup therapy does cause a distal rotation of the mandible. Therefore, the chin cup may be useful for managing mild mandibular protrusion in which the vertical proportions are short to normal.

Functional appliances designed for the management of class III mandibular excess show the same minor changes as those occurring in class III maxillary deficiency.

## Growth Modification Applied to Transverse Problems

The most common transverse problem in the preadolescent is maxillary constriction with a posterior crossbite. Management of maxillary constriction can begin as soon as the problem is discovered if the child is mature enough to accept treatment. Treatment has the potential to eliminate crossbites of the succedaneous teeth, increase arch length, and simplify future diagnostic decisions that can be complicated by functional shifts. Most clinicians agree with the philosophy of early correction if there is a mandibular shift. Generally, it is believed that long-term facial asymmetry attributable to soft tissue enlargement can result from untreated mandibular shifts. Regardless of philosophy, treatment prior to

adolescence and midpalatal suture bridging is recommended.

Three appliances can be used to correct the constriction, but the appliances are not interchangeable. In Chapter 27, the quad helix and the W arch for management of maxillary constriction are described. The appliances provide both skeletal and dental movement in the 3- to 6-year-old child.[5] As the patient gets older, more dental change and less skeletal change occur. This is true because the midpalatal suture, which was open at an early age, has developed bone interdigitation that makes it difficult to separate. More force is required to separate the suture after initial interdigitation of the suture to obtain true skeletal correction than a quad helix or W arch can deliver.

In the older preadolescent patient, in whom there is a chance that the midpalatal suture is closed, an appliance that can deliver large amounts of force is necessary to correct the skeletal constriction.[18] Rapid palatal expansion is the term given to the procedure in which an appliance cemented or bonded to the teeth is opened 0.5 mm/day to deliver 2000 to 3000 g of force (Fig. 35-6). In the active phase of treatment, there is little dental movement because the periodontal ligament has been hyalinized, which limits dental movement, and the force is transmitted almost entirely to the skeletal structures. During retention, however, the skeletal structures begin to relapse toward the midline. Because the teeth are held rigidly by the appliance, they move relative to the bones. Depending on the amount of expansion needed, active treatment normally takes 10 to 14 days. Another approach to skeletal expansion is slow rather than rapid palatal expansion.[20] Essentially the same appliance is used as in rapid palatal expansion, although force levels are calibrated to provide only 900 to 1300 g of force. Coupled with a slower activation rate, slow palatal expansion widens the palate by dental and skeletal movement. Although the final position of the teeth and supporting structures is approximately the same in rapid and slow expansion, proponents of slow expansion maintain that slower expansion is more physiologic and stable. Transverse growth modification also can be accomplished by means of acrylic or wire buccal shields attached to functional appliances or lip bumpers. The buccal shields relieve the teeth and alveolar structures from the resting pressure of the cheek muscles and soft tissues. Transverse

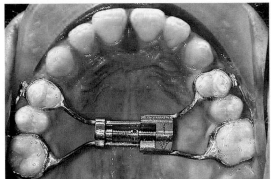

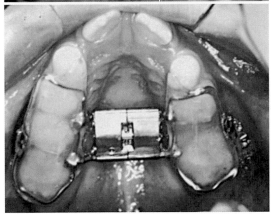

**Figure 35-6**   Rapid palatal expansion is used to treat maxillary constriction and posterior crossbite when there is a chance that the midpalatal suture is partially closed. The jackscrew in the appliance provides approximately 2000 to 3000 g of force when it is opened 0.5 mm/day. Depending on the amount of expansion needed, the appliance is normally activated two times each day for 10 days to 2 weeks. The appliance can be either (**A**) cemented on the teeth with orthodontic bands or (**B**) bonded to the teeth.

expansion of 3 to 5 mm can be achieved, although the changes vary considerably. Whether the movement is dental or skeletal and whether it will remain stable remains in question because there are no controlled experimental studies to provide answers.

## Growth Modification Applied To Vertical Problems

Vertical skeletal problems are manifested as long and short facial heights and usually are located below the palatal plane.[14] The short-faced person has a reduced mandibular plane angle and under-erupted teeth. In the long-faced patient, the mandibular plane angle, lower facial height, and amount of dental eruption are increased in comparison with the patient with a normal face. Vertical skeletal problems can be managed with growth modification techniques, and some can be managed successfully; however, even when the treatment has been successful, maintaining the correction is extremely difficult. The face grows vertically for a long time, and there is a tendency for the original growth pattern and problem to recur.

### Vertical Excess
Vertical skeletal excess may be managed with extraoral force, intraoral force, or a combination of the two. Extraoral force is delivered by means of a high-pull headgear through the maxillary first molars. The force is applied in a superior and distal direction and is designed to inhibit vertical development of the maxilla and eruption of the posterior maxillary teeth[16] (Fig. 35-7). Because no force is applied to the mandibular teeth, they are free to erupt and compensate for the reduced vertical development in the maxilla. In some cases, this compensatory eruption can eliminate all the positive effects of the high-pull headgear and lead to downward and backward rotation of the mandible instead of forward mandibular projection.

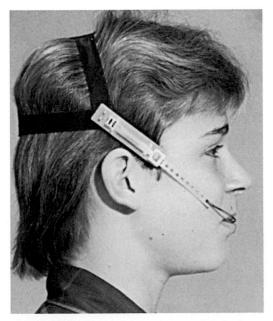

**Figure 35-7**   The patient with vertical skeletal excess is often treated with high-pull headgear. The force, generated by the strap resting on the head, is applied in a superior and distal direction and is intended to inhibit vertical development of the maxilla and eruption of the maxillary posterior teeth.

An alternative method for controlling vertical development is to block the eruption of the maxillary and mandibular teeth. A functional appliance can be designed that will force the mandible open to an increased vertical rest position. The force of the mandible attempting to return to its original vertical rest position is transmitted to the maxilla and the teeth in both arches. This results in mandibular growth being directed forward because no dental eruption has occurred to increase the vertical dimension and less increase in lower and total face height[22] (Fig. 35-8). To supplement the skeletal treatment effect on the maxilla, headgear can be attached to the functional appliance so that the headgear and the functional appliance can be worn at the same time[30,40] (Fig. 35-9). Developments in rare-earth magnets may also prove to be of value in restricting vertical facial development. Magnets placed to repel each other in each arch may provide enough force to restrict vertical eruption and skeletal growth.[29] By whatever means with which vertical excess is managed, excellent patient cooperation is necessary because treatment must be continued or retained as long as the patient is growing.

### Vertical Deficiency

Vertical skeletal deficiencies can be managed with either headgear or functional appliances, depending on the accompanying anteroposterior rela-

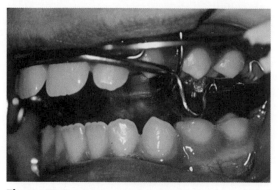

**Figure 35-9**    In some cases, a headgear tube is added to a functional appliance such as the one described in Figure 35-7. This tube allows the patient to wear the functional appliance and the high-pull headgear at the same time to further restrict vertical skeletal and dental growth.

tionships. The force vector from the headgear should direct the maxilla distally and extrude the maxillary posterior teeth, which would require cervical pull headgear. Because functional appliances are typically designed to inhibit eruption of upper and lower anterior teeth and promote eruption of the posterior teeth, they can also increase vertical facial height. As in vertical skeletal excess, the original growth pattern tends to recur until growth is complete, and retention should be designed to prevent this recurrence.

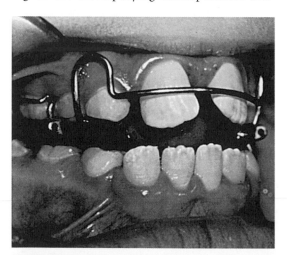

**Figure 35-8**    Vertical skeletal excess also can be managed with a functional appliance designed to inhibit eruption of the maxillary and mandibular teeth. The appliance is constructed in such a way that the mandible is placed in an open posture in an increased vertical position. The force of the mandible attempting to return to its normal, more closed vertical position is transmitted to the maxilla and to the teeth in both arches.

## DENTAL PROBLEMS

### Space Maintenance

A philosophy for space maintenance and the appliances recommended for the primary dentition are discussed in Chapter 25. The same philosophy and appliances apply to space maintenance in the 6- to 12-year-old age group. However, treatment for early loss of primary teeth in the mixed dentition requires some additional thought and consideration. Loss of posterior teeth in the primary dentition is a nearly universal indication for space maintenance therapy. In the mixed dentition, the timing of permanent tooth eruption, timing of tooth loss, presence of succedaneous teeth, and extent of crowding must also be taken into account.

Premature loss of a primary molar at a very early age delays the eruption of the permanent tooth. On the other hand, premature loss of a primary molar at an age near the time of normal eruption of the succedaneous tooth may actually accelerate the eruption of the permanent tooth and make space maintenance unnecessary. In general, eruption of the permanent premolar will be delayed if the primary molar is lost before age 8, whereas the premolar will tend to erupt earlier than normal if the primary molar is lost after age 8. A more accurate method of determining delayed or accelerated eruption of permanent teeth is to examine the amount of root development and alveolar bone overlying the unerupted permanent tooth from panoramic or periapical films. The succedaneous tooth begins to actively erupt when root development is approximately one half to two thirds completed. In terms of alveolar bone coverage, roughly 6 months should be anticipated for every millimeter of bone that covers the permanent tooth. If it is apparent that the tooth will be delayed in erupting and the space is adequate, space maintenance is absolutely indicated. Because space loss usually occurs within the first 6 months after the premature loss of a primary molar, space maintenance should be undertaken unless the tooth is expected to erupt within 6 months or unless there is enough space in the arch that a 1- or 2-mm space reduction will not compromise eruption of the permanent tooth.

A second factor to consider is the amount of time that has elapsed since the primary tooth was lost. At one extreme is the case of a primary molar scheduled for extraction. At the other extreme is a primary molar already missing for 6 months or longer. In the first case, space maintenance is certainly indicated to prevent space loss when the tooth is extracted. In the second case, the majority of space loss has already occurred, and space maintenance may not be indicated. The clinician should complete space and profile analyses and make a decision based on those findings. If there is excess space in the arch or if so much space has been lost that extraction of permanent teeth is inevitable, space maintenance is contraindicated. A space maintainer is indicated to prevent any more space loss if the space remaining is only marginally adequate to allow the permanent tooth to erupt. As always, there is little if any rationale for maintaining inadequate space.

The absence of a permanent successor also complicates space maintenance in the mixed dentition. The second premolar is the most commonly missing posterior tooth in the permanent dentition, excluding the third molars. If the primary second molar is lost prematurely, the clinician must make a decision about the space that would have been occupied by the missing second premolar. Two choices can be made. One alternative is to maintain space in the arch and eventually construct a fixed prosthesis or have an implant placed and restored. This is most feasible if the skeletal and dental relationships are class I, there is no crowding, and there is good interarch occlusion. This is an even more inviting alternative if only one of the premolars is missing (i.e., a unilateral missing premolar). The advent of resin-bonded bridges and intraosseous implants has made this option more popular. Another alternative is to allow or encourage the space to close. Factors that favor this solution include crowding in the arch, protrusive incisors and lips, bilateral missing premolars, and possibly other missing teeth. This topic is addressed in more detail later in this chapter.

The amount of crowding in the arch is an important factor in the decision about space maintenance, and it is predicted from the space analysis and put in perspective by the facial form analysis. If the incisor position is normal and there is adequate space or minor crowding in the arch, space maintenance should be initiated. However, early loss of a primary molar in an arch with substantial crowding must be considered carefully. Space maintainers alone will not solve a problem of this magnitude. Either permanent teeth will have to be extracted or the arches will have to be expanded. Expansion is possible only if the incisor position is normal or retrusive and the periodontal health is good enough to allow the incisors to be moved facially. If expansion is contemplated, space maintainers should be placed. In some cases, however, crowding of this magnitude is managed by extracting two first premolars and closing the remaining space orthodontically.

If no space maintenance is implemented and tooth movement results from drifting prior to first premolar extractions, less space remains to be closed later. Consultation with a specialist is usually desirable before this type of decision is made. If the crowding approaches 10 mm/arch, space maintainers may be needed even though permanent tooth extraction is inevitably required. The average width of a premolar is approximately 7 mm; therefore, the extraction of two premolars would effectively result in a gain of 14 mm of arch length. If more space is lost in an arch that is already severely crowded, a two-premolar extraction may not resolve all of the crowding. Space maintainers would ensure that no further decrease in arch length occurs. In some instances, timed extraction (called serial extraction) can alleviate the crowding and relieve the demands of subsequent orthodontic treatment.

Probably the most significant difference between space maintenance strategy in the mixed dentition and that in the primary dentition is bilateral loss of teeth in the mandibular arch. In the primary dentition, two band and loop appliances are indicated; in the mixed dentition, the lingual arch is preferred if all lower incisors have erupted. Primary second molars or permanent first molars may be used as abutment teeth. If oral hygiene is a problem, it is recommended that primary second molars be banded. This is done so that if decalcification under bands occurs as a result of poor oral hygiene, it occurs on teeth that will eventually exfoliate.

Space maintenance in the mixed dentition requires close supervision as permanent teeth erupt and primary teeth exfoliate. When primary abutment teeth exfoliate, an appliance may have to be remade, using permanent teeth as abutments. Space-maintaining appliances obviously should be removed when the permanent tooth erupts into its proper position.

## Potential Alignment and Space Problems

### Ectopic Eruption

Problems associated with ectopic eruption of the permanent first molar have been discussed previously in Chapter 30. A 3- to 6-month observation period usually is the best initial therapy if the resorption is not too severe because there is a possibility that the molar will self-correct spontaneously or "jump" distally and erupt into its normal position (Fig. 35-10). Intervention is necessary if the molar is still blocked from erupting at the end of the observation period or if the permanent molar is severely impacted.[25] The goal of treatment is to move the ectopically erupting tooth away from the tooth it is resorbing, allow it to erupt, and retain the primary second molar.

If a small amount of movement is needed and little or none of the permanent molar is clinically visible, a piece of 20-mil brass wire can be passed around the contact between the permanent molar and the primary second molar. The brass wire is tightened every 2 weeks. When the wire is tightened, the periodontal ligament space is com-

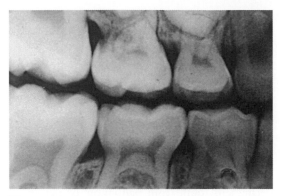

**Figure 35-10**    This radiograph illustrates the ability of an ectopically erupting permanent first molar to self-correct spontaneously. Note that the distal root of the primary maxillary second molar has been resorbed. Usually this type of resorption is the result of an erupting permanent molar that is caught on the distal aspect of the primary molar. If the resorption does not progress too far, the permanent molar usually "jumps" past the resorptive defect in 3 to 6 months.

pressed and the molar is forced distally until it can slip past the primary molar and erupt (Fig. 35-11). In some cases, a steel spring clip separator may be used to dislodge the molar, but only in cases in which there is minimal resorption of the primary molar. It may be difficult to seat the spring if the contact point between the molars is below the cementoenamel junction of the primary molar. Some authors advocate elastomeric separators, but they must be carefully supervised because they may dislodge in an apical direction, causing a periodontal abscess. Some elastomeric separators are not radiopaque and can be difficult to locate in the gingival sulcus.

A second method of moving the permanent molar distally is to band the primary second molar and apply a distal force to the permanent molar through a helical spring or elastomer (Fig. 35-12). In fact, a type of band-and-spring appliance can be constructed at chairside using the orthodontic archwire tube on a molar band and easily activated intraorally at subsequent appointments. These methods require that the occlusal surface of the permanent molar be visible so that force can be applied to move the tooth distally. A small ledge of resin or a metal button can be bonded to the occlusal surface to serve as the point of force application, or the end of the spring can be bonded directly to the impacted tooth. However, salivary contamination of the occlusal surface sometimes makes bonding a frustrating

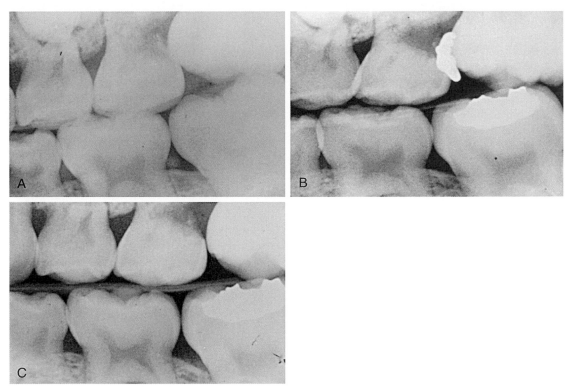

**Figure 35-11    A,** This radiograph shows an ectopically erupting permanent maxillary left first molar. **B,** Because only a small amount of movement is required to correct the ectopic eruption, a piece of 20-mil brass wire is slipped around the contact point between the permanent molar and the primary second molar and is tightened. **C,** After the wire has been tightened three times at 2-week intervals, the molar is dislodged and begins to erupt into a normal position. (From Fields HW, Proffit WR: Orthodontics in general practice. In: Morris AL, Bohannan HM, Casullo DP, editors. *The Dental Specialties in General Practice.* Philadelphia, Saunders, 1983.)

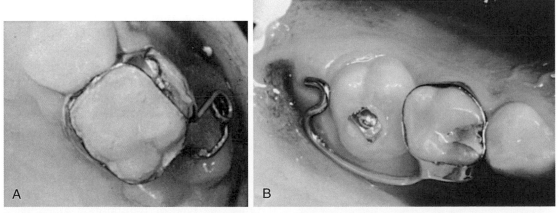

**Figure 35-12    A,** A band and helical spring appliance is used to treat an ectopically erupting permanent molar that requires a large amount of movement. The primary second molar is banded, and a helical spring is soldered to the band. A small ledge of composite resin, a metal button bonded to the occlusal surface of the permanent molar, or a small preparation can serve as a point of force application. The spring is reactivated at monthly intervals until the permanent molar is dislodged. (From Fields HW, Proffit WR: Orthodontics in general practice. In: Morris AL, Bohannan HM, Casullo DP, editors: *The Dental Specialties in General Practice.* Philadelphia, Saunders, 1983.) **B,** Another band and spring design with a metal button bonded to the occlusal surface of the erupting permanent molar. Elastomeric chain or thread is attached from the button to the distal hook on the wire and changed monthly to provide the distal force to dislodge the molar.

and difficult procedure. Such a band-and-spring appliance should be evaluated every 2 weeks and can work effectively in a short time because of the minimal root development on the permanent molar.

Occasionally, the primary second molar must be removed if the permanent molar has caused extensive resorption of the primary root structure. In these cases, loss of arch length is certain, and some plan of treatment for the impending space deficiency should be considered in advance (Fig. 35-13). If there is a congenitally missing second premolar or premolar extraction followed by space closure is being considered because of the crowding, then reduction in arch length by mesial movement of the molars is advantageous. To manage the space after extraction of the primary molar, a distal shoe can be placed to guide eruption of the permanent molar (see Figs. 25-8 and 25-9). A distal shoe maintains space but does not regain much space lost prior to the primary molar extraction. An alternative plan is to allow the permanent molar to erupt and then regain the space with a space-regaining appliance (described subsequently). After the space is regained, a space maintainer should be placed.

Ectopic eruption of lateral incisors is usually an early indication of crowding but may only be the result of aberrant tooth positioning. If a

primary canine exfoliates prematurely as a result of ectopic eruption, the lower incisors typically drift to that side of the arch, creating a midline discrepancy. If the laterals cause resorption and exfoliation of both primary canines, the incisors usually tip lingually and decrease arch length. When this happens and the incisors align, it appears that the space problem is corrected because the incisor alignment usually improves, but this is only temporary, and the space shortage will become apparent again when the permanent canines begin to erupt. Whether the loss of primary canines is unilateral or bilateral, the clinician should determine whether there is an arch length inadequacy and assess anteroposterior lip and incisor position. This information helps determine whether space maintenance, space regaining, or more extensive treatment is needed.

The goal of treatment should be to prevent a midline shift and manage the space according to the long-term plan. This can be accomplished by placing a lingual arch with a soldered spur distal to the lateral incisor to hold the midline if adequate space is present and the incisors are in a good position. If the midline has already shifted, the contralateral primary canine can be removed to promote spontaneous midline correction. If space loss cannot be tolerated due to lingual incisor tipping, a lingual arch should be placed following extraction. If there is sufficient crowding so that space maintenance is contraindicated, or if the incisors are considered too protrusive to be maintained in this position, no lingual arch should be placed following the extraction of the contralateral primary canine. In situations in which both canines exfoliate prematurely because of ectopic eruption, similar treatment decisions should be made, although the clinician does not normally have to worry about a midline shift.

### Transposition

Early transposition can be addressed during the mixed dentition and provides an opportunity to intercept a developing problem. As mentioned earlier, the type of transposition amenable to early treatment is most commonly encountered in the mandibular arch. The lateral incisors resorb either the primary canine or primary canine and first molar (Fig. 35-14, A). They rotate as they erupt, so treatment includes repositioning them mesially and derotating them. If this is accomplished prior to canine eruption, transposition can be avoided (Fig. 35-14, B).

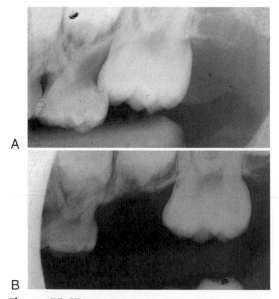

A

B

**Figure 35-13** **A,** In some cases, ectopic eruption causes extensive resorption of the primary tooth root. **B,** That can lead to tooth loss and mesial migration and reduced arch length. Treatment planning might include space regaining or permanent tooth extraction.

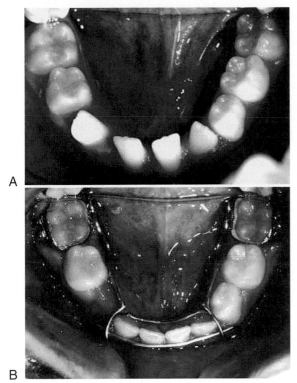

A

B

**Figure 35-14** **A,** Early transposition can cause loss of the primary canine and primary canine and first molar as it has in this patient. **B,** Correction with banded and bonded appliances has prevented true transposition.

### Impacted Teeth

The most common site of impacted teeth in the mixed dentition is in the maxillary canine region. These teeth often erupt in a mesial direction and become impacted in the palate or resorb the permanent canine roots.[12] This problem is often diagnosed because there is no bulge on the facial alveolus in the canine area at approximately 9 or 10 years of age.[28] If this finding is followed up with an occlusal radiograph, the true position of the canines relative to the lateral incisors is evident. This radiographic method appears to provide a better gauge of the true canine position than a panoramic radiograph but in conjunction with a panoramic radiograph will help localize the canine facial or lingual relative to the adjacent teeth (see Chapter 30 for details). If the permanent canine overlaps less than half of the lateral incisor root, there is some hope of redirecting the canine distally simply by timely extraction of the primary canines[13] (Fig. 35-15). If there is more than this amount of overlap, redirection is less likely.

### Missing Permanent Teeth

The absence of permanent teeth creates many treatment problems for the clinician, and most treatment decisions of this nature are best made

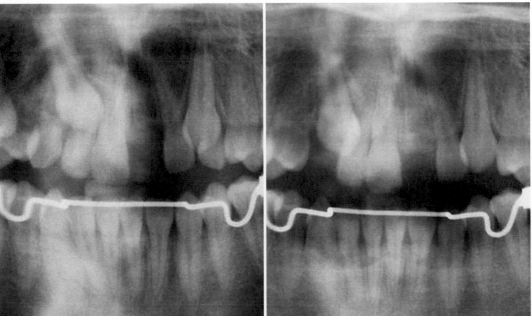

A                                                                      B

**Figure 35-15** **A,** Even though this patient has considerable mesial migration of the permanent maxillary right canine and it overlaps the entire lateral root, the primary canine was extracted in an attempt to redirect its eruption path. **B,** Note the distal movement of the permanent right canine with little overlap of the lateral incisor at follow-up.

by a specialist. The maxillary lateral incisor and the mandibular second premolar are the most common congenitally missing teeth in the permanent dentition, whereas anterior teeth, specifically the incisors, are often lost to trauma. Treatment decisions are based not only on which tooth is missing but also on arch length, adjacent tooth morphology and color, incisor position, and lip and profile aesthetics.

Treatment of congenitally missing maxillary lateral incisors varies depending on whether one or both incisors are absent and on the position of the permanent canine when it erupts into the arch. The canine either erupts into the normal canine position or resorbs the primary lateral incisor and spontaneously substitutes for the missing lateral incisor. If the canine erupts into its proper position, the primary lateral incisor will eventually have to be removed because it does not make an aesthetically pleasing substitute for the permanent lateral incisor and because the root will eventually be resorbed. The missing lateral

incisor can be replaced with a resin-bonded bridge, a conventional bridge, or an implant. A bridge or an implant is the treatment of choice when the occlusion, incisor position, and profile are nearly ideal and when closing space orthodontically is not appropriate (Fig. 35-16).

If the permanent canine erupts into the lateral incisor position, the primary canine must be extracted and the space closed, or the permanent canine moved back to the correct position and a bridge constructed or an implant placed for the missing lateral incisor. Crowding or protrusive incisors usually call for space closure and substitution of canines for lateral incisors (Fig. 35-17). These canines require recontouring by enamel removal and resin addition to improve the aesthetic appearance of the teeth. Canine substitution cases are considered difficult to treat well. A normal pretreatment occlusion favors canine retraction and bridge or implant placement as does short or wide canine crown morphology and dark canine color. These elements reduce the

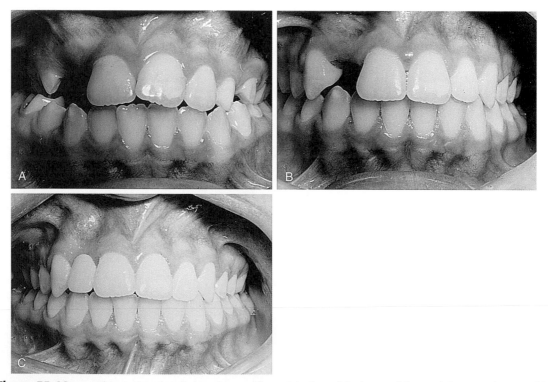

**Figure 35-16** **A,** This patient is missing the maxillary right lateral incisor and has a right posterior crossbite. Because the patient has class I molars and relatively good alignment, a decision was made to replace the missing lateral incisor prosthetically. **B,** At the end of treatment, a space identical in size to the left lateral incisor was created to replace the right lateral incisor. **C,** A right lateral incisor pontic was created by shaping a denture tooth to the appropriate width and length. Orthodontic wire is inserted into the pontic on the lingual surface and bent to fit the lingual surface of the canine and central incisor. The wire is bonded with resin to each abutment tooth. This type of restoration does not work with a deep bite because of the shearing force of occlusion on the lingual surface.

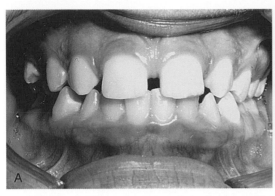
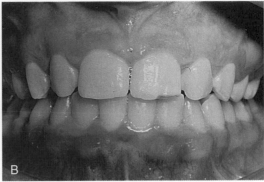

**Figure 35-17** **A,** This patient was missing both maxillary lateral incisors. A treatment plan was developed to bring the canines forward to substitute for the missing lateral incisors. **B,** At the end of treatment, the patient had class II molar and canine relationships because of the substitution. The patient elected not to reshape the canines to resemble lateral incisors.

chances of providing an aesthetic canine substitution for the lateral incisor. Even if the canine must be retracted, this is not without some virtue. The canine brought bone with it during its eruption, and this bone will enhance future aesthetics and potential implant placement.

When incisors are lost to trauma, usually the space is maintained and ultimately restorative or implant solutions are used when growth is completed and the risk of traumatic injury from sports is reduced.[47]

Another possibility is the use of transplanted posterior teeth, usually a premolar, into the position of the maxillary central incisor. With reshaping and either resin or veneer restoration, this option can be quite successful. Although not widely adopted in North America, in Scandinavian countries posterior tooth transplantation is a real option.[11]

Arch length, incisor position, and facial appearance must be thoroughly evaluated before a treatment plan is generated when a premolar is congenitally missing. Unlike primary canines and laterals, a primary molar may be a reasonable substitute for a missing premolar. The size, shape, and restorative status of the primary molar give some indication of the possibility of maintaining the tooth for a period of time (Fig. 35-18). Ankylosis and advanced root resorption indicate that the primary molar should be removed. Most clinicians favor removing the primary molar and closing the space orthodontically (Fig. 35-19), but in certain situations a resin-bonded bridge, conventional bridge, or implant may be a more ideal treatment (Fig. 35-20). These situations occur most likely in class I skeletal and dental patients with ideal or nearly ideal occlusions or when a tooth is missing unilaterally.

If the arch is so crowded that teeth must be extracted, or if the incisors are too protrusive or the profile too full, the retained primary molar should be removed and the case treated in a manner similar to that for a four-premolar extraction case. Typically, first premolars are removed in an extraction case, but the majority of congenitally missing premolars are second premolars. If it can be determined that the second premolar is missing and that extractions are necessary to resolve the arch length inadequacy, the primary molar can be removed early, allowing the space to close by mesial drifting of the permanent first molar and distal drifting of the anterior teeth. Unfortunately, congenital absence of the second premolar may not be definitively determined at an early age, and this delays the extractions. The longer the extractions are delayed, the less drifting and spontaneous space closure will occur. Using the space of the missing second premolars to reduce protrusion is much more complicated and requires the teeth to be retracted into the space of the missing teeth. This precludes dental drifting and should be planned by the specialist.

One further word of caution. If the primary molars are ankylosed and the permanent successor missing, then the primary molars should be extracted before the vertical bony discrepancy of the alveolus becomes too great (Fig. 30-21). This may require subsequent space maintenance, but the loss of bony ridge will be minimal and the maintenance of good bony contours for the adjacent teeth without periodontal defects will be

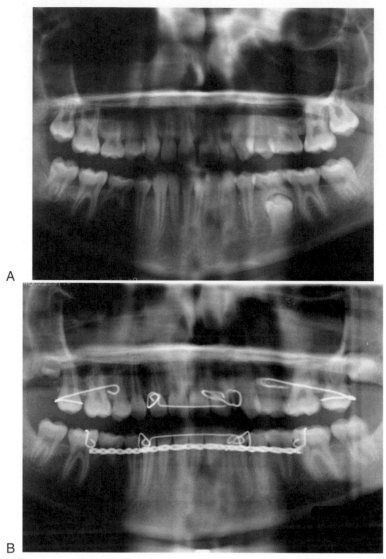

A

B

**Figure 35-18** In some cases retaining primary molars as an interim replacement for missing premolars is acceptable. Usually, the primary molars ultimately will require replacement. **A,** Patient with missing mandibular right second premolar and maxillary left second premolar. **B,** The mandibular right primary molar was retained, and the maxillary left space was closed orthodontically. Treatment took advantage of the predominant mesial drift in the maxillary arch. The radiopacities are the wires on the retainer.

improved. Later, implants or restorations can be placed, and in some cases the space can be closed orthodontically.

### Supernumerary Teeth

A supernumerary tooth may create space and eruption problems. It can cause permanent teeth to erupt into malalignment or even prevent eruption. Treatment is directed at minimizing the effect of the supernumerary tooth by immediate removal or observation and later removal. Management of the supernumerary varies depending on the size, shape, and number of supernumeraries and the dental development of the patient. Typically, the supernumerary is detected on a panoramic radiograph or an anterior occlusal film unless there is clinical evidence of an extra tooth at an earlier age. If the supernumerary is conical and is not inverted, there is a reasonable chance that it will erupt, at which time it should be removed (see Fig. 35-21). If the supernumerary is inverted, it may migrate superiorly away from the teeth and possibly into the nose. A tubercular-shaped tooth will not migrate but may, as with

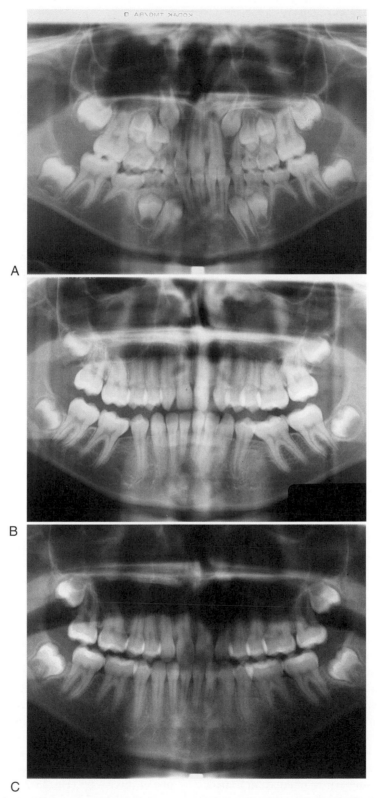

**Figure 35-19**   Closing the spaces that accompany missing teeth and avoiding prosthetic replacements are sometimes advantageous. **A,** This patient is missing maxillary lateral incisors and mandibular second premolars. **B,** The remaining primary teeth were extracted and allowed to drift. **C,** Orthodontics was completed and the teeth were finally positioned.

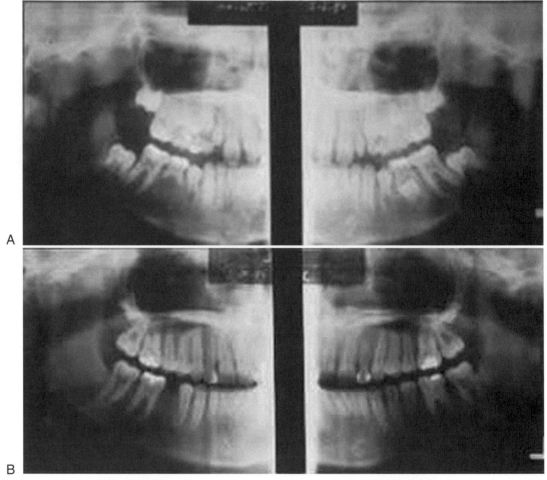

**Figure 35-20**  When permanent teeth are missing, often unilaterally, the best solution is to adjust the space and plan for prosthetic replacement. **A,** Due to the short roots and restorative status, the primary mandibular right second molar was extracted. **B,** The space was adjusted to accommodate a prosthetic replacement.

any supernumerary tooth, significantly impede eruption of the adjacent teeth. When multiple supernumerary teeth are present or if the supernumerary tooth fails to erupt, there is an increased chance of impeding the eruption of at least one tooth. In these cases, surgical removal makes sense (Fig. 35-22). Ideally, the surgery is timed so that removal of the supernumerary tooth does not interfere with permanent tooth development. The earlier the supernumerary can be removed, however, the more likely it is that the permanent teeth will erupt normally. Surgery to remove a supernumerary is often complicated, especially if there are multiple supernumerary teeth or if access to the supernumerary tooth is limited. These patients are appropriately referred to a specialist.

## Tooth Size Discrepancies

Isolated tooth size discrepancies can cause alignment problems. The maxillary lateral incisor commonly creates this type of problem because it is undersized or pegged in shape. Occasionally the lateral incisor can be restored to its normal size with composite resin and requires no other treatment. As discussed in Chapter 30, sometimes the pegged lateral needs a combination of tooth movement and restorative dentistry to achieve normal occlusion. Depending on the size of the discrepancy, the pegged lateral can be treated in one of three ways (Fig. 35-23).

If the lateral incisor is only slightly smaller than normal, the entire space can be closed (see Fig. 35-23, *A*). An alternative method for a marginally small incisor is to move the lateral incisor

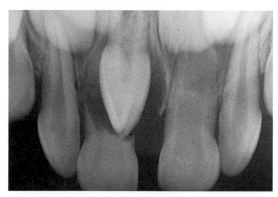

**Figure 35-21** A conical supernumerary in the maxillary central incisor region was detected during a radiographic examination after a traumatic injury to the maxillary anterior region. This supernumerary was not interfering with the normal eruption of the permanent incisors and was allowed to erupt before it was removed.

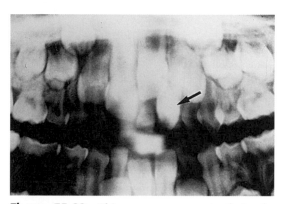

**Figure 35-22** This supernumerary tooth in the maxillary anterior region significantly affected the eruption of the permanent maxillary left central incisor. The supernumerary tooth was surgically removed, and the central incisor was moved orthodontically to the correct position.

orthodontically until it contacts the central incisor and leave space distal to the lateral (see Fig. 35-23, *B*). This solution is generally not aesthetically pleasing unless only a small space is left distal to the lateral and requires retention to hold the space. The canine usually is not brought forward to close the space because this would put the canine in an end-to-end relationship and disrupt the previously normal occlusion. A third solution, usually reserved for incisors that are considerably undersized, is a combination of orthodontic tooth movement and resin bonding to reshape the crown (see Fig. 35-23, *C*). The lat-

eral incisor should be positioned so that the resin addition will be cosmetically pleasing and will restore near-normal crown anatomy. This type of treatment is best performed by a specialist who has completed a diagnostic set up as described in Chapter 37 to plan the tooth movement and restorative requirements.

Occasionally, a single tooth will be extremely large, which will result in crowding and malpositioning of the teeth. In these cases, the tooth often can be reduced to match the contralateral tooth and repositioned.

Fusion and gemination in the permanent dentition are even more difficult to treat and should also be referred to a specialist. It is possible in some cases to divide fused permanent teeth, move one or both of the resulting teeth into good position, and then restore the remaining tooth or teeth.[49] It is quite possible that endodontic treatment will be required for the resulting teeth.

Dens evaginatus and incisor talon cusps provide interesting challenges in securing an ideal occlusion (Fig. 35-24). In most cases of dens evaginatus, a fine, thread-like pulp extends from the main pulp chamber into the evagination, and the location of this pulp tissue extension should be determined radiographically. Most such teeth in the posterior region do not require treatment because the force of mastication slowly wears the evagination down, and reparative dentin is formed. In the anterior region, however, the attrition must be accomplished mechanically with a hand piece and bur. A small amount of tooth structure is removed at each appointment, and after each session calcium hydroxide paste is applied to the exposed dentin to stimulate the reparative process. Usually the tooth can be treated at monthly appointments without permanent injury to the pulp. When treatment is complete, the exposed dentin is covered with a calcium hydroxide base and a resin restoration is placed.

### Alignment Problems

Anterior and posterior tooth irregularities with adequate space should be regarded as different from anterior and posterior space shortages. Tooth irregularity alone consists simply of rotated and tipped teeth in which there is no shortage of arch length when the leeway space is considered. Arch length discrepancies, that is, a true lack of space, also result in tooth irregularities, but are a

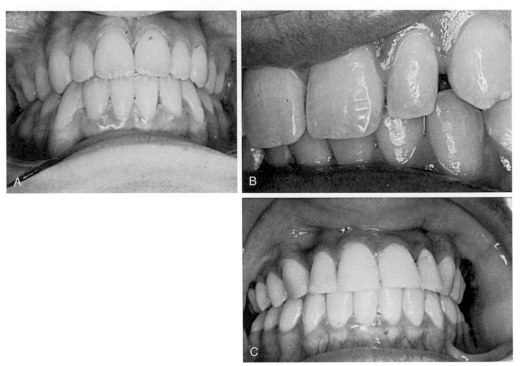

**Figure 35-23**  Isolated tooth size discrepancies such as a maxillary peg lateral can cause alignment problems that can be treated in one of three ways. **A,** If the lateral incisor is only slightly smaller than normal, the entire space is closed orthodontically. This leaves the patient with minimal overjet and overbite. **B,** An alternative is to move the lateral incisor until it contacts the central incisor and to leave space distal to the lateral incisor. The canine is not moved forward to close the space because it would place the canine in an end-to-end relationship and disrupt the occlusion. This alternative is generally not aesthetically acceptable unless only a small amount of space is left distal to the lateral incisor. **C,** A third solution is a combination of orthodontic tooth movement and resin bonding to reshape the crown of the tooth. The lateral incisor is positioned so that the resin addition is a aesthetically pleasing and restores near-normal crown anatomy. In this patient, two peg laterals were treated with orthodontic tooth movement and resin addition.

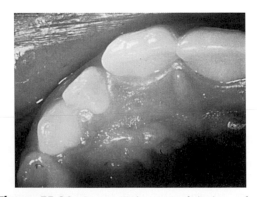

**Figure 35-24**  Dens evaginatus and incisor talon cusps create problems in the development of good occlusion. The talon cusp on this maxillary right lateral incisor has interfered with the normal positioning of the mandibular right lateral incisor.

different situation and require different management and timing.

*Appliance Considerations*
Tooth irregularities can be managed with either fixed or removable appliances. If a simple tipping force and no rotation are required to align the tooth, a removable appliance with a finger spring is an appropriate choice. A great variety of removable appliances exist; however, several essential components must be included in the design. The appliance must be retentive so that the force applied to the tooth will not dislodge the appliance. Adams clasps are often prescribed and are very retentive, although they require careful adjustment and may interfere with the occlusion. Other types of clasps, such as ball clasps and "C"

clasps, are also popular but provide distinctly less retention and flexibility. Multiple clasps should be used to enhance the retention. Additional retention and stability are gained from the palatal acrylic in maxillary appliances. A 22-mil helical finger spring incorporated into the palatal acrylic delivers a light, continuous force. The spring should be activated 2 mm to move the tooth approximately 1 mm/month (Fig. 35-25).

Fixed appliances can be used to correct irregularities and are indicated when bodily movement of teeth or rotational control is necessary. Orthodontic appliances have evolved to a point where specific brackets are designed for specific teeth. The brackets are constructed to provide proper crown and root positioning when they are precisely placed on the teeth. Before the appliances can be placed, the facial surfaces of the teeth selected for treatment are thoroughly cleaned with a prophy cup and fine pumice or pumice and a cotton roll (Fig. 35-26, A). Then the teeth are isolated with either cotton rolls or specially designed retractors to provide a field free of salivary contamination with optimal access (Fig. 35-26, B).

The conventional acid-etch technique can be used where etching solution or gel is painted on or applied to the facial surfaces of the teeth (Fig. 35-26, C). The solution is restricted to the area

that will eventually be covered by the bracket. After the enamel has been etched for 1 minute, the facial surfaces are thoroughly washed with water and dried (Fig. 35-26, D). If the enamel surfaces appear to be well etched (Fig. 35-26, E), a bonding agent is applied to the teeth, and the excess is blown away with an air syringe (Fig. 35-26, F). A composite resin designed specifically for orthodontic use is placed on a single bracket pad (Fig. 35-26, G). The resin may be an autopolymerizing two-paste system; a no-mix, one-step system; or a light-cured system. Currently light-cured resins provide the best control of the bonding process.

The bracket is placed on the tooth and moved into proper position (Fig. 35-26, H). Proper position is dictated by the manufacturer's specifications and is based on the long axis of the crown, the long axis of the root, or the incisal edge (Fig. 35-26, I). After the bracket is in position, it is firmly seated against the enamel surface with a scaler or explorer. The excess composite resin expressed from beneath the bracket pad is carefully removed (Fig. 35-26, J) before it is fully polymerized (Fig. 35-26, K). Removal of this excess flash ensures that the bracket slots can be fully engaged and also eliminates a source of plaque retention. This process is repeated until all the brackets have been properly placed. The archwire is place and ligated with steel ligatures or elastomeric modules to complete the bonding procedure (Fig. 35-26, L).

Recent development can lead to time savings when etch/conditioners are used. This one-step method achieves all tooth preparation in one step. The teeth are cleaned of debris and isolated as with the acid-etch method. The etch/conditioner liquid is mixed, dispensed from the package, and applied with an applicator (Fig. 35-27, A). The liquid is rubbed (as compared to painting with the acid etch method) with the applicator on the tooth surface for 5-7 seconds (Fig. 35-27, B) and gently air dried (Fig. 35-27, C). The next steps are similar to the acid-etch sequence for bracket placement, positioning, clean-up, polymerization, and archwire placement. The light-cured resin is applied on the bracket base, the bracket positioned, the excess removed and light cured. Using these newer methods and high-intensity curing lights greatly reduces bonding time.

The clinician should understand the physical properties of wires because a wire must be selected that is strong enough to withstand the

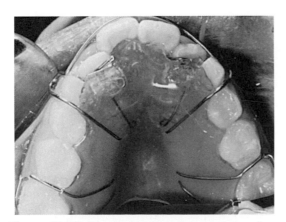

**Figure 35-25** Removable appliances can be used to manage alignment problems but are more effective for some problems than for others. Notice that the maxillary right lateral incisor can easily be tipped facially, but it is more difficult to rotate the left lateral incisor and requires use of the lingual finger spring and the labial bow in concert to create a movement. Generally, this type of movement is more efficient with a fixed banded and bonded appliance.

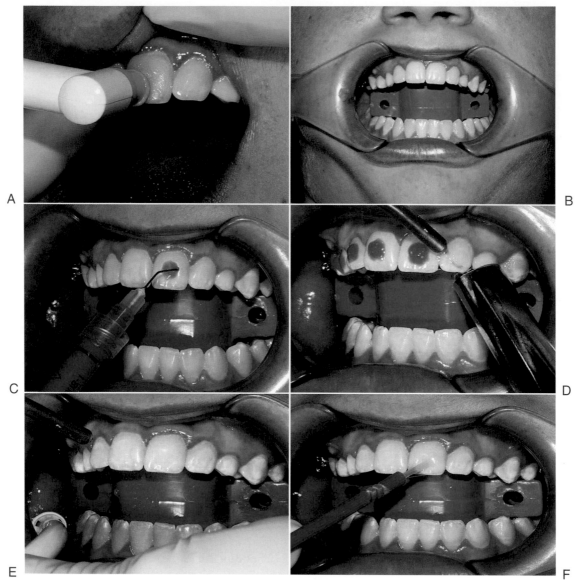

**Figure 35-26** Orthodontic appliances are designed to provide proper crown and root positioning when they are precisely placed on the teeth. Therefore, it is imperative to follow the appropriate sequence when placing the appliances. This is the sequence of steps when using an acid-etched and light-cured resin. **A,** Before the appliances are placed, the teeth selected for treatment must be thoroughly cleaned, preferably with pumice. **B,** After the teeth have been cleaned, they are isolated to provide a field free of salivary contamination. **C,** An etching solution or gel as shown here is painted on the facial surface of the teeth. **D,** The tooth is rinsed with water and dried (**E**) . **F,** The tooth is painted with a bonding agent.                                                                          *Continued*

force of occlusion in the posterior segments yet flexible enough in the anterior region to be deflected into the brackets and deliver a light, continuous force. Small stainless steel wires, some titanium alloys, and braided stainless steel wires usually provide ample strength and flexibility as an initial archwire. Occasionally, loops should be bent into the archwire to produce anterior flexibility and posterior strength. Retention is essential

after the correction of irregularity because the teeth have a strong propensity to relapse.

Gingival fibers reorganize very slowly following these types of movements, and in some cases irregularity returns even if retention is well conceived. Some clinicians have suggested that if the periodontium is healthy, a circumferential supracrestal fiberotomy may be performed to reduce relapse.

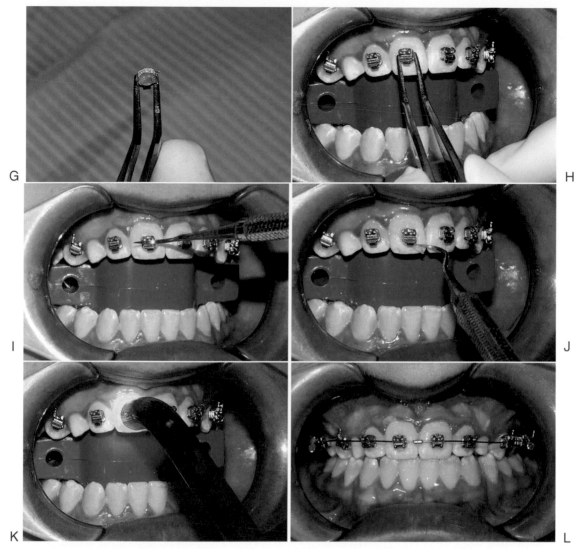

**Figure 35-26—cont'd**    (**G**) A small amount of resin is placed on the bracket pad. (**H**) The bracket is placed on the tooth. (**I**) The bracket is adjusted to the proper orientation with the tooth based on the long axis of the crown and root and height from the incisor edge. (**J**) The excess resin is cleaned up. (**K**) The resin is light cured. (**L**) An archwire is placed in the bracket and ligated with steel ligature ties or elastomeric ties.

When treatment is complete or nearly complete, the supracrestal gingival fibers are cut with a scalpel and a no. 12B blade under local anesthesia. Theoretically, the stretched gingival fibers will not need to reorganize but will reattach in a new position after being cut. Care should be taken if this procedure is used in patients with a thin gingival covering.

## Crowding Problems

The first sign of crowding in the mixed dentition usually coincides with eruption of the permanent incisors. Arch length insufficiency may manifest in several ways, ranging from slight incisor rotation and irregularity to gross incisor malalignment. The first step should be to perform a space analysis and determine the extent of the arch length inadequacy. This finding is then placed in the context of the facial profile analysis.

### Mild Crowding

Many children have a midline diastema in the mixed dentition, and this is considered a normal stage of development. Occasionally, a large midline diastema is present that is due to a mesiodens or other midline intrabony pathologic process, protruding incisors, or a tooth size problem. A

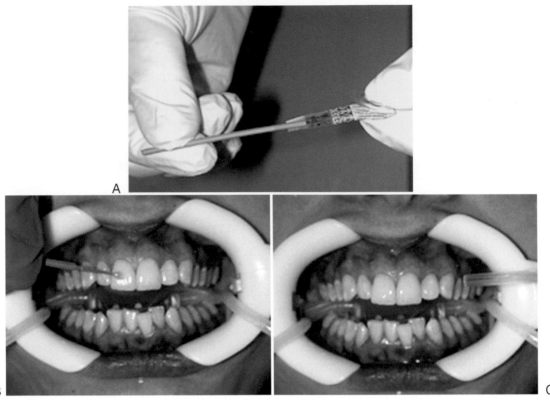

**Figure 35-27**  Recently, one-step tooth preparation has been developed to save time in the bonding process. This replaces the etch, rinse, dry steps. After the tooth is cleaned and dried, an etch/primer is used. **A,** The etch/ primer is combined in a special bubble "pop" dispenser. **B,** The one-step liquid etch/primer is rubbed on the tooth for several seconds. **C,** The preparation is lightly air dried. The tooth is now ready for the bracket and bonding resin to be applied.

diastema caused by a midline supernumerary tooth or abnormality is managed by removal of the supernumerary tooth or the abnormality. The supernumerary tooth should be removed as early as possible without causing injury to the adjacent permanent teeth. Early removal of the mesiodens allows the permanent teeth to erupt normally, and the space usually closes spontaneously.

In some cases, a large diastema may be due to faciolingual rather than mesiodistal positioning of the incisors. Flared incisors are cosmetically unappealing and are at greater risk of traumatic injury.[1] If the teeth can be tipped back into an ideal position to close the diastema and if the overbite will not hinder tooth movement, a removable appliance is recommended. The appliance is designed to include at least two clasps for retention: palatal acrylic and a 28-mil labial bow with adjustment loops (Fig. 35-28). The labial bow is activated to tip the incisors lingually by closing the adjustment loops. At the same time, acrylic must be removed from the lingual side of the appliance to permit tooth movement and

excess gingival tissue. The labial bow is activated approximately 2.0 mm/month until the diastema is closed and the teeth are in ideal position.

Fixed orthodontic appliances are suggested if the incisors are so protrusive that bodily movement is required to close the diastema or if the teeth are rotated. The molars are banded, and the incisors are bonded with orthodontic brackets (Fig. 35-29). The teeth are aligned initially if necessary with small, round archwires and then are retracted via a larger rectangular wire with closing loops or elastomeric chain (Fig. 35-30). Rectangular archwires are necessary to provide full control of tooth position during retraction. Headgear may be necessary to reinforce the molar anchorage at the same time because the molars have a strong tendency to come forward while the incisors are retracted. The choice of headgear is based on the vertical dimensions of the face.

If the diastema is due to a relative discrepancy between the upper and lower teeth of mandibular anterior excess tooth size, treatment usually requires the addition of resin to the interproximal

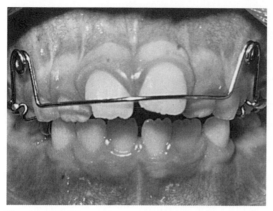

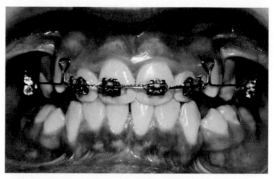

**Figure 35-29** When rotations are present or bodily movement is required to close space and retract incisors, the best alternative is a fixed appliance. The space closure is being accomplished using a looped archwire to provide the force to move the teeth.

**Figure 35-28** A large diastema that is due to excessively protruding incisors is sometimes managed with a removable appliance if the overbite will not interfere with retraction of the incisors. The appliance incorporates a labial bow with adjustment loops that are activated to tip the incisors lingually. By tipping the incisors lingually, both the diastema and the incisor protrusion are corrected.

surfaces of the maxillary incisors. Closing the space by means of orthodontic procedures only will eventually result in relapse because the occlusion will force the space open again.

Treatment to close a midline diastema not associated with an anteroposterior position or a tooth size problem is usually initiated if the diastema is significantly aesthetically objectionable, greater than 3 mm, or still present after the permanent canines have fully erupted. A diastema larger than 3 mm usually inhibits or disturbs eruption of the lateral incisors and should be closed before these teeth emerge. Both of these types of diastema are due to faulty mesiodistal

positioning of the incisors, but the choice of appliance is still based on the type of tooth movement required to close the space. If the central incisors can be tipped together to close the diastema, a removable appliance should be used. Finger springs are either incorporated into the palatal acrylic or soldered to the labial bow to engage the distal edge of the incisor crown (Fig. 35-31). The springs are activated at a rate of 2 mm/month, and closure should not take more than 2 months.

Brackets are bonded on the facial surface of the central incisors if the teeth require bodily mesiodistal movement or rotational control to close the diastema. After initial alignment, a large segmental or full rectangular archwire is placed in the brackets, and the teeth are moved together via elastomeric chain. The chain is attached only to the mesial wings of each bracket while the distal

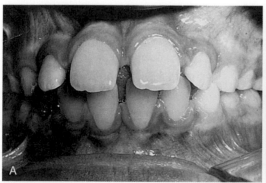

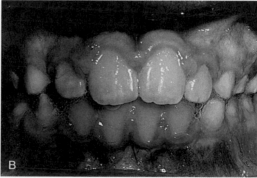

**Figure 35-30** **A,** Space, such as that shown here, is closed with either closing loops or elastomeric chain to retract the teeth. **B,** Retention is necessary to maintain space closure and is usually accomplished with a removable appliance. If the frenal attachment is thought to be the cause of the diastema, frenectomy can be completed at the end of the active appliance phase or during the retention phase.

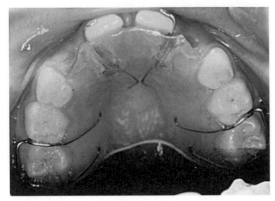

**Figure 35-31**    In this case, a midline diastema is due to the mesiodistal positioning of the maxillary central incisors. A removable appliance with finger springs incorporated into the palatal acrylic closes the space, tipping the teeth together. (From Fields HW: Treatment of nonskeletal problems in preadolescent children. In Proffit WR et al, editors. *Contemporary Orthodontics*. St Louis, Mosby, 1999.)

wings are ligated separately. This prevents the teeth from rotating when the space is closing (Fig. 35-32).

No matter which type of treatment is used to close a midline diastema, retention can be a problem and should be planned. In most cases, a removable appliance maintains the space closure. The appliance should be adjusted periodically if the diastema is closed before the lateral incisors and canines have erupted fully. If the diastema reopens during or following retention, the incisors should be realigned. At that time, a

surgical procedure, frenectomy, can be performed if the frenum is thought to be the cause of the diastema's reopening. The frenectomy is performed after the space is closed because the scar tissue created by the procedure may actually impede closure if the surgery is accomplished first. If the diastema again reopens following retention and the surgical procedure, a 17.5-mil multistranded wire can be bonded to the lingual surface of the incisors to keep the teeth together (Fig. 35-33). The only contraindications to a bonded wire retainer are an excessively deep bite and poor oral hygiene.

As mentioned earlier, children can have various amounts of irregularity without any real arch length shortage when the leeway space is included. Mild irregularity is even considered normal in patients who have no arch length discrepancy. Longitudinal studies of persons with ideal occlusions show that there is a period when up to 2 mm of transitional irregularity occurs early in the mixed dentition and eventually resolves.[36] Observation is usually the best course. Some patients have little or no overall arch length shortages and demonstrate noticeable crowding during incisor eruption. This is due to the larger permanent incisors and the transitional crowding they cause during the transition from the primary to mixed dentitions. Gianelly[17] has described these conditions and noted that a large percentage of patients with irregularity can be treated simply by protecting the leeway space with a lingual arch. If, on the other hand, the leeway space is left unattended, the molars will move anteriorly into

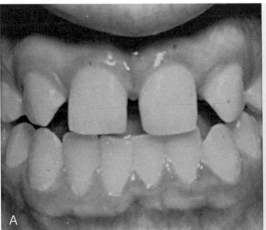
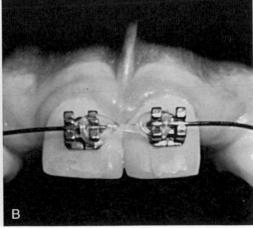

**Figure 35-32**    **A,** If bodily mesiodistal movement is needed to close a diastema, fixed appliances are placed on the teeth. **B,** After initial alignment, either a segmental or a full archwire is placed in the brackets, and the teeth are moved together with an elastomeric chain.

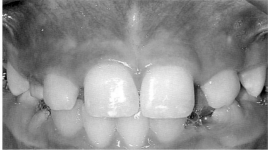

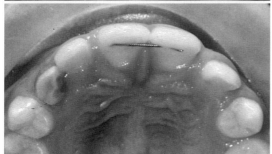

A

B

**Figure 35-33** **A,** Following diastema closure, retention is required. **B,** One method that reduces the need for patient cooperation is the light, multistranded bonded wire. The wire must be placed far enough gingivally to avoid occlusal interferences. In addition, the patient must clean the area carefully and avoid direct contact with hard foods.

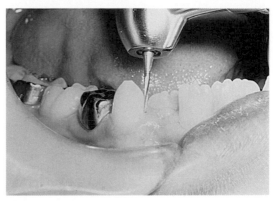

**Figure 35-34** When the arch length discrepancy is determined to be 2 mm or less and the lateral incisor is erupting lingual to its proper position, the primary canine can be disked with either a high- or low-speed handpiece or a hand-held strip. In this case, a tapered fissure bur in a high-speed handpiece is being used to disk the mesial surface of the primary canine.

the leeway space and a true arch length shortage will exist.

The clinical management of irregularity without a true arch length shortage can take several forms depending on the amount of irregularity. Generally, if the irregularity is minor, no treatment is indicated. If the irregularity is slightly more severe, interproximal stripping or disking of the primary teeth (usually the incisors and canines) can be accomplished to provide temporary space (Fig. 35-34). Disking may be accomplished with a hand-held strip, a sandpaper disk in a low-speed handpiece, or a tapered bur in a high-speed handpiece. The enamel-reducing instrument must be held vertically to reduce the true mesiodistal dimension of the tooth even subgingivally to be successful. The procedure is performed without anesthesia so that the child can indicate any discomfort. Extreme discomfort usually indicates that sufficient enamel has been removed to cause the pulpal tissues to react. Typically, careful disking yields 2 to 4 mm of space. A professional-strength topical fluoride preparation can be applied to the canines after disking and may reduce postoperative sensitivity. Note that in the mixed dentition, interproximal

reduction of permanent teeth before the eruption of the permanent canines and evaluation of the patient's tooth size is contraindicated. If teeth are prematurely reduced, an iatrogenic tooth size problem may be created.

If it is apparent that disking will not alleviate the anterior irregularity, it may be appropriate to extract the primary canines and place a lingual arch so that the available space can be used by the larger incisors for alignment and later the smaller premolars can erupt in the remaining space. For the most part, this therapy is undertaken in the mandibular arch, although there are a few situations in which it is indicated in the maxilla. A lingual arch is necessary because the lower incisors tend to tip lingually without the support of the primary canines. This results in shortening of arch length. In this situation, the lingual arch is placed in a passive state, that is, the arch exerts no force to move the incisors and increase the space. The clinician should communicate to the parent that this treatment requires close supervision and that the primary first molars may have to be disked or extracted when the permanent canines erupt. The lingual arch remains in place until the second premolars have erupted or until it is evident that there will be sufficient space for all the permanent teeth to erupt. Essentially, one is using the leeway space and controlling all available arch length to achieve alignment of the teeth (Fig. 35-35). In some cases, this means that the molars (those that are end-to-end) will not achieve a

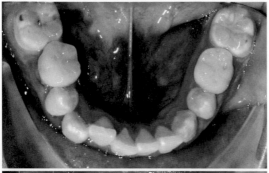

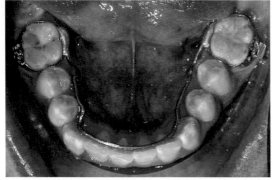

**Figure 35-35** Space that is available in the arches (leeway) can be used to alleviate crowding by maintaining space when crowding is present and allowing alignment when the larger primary second molars exfoliate or are extracted. **A,** This patient shows some crowding with the primary second molars in place. **B,** A lower lingual arch was placed so the leeway space could be used for spontaneous alignment.

class I relationship because the mandibular mesial molar shift has been prevented. Either headgear or interarch mechanics such as elastics will need to be used to achieve the correct occlusal relationships. In other situations, a class I molar relationship may have already been present and this is not a concern.

A true arch length discrepancy of 0 to 2 mm may not be apparent or may be manifested as a mild irregularity, most likely in the incisor region. Treatment may be indicated for these children if the lateral incisors erupt lingual to their proper position or in very irregular positions. If treatment is deemed necessary, interproximal stripping of primary teeth as described above may be used. With true, small arch length shortages, ultimately minor crowding will have to be accepted, permanent teeth will have to be reduced in the mesiodistal dimension, or the arch will have to be expanded with the appropriate fixed or removable appliances as described in the next section.

*Moderate Crowding*

Treatment for a moderate arch length discrepancy of less than 5 mm is based on the facial profile, incisor position, crowding, and the amount of facial keratinized tissue. If the profile is straight, with good anteroposterior or slightly retrusive position of the lips and incisors, a small amount of expansion can be tolerated to accommodate all the teeth. Expansion is not a good treatment option if the incisors are already protrusive. The clinician must always keep in mind the interaction between crowding, incisor position, and profile because they are essentially part of the same problem, expressed in a different way.

Moderate crowding may be localized or generalized. Localized crowding may be the result of space loss after extraction or premature exfoliation of a primary tooth. If space loss is 3 mm or less, the adjacent tooth usually can be tipped into proper position with a removable appliance, an active lingual arch, or a fixed banded and bonded appliance. For example, a removable appliance with a finger spring can tip a permanent maxillary first molar distally after removal of a primary second molar compromised by ectopic eruption (Fig. 35-36). Numerous other fixed appliances such as lingual holding arches or a Nance lingual arch supporting segmental arches and compressed coil springs can be used to move posterior teeth distally (Fig. 35-37). Regardless of the appliance configuration, the method is basically the same,

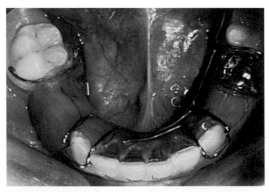

**Figure 35-36** Localized crowding is often the result of prematurely exfoliating primary teeth. In this case, the primary mandibular right second molar was lost prematurely, allowing the permanent first molar to drift mesially. A removable appliance has been designed to tip the permanent first molar back with a finger spring. The spring is activated until the molar is correctly positioned. Then a band and loop or lingual arch can be placed.

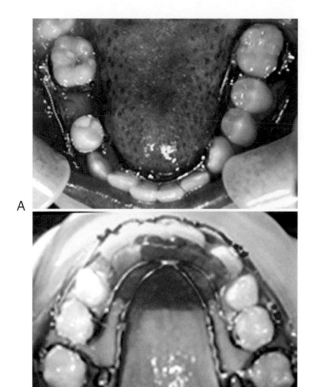

**A**

**B**

**Figure 35-37** A fixed appliance can be used to distalize molars in either arch. **A,** In this patient a lower lingual arch was used to support distal movement of the permanent molar with a coil spring. **B,** Bilateral distal molar movement can be used with palatal support. This fixed appliance uses a modified Nance palatal coverage and NiTi springs to generate the tooth moving force. Generally, some anterior incisor movement also occurs.

and these appliances can be used either unilaterally or bilaterally. The distal molar movement is accompanied by an anterior movement of the anchor or anterior segment.[7,8] Alternatively, headgear can be used if bilateral space regaining is desired. After the space has been regained, arch length should be near ideal and can be maintained. A band-and-loop appliance or a lingual arch type of appliance can be placed to maintain the space.

If localized crowding is not due to terminal molars drifting anteriorly but is located in the anterior or midportions of the arch, permanent tooth impaction is likely. Orthodontic tooth movement is necessary to increase the space and allow room for eruption (Fig. 35-38, *A, B*). Fixed orthodontic appliances are placed on a portion or the entire arch, and the arch is aligned with light, flexible archwires. After alignment, a heavy arch-

wire is placed to maintain good arch form during space-regaining movements. A compressed coil spring provides the force necessary to open the space. After the space has been opened, the tooth can erupt or it may be necessary to expose the crown of the tooth surgically if it does not erupt within a 6-month period. Surgical exposure of the crown requires the elevation and repositioning of soft tissue to provide adequate keratinized tissue around the impacted tooth. Adequate attached gingiva is essential for good periodontal support and aesthetic appearance. If the clinician is not well versed in surgical exposure, the patient is best referred to a specialist. When the crown is exposed, the tooth can be allowed to erupt or an orthodontic attachment is bonded to the crown, and the tooth is moved with traction into the arch (Fig. 35-38, *C–F*). Several methods can be used to generate the force to move the tooth occlusally, but using an overlay flexible wire (usually NiTi) is simple and effective. The overlay wire technique is an especially applicable technique for extruding traumatically intruded incisors so that they can be assessed and/or accessed for endodontic treatment because the method is simple, does not impinge on the adjacent tissue, permits easy cleaning, and allows reasonably efficient movement of teeth (Fig. 35-38, *G*).

Patients characterized by anterior or generalized crowding of less than 5 mm present difficult treatment decisions. As stated earlier, incisor and lip position provide important guides to whether arch length can be created by expansion. Upright or lingually inclined incisors may be moved facially into correct alignment if the lips are retrusive. However, the risk associated with generalized arch expansion is instability of the new position.[32,33] Movement of teeth facially may upset the existing equilibrium and cause relapse after the appliances are removed. Relapse does not occur in all cases; some patients maintain increased arch dimensions and remain stable after treatment is complete. However, there does not seem to be a good method for predicting stability.[31] Unfortunately, clinical judgment and long-term retention must be relied on in many cases.

If the clinician elects to alleviate arch length inadequacy by expansion (because the leeway space will not supply enough needed space), several approaches can be taken. An active lower lingual arch can be constructed with adjustment loops to tip the incisors facially if the overbite is not prohibitively deep to prevent movement of

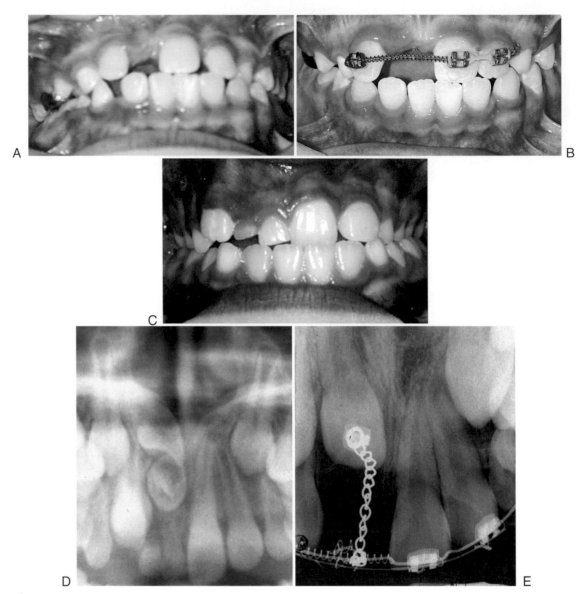

**Figure 35-38**    Many situations rely on the same principles for treatment of crowding in the anterior segment. Generally, the first step is to align and open space. **A,** This patient lost the maxillary right central incisor to trauma and subsequently space redistributed. **B,** The teeth were aligned with a segmental arch in the first phase of treatment and then a coil spring was used to open the space for the prosthetic replacement. **C,** The next step is surgery to remove any pathologic structures and gain access to the unerupted tooth. This patient has retained primary maxillary incisors, an unerupted central incisor, and supernumerary teeth. **D,** This radiograph confirms the problem. Note supernumerary central and lateral incisors. **E,** The next step is extrusion. Following removal of the supernumerary teeth, the unerupted tooth has a bonded bracket and chain attached so the forces can be delivered by the light overlay wire. *Continued*

the facial incisors (Fig. 35-39) and perhaps to move the molars distally a small amount. The adjustment loops, located mesial to the molars, should not be activated beyond 1 mm because the activation of such a large wire (36 mil) places extremely large forces on the teeth. When the appliance is properly activated, the wire contacts the tooth high on the cingulum of the incisors. The direction of force is apical, but it tips the incisors facially because of the inclination of the lingual surface of the teeth. In 4 to 6 weeks, the appliance can be activated another millimeter. This process is repeated until arch length is adequate for the permanent dentition. Primary

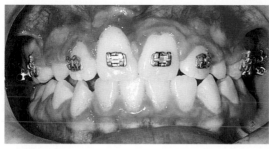
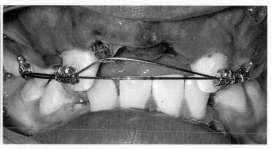

F        G

**Figure 35-38—cont'd**   **F,** The tooth in final position. Note the more gingival attachment on the extruded tooth. These levels should approximate one another with time. **G,** Extrusion with overlay wires can be used successfully following traumatic intrusion injuries. The overlay archwire, which is a light and flexible wire and now usually NiTi, is ligated with a stiffer supporting archwire, usually stainless steel. The light wire is engaged in the bracket and provides light continuous forces over a large range to rapidly and physiologically extrude the tooth.

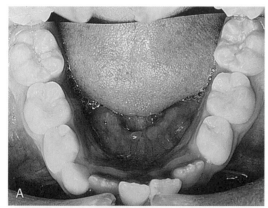

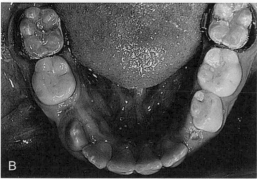

**Figure 35-39**   **A,** Generalized crowding of less than 5 mm is occasionally managed with an adjustable lingual arch if the overbite is not too deep to prevent facial movement of the mandibular incisors. The appliance is activated by opening the adjustment loops. In this case, a lingual arch was inserted after removal of the mandibular primary right canine. The canine was removed to keep the midline from shifting any further to the left. **B,** The same patient after 3 years of lingual arch therapy. The midline has shifted back to the right. The crowding is being managed by facial movement of the incisors and by use of the leeway space.

canines may have to be disked or removed as discussed previously if the crowding is in the anterior region.

A lip bumper, a wire appliance inserted in tubes on the lower molars, may be used to decrease lower lip pressure and achieve generalized arch expansion in the incisor, canine, and premolar regions (Fig. 35-40). The location of the expansion depends on the location of the lip bumper. The lip bumper removes resting pressure of the lips and cheeks from these teeth. The teeth move facially as a result of lack of lip pressure and the force of resting tongue pressure. The pressure from the lower lip may tip the molar distally.[37] Remember that ultimately both arches must be coordinated.

Arch expansion may also be accomplished via a functional appliance with buccal shields in the vestibule.[39] The buccal shields disrupt the equi-

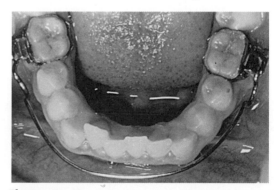

**Figure 35-40**   A lip bumper is also used to treat generalized crowding of less than 5 mm. The lip bumper is designed to decrease lower lip pressure on the teeth and to allow generalized expansion by facial movement of the teeth.

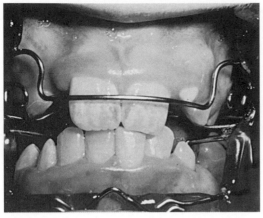

**Figure 35-41**    Generalized arch expansion can also be accomplished via a functional appliance with buccal shields. The buccal shields disrupt the equilibrium between the facial musculature and the tongue and allow the teeth to move facially.

librium between the tongue and the cheek and allow the teeth to move facially (Fig. 35-41). Some investigators claim that properly constructed buccal shields actually stretch the underlying periosteum of the bone and cause skeletal remodeling in the transverse dimension. Although this claim has not been substantiated by careful inves-

tigation, there is no doubt that enough expansion can be created in this manner to relieve minor to moderate crowding.

Like removable appliances, fixed (banded and bonded) appliances can be used to tip teeth. Fixed orthodontic appliances are necessary to increase arch length when bodily movement of teeth is required to alleviate crowding and align the teeth. Banded and bonded appliances also offer the opportunity to efficiently control rotational problems of teeth. A variety of archwire designs can be used to expand the arch depending on the number of teeth with attachments (Fig. 35-42). Clearly, any dimension of the arch can be altered with this method. After the expansion has been completed, a lower lingual arch is placed to retain the expansion.

In most cases, further treatment is necessary to align the remaining permanent teeth when they erupt. In addition, distal movement of the maxillary molars may be required if some of the leeway space was used to align the mandibular teeth and cannot be used for the mesial molar shift. When a class I molar relationship is present initially, this is not an issue. Therefore, multibonded appliances should be used sparingly, generally only in cases in which the molars are

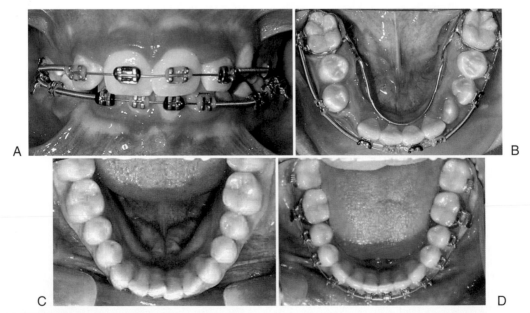

**Figure 35-42**    Expansion of the dental arches to reduce crowding can be accomplished with fixed appliances and is usually indicated when there are rotations or bodily tooth movement is required. **A,** Expansion during the mixed dentition using fixed appliances. **B,** The mechanics often are a combination of coil springs and elastomeric chains to move teeth and increase arch dimensions. A lingual arch can be used for maintenance of the intermolar dimension. **C,** Arch expansion can be accomplished during the permanent dentition years too. **D,** The anterior irregularities, mostly rotations, were managed with a fixed appliance.

already class I and there is some increased overjet, unless one is prepared to complete the case appropriately by adjusting the interarch relationships. Regardless of which appliance is selected, expansion is achieved at the expense of incisor position and profile.

### Severe Crowding

Crowding of more than 5 mm is considered severe. This amount of crowding is managed either with generalized arch expansion or with removal of selected permanent teeth. This degree of generalized arch expansion can be accomplished with different appliances but usually requires bodily tooth movement with fixed appliances. Achieving considerable expansion often is difficult. Incisor position, profile, and periodontal status all influence whether the patient should be treated without extraction. Patients with this degree of crowding are most appropriately referred to a specialist.

The decision to extract teeth is based on the factors listed previously and is further influenced by the location of the crowding, the position of the dental midline, and the dental and skeletal relationships of the patient. After careful case analysis, appropriate teeth may be removed to make subsequent tooth movement easier to accomplish and to minimize the effects of extraction on the profile. The permanent first premolar is most often selected for extraction because it is located at a midpoint in the arch and because the space it occupies can be used to correct midline problems, incisor protrusion, molar relationship problems, or crowding. Other teeth can be removed depending on the specifics of the case and the type of therapy used. Management of extraction cases is best performed by a specialist.

In some children, crowding is so severe in the mixed dentition that expansion is not feasible, and extractions are necessary to obtain a suitable occlusion that is in harmony with the supporting structures and the facial profile. In these cases, a planned sequence of extractions of primary and permanent teeth can benefit the patient by reducing incisor crowding and irregularity in the early mixed dentition, which will make subsequent orthodontic treatment easier and quicker. The extractions also make room for teeth to erupt over the alveolus and through keratinized tissue rather than being forced buccally or lingually into positions that may affect the periodontal health of the teeth. Guidance of eruption and serial extrac-

tion are terms used to describe this sequence of extractions.[21,27] Guidance of eruption was originally developed to manage severe crowding without orthodontic appliances but now is viewed as the first step in treatment culminating in fixed orthodontic appliance therapy. For this reason, the clinician should consult with a specialist before embarking on a planned extraction sequence.

Guidance of eruption should be considered an option when crowding is greater than 10 mm per arch, a measurement that should be confirmed by space analysis after the permanent lateral incisors have erupted. In addition, the patient should have a class I dental and skeletal pattern with good lip and incisor position (unless one is prepared to address these problems) because guidance of eruption does not correct skeletal problems. Guidance of eruption begins in the early mixed dentition with the eruption of the lateral incisors. If a significant arch length discrepancy is predicted, the primary canines should be removed. This allows the incisors ample room to erupt and align. Typically, the incisors also tip lingually and upright, causing the bite to deepen. Faciolingual incisor displacement usually improves, but rotations are more resistant to spontaneous correction.

The child is then observed for 2 years or until it appears that the canines and premolars are ready to erupt. At that time, another space analysis should be completed to ensure that the arch length deficiency is still great enough to warrant permanent tooth extraction, and a radiograph should be obtained to determine the position of the unerupted teeth. The goal of treatment is to encourage the eruption of the permanent first premolar so that it can be extracted before the permanent canine erupts. Unfortunately, the mandibular canine erupts first nearly half the time in the mandibular arch. If it appears that the canine is ahead of the premolar and will erupt facially, the primary first molar should be removed when half to two thirds of the first premolar root is formed. At this stage of root development, premolar eruption will be accelerated, and the premolar will erupt before the canine enters the arch. This makes removal of the first premolar much easier. In the maxillary arch, the first premolar normally erupts before the canine, and this is not a problem. In some cases, the primary first molar is removed, but the permanent canine still erupts before the first premolar. This can lead to impaction of the first premolar, requiring surgical removal. Similarly, it may become apparent that the permanent canine will erupt before the first premolar regardless of the extraction sequence. In this situation, the primary first molar and first premolar are removed at the same time. This procedure is called *enucleation* because the premolar is removed from within the alveolar bone.

Surgical removal of teeth from within the alveolar bone should be avoided if possible because it carries the potential for creating bone and soft tissue defects. These occur if the alveolar bone is fractured or removed. New alveolar bone will not be stimulated to form because no tooth will erupt through this area. Surgical soft tissue defects resolve infrequently.

An alternative extraction sequence has been advocated to prevent lingual tipping of the lower incisors and the subsequent increase in overbite, but this sequence is recommended only when incisor crowding is limited. The primary canine is not removed when the lateral incisor erupts. Instead, the primary canine is retained, and the primary first molar is extracted to accelerate the eruption of the permanent first premolar. This allows some anterior crowding to resolve. The premolar is extracted when it erupts into the arch. The primary canine is often extracted at the same time as the premolar or is left to exfoliate when the permanent canine erupts. The drawback of this alternative is that substantial incisor crowding is not readily resolved, which somewhat defeats the goal of selective tooth removal to encourage good dental alignment.

### Anteroposterior Dental Problems

#### Anterior Crossbite

Anterior crossbite in the mixed dentition is not an uncommon finding. The clinician should determine whether the crossbite is skeletal or dental in origin from the profile analysis and intraoral findings. Skeletal problems should be referred to a specialist, whereas dental problems can be addressed immediately. The most common cause of nonskeletal crossbite is a lack of space for the permanent maxillary incisors to erupt. A space analysis verifies the space shortage. Anterior crossbite develops because the permanent tooth buds form lingual to the primary teeth. When space is inadequate, the incisors are forced to erupt on the lingual side of the arch. If it is apparent that the permanent incisors are beginning to erupt lingually, the adjacent primary teeth

should be disked or removed to provide space for the permanent incisors. If space is provided as the incisors are just beginning to erupt, they will migrate facially out of crossbite, and appliance therapy may not be necessary.

If the incisor fails to erupt facially or if the anterior crossbite is not diagnosed early in the mixed dentition, appliance therapy is needed to correct the crossbite. Space for the incisors is gained by disking or extracting the adjacent primary teeth. At this point, a decision must be made as to whether the teeth should be tipped into position or bodily moved into place. If tipping will accomplish treatment goals, either a removable appliance or a fixed appliance can be used to correct the crossbite. As described earlier, a removable appliance can be used to tip one or more teeth into proper alignment. The appliance is constructed of palatal acrylic with at least two Adams clasps for retention and a 22-mil finger spring to move the teeth (Fig. 35-43). The spring is a double-helix design that provides a physiologic amount of force over an extended range of action. The spring is activated 2 mm to provide 1 mm of tooth movement per month. As with all removable appliances, the child must cooperate by wearing the device full time (except during eating) to allow the appliance to accomplish the desired tooth movement.

An anterior crossbite with an accompanying deep overbite does not necessarily require a biteplane or bite-opening device during treatment. Most persons habitually keep the mandible open and occlude it only during swallowing and parafunctional movements. If the crossbite has

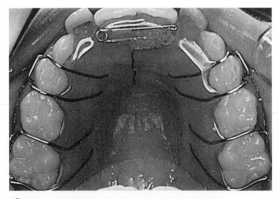

**Figure 35-43** If an anterior crossbite can be corrected by tipping the teeth facially, a removable appliance will accomplish this goal. In this case, a single finger spring is tipping both maxillary central incisors out of crossbite.

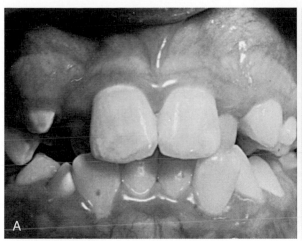
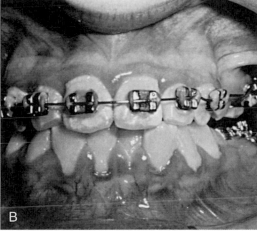

**Figure 35-44** **A,** Fixed appliances also can be used to tip teeth out of anterior crossbite. In this patient both maxillary lateral incisors were in anterior crossbite. **B,** After the brackets were placed, progressively larger round wires were used to tip the teeth out of crossbite. A rectangular archwire will be used to achieve proper crown and root position.

not improved after 3 months of active treatment, it may be necessary to open the bite by adding acrylic to the appliance to cover the occlusal surfaces of the posterior teeth. This limits closure and keeps the anterior teeth apart, which allows uninhibited incisor movement. In most cases, the crossbite will correct quickly and the biteplane can be removed. Extended use of a biteplane is discouraged because the teeth not in contact with the appliance will continue to erupt, creating a vertical occlusal discrepancy.

Fixed appliances also can tip teeth out of crossbite and do not require as much cooperation from the child. A fixed appliance also provides precise control of tooth movement in all three planes of space by using rectangular wires (Fig. 35-44). The disadvantage of either a labial or a lingual fixed appliance is the patient's inability to clean around the teeth and appliance thoroughly, which can result in marginal gingivitis and caries. A maxillary lingual arch is a suitable appliance to correct an anterior crossbite if the teeth require tipping. The maxillary arch is constructed of 36-mil wire and has adjustment loops similar to those used in a lower lingual arch. Finger springs made of 22-mil wire provide the tooth-moving force. The springs are usually soldered on the opposite side of the arch from the tooth being moved so as to increase the length and range of the spring (Fig. 35-45). The springs are activated approximately 3 mm before the appliance is cemented in place. During cementation, the springs are tied with steel ligatures to the lingual arch so that they will

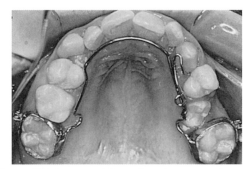

**Figure 35-45** Fixed lingual appliances can be used to tip the teeth out of anterior crossbite. This patient required facial movement of the maxillary left canine to correct the crossbite. A small finger spring was soldered to the base lingual arch and was activated to provide the force necessary to move the tooth.

not interfere with the seating of the appliance. After the excess cement has been cleaned away, the ligature is cut away to activate the springs. In some cases, the spring slips over the incisal edge of an incisor that is not fully erupted. In these cases, a stainless steel guide wire is soldered to the lingual arch at the midline to prevent the spring from slipping incisally. Three millimeters of activation provides 1 mm of tooth movement per month. The appliance should be removed, reactivated, and recemented at 4- to 6-week intervals until the crossbite is corrected.

In older patients, space may need to be created for crossbite correction by arch expansion because there are no primary teeth to disk or extract. In this situation, the permanent molars should be banded and the incisors bonded with orthodontic brackets.

An anterior crossbite that requires bodily movement of teeth to correct the problem is best managed with bonded brackets and a planned sequence of archwires. Initially, teeth can be tipped out of crossbite. Usually an archwire is selected that is strong enough to withstand the force of occlusion in the posterior segments yet flexible enough in the anterior region to engage the brackets of the malaligned teeth. This may require a stainless steel archwire with loops bent mesial and distal to the tooth in crossbite. Loops in the anterior region are designed to provide horizontal or vertical tooth movement and exert optimal force to move the teeth out of crossbite while stabilizing those that are in the correct position. Alternatively, a flexible titanium alloy wire can be used for alignment. This requires no wire bending or loop forming but moves both the teeth in crossbite and those not in crossbite.

After alignment is completed by either method, a rectangular archwire is inserted into the brackets that is capable of delivering a root-positioning force to the tooth previously in crossbite. The purpose of such a force is to move the root into proper position so that the entire tooth essentially moves forward out of crossbite.

Retention must be planned in all cases, regardless of the appliance selected. Active tooth movement is usually continued until the crossbite is slightly overcorrected. The correction should be retained with a passive fixed or removable appliance for 2 months if there is a positive overbite. If there is not adequate overbite, retention should be continued until adequate overbite develops. Circumferential supracrestal fiberotomy should also be considered if rotational movement was made during treatment. In a small number of cases, the anterior crossbite is caused by excessive spacing and flaring of the mandibular incisors. A removable appliance can be constructed with an adjustable 28-mil labial bow to retract the lower incisors and close the space. The appliance should be activated 2 mm/month, and treatment should be continued until the space is closed and there is positive overbite and overjet. The tooth movement can be retained with the same removable appliance, which is made passive.

### Incisor Protrusion

Incisor protrusion in the mixed dentition is a serious aesthetic problem for the preadolescent patient. Protrusive incisors not only are unattractive but also are more prone to dental injury than incisors with a normal angulation. For these reasons, treatment is usually undertaken to move the incisors lingually into a more suitable position if the overbite is not prohibitively deep and the overjet will allow lingual movement. This treatment is used for a dental problem, not a skeletal problem. Skeletal problems should be referred to a specialist for growth modification.

Treatment of incisor protrusion has already been discussed in the earlier section on management of diastemas in the mixed dentition (see Figs. 35-28 and 35-29). To summarize, teeth that can be tipped back into ideal alignment should be treated with a removable appliance that incorporates an active labial bow. The bow is activated by means of an adjustment loop to provide a lingual tipping force to the flared incisors. One to two millimeters of palatal acrylic is removed from the appliance to allow the crown to move lingually and to accommodate the palatal tissue that tends to bunch up behind the tooth being moved. The retention schedule should be full-time wear for 3 months.

In some cases, bodily movement of teeth is necessary to correct incisor protrusion. The maxillary first molars should be banded, and brackets should be bonded to the anterior permanent teeth. A small, round, flexible archwire is placed in the brackets to align the teeth initially. Anterior tooth retraction is accomplished by means of a rectangular archwire with a closing loop or elastomeric chain. A headgear device or a transpalatal arch is usually used during retraction to supplement anchorage. The choice between cervical, combination, or high-pull headgear is based on the patient's vertical facial dimensions. Cervical headgear is generally used when the patient has normal vertical facial proportions, whereas high-pull headgear is indicated when the patient has increased lower facial height. The clinician should follow the progress of a patient undergoing incisor retraction carefully to prevent problems associated with retraction. A complication encountered during incisor retraction is movement of the root of the permanent lateral incisor into the path of the unerupted permanent canine. The lateral incisor root either impedes eruption of the canine or may be resorbed. To avoid this complication, the wire should be bent or the bracket placed so that the lateral incisor root is upright or even tipped slightly mesially.

## Transverse Dental Problems

Posterior crossbite correction in the mixed dentition can be difficult and confusing. The clinician must rely on a well-documented database to determine whether skeletal or dental correction is necessary. The presence of a mandibular shift also is an important finding. A posterior crossbite with an associated mandibular shift should be managed as soon as possible to prevent soft tissue and dental compensation. Crossbites can be corrected with a W arch or a quad helix in the primary and early mixed dentitions. Both skeletal and dental movements occur with these appliances, and it is difficult to affect only one or the other. In the late mixed dentition, the midpalatal suture may be more interdigitated, and the clinician can make primarily dental or skeletal changes depending on the appliance selected to treat the patient. Skeletal problems should be referred to a specialist for treatment with a rapid palatal expander (RPE) (see Fig. 35-6), but dental problems can be managed without referral.

Posterior dental crossbites are either generalized or localized. Generalized crossbites of dental origin are usually bilateral and are corrected with a W arch or a quad helix (Fig. 35-46). If the crossbite is due to a unilateral dental constriction, an unequal W arch (made of 36-mil wire) or a quad helix (made of 38-mil wire) can be used to expand the arch. Alternatively, a lower lingual arch can be used to stabilize the lower teeth, and cross-elastics can be worn to the maxillary arch to correct the crossbite unilaterally. These appli-ances have been discussed in previous sections. Localized crossbites are usually due to displacement of single teeth in one or both arches. For example, a maxillary lingual crossbite involving the permanent first molars is usually the result of lingual displacement of the maxillary molar or the facial displacement of the mandibular molar. If teeth in opposing arches are at fault, it is easy to correct the problem using a simple crossbite elastic. The offending teeth are fitted with orthodontic bands without attachments. After the bands are fitted, they are removed, and a button is welded to the opposite surface of the band from the direction in which the tooth is to be moved.

In the example just noted, a button is welded to the lingual surface of the maxillary band and to the buccal surface of the mandibular band. After the bands have been welded and cemented, a medium weight (3/16-inch, 6-ounce elastic) is attached from button to button through the occlusion (Fig. 35-47). The elastic should be worn full time, except when the patient is eating, and should be changed at least once per day. The elastic should be worn until the crossbite is slightly overcorrected. It may be prudent to leave the

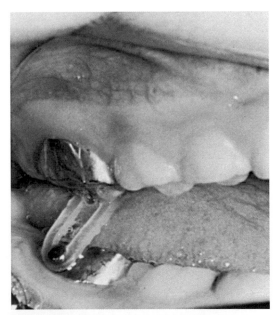

**Figure 35-47** If teeth are at fault in both arches, a simple crossbite elastic is used to correct the crossbite. Bands can be placed on both permanent right first molars, and buttons can be welded to the lingual side of the maxillary band and to the facial side of the mandibular band. A medium-weight elastic (4- to 6-ounce) is attached from one button to the other to provide the force required to correct the crossbite.

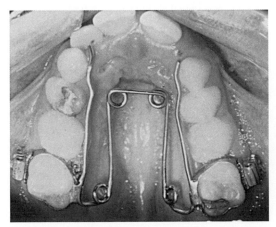

**Figure 35-46** Posterior crossbites of dental origin in the mixed dentition can be treated with either a W arch or a quad helix. In this patient, a quad helix is being used to correct a bilateral posterior crossbite.

bands in place and discontinue the use of elastic for 1 month to ensure that the teeth do not relapse into crossbite. When the occlusion is stable after 4 to 6 weeks without elastic force, the bands can be removed. Buttons are now available that can be bonded directly to the tooth, making bands unnecessary, but there is a risk of bond failure and appliance aspiration.

## Vertical Dental Problems

Vertical problems in the mixed dentition are primarily open bite or deep bite malocclusions. Dental open bite is most often the result of an active digit habit that has impeded eruption of the anterior teeth. In some cases, the digit habit has been discontinued but the open bite has been maintained because the tongue rests between the teeth and prevents eruption. Treatment is essentially the same as that described for digit habits in the late primary and early mixed dentitions. If therapy without an appliance is unsuccessful, a palatal crib (see Fig. 26-6) is effective if the patient desires to stop the habit. The crib reminds the child to refrain from the habit and blocks the tongue from being placed forward. Therapy is successful in the majority of cases unless the child is unwilling to abandon the habit.

In some cases of open bite, the anterior teeth are encouraged to erupt. This is accomplished by opening the bite and preventing the posterior teeth from erupting with acrylic stops between the teeth, while allowing the anterior teeth to erupt (Fig. 35-48). Skeletal open bite treatment has been described previously, and these patients should be referred to a specialist.

Dental deep bite is caused by overeruption of the anterior teeth or undereruption of the posterior teeth. It should be distinguished from skeletal deep bite, which is characterized by a flat mandibular plane angle and a short vertical dimension as well as by over- and undererupted teeth. In a normal incisor-to-lip relationship, 2 mm of the maxillary central incisor is exposed when the lip is at rest. If more than 2 mm of incisor is exposed, maxillary anterior overeruption must be considered. In the mandibular arch, overeruption is difficult to diagnose; however, the curve of Spee may provide some clue. An excessive curve of Spee (2 mm or more) suggests mandibular incisor overeruption.

Management of deep bite in a growing patient can usually be incorporated into comprehensive orthodontic treatment. Occasionally, treatment in a mixed dentition is aimed at preventing further anterior eruption and encouraging or allowing posterior eruption. In these cases, the incisor teeth are placed in contact with a biteplane and the appliance is constructed so that acrylic touches the upper and lower incisors but allows the posterior teeth to erupt. This is a variation of the appliance shown in Fig. 35-48. The appliance must be worn full time to enable correction to take place and then must be worn as a retainer to maintain the correction until the patient stops growing vertically.

If the deep bite is deemed to be the result of maxillary incisor overeruption or a combination of maxillary and mandibular overeruption, fixed orthodontic appliances are placed on the teeth. An intrusion arch, a wire that connects the permanent first molars to the incisors, is constructed to exert a light intrusive force on the incisors (Fig. 35-49). Because there is an equal and opposite reaction to every force placed on the teeth, the molars experience an extrusive force. Specifically,

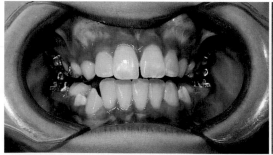
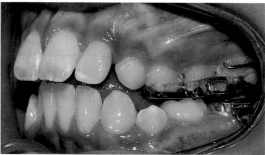

A                                                                            B

**Figure 35-48**   A removable bite plane can allow eruption of posterior teeth or anterior teeth to increase or reduce overbite. **A,** This bite plane prevents eruption of posterior teeth while encouraging anterior teeth to erupt. **B,** The bite plane is retained with the clasps around the molar tubes. For posterior eruption to occur, the acrylic would open the bite and be placed between the anterior teeth.

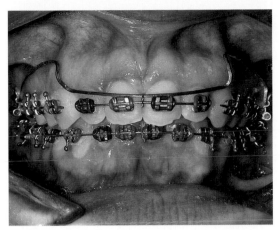

**Figure 35-49**  The intrusion arch can be used to lift the maxillary teeth and reduce overbite. The auxiliary arch, shown here extending from the molars to the incisors gingival to the brackets, is inserted in the auxiliary molar tube. The molar is tied to the segmental archwires so it uses the anchorage of the molars, premolars, and canines.

the molar erupts and tips distally and facially. Facial movement of the molars can be counteracted by a transpalatal arch or a lower lingual arch, but neither will prevent the distal crown tipping. In the maxillary arch, headgear that delivers distal root tip to the molars can offset the extrusive and distal crown tipping forces of intrusion arches. Often overbite reduction is the first phase of comprehensive orthodontic treatment, and consultation with a specialist is appropriate.

# REFERENCES

1. Andreason JO, Ravn JJ: Epidemiology of traumatic dental injuries to primary and permanent teeth in a Danish population sample. *Int J Oral Surg* 1:235-239, 1972.
2. Baik HS: Clinical results of the maxillary protraction in Korean children. *Am J Orthod Dentofac Orthop* 108:583-592, 1995.
3. Baumrind S, Korn EL: Patterns of change in mandibular and facial shape associated with the use of forces to retract the maxilla. *Am J Orthod Dentofac Orthop* 80:31-47, 1981.
4. Baumrind S, Korn EL, Isaacson RJ et al: Quantitative analysis of the orthodontics and orthopedic effects of maxillary traction. *Am J Orthod Dentofac Orthop* 84:383, 1983.
5. Bell R, LeCompte E: The effects of maxillary expansion using a quad helix appliance during the deciduous and mixed detentions. *Am J Orthod Dentofac Orthop* 79:152-161, 1981.
6. Bookstein FL: On the cephalometrics of skeletal change. *Am J Orthod Dentofac Orthop* 82:177-198, 1982.
7. Bussick TJ, McNamara JA Jr: Dentoalveolar and skeletal changes associated with the pendulum appliance. *Am J Orthod Dentofac Orthop* 117:333-43, 2000.
8. Byloff FK, Darendeliler MA: Distal molar movement using the pendulum appliance. Part 1: Clinical and radiological evaluation. *Angle Orthod* 67:249-260, 1997.
9. Cha KS: Skeletal changes of maxillary protraction in patients exhibiting skeletal class III malocclusion: a comparison of three skeletal maturation groups. *Angle Orthod* 73:26-35, 2003.
10. Chertkow S: Tooth mineralization as an indicator of the pubertal growth. *Am J Orthod Dentofac Orthop* 77:79-91, 1980.
11. Czochrowska EM, Stenvik A, Bjercke B, Zachrisson BU: Outcome of tooth transplantation: survival and success rates 17–41 years posttreatment. *Am J Orthod Dentofac Orthop* 121:110-119, 2002.
12. Ericson S, Kurol J: Incisor resorption caused by maxillary cuspids: a radiographic study. *Angle Orthod* 57:332-346, 1987.
13. Ericson S, Kurol J: Early treatment of palatally erupting maxillary canines by extraction of primary canines. *Eur J Orthod* 10:283-295, 1988.
14. Fields HW, Proffit WR, Nixon WL et al: Facial pattern differences in long-faced children and adults. *Am J Orthod Dentofac Orthop* 85:217-223, 1984.
15. Fields HW, Lowe BF, Phillips C et al: Evaluation of anteroposterior skeletal classification methods in children and adults. AAO Annual Meeting Program, Seattle, Wash., 1991.
16. Firouz M, Zernik J, Nanda R: Dental and orthopedic effects of high-pull headgear in treatment of class II, division 1 malocclusion. *Am J Orthod Dentofac Orthop* 102:197-205, 1992.
17. Gianelly AA: Treatment of crowding in the mixed dentition. *Am J Orthod Dentofac Orthop* 121:569-571, 2002.
18. Haas AJ: The treatment of maxillary deficiency by opening the mid-palatal suture. *Angle Orthod* 35:200, 1965.
19. Hagg U, Pancherz H, Taranger J: Pubertal growth and orthodontic treatment. In: Carlson DS, Ribbens KA, editors. *Craniofacial Growth During Adolescence.* Monograph 20, Craniofacial Growth Series, Center for Human Growth and Development, University of Michigan, Ann Arbor, 1987.
20. Hicks E: Slow maxillary expansion: a clinical study of the skeletal versus the dental response to low magnitude force. *Am J Orthod Dentofac Orthop* 73:121-141, 1978.
21. Hotz RP: Guidance of eruption versus serial extraction. *Am J Orthod Dentofac Orthop* 58:1-20, 1970.

22. Iscan HN, Sarisoy L: Comparison of the effects of passive posterior bite-blocks with different construction bites on the craniofacial and dentoalveolar structures. *Am J Orthod Dentofac Orthop* 112:171-178, 1997.

23. Keeling SD, Wheeler TT, King GJ et al: Anteroposterior skeletal and dental changes after early class II treatment with bionators and headgear. *Am J Orthod Dentofac Orthop* 113:40-50, 1998.

24. Kelson A, Fields H, Beck M et al: Concordance of multiple a-p cephalometric methods in long, normal and short-face individuals at varied treatment stages. *J Dent Res* 82:1490, 2003.

25. Kennedy DB, Turley PK: The clinical management of ectopically erupting first permanent molars. *Am J Orthod Dentofac Orthop* 92:336-345, 1987.

26. Kim JH, Viana MA, Graber TM et al: The effectiveness of protraction facemask therapy: a meta-analysis. *Am J Orthod Dentofac Orthop* 115:675-685, 1999.

27. Kjellgren B: Serial extraction as a corrective procedure in dental orthopedic therapy. *Trans Eur Orthod Soc* 134-160, 1947.

28. Kurol J: Early treatment of tooth-eruption disturbances. *Am J Orthod Dentofac Orthop* 121:588-591, 2002.

29. Kuster R, Ingervall B. The effect of treatment of skeletal open bite with two types of bite-blocks. *Eur J Orthod* 14:489-499, 1992.

30. Lagerstrom LO, Nielsen IL, Lee R et al: Dental and skeletal contributions to occlusal correction in patients treated with the high-pull headgear/activator combination. *Am J Orthod Dentofac Orthop* 97:495-504, 1990.

31. Little R: The effects of eruption guidance and serial extraction on the developing dentition. *Pediatr Dent* 9:65-69, 1987.

32. Little RM, Riedel RA, Artun J: An evaluation of changes in mandibular anterior alignment from 10 to 20 years postretention. *Am J Orthod Dentofac Orthop* 93:423-428, 1988.

33. Little RM, Riedel RA, Stein A: Mandibular arch length increase during the mixed dentition: postretention evaluation of stability and relapse. *Am J Orthod Dentofac Orthop* 97:393-404, 1990.

34. McNamara JA, Bookstein FL, Shaughnessy TG: Skeletal and dental changes following functional regulator therapy on class II patients. *Am J Orthod Dentofac Orthop* 88:91-110, 1985.

35. Merwin D, Ngan P, Hagg U et al: Timing for effective application of anteriorly directed orthopedic force to the maxilla. *Am J Orthod Dentofac Orthop* 112:292-299, 1997.

36. Moorrees CFA, Gron AM, Lebret LML et al: Growth studies of the dentition: a review. *Am J Orthod Dentofac Orthop* 55:600-616, 1969.

37. Nevant CT, Buschang PH, Alexander RG et al: Lip bumper therapy for gaining arch length. *Am J Orthod Dentofac Orthop* 100:330-336, 1991.

38. O'Brien K, Wright J, Conboy F et al: Effectiveness of treatment for class II malocclusion with the Herbst or Twin-block appliances: a randomized, controlled trial. *Am J Orthod Dentofac Orthop* 124:128-137, 2003.

39. Owen AH III: Morphologic changes in the transverse dimension using the Frankel appliance. *Am J Orthod Dentofac Orthop* 83:200-217,1983

40. Ozturk Y, Tankuter N: Class II: a comparison of activator and activator headgear combination appliances. *Eur J Orthod* 16:149-157, 1994.

41. Pileski RCA, Woodside DG, Gavin JA: Relationship of the ulnar sesamoid bone and maximum mandibular growth velocity. *Angle Orthod* 43:162-170, 1973.

42. Proffit WR, Fields HW: *Contemporary Orthodontics*, 3rd ed. St Louis, Mosby–Year Book, 2000.

43. Proffit WR, White RP, Sarver DM: *Contemporary Treatment of Dentofacial Deformity*. St. Louis, Mosby–Year Book, 2003.

44. Remmer HR, Manandras AN, Hunter WS et al: Cephalometric changes associated with treatment using the activator, the Frankel appliance, and the fixed appliance. *Am J Orthod Dentofac Orthop* 88:363-372, 1985.

45. Sakamoto T, Iwase I, Uka A et al: A roentgenocephalometric study of skeletal changes during and after chin cap treatment. *Am J Orthod Dentofac Orthop* 85:341-350, 1984.

46. Sugawara J, Asano T, Endo N et al: Long-term effects of chincup therapy on skeletal profile in mandibular prognathism. *Am J Orthod Dentofac Orthop* 98:127-133, 1990.

47. Thilander B, Odman J, Lekholm U: Orthodontic aspects of the use of oral implants in adolescents: a 10-year follow-up study. *Eur J Orthod* 23:715-31, 2001.

48. Thompson GW, Popovich F, Anderson DL: Maximum growth changes in mandibular length, stature, and weight. *Hum Biol* 48:285-293, 1976.

49. Tsurumachi T, Kuno T: Endodontic and orthodontic treatment of a cross-bite fused maxillary lateral incisor. *Int Endod J* 36:135-142, 2003.

50. Tulloch JFC, Phillips C, Proffit WR: Benefit of early class II treatment: progress report of a two-phase randomized clinical trial. *Am J Orthod Dentofac Orthop* 113:62-72, 1998.

51. Turley PK: Orthopedic correction of class III malocclusion with palatal expansion and custom protraction headgear. *J Clin Orthod* 22:314-325, 1988.

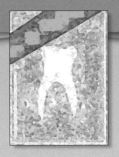

# PART 5

## ADOLESCENCE

Adolescence represents an extremely important time in the dental care of the pediatric patient. Certainly, prevention of dental diseases is one of the pivotal concerns of the dentist who cares for adolescents. Adolescence marks a time in which the role of the parent in the child's dental home care needs to be minimized, and the responsibility of the adolescent for managing his or her own oral health program must be emphasized. Some adolescents are able to do this easily and seem to be inherently motivated to practice proper oral hygiene on a day-by-day basis. However, there are exceptions, and some of these exceptions can be extremely stubborn! The dentist must play a role in educating and motivating such patients, for not only is caries a problem but so is periodontal disease and its unfortunate implications that become increasingly important as the child proceeds to the later years of adolescence.

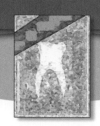

# CHAPTER 36
## The Dynamics of Change

## PHYSICAL CHANGES

### Body

*Jimmy R. Pinkham*

Adolescence in some societies is a very short transitional period that marks the arrival of a child to full citizenship within his or her respective tribe and culture. In a technologic society such as Europe or North America today, adolescence is a time of enormous transition and is certainly not of short duration. Hence, the term *teenager* has become synonymous with the term *adolescent* in our society. Literature describing adolescents may portray them as old children or young adults. Certainly, adolescence is an in-between age in our society and must be understood as something separate from childhood or adulthood.

Critical to the definition of adolescence regardless of culture and to the understanding of the adolescent physically is the concept of puberty. Puberty is the landmark in physical development when an individual becomes capable of sexual reproduction. In common law, this has been established historically in our society as age 14 for boys and age 12 for girls. The advent of puberty is paralleled by the development of genital tissue and secondary sexual characteristics, such as the development of hair in the genital area.

It is also a time when there is an increase in the mass of muscles, a redistribution of body fat, and an increase in the rate of skeletal growth. A growth spurt is associated with this time of life. This growth spurt follows two different forms, depending on gender. It appears earlier in females than in males. The average onset in males is 2 years later than that in females. The fact that males experience their growth spurt later than females and therefore have a longer maturation period before the growth period is one of the reasons why the height of males generally exceeds the height of females. The earlier growth spurt of females also accounts for the period of time during which mean height of a group of young female adolescents may exceed that of males. It is important to realize also that in females menarche serves as a signal that growth is ending, but for males there is no such marker. The magnitude of the velocity of change during the growth spurt also differs between the sexes. In 1975, Tanner and colleagues concluded that the growth spurt in females peaks at 9 cm change per year at age 12, and that in males it peaks at just over 10 cm at age 14.[1]

## REFERENCE

1. Tanner JM, Whitehouse RH, Marshall WA et al: *Assessment of Skeletal Maturity and Prediction of Adult Height: TW 2 Method.* New York, Academic Press, 1975.

### Craniofacial Changes

*Jerry Walker*

During and following adolescence, continued changes in the skeletal growth of the face and skull take place because the facial sutures are still open and viable[6] and mandibular growth can potentially continue. These changes not only cause variation and individuality in facial appearance[5] but affect the dental structures as well. The continued changes make a final and nonchanging dentition and occlusion a difficult concept to imagine, much less attain. There is a slow increase in facial height accompanied by an increase in prognathism in males.[1,2]

Profile changes occur as changes in specific locations take place. The brow area becomes larger as a result of pneumatization of the frontal sinuses and apposition on the glabella.[7] Also, appositional changes during adolescence and early adult life in the frontal bone area and brow result in this area's becoming more prominent.[1] In adolescence the nose and chin also become more prominent. The tip of the nasal bone lies well ahead of the basal bone of the premaxilla. Soft tissue changes also contribute to the growth in the length of the nose and can affect the harmony existing between the nose, lips, and chin. The mandible shows a greater prognathism than the maxilla because of the circumpubertal growth spurt, which has more effect on the mandible than on the maxilla, especially in males. The chin also becomes more prominent owing to local bone deposition. Lip prominence is reduced by these changes in adjacent structures.

Underlying maxillary changes also occur. The maxillary sinuses, which have since birth expanded laterally and vertically, occupy the space left by the permanent teeth as they erupt. By puberty, the sinuses are usually fully developed, although they may continue to enlarge. There is considerable individual variation in the size of the maxillary sinuses, and they often lack symmetry. Lowering of the palatal vault continues because of remodeling. In 1966, Bjork concluded that sutural growth as well as appositional growth of the maxilla contributed significantly to the increase in the height of the maxillary body (Fig. 36-1).[3] This can be an example of sexual dimorphism in skeletal growth (Table 36-1). Vertical maxillary facial growth is often greater in females. Because the mandible does not continue to grow as much in females, marked vertical changes in the maxilla can result in downward and backward positioning of the mandible and an increase in facial convexity (Fig. 36-2).[1]

Mandibular growth contributes more than profile changes. This growth may be sufficient to provide room for the third molars. In many cases growth is inadequate, and these molars become impacted (Fig. 36-3). The marked mesial inclination of the posterior permanent teeth diminishes somewhat as the mandible completes its growth from under the maxilla, and the lower incisors tend to become upright. Often this is accompanied by crowding of the lower incisors.[7]

Late mandibular growth imparts an increase in the vertical height of the mandibular ramus, which becomes more upright. The elongation of the ramus accommodates the massive vertical expansion of the nasal region and the lowering of the palate, which is accompanied by dental eruption. Usually the maxillary and mandibular growths are compatible and coordinated. If they are not, significant orthodontic problems can result. Particularly in males, there can be late anterior growth that is undesirable.[1]

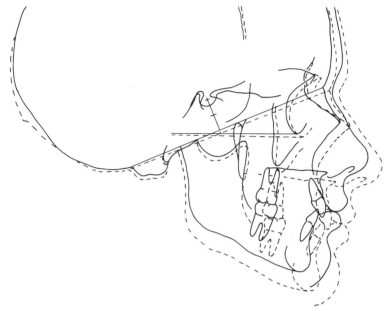

**Figure 36-1**    This anterior cranial base superimposition of the Bolton Standard 12- and 18-year-olds (solid line and broken line, respectively) demonstrates the magnitude of anteroposterior and vertical skeletal growth during this period as well as the soft tissue change. (Redrawn from Broadbent BH Sr, Broadbent BH Jr, Golden WH: *Bolton Standards of Developmental Growth.* St Louis, Mosby, 1975.)

## TABLE 36-1
### Growth of the Aging Skeleton: Sexual Dimorphism in Craniofacial Growth

|  | FEMALES | MALES |
|---|---|---|
| Circumpubertal growth spurt | 10–12 years | 12–14 years |
| Mature size | Growth plateaus at 14 with increases to 16 years | Active growth to 18 years |
| Supraorbital ridges | Absent | Well developed |
| Frontal sinuses | Small | Large |
| Nose | Small | Large |
| Zygomatic prominences | Small | Large |
| Mandibular symphysis | Rounded | Prominent |
| Mandibular angle | Rounded | Prominent lipping |
| Occipital condyles | Small | Large |
| Mastoid processes | Small | Large |
| Occipital protuberance | Insignificant | Prominent |

From Behrents RG: *Growth in the Aging Craniofacial Skeleton.* Ann Arbor, MI, Center for Human Growth and Development, University of Michigan, 1985.

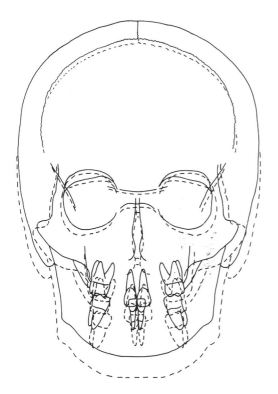

**Figure 36-2** This anterior cranial base superimposition of the Bolton Standard 12- and 18-year-olds (*solid line* and *broken line,* respectively) demonstrates the magnitude of transverse and vertical skeletal growth during this period. (Redrawn from Broadbent BH Sr, Broadbent BH Jr, Golden WH: *Bolton Standards of Developmental Growth.* St Louis, Mosby, 1975.)

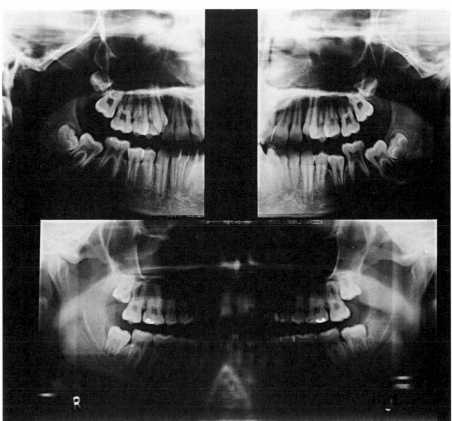

**Figure 36-3** These two panoramic radiographs show the changes that occur during adolescence. Some eruptive and mesial drift is expected, combined with distal incisor movement. Third molar eruption often occurs at the end of this age period.

## REFERENCES

1. Behrents RG: *Growth in the Aging Craniofacial Skeleton.* Monograph 17, Craniofacial Growth Series. Ann Arbor, Center for Human Growth and Development, 1985.
2. Bjork A: The face in profile. *Sven Tanalak Tidskr* 40:Suppl 5B, 1947.
3. Bjork A: Sutural growth of the upper face studied by the implant method. *Acta Odontol Scand* 24:109-127, 1966.
4. Broadbent BH Sr, Broadbent BH Jr, Golden WH: *Bolton Standards of Developmental Growth.* St Louis, Mosby, 1975.
5. Enlow DH: *Handbook of Facial Growth.* Philadelphia, Saunders, 1990.
6. Kokich VG: Age changes in the human frontozygomatic sutures from 20 to 95 years. *Am J Orthod* 60:411-430, 1976.
7. Ranly DM: *A Synopsis of Craniofacial Growth.* New York, Appleton-Century-Crofts, 1980.

### Dental Changes

*Clemons A. Full*

All of the permanent teeth generally have erupted by age 12, except possibly the four second molars, which may erupt as late as age 13, and the third molars, which usually erupt between the ages of 17 and 21.

Except for the third molars, the dentist should be concerned about any unerupted permanent tooth after age 13 and should examine the area in question radiographically.

The roots of all teeth are considered to have been completed by age 16 except for those of the third molars, which can achieve completion as late as age 25.

## COGNITIVE CHANGES

*Jimmy R. Pinkham*

The adolescent continues his or her cognitive development and by middle to late adolescence is capable of extremely sophisticated intellectual tasks. High ability at abstract thinking allows the adolescent to deal with complex and difficult vocational and educational challenges. Formal operational thinking and the ability to store information in the memory after perceiving it are hallmarks of the maturation of cognitive ability in adolescents.

The new information available to the adolescent, along with more sophisticated ways of analyzing this information, often makes him or her appear to be a rebel, a complainer, or an accuser. Persons of this age often ascertain the possible and become discontented, even angry, with the real. Kiell[1] pointed out in 1967 that Aristotle, more than 2000 years ago, concluded that adolescents "are passionate, irascible, and apt to be carried away by their impulses." It has been noted that the thoughts of adolescents are both *introspective* and *analytic.* They are also *egocentric.* This dwelling on one's self may make an individual overly self-conscious. Clothes, cars, hairstyle, tastes in music, and identification with certain people or groups probably reflect the adolescent's involvement in self-consciousness.

In summary, by mid- to late adolescence, most young people are capable of formal operational thinking and can, both in and out of school, master subject material that is extensive, difficult, and abstract. Many have matured into skillful, enthusiastic communicators and conversationalists. Many are also opinionated and perhaps argumentative. These last two characteristics may make for some trying times for parents, teachers, and dentists.

## REFERENCE

1. Kiell N: *The Universal Experience of Adolescence.* Boston, Beacon, 1967.

## EMOTIONAL CHANGES

*Jimmy R. Pinkham*

The very rapid and dramatic changes that occur in adolescents may be paralleled by many emotional circumstances. The self-confidence and personal identity of an adolescent may be compromised if his or her feelings about body image are negative. In 1984, Mussen and colleagues noted that the following issues create the possibility of misinterpretation and anxiety for this age group:[1]

- Being attractive or unattractive
- Being loved or unloved
- Being strong or weak
- Being masculine or feminine

For females, the onset of menstruation may also present circumstances that can be anxiety provoking. This is not necessarily the rule, but the chances of anxiety rise if there is a prevailing negative reaction to the menstrual process by family and peers, if the child is showered with sympathy, or if there is considerable pain before and during menses. Anyone who works with post-menarchal females should be aware that some of them will display irritability or depression at times.

The advent of puberty and the hormones associated with puberty lead to sexual feelings and urges. The timing of this process, its nature and magnitude, and the choice of what to do about these feelings and urges are handled differently from one adolescent to another. Family guidance, the adolescent's own values, the values of peers, and the value system of the person that the adolescent first loves are just a few of the factors that ultimately predict how he or she will deal with these new feelings.

One last emotion is critical to understanding adolescents. This is the emotion of love. Adolescents are capable of great commitment to one another, and some of these relationships can become long-term commitments. Unfortunately, many such relationships do not last, as one partner becomes uninterested. This can lead to genuine depression for the abandoned partner. The term "puppy love" is a terrible misnomer and belies exactly how painful these broken relationships can be.

## REFERENCE

1. Mussen PH, Conger JJ, Kagan J et al: *Child Development and Personality,* 6th ed. New York, Harper & Row, 1984.

## SOCIAL CHANGES

*Jimmy R. Pinkham*

Adolescence represents the final transition socially from childhood to adulthood. When it is over, if everything proceeded as it should, the emerging young adult will be able to establish and maintain loving and sexual relationships with a partner, be independent of the parents, be capable of working with peers, and be self-directed. These are formidable social challenges, and some adolescents cannot master them. Delinquency, attempted or successful suicide, alcohol and drug use and abuse, running away from home, teenage prostitution, and dropping out of school are some of the frequently cited instances of adolescent failure to socialize properly.

Peers are important social agents in large technologic societies, in which children of the same age group are often kept together. It can be argued that as relationships and dependencies on parents start to decline, the importance of peers escalates. Increasingly, the adolescent may find that it is difficult to share secrets, thoughts, and fantasies with his or her parents. In these situations, the close friend becomes the adolescent's confidant(e), and the peer is a valuable and useful audience.

Despite the obvious value of peers, there are peer relationships that are not so fortunate for the involved adolescent. For example, to avoid rejection or ridicule from peers an adolescent may experiment with drugs, participate in criminal acts, or defy authority.

Another important social change in the adolescent is an increase in the size and range of acquaintances. Children younger than adolescence tend to limit their friends to those of their neighborhood, school, and perhaps church. Adolescents, on the other hand, may have individual friends, belong to a clique of friends, and can identify with larger groups such as an Explorer troop or a football team. An adolescent's ability to sustain relationships with all three of these groups indicates good social skills and is a sign that the socialization process is going well.

Popularity is an important desire in adolescents. There are few adolescents who are not preoccupied with acceptance by peers. The following qualities in an adolescent seem to correlate with social acceptance by peers:

- Friendly, likes other people
- Energetic and enthusiastic
- Flexible and forgiving
- Laughs, good sense of humor
- Outgoing
- Self-confident but not conceited
- Appears natural
- Tolerant of the shortcomings of others
- Shows leadership qualities
- Others feel good when this person is around

The adolescent who gets along with his or her peer group seems to relate successfully to adults. Those who do not achieve peer acceptance seem to have more difficulty with adults and grow up to have a variety of social and emotional difficulties.[1]

## REFERENCE

1. Hartup WW: The peer system. In: Mussen PH, editor. *Handbook of Child Psychology*, 4th ed. Volume 4 in Socialization, Personality, and Social Development (Hetherington EM, editor). New York, John Wiley, 1983.

## EPIDEMIOLOGY AND MECHANISMS OF DENTAL DISEASE

*Steven M. Adair*

Adolescents have benefitted from the reduction in the prevalence of dental caries in the United States during the latter part of the 20th century. However, data from the large-scale survey in 1987–1986[4] indicated that almost 85% of 17-year-olds were affected to some degree by dental disease. Even though this was an improvement over a similar 1979–1980 survey,[8] the data suggest to some that the development of tooth decay is merely postponed and not truly prevented in younger children. This section will explore data on caries prevalence in teenagers. The reasons for the significant reductions in caries prevalence are discussed in Chapter 29 under "Epidemiology and Mechanisms of Dental Disease," but this section also will discuss the major basis for the control of caries in the United States in the latter half of the 20th century, that is, water fluoridation.

### Epidemiology of Caries in the Adolescent Years

The most comprehensive data on the caries experience of United States schoolchildren were compiled by the Epidemiology and Oral Disease Prevention Program of the National Institute of Dental Research (NIDR) in a nationwide study conducted in 1986–1987.[4] More than 39,000 children, ages 5 to 17, were examined using visual-tactile criteria.

Figure 36-4 demonstrates the mean number of decayed, missing, and filled permanent tooth surfaces (DMFS) for adolescent children by age and sex. The DMFS for 12-year-olds, who may

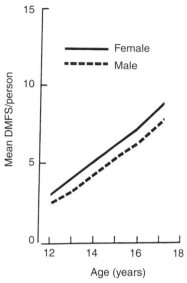

**Figure 36-4** Mean decayed, missing, filled tooth surfaces (DMFS) for children aged 12 to 17 in the United States by age and sex. (Redrawn from Epidemiology and Oral Disease Prevention Program, National Institute of Dental Research: *Oral Health of United States Children. The National Survey of Dental Caries in U.S. School Children: 1986–87*. NIH Publication 89-2247, 1989.)

not have erupted all permanent teeth, was 2.66. For 14-year-olds, who would generally have all permanent teeth erupted with the exception of third molars, the DMFS was 4.68 (about 75% higher). At the time of the survey, 17-year-olds demonstrated a mean DMFS of slightly over 8. These increases reflect the effects of time on a somewhat increasing number of permanent tooth surfaces susceptible to decay during adolescence. As was true in the transitional dentition, females had slightly higher DMFS scores than males.

The 1986–1987 survey found that the DMFS of whites was somewhat lower than that of non-whites. This difference was about 17% for children ages 5 to 13. For 12- to 17-year-olds, the difference was maintained, but for 17-year-olds alone it was more than 22%. A more telling statistic is the percentage of the DMFS score that is attributable to decay. For whites ages 5 to 17, that figure was 10.6%. For nonwhites, 23.8% of the DMFS was represented by decayed surfaces. Clearly, nonwhites suffered more dental disease and, as a group, presented higher treatment needs than whites.

Data from the 1971–1974[9] and 1988–1994[10] National Health and Nutrition Examination

## TABLE 36-2

### Decayed, Missing, and Filled Teeth in Children Ages 12 to 18 Reported by NHANES I* and NHANES III[†]

|  | NHANES I | NHANES III | DIFFERENCE |
|---|---|---|---|
| Overall DMFS | 6.65 | 3.08 | −3.57 |
| At or below FPL[‡] | 6.68 | 3.20 | −3.48 |
| Above FPL | 6.65 | 3.04 | −3.61 |

*NHANES I: National Health and Nutrition Examination Survey, 1971-1974.[9]
[†]NHANES III: National Health and Nutrition Examination Survey, 1988-1994.[10]
[‡]FPL: Federal poverty level.
All differences are statistically significant.

Surveys (NHANES I and III) indicate a significant reduction in decayed, missing, and filled permanent teeth (DMFT) between the two surveys in adolescents ages 12 to 18 years (Table 36-2).[2]

In addition, the surveys demonstrate a clear link between lower socioeconomic status and increased dental disease burden.

## Basis for Caries Reductions

The basis for the striking reductions in caries prevalence in U.S. children has been explored in more detail in Chapter 29 under "Epidemiology and Mechanisms of Dental Disease." There seems to be no change in the disease process itself, and per capita consumption of sugars in this country has not changed appreciably over the past 30 years. The best explanation appears to be the more widespread exposure to fluoride in various forms. In addition to optimally fluoridated water supplies, exposure to fluoride has increased through therapeutic products (dentifrices, mouth rinses, and other topical and systemic agents), some of which are ingested by younger children. Residents of fluoride-deficient communities also ingest foods processed in fluoridated communities. This increased fluoride ingestion in fluoride-deficient communities has been termed the "halo effect," and has led to lower caries rates and higher enamel fluorosis prevalence than would have been expected from the original studies of artificial fluoridation. The best example of this phenomenon was demonstrated in the 1986–1987 NIDR survey. The mean DMFS of 5- to 17-year-old children residing in fluoridated communities was 2.79, compared with 3.39 for children from fluoride-deficient communities. This represents a difference of only 17.7%.

## Water Fluoridation

No single preventive dentistry measure has had the impact and success in reducing disease than the adjustment of the fluoride concentration in community drinking water supplies. In addition to providing caries reductions in the range of 50% to 70% at the time of the trials, water fluoridation is the most cost-effective means of caries prevention. It has been estimated that the annual per capita cost of water fluoridation in the United States is between $0.12 and $5.41, depending on the size of the community, with the annual mean cost being $0.51.[11]

### History

In 1901, Dr. Frederick S. McKay began practicing dentistry in Colorado Spring, Colorado. He noticed staining in the enamel of many of his patients. Further investigation led him to the conclusion that this "Colorado brown stain," as it came to be known (Fig. 36-5), followed a distinct geographic pattern. McKay invited Dr. G. V. Black of the dental school at Northwestern University to

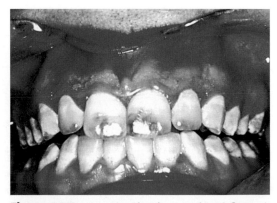

**Figure 36-5**   An example of severe dental fluorosis, termed "Colorado brown stain" by Dr. F. S. McKay.

join in the investigation. The result was a full report of their clinical and histologic findings, published in 1916.[1] The term "mottled enamel" was used to describe an endemic condition affecting 87.5% of the population in specific regions. McKay and Black advanced the idea that the causative factor, still undetermined at that time, was present during the development of the enamel, and further, that in children who resided in these locations for specific periods of time, only certain groups of teeth were affected.

Black and McKay described the appearance of affected teeth as ranging from paper white, to brown, to black, with every conceivable intermediate degree represented. They noted that the general morphology of the teeth was normal. Perhaps their most important observation was that these teeth seemed remarkably resistant to decay.

The histologic analysis of the teeth showed that the abnormal enamel was generally confined to the outer one third, with less involvement of the inner layers and dentin. Both the enamel interprismatic substance and the enamel rods were found to be affected. Some dentin involvement was noted.

Although McKay and others had speculated on the possible causative factors, it was not until 1926 that McKay[7] openly implicated drinking water supplies. However, he was unsure as to what substances (or their absence) might contribute to mottling. It is interesting to note that in 1925 a study was published[6] in which it was found that rats on high-fluoride diets developed staining in

their incisors. This fact was not related to human enamel mottling for years.

In 1930, Kempf and McKay[5] demonstrated that enamel mottling in people living in Bauxite, Arkansas, disappeared only after the town changed its community water supply. There followed several studies in the 1930s conclusively linking water-borne fluoride with both enamel mottling and resistance to decay. The character of the studies of mottling, which now was termed "dental fluorosis," began to change, emphasizing whether a fluoride concentration could be found that would balance the benefits of caries protection with the risk of enamel discoloration

By employing a system of fluorosis classification, Dean[3] and others determined that in communities with about 1.0 part per million (ppm) fluoride in the drinking water, fluorosis was not an aesthetic problem. Moreover, these communities had a lower caries prevalence than similar communities without fluoride. The relationship between fluoride content of the drinking water, caries prevalence (DMFT), and dental fluorosis is demonstrated in Figure 36-6.

At this point, fluoride research took a logical but dramatic turn. The emphasis now was placed on whether fluoride could be added to community water supplies to effect caries reductions. Between 1945 and 1947, large independent clinical studies were undertaken in four pairs of North American cities to test the results of fluoridation. These studies constitute some of the best designed and controlled public health trials ever undertaken. In most cases, each city was paired with a

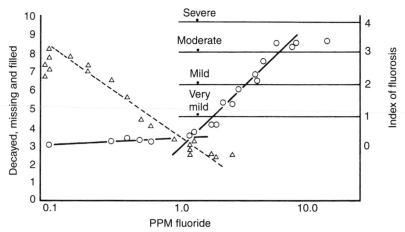

**Figure 36-6**    Relationship between the fluoride content of the drinking water, caries prevalence, and the index of dental fluorosis. (Redrawn from Hodge HC, Smith FA: Some public health aspects of water fluoridation. In: Shaw JH, editor. *Fluoridation as a Public Health Measure.* Washington, DC, AAAS, Publication 38, 1954, p 88.)

## TABLE 36-3

### Comparison of Caries Scores and Percent Reduction in 12- to 14-Year-Old Children in Communities With and Without Water Fluoridation

| City | Fluoride Status | Year | DMFT per Child | Percent Caries Reduction |
|------|-----------------|------|----------------|--------------------------|
| Kingston | No F | 1960 | 12.46 | |
| Newburgh | F | 1960 | 3.73 | −70.1 |
| Sarina | No F | 1959 | 7.46 | |
| Brantford | F | 1959 | 3.23 | −56.7 |
| Grand Rapids | No F | 1945 | 9.50 | |
| | F | 1959 | 4.26 | −55.2 |
| Evanston | No F | 1946 | 9.03 | |
| | F | 1959 | 4.66 | −48.4 |

From Newbrun E, editor: *Fluorides and Dental Caries,* 3rd ed. Springfield, IL, Charles C Thomas, 1986.

neighboring city, similar in almost all respects except for the lack of fluoride in the water supply. Table 36-3 illustrates the results of follow-up examinations of children 12 to 14 years of age conducted about 15 years after fluoridation was begun. Children residing in the trial cities had DMFT scores 50% to 70% lower than their counterparts in the control cities.

Further studies of water consumption led to the recognition that fluid intake is directly proportional to the average maximal daily air temperature of the community. Thus, a range of water fluoride concentrations from 0.7 to 1.2 ppm was developed by the Public Health Service to reflect the climate of various communities. The water fluoride concentration should vary inversely with the population water consumption.

Today more than 62% of the population in the United States is served by fluoridated public water supplies.[12] Thus, about 182 million people in the United States benefit from drinking water with sufficient fluoride to provide significant caries protection.

### Summary

Caries prevalence among adolescents in the United States has declined over the past 30 years, though the decline has not been equal across all racial/ethnic and socioeconomic groups. The initial reductions brought about by water fluoridation have been improved further by the widespread availability of fluoride in other forms: dentifrices, mouth rinses, systemic supplements, and professionally applied topical agents. In addition to this, the "halo effect" of exposure to foods and beverages processed in fluoridated communities has substantially improved the dental health of persons residing in fluoride-deficient areas. Caries has not yet disappeared, and attempts at further reductions may reach a point of diminishing returns. Nevertheless, the goal of maintaining an individual patient free of caries into young adulthood is certainly achievable, but only for those with access to dental care.

## REFERENCES

1. Black GV, McKay FS: Mottled teeth: an endemic developmental imperfection of the enamel of teeth heretofore unknown in the literature of dentistry. *Dent Cosmos* 58 (part I) 477, (part II) 627, (part III) 781, (part IV) 894, 1916.
2. Brown LJ, Wall TP, Lazar V: Trends in total caries experience: permanent and primary teeth. *JADA* 131:223, 2000.
3. Dean HT: Classification of mottled enamel diagnosis. *JADA* 21:14216, 1934.
4. Epidemiology and Oral Disease Prevention Program, National Institute of Dental Research: *Oral Health of United States Children. The National Survey of Dental Caries in U.S. School Children: 1986–87.* NIH Publication 89-2247, 1989.
5. Kempf GA, McKay FS: Mottled enamel in a segregated population. *Public Health Rep* 45:2923, 1930.
6. McCollum EV, Simmonds N, Becker JE, Bunting RW: The effect of additions of fluoride to the diet of the rat on the quality of the teeth. *J Biol Chem* 63:553-562, 1925.

and family pressure are some of the challenges that today's adolescent must face. Perhaps the most poignant statement on this aspect of the teenage years is that accidental death is the leading cause of mortality. Dental professionals see trauma, oral manifestations of sexual activity, hormonal gingivitis, smokeless tobacco–induced hyperkeratosis, noncompliance with dental recommendations, and drug-related behaviors, to mention a few examples.

3. *The need to learn to cope, make decisions, and become independent.* It isn't surprising that primitive cultures associated emerging adulthood with rituals and great significance. Adolescence has always been a time to make decisions, seek independence from families, deal with sexuality, and choose a career. The dentist often sees this turmoil reflected in poor compliance with oral hygiene or refusal to accept treatment. The missed appointment is just one of many ways to say, "I am too involved in my search for self, my changing values, and handling my environment to worry about my teeth."

## THE PATIENT HISTORY

The health history of the adolescent is constantly changing and must be kept current. An adult history format captures both of these elements. Perhaps more important from the standpoint of accuracy is the process of obtaining information from the teenager. The following are some of the topics that should be considered when taking a history from an adolescent patient.

The health history should address the issues of smoking, recreational drugs and alcohol, birth control, pregnancy, and sexually transmitted diseases. The controversy over inclusion of these issues is easily quieted by the simple realities of adolescent life in the United States. Consider the facts:

- Every day, approximately 3000 teenagers start smoking.
- Out-of-wedlock births have increased by 50% in recent years.
- Radiation and medications used in dentistry can be dangerous to a fetus.
- The majority of adolescents now try drugs or alcohol before leaving high school. Untoward interactions between prescribed and illicit medications can be fatal.

- Sexually transmitted diseases are epidemic in the adolescent age group.

Inadequate surveying of these elements of the health history puts both dentist and patient at risk. These issues can be addressed forthrightly by including them as choices interspersed with others on a health history form. A less threatening approach is to phrase these questions in the past tense or to associate a risk with them in order to alert the patient to their importance.

The history-taking process should allow privacy and encourage disclosure. Taking an accurate history may mean allowing the adolescent to assume greater participation in the process. The desired yield on the adolescent history from this perspective is information that might not be available from or known to a parent, such as those items described previously. The dentist may be caught in a double bind by providing an environment that fosters disclosure if pregnancy or illicit drug use is uncovered and the parents are unaware of it. This is a risk that requires counseling and resolution prior to dental treatment, and the dentist's responsibility is to help direct the family to address the issue. Unfortunately, the adolescent may see this as betrayal or breach of confidence, and the relationship between the dentist and patient may be jeopardized. There is no easy way to deal with this type of problem, but the dentist who treats adolescents should be aware of the responsibilities of the situation. It also may mean delaying treatment until the problem is resolved.

The dentist can take some actions that both facilitate an accurate history and deal consistently with identified problems of a serious nature:

- Encourage parents to complete histories with adolescents, not for them.
- Allow the adolescent the opportunity to contribute to the history alone, which can be done in the context of a final check prior to treatment at chairside.
- Never treat an adolescent without a consenting parent available. Dental care would be considered nonurgent care and most jurisdictions require adult consent.
- Explain suspicions or concerns to both parent and adolescent.
- Establish a policy on deferring treatment and dealing with identified problems of a

serious nature that is medicolegally consistent and sound.

- Have resources available in case consultation with a specialist is needed. It is far better to have an established professional relationship than to seek help from a stranger.

## THE EXAMINATION

The techniques of clinical examination remain the same for the adolescent, but closer attention is paid to identification of problems specific to this group, such as occlusal disharmonies, periodontal conditions, and temporomandibular joint disorders. Table 37-1 lists some of the clinical findings peculiar to adolescent patients.

## Behavioral Assessment

The access to dental care available to most healthy Americans has made it unlikely that a teenager will present for a first visit at that period in life, although first visits during adolescence are possible. Most people have made at least one visit to a dentist before they reach adolescence. Personality changes and other behavioral aberrations can suggest problems for the adolescent. Extremes in behavior, such as depression or overt flirting, may indicate sexual abuse in the adolescent girl, especially if the child demonstrates a reluctance to allow oral examination. Depression, manifested by severe introversion, can also be a sign of suicidal tendency, family dysfunction, or even drug use. It is not the dentist's responsibility to diagnose or manage these kinds of problems,

## TABLE 37-1
### Possible Clinical Findings in Examination of the Adolescent

| STRUCTURE | FINDING | COMMENT |
| --- | --- | --- |
| **Extraoral Evaluation** | | |
| Skin | Acne | May be painful locally |
| | | Adolescent may take antibiotics |
| | | Can show up as radiopacity on some radiographs if calcification occurs |
| | Cosmetic use | Can complicate evaluation of skin |
| | | Can cause local allergic response |
| Neck | Hematoma | From suction; indicates sexual activity |
| Ears | Healing or scarred punctures | Multiple ear piercing common in both sexes |
| Hair | Coloring and preparation | Can complicate examination of scalp |
| **Intraoral Examination** | | |
| Mucosa | Generalized erythema | Effect of smoking |
| | | Sexually transmitted disease |
| Buccal mucosa | Erythema, hyperkeratosis | Use of smokeless tobacco |
| Tongue | Coating, odor | Smoking; poor hygiene; fungal overgrowth from medication |
| Breath | Acetone; alcohol | Excessive dieting; alcohol abuse; metabolic disorders (e.g., diabetes) |
| Gingiva | Inflammation | Hormonal change |
| | Pregnancy tumor | Use of oral contraceptives |
| | | Pregnancy |
| Teeth | Erosion | Bulimia |
| | Wear facets | Temporomandibular joint disorders/bruxism |
| | Excessive stain | Tobacco use |
| | Discoloration | Existing pulpal pathosis from trauma |

but the dentist should be aware of the impact of the problem on the child and comment to parents about noticeable changes in behavior. Few behavioral problems should be encountered that will preclude delivery of care, but exceptions do occur. The following are situations that may require behavioral management:

1. *Sexual abuse.* The young adolescent girl or boy who has been sexually abused with oral penetration may be reluctant to accept dental care from a dentist of the same sex as the perpetrator. Aids in uncovering this situation are a good history of previous compliance, behavioral cues such as depression, and overt refusal of care when oral contact is made. Nonetheless, confirmation is difficult because the parents may be unaware of the abuse. It may be the limit of the dentist's role to recommend counseling for such a child in the hope that intervention may uncover the cause.

2. *Rampant caries.* Clinicians have noted that rampant caries, a condition of rapid onset and progression of decay in an adolescent (more often a girl), is often associated with personality problems (Fig. 37-1). The typical manifestation is a shy, reluctant, introverted person who is passive about treatment. The behavioral signs can be varied, with the girl crying silently or not saying a word during the appointment. In some cases, appointments can degenerate as the child whimpers and finally loses her composure. Time and engagement in conversation are often the most successful behavioral management keys in dealing with these adolescents. Dramatic changes in behavior can occur with the dentist's verbal reinforcement of improved hygiene and provision of

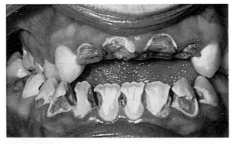

**Figure 37-1** This 14-year-old girl has rampant caries, which is a distinct clinical entity with rapidly progressing decay, multiple pulpally involved teeth, and short onset. Patients may give a history of minimal caries prior to development of overt signs of decay.

even temporary aesthetic anterior restorations that allow the patient to smile and experience a more positive self-image.

3. *Extreme anxiety.* Pinkham and Schroeder[21] described the behavioral management of the child who shows extreme anxiety at the prospect of dental treatment. Desensitization by psychological intervention may be the key to development of acceptable clinical behavior in such children. Tools available to the dentist are the use of noninvasive therapies at first, reinforcement of positive accomplishments, positive peer interaction, and involvement with a psychologist. The poorly treated or untreated adolescent phobic may become the adult dental phobic.

4. *Anorexia nervosa.* Treatment of the child with an eating disorder can be difficult. Experience indicates that these patients, mostly girls, tend to develop dependency on a male authority figure. They also require a dentist's full attention during office visits and, unless counseled, may demand time outside scheduled appointments.

5. *Illicit drug use.* Clinicians have noted bizarre behavior on the part of adolescents and young adults who present for treatment after taking nonprescription medications. A number of untoward reactions to dentist-administered medications have been associated with prior ingestion of drugs or alcohol by a young patient. Manifestations of drug ingestion may vary from a slight mental dissociation or drifting to outright verbal aberrations or extreme changes in personality.

Management of behavioral problems in the adolescent can be complex and often involves parents and other professionals. On the other hand, a number of adolescents show age-appropriate behavior that may be disruptive to delivery of care. Most practitioners treating adolescents try to treat these patients alone rather than in a setting in which other peers are present. This one-on-one relationship provides the necessary attention to the patient and prevents disruptive interactions. Any dentist who has worked with a group of seventh- or eighth-grade students will appreciate this recommendation. The teenager who is acting up but is simply expressing healthy emotions should respond to reason and provide compliance.

An important part of behavior management in this age group involves the simple transfer of information. A good communicator is aware of the characteristics of adolescence, which enhances his or her ability to relate to teenagers. These characteristics are as follows:

1. *Peers are important.* The adolescent's relationship to those outside the nuclear and extended family becomes important. Friends, classmates, teammates, and popular persons of similar age are all involved in the life of the teenager. A dentist can enhance his or her ability to communicate with adolescents by asking about peer interaction and by knowing who is involved in the teen's life.

2. *Fads and experimentation are part of adolescence.* Successful adolescent practitioners are those who are aware of the trends, popular fads, and celebrities that are of interest to teens. A clear demonstration of this to teens is the presence of posters or contemporary music in the operatory. The dentist who knows the trends and interests of the adolescent has an edge in establishing communication and in reaching the teen on a nonauthoritarian basis. These are an entree into the teen's world that can be fostered and can lead to discussion of more significant issues with a sense of relationship. Contrast that access to the barrier that arises when both teen and dentist see themselves as worlds apart.

3. *Teens are trying to establish independence, searching for identity, making educational or career choices, and experimenting with sexuality.* All of these involve a certain degree of stress. Within that stressful period are times of anxiety, satisfaction, anger, excitement, and a host of other emotions. The dentist is a small part of the adolescent's world but is a mirror of it. How the practitioner fosters the healthy development of personality in a child and counsels him or her toward independence and career may be important in terms of both the teen's life and his or her dental health. In talking with teens, it is helpful to remember their "problem list" and to empathize about the stress of their lives, which is real to them. The office visit should be a mirror of life. It should provide a respite from pressures and be a cameo of the role that the adolescent plays as an adult patient. The relationship that the dentist would like to have with the adolescent as an adult should be fostered.

4. *The basis of success in adolescent-adult interactions is a good relationship.* The most significant factor in successful compliance and communication is the quality of the relationship between the dentist and the adolescent. In earlier periods of life, the child could be successfully motivated with reason, praise, or other approaches. The changing values and their short-term intensity in adolescence belie the use of these approaches in fostering long-term motivation. A feeling of trust, good communication, and a perception by the teenager of the dentist's sincere interest provide a strong motivation for compliance.

## General Appraisal

The general appraisal of the adolescent is confounded by the timing of physical growth changes, especially in the early teenage years. Within a group of young teenagers, girls can tower over boys and look far more like adults than their male peers. Similarly, within a group of boys, variations in voice tone, skin condition, amount and distribution of fat, and skeletal proportion are often remarkable. Differentiation of growth disorders is difficult at best.

### Determination of Developmental Status

Patients in early adolescence are clearly growing, but in the later stages growth slows dramatically and at some point nearly ceases. Extremely slow growth proceeds after that into early adulthood. The same is roughly true for facial growth. When patients are clearly growing, growth modification can be attempted. The question does arise in late adolescence regarding whether growth is continuing. At that point, growth modification should not be attempted and camouflage or surgical intervention should be considered.

This judgment on treatment method would be much easier if a biological marker could be identified that provided definitive information about the developmental status of the patient. Growth modification could be started if the marker indicated that sufficient growth remained to alter skeletal relationships. To be clinically useful, this biological marker would have to be reliable, easily identified, recognized in both sexes, and closely correlated with the growth of the facial bones. Unfortunately, a single biological marker of this description is not available. A number of clinical markers have been identified. However, studies have indicated that the relationship between the markers and facial growth, although statistically significant, is not so precise that growth can be predicted accurately. Because of the limited predictive value of the markers, one marker or another may be used to determine whether there is remaining growth, but it is extremely difficult to determine the extent of any remaining growth.

Height and weight measurements are often used to determine the patient's growth status. Measurements are plotted on standardized growth charts, which indicate the relative size of the patient. An average-sized child is located near the 50th percentile, and a large child is somewhere near the 90th percentile. A single measurement does not provide the clinician with all pertinent growth information, but it does give some idea about where the patient is developmentally compared with other children at this age.

A series of measurements, which may be available from the patient's physician or school nurse, provides much more information. The measurements can be plotted in one of two ways. The first way is to plot the measurements on a cumulative growth chart (Fig. 37-2). This provides information about the patient's total amount of growth up to the last measurement. The normal growth curve is sigmoidal, and the pubertal growth spurt corresponds to the steepest portion of the slope. Because growth charts are based on mean growth rates, the individual patient may show an accelerated or delayed growth spurt if his or her growth rate is not coincident with the mean growth rate. More importantly, some concern should be expressed if the patient is not following the percentiles (e.g., dropping from the 50th to the 40th to the 30th percentile over time). This suggests there may be a physical or psychological problem requiring medical attention.

Height and weight measurements can also be plotted as yearly growth increments rather than as total growth achieved up to that point (Fig. 37-3). By plotting measurements this way, changes in the growth rate can be easily identified. A sharp rise in height usually signals the start of the pubertal growth spurt, and growth modification treatment should be initiated immediately if it is required.

Height and weight measurements also can be compared with the height and weight of the patient's natural parents and siblings. Although the interaction between environment and heredity is not clearly understood, there is some familial influence on ultimate size, and it may be possible to glean useful information from the comparison.

Hand-wrist radiographs are used by some investigators to judge the skeletal age and development of the patient (Fig. 37-4). The size and maturational stage of certain hand and wrist bones are compared with published standards of normal bone development and skeletal age.[11] Unfortunately, the correlation between the appearance of reliable bone markers (skeletal growth status) and mean maximal mandibular growth velocity is not perfect and should not serve as the only index of facial growth. The ability to reliably read hand-wrist radiographs requires consistent practice. These radiographs should be used when growth is clearly a significant question. A hand-wrist radiograph for an 8-year-old invariably indicates future growth potential. But these radiographs are appropriate to determine the potential for remaining growth when skeletal problems remain to be corrected or are becoming a significant problem.

Another radiographic method that does not require additional radiation exposure is the use of cervical vertebral maturation from routine cephalometric radiographs (Fig. 37-5). This method uses the maturation stages of the second through fourth cervical vertebrae (Fig. 37-6) to evaluate mandibular growth potential. It is claimed that the peak mandibular growth occurs between stages 2 and 3.[2] Timing treatment for growth modification during this period of growth, according to some, could enhance the treatment effects.[3]

Secondary sexual characteristics provide some information about the amount of growth the patient has yet to experience. In females, breast stage development and menarche are markers that can be used to assess developmental status. Breast development determination as an objective clinical evaluation is obviously not practical in the dental office and is of little clinical use. Menarche, however, can be determined from the health history questionnaire or from an interview at the initial patient examination. Unfortunately, the pubertal growth spurt precedes menarche by more than 1 year.[28] Therefore menarche is basically used to decide whether growth modification is still feasible.

In the male, there is no single indicator such as menarche by which to judge developmental status. The amount and texture of facial hair and the patient's general physical appearance are two highly variable indicators of male developmental status and maturity. Facial hair usually appears near or following peak statural growth.

For a person with an obvious skeletal problem, more than one cephalometric head film of the patient may be available. These head films can be

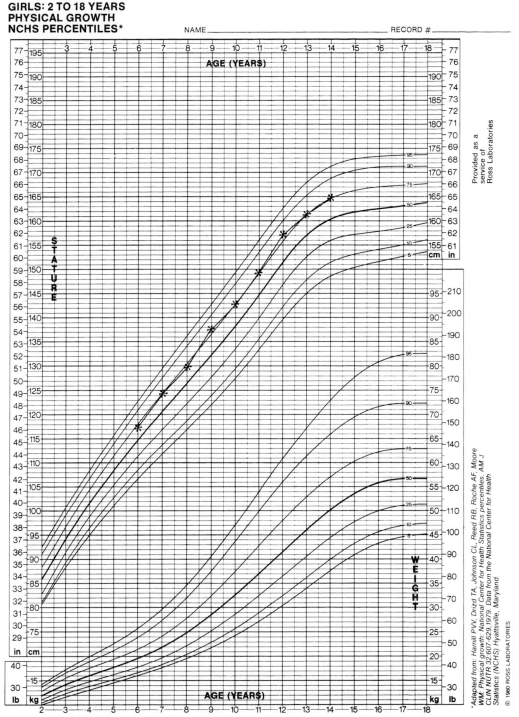

**Figure 37-2**   A standardized growth chart is used to indicate the relative size of the patient. A single measurement does not provide the clinician with all pertinent growth information, but it does give some idea of the developmental level of the patient compared with other children at a particular time. A series of measurements plotted on a standardized growth chart provides much more information than a single measurement. The measurements may be plotted in two ways. In the cumulative growth chart method, illustrated here, asterisks plot the measurements. This chart shows the patient's total growth up to the last measurement. This female patient has been measured yearly, starting at age 6, and is roughly following the 75th percentile line. (Adapted from Hamill PVV, Drizd TA, Johnson CL et al: Physical growth: National Center for Health Statistics percentiles. *Am J Clin Nutr* 32:607-629, 1979. Data from the National Center for Health Statistics, Hyattsville, Md. Courtesy of Ross Laboratories.)

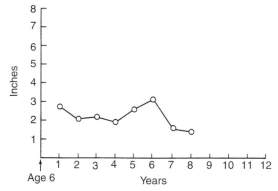

**Figure 37-3** Growth information also can be plotted as yearly growth increments rather than as total growth achieved to a certain point. The growth data for the female patient described in Fig. 37-2 are plotted here incrementally, beginning at age 6. By plotting measurements this way, changes in the growth rate can be easily identified. A sharp rise usually signals the start of the pubertal growth spurt.

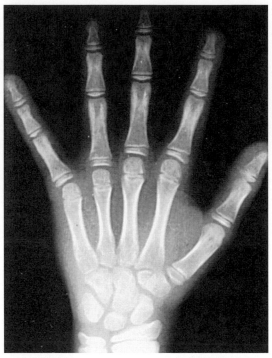

**Figure 37-4** A hand-wrist film is used occasionally to judge the skeletal age and skeletal development of a patient. The size and stage of certain bones are compared with published standards for known normal bone development and skeletal age. Reliable and accurate reading of the films requires considerable practice.

superimposed on each other to provide information about the amount and direction of growth that has occurred over time (Fig. 37-7). Although past growth tendencies do not guarantee that the patient will continue to grow or will grow according to the same pattern, comparing head films provides a great deal of information about the patient. However, it is unlikely for the average

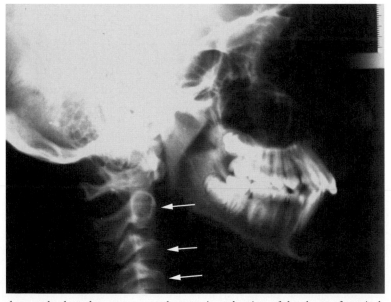

**Figure 37-5** Another method used to gauge growth status is evaluation of the shape of cervical vertebrae 2, 3, and 4 *(arrows)*. These images are available on routine cephalometric radiographs and require no additional radiation. It appears they can be reliably read, and are interpreted according to the stages described in Fig. 37-6.

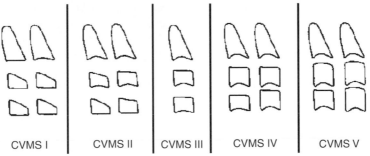

CVMS I     CVMS II     CVMS III     CVMS IV     CVMS V

**Figure 37-6**   The five stages of cervical vertebrae maturation are described in this diagram. These stages are equated with physical maturation, somatic growth, and mandibular growth. According to the reported data, peak mandibular growth is experienced prior to stage 3. A concavity develops on the lower border of the third vertebra during stage 2 and a similar one develops on the lower border of the fourth vertebra during stage 3. Vertebrae 3 and 4 undergo gradual transformation from horizontally rectangular shape to square to vertically rectangular shape during the maturation process. (From Baccetti T, Franchi L, McNamara JA Jr: An improved version of the cervical vertebral maturation (CVM) method for the assessment of mandibular growth. *Angle Orthod* 72:316-23, 2002.)

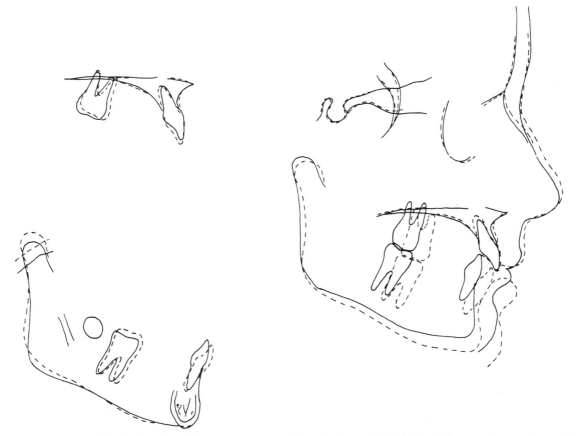

**Figure 37-7**   If more than one cephalometric head film of a patient is available, the head films can be superimposed on each other to provide information about the amount and direction of growth that has occurred over time. Although past growth tendencies do not guarantee that growth will continue in the same amount or in the same pattern, superimposed films provide substantial information about facial growth. The superimposition of the whole face registering on the anterior cranial base *(above right)* demonstrates changes of the maxilla, mandible, and profile. The maxillary superimposition registered on the ANS-PNS line, and internal architecture *(upper left)* shows maxillary dental changes. The mandibular superimposition registered on the inferior alveolar nerve canal, unerupted third molar crypt, and the inner aspect of the symphysis *(lower left)* shows mandibular dental changes and condylar growth.

patient to have a series of head films available for pretreatment review.

The patient's developmental status can also be judged from the developmental stage of the dentition. Panoramic or periapical radiographs can be used to determine the stage of development of individual permanent teeth. The results can be compared with standards relating dental development to chronologic age.[16] However, studies indicate that the relationship between dental age and skeletal maturation is weak and clinically useless.[7]

In summary, a number of biological markers are available by which the clinician can assess the developmental status of the patient. Unfortunately, no one marker by itself provides definitive information about the patient's growth potential. The most logical approach is to gather all available information and then make a judgment regarding the patient's growth potential and suitability for growth modification.

## Head and Neck Examination

The principles of the head and neck examination of the teenager are similar to those applied to the adult or child. Variations from normal can be caused by a variety of factors, the most notable of which are growth and developmental changes and the effects of the adolescent's environment.

The physical changes and habits in the teen require modification of the procedures used in children. On the positive side, the loss or redistribution of body fat and the elongation of the neck allow one to perform a better lymph node evaluation. These changes facilitate a thorough head and neck and cancer examination.

## Facial Examination

In the facial examination the dentist analyzes the soft tissue profile and the frontal face. During adolescence the face is beginning to assume adult-like features, and treatment decisions can be based more on current rather than on projected facial appearance. This does not mean that growth is complete, only that it has slowed considerably from its previous pace during the early adolescent growth spurt. The adult profile tends to be straighter than the adolescent's because of continued mandibular skeletal growth. In addition, the soft tissue of the chin increases

slightly in thickness. The nose also continues to grow, both horizontally and vertically. Most of this growth is horizontal, but the nasal tip tends to drop down a small amount. The lips are less protrusive in the adult because of these nasal and chin changes combined with a slight thinning of the soft tissue thickness of the lips.

For patients with class I skeletal and dental characteristics, the facial profile examination should provide an adequate basis for analysis when minor orthodontic treatment is considered. For the patient with a skeletal problem, a cephalometric radiograph and analysis are required to diagnose the problem definitively and prescribe treatment. When physical growth is occurring, facial growth usually is also occurring.

Treatment for skeletal orthodontic problems during preadolescence or early adolescence, when the adolescent growth spurt is still active, can result in growth modification. The preadolescent patient is assumed to be growing and is expected to experience a pubertal growth spurt. The young adolescent, especially the male, still has enough growth remaining to allow significant skeletal changes to occur with treatment. The adolescent by definition has experienced the pubertal growth spurt and is on the down side of the growth rate curve. Adults, on the other hand, have such limited facial growth that it is of little therapeutic potential.

These differences in growth potential have a large impact on how skeletal malocclusion is managed in the adolescent. The point is that as the individual becomes more skeletally mature, less skeletal growth modification can be accomplished. Therefore, as noted earlier, it is essential to establish the growth or developmental status of the patient in order to plan sensible treatment.

## Intraoral Examination

The larger oral cavity of the adolescent permits good visualization. Also, normal intellectual status and reasonable behavior provide cooperation in functional assessment of the occlusion and the temporomandibular joint. On the negative side, there are more teeth to evaluate, gingival and periodontal issues are present that were not critical in early childhood, and unpredictable growth changes can occur. The clinician should approach the adolescent as an adult, especially in the later teen years. For the first visit, the dentist may choose to "walk" the adolescent through the examination, using a hand mirror to explain procedures and normal findings.

## Periodontal Evaluation

In the adolescent more emphasis is placed on the periodontal examination. The prevalence of periodontal disease begins to increase in this age group.[22] The reason for this increase in periodontal disease is unknown at this time. Therefore, a thorough evaluation of the supporting structures is an absolute necessity. A periodontal probe is used to measure pocket depths, the width of keratinized gingiva, and the amount of attached gingiva, and to establish a bleeding index (Fig. 37-8). Periodontal probing should be confined to fully erupted teeth. Mobility tests may reveal slightly increased mobility in erupted teeth without complete root formation. The use of disclosing agents to reveal plaque, though helpful, may be discontinued at the patient's request. If a panoramic radiograph is used for diagnosis, selected periapical films may be needed if the clinical examination exposes any unusual periodontal findings. Referral to a specialist is suggested if significant periodontal disease is evident. During orthodontic treatment, gingival, plaque, and bleeding indices should be established at regular intervals to detect newly active periodontal disease.

## Related Hard and Soft Tissue Problems

A number of pathologic conditions may occur in adolescence and may be first noticed in this period. One is temporomandibular joint disorder (TMD), described in more detail later in this

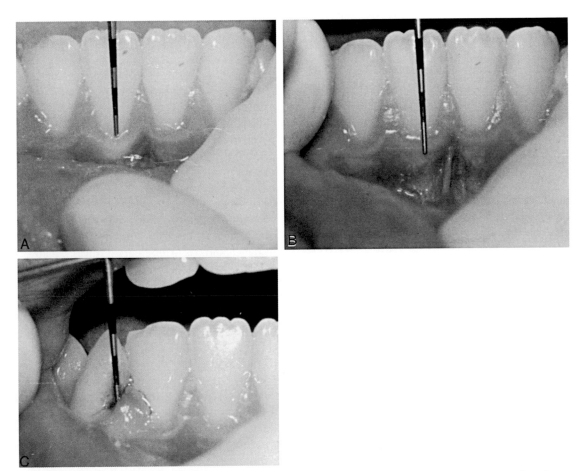

**Figure 37-8** The prevalence of periodontal disease begins to increase in the adolescent patient; therefore, a thorough evaluation of the periodontium is absolutely necessary. A periodontal probe is used to measure pocket depth (**A**) and the width of the keratinized gingiva (**B**) and to probe to establish a bleeding index (**C**). The amount of attached gingiva is determined by subtracting the pocket depth from the width of the keratinized gingiva.

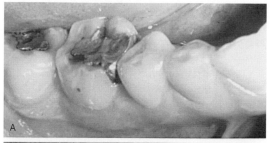

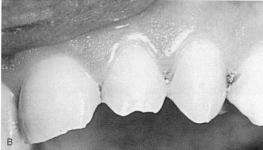

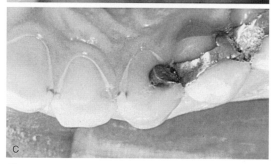

**Figure 37-9** Common intraoral findings for a bulimic patient are as follows: **A,** loss of occlusal enamel with exposure of dentin; **B,** ragged incisal edges as a result of fracturing of enamel; and **C,** lingual exposure of dentin highlighted by outlines of remaining enamel and exposed surfaces of restorations. (From Casamassimo P, Castaldi C: Considerations in the dental management of the adolescent. *Pediatr Clin North Am* 29:648, 1982.)

chapter. Anorexia nervosa often shows up in enamel erosion of all teeth if vomiting is a regular component of this psychiatric disorder.[4] Bulimia is the term given to those who vomit regularly to purge themselves of food in a misdirected attempt to control their weight. Bulimia affects far more girls than boys, but boys can exhibit similar behavior. The regurgitated stomach contents, which are highly acidic, erode the enamel of teeth in a process called perimyolysis (Fig. 37-9). Dentin is exposed, making teeth sensitive and encouraging decay. Enamel flakes off, leaving sharp edges. Restorations may appear to have grown out of their preparations as enamel and dentin dissolve around them. During clinical examination, these

problems speak for themselves; however, in the early bulimic, they may be absent. It may help to air dry the teeth to look for etching of surfaces.

Management of bulimia is a psychiatric problem. Treatment of the teeth is equally difficult and expensive. Pulpal pathosis, elongated clinical crowns, gingival recession, and loss of vertical dimension are a few of the treatment issues noted in bulimia. Unless the vomiting is stopped, extensive treatment may be futile. The dentist should work with a psychotherapist to deal with this problem.

Another pathologic problem is dental trauma. The clinical and radiographic examination should address tooth crazing, chips, or discoloration with adjunctive radiographs to clarify the status of teeth. Not all teeth that appear sound clinically are healthy (Fig. 37-10), and not all trauma is to hard tissues. The effects of smoking and oral sexual activity (Fig. 37-11) may be identified during the examination. Oral piercing has become popular in teenagers and young adults, but it is associated with risks of systemic infection and tissue damage during placement and deferred risks of tooth fracture and localized infection while the item is being worn (Fig. 37-12).

Evaluation of third molars is usually completed during mid- to late adolescence. Parents commonly ask about treating these teeth. The reasons for extraction of third molars include impaction or failure to erupt; potential or existing pathosis such as cysts or ameloblastoma; decay; posteruption malposition; nonfunction as a result of an absent opposing tooth; difficulty with hygiene; and recurrent pericoronitis. If any of these are considerations, third molars should be removed during adolescence.

The concept of anterior crowding as the result of forward pressure from third molars is currently unproved and is not a reason to extract. Surgical access and root development are important issues in determining when to extract. Some root development is desired to stabilize teeth, but complete root development can make extraction more difficult and may increase the likelihood of root fractures. Females using oral contraceptives and smokers may also run a high risk of postsurgical dry socket.

### Occlusal Evaluation

Evaluation of the occlusion in three spatial planes is similar to the intraoral examination described in previous chapters. The major difference is that

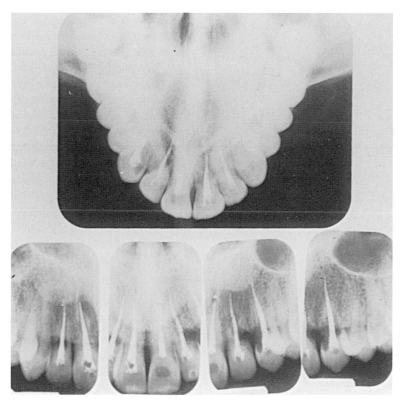

**Figure 37-10** Severe resorption of roots secondary to trauma is evident on radiographic examination. These teeth were remarkably stable clinically despite the amount of root resorption.

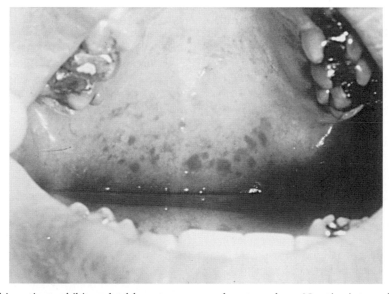

**Figure 37-11** This patient exhibits palatal hematomas secondary to oral sex. Negative intraoral pressures cause blood to be pulled to the surface of the palatal tissue.

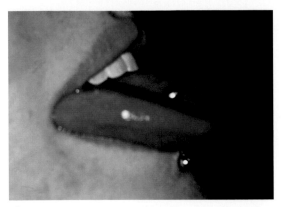

**Figure 37-12** An example of a tongue piercing, known as a dumbbell, that is common among teenagers and young adults but that has been shown to fracture enamel.

arch length deficiencies are no longer predicted from space analyses but are measured directly from the casts because all permanent teeth usually have erupted by this age. The first step is to measure the arch circumference by dividing the arch into segments extending from the mesial of the permanent first molar to the mesial of the contralateral first molar (Fig. 37-13, *A*). Each segment is measured over the contact points and incisal edges of the teeth. The segments are added together to yield the total arch circumference. Next, the mesiodistal width of each individual permanent tooth is measured, and the widths are added together (Fig. 37-13, *B*). The difference between the arch circumference and the sum of the mesiodistal widths indicates the amount of

---

# Smoking and Smokeless Tobacco
*Henry W. Fields*

The use of tobacco by children and adolescents is a complex issue. The data appear clear that the impact of tobacco on the body is both systemic and local. With regard to smoking, cardiovascular (stroke, heart attack, and hypertension) as well as lung disease and cancer of the oral and respiratory tree are well known sequelae.[1] Periodontal disease also is more prevalent in smokers.[2] Although most oral cancer occurs after 30 years of age, it can occur earlier.[3] An oral cancer examination should be routine for all patients with examination of all mucosa, tongue, palatal, and oropharyngeal surfaces.

Smoking cessation is difficult at best. The social and environmental cues that reinforce the smoking habit, combined with the potential nicotine addiction, make this a tough problem to conquer. This may be compounded in youth where both the habit and the search for help are often clandestine. Certainly educating children and adolescents and preventing tobacco use is the preferred approach. When the habit has been acquired, the best cessation results appear to be those where behavioral support is combined with nicotine replacement therapy (NRT).[4] Clinicians should attempt an intervention because they provide great impact.[5] The options are: patients *willing* to try to quit tobacco use should be provided treatments identified as effective or patients *unwilling* to try to quit tobacco use should be provided a brief intervention designed to increase their motivation to quit.[4] The latter can be an unstructured and informal discussion of the reasons to quit and the barriers that the patient might encounter. Working with parents and children in a cessation regimen incorporating NRT requires parental consent because although those under 18 years of age have ready access on most occasions, it is a violation of Food and Drug Administration regulations.[6]

Smokeless tobacco appears to be an increasingly popular alternative to smoking, especially among young men where it has increased from 0.7% in 1970 to 7.5% in 1991.[7] More distressing, among high school students the prevalence is approximately 9% with 20.6% among white high school males.[8] Smokeless tobacco is easier to consume without impinging on family, friends, and smoke-free environments while at the same time achieving a substantial nicotine impact. Whether smokeless tobacco is implicated in oral cancer is important because since 1970 the 5-year survival rate of oral cancer victims has increased, but only by about 3%.[9] Like smoking, the environment (e.g., certain social situations) can provide behavioral cues that stimulate the desire to use smokeless tobacco.[10]

Aside from the unsightly necessities that accompany some smokeless spit tobaccos, there are other side effects that make it a questionable health practice. The potential for nicotine addiction is high with all types of tobacco products.[11] Certainly, long-term use of nicotine in any form carries the risk of hypertension. Blood pressure monitoring indicates that such changes follow tobacco users of any type.[12] Furthermore, it appears to some that

## Smoking and Smokeless Tobacco—cont'd

smokeless tobacco is a gateway drug to cigarettes.[13]

When oral health is considered, there appears to be greater risk of localized periodontal attachment loss in the form of gingival recession in smokeless tobacco users, commonly adjacent to where the tobacco is placed.[14] There also appears to be a greater risk of leukoplakia among smokeless tobacco users,[15] even when they are adolescents.[16] But there is good evidence that smokeless tobacco keratosis is largely reversible.[17] The major dispute in this area is whether smokeless tobacco is a likely cause of oral cancer. The evidence is not decisive but points in that direction.[15] It is not unreasonable to counsel your patients and help them with cessation programs so that they can avoid the transient and possibly more morbid potential effects of smokeless tobacco as well as the potential systemic side effects.

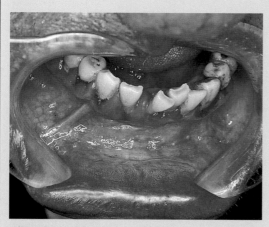

Clinical appearance of a white lesion associated with smokeless tobacco (tobacco pouch keratosis). (From Ibsen O, Phelan J: *Oral Pathology for the Dental Hygienist*, 4th ed. Philadelphia, Saunders, 2004.)

As mentioned earlier, cessation programs can and should be initiated by dentists for their patients who use smokeless tobacco using a combined behavioral and pharmacologic approach. These can be self-help programs or those with more personal interactions. Data indicate some substantial success with these types of cessation interventions.[18] Some of these methods may be difficult without parental involvement given the restrictions for NRT. Enhancing this difficulty is the fact that most smokeless tobacco users do not associate their tobacco use with nicotine addiction.

1. Mitchell BE, Sobel HK, Alexander MH: The adverse effects of tobacco and tobacco-related products. *Tobacco Use and Cessation* 26:463-499, 1999.
2. Linden GJ, Mullally BH: Cigarette smoking and periodontal destruction in young adults. *J Periodontol* 65:718-723, 1994.
3. Ries LAG, Eisner MP, Kosary CL et al, editors. *SEER Cancer Statistics Review, 1975–2001*, Bethesda, MD, National Cancer Institute. Available at http://seer.cancer.gov/csr/1975_2001/, 2004.
4. Fiore MC, Bailey WC, Cohen SJ et al: *Treating Tobacco Use and Dependence.* Clinical Practice Guideline. Rockville, MD, US Department of Health and Human Services, Public Health Service, June 2000.
5. Demers RY, Neale AV, Adams R et al: The impact of physicians' brief smoking cessation counseling: a MIRNET study. *J Fam Pract* 31(6):625-629, 1990.
6. Johnson KC, Klesges LM, Somes GW et al: Access of over-the-counter nicotine replacement therapy products to minors. *Arch Pediatr Adolesc Med* 158(3):212-216, 2004.
7. Giovoni G, Schooley M, Zhu B et al: Surveillance for selected tobacco-use behaviors: United States, 1900–1994. Centers for Disease Control and Prevention. *MMWR Morb Mortal Wkly Rep* 43:1-43, 1994.
8. Centers for Disease Control and Prevention: Tobacco used among high school students: United States. *MMWR Morb Mortal Wkly Rep* 43:229-233, 1998.
9. American Cancer Society. Cancer Facts and Figures 2003. Available at http://www.cancer.org/downloads/STT/CAFF2003PW/Secured.PDF; June 2004.
10. Coffey SF, Lombardo TW: Effects of smokeless tobacco–related sensory and behavioral cues on urge, affect, and stress. *Exp Clin Psychopharmacol* 6(4):406-418, 1998.
11. Benowitz NL: Pharmacology of nicotine: addiction and therapeutics. *Annu Rev Pharmacol Toxicol* 36:597-613, 1996.
12. Bolinder G, de Faire U: Ambulatory 24-h blood pressure monitoring in healthy, middle-aged smokeless tobacco users, smokers, and nontobacco users. *Am J Hypertens* 11(10):1153-1163, 1998.
13. Haddock CK, Weg MV, DeBon M et al: Evidence that smokeless tobacco use is a gateway for smoking initiation in young adult males. *Prev Med* 32(3):262-267, 2001.

*Continued*

## Smoking and Smokeless Tobacco—cont'd

14. Robertson PB, Walsh M, Greene J et al: Periodontal effects associated with the use of smokeless tobacco. *J Periodontol* 61(7):438-443, 1990.
15. Waterbor JW, Adams RM, Robinson JM et al: Disparities between public health educational materials and the scientific evidence that smokeless tobacco use causes cancer. *J Cancer Educ* 19(1):17-28, 2004.
16. Creath CJ, Cutter G, Bradley DH, Wright JT: Oral leukoplakia and adolescent smokeless tobacco use. *Oral Surg Oral Med Oral Pathol* 72(1):35-41, 1991.
17. Martin GC, Brown JP, Eifler CW, Houston GD: Oral leukoplakia status six weeks after cessation of smokeless tobacco use. *JADA* 130(11):1558, 1999.
18. Severson HH, Akers L, Andrews JA et al: Evaluating two self-help interventions for smokeless tobacco cessation. *Addict Behav* 25:465-470, 2000.

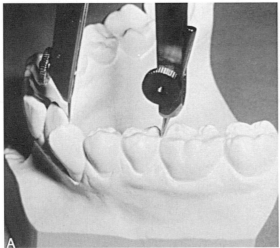
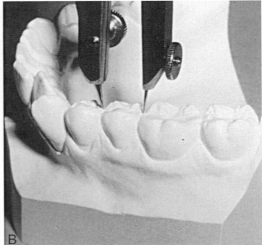

**Figure 37-13    A,** Arch length analysis in the adolescent patient is measured directly from casts rather than by using prediction tables of mixed dentition space analysis because all permanent teeth usually have erupted by this age. The first step is to measure the arch circumference by dividing the arch into segments extending from the mesial of the permanent first molar to the mesial of the contralateral first molar. **B,** Next, the mesiodistal width of each individual permanent tooth is measured, and the widths are added together. The difference between the arch circumference and the sum of the mesiodistal width indicates the amount of crowding or spacing within the arch.

crowding or spacing in the arch. If one or two primary teeth have not exfoliated, the width of the contralateral erupted permanent tooth can be substituted for the unerupted permanent tooth.

Careful attention should be paid to teeth adjacent to edentulous areas because these teeth may need to be repositioned orthodontically prior to restorative treatment. The pulpal and restorative status of these teeth helps to determine the direction of treatment.

Once again, the interaction between the facial profile and dental crowding should be considered. Committing the patient to treatment based solely on dental characteristics can have a disastrous effect on the facial profile.

The anteroposterior, transverse, and vertical occlusal components should be evaluated as described in Chapter 30.

### Radiographic Evaluation

The adolescent radiographic examination ranges from a transitional to an adult multifilm survey, depending on the child's dentition. The issues surrounding radiographic examination in the adolescent are related to the type and frequency of exposure. The types of films used in adolescent radiography should be determined by the number of teeth present and the reason for radiographic examination. For the new adolescent patient with major dental care needs, a survey should include, at the minimum, three to five anterior maxillary periapical films, three mandibular anterior films, a periapical film of each posterior quadrant, and right and left bitewing films. The anterior films should be adult size no. 1, whereas posterior films should be no. 2 films. It is also recommended that all tooth-bearing areas be surveyed within 2 years of the eruption of the permanent second molars. This can be achieved with a full-mouth survey or a panoramic radiograph combined with bitewing radiographs.

The radiographic examination in this age group should address mainly growth and development issues: the eruption status of unerupted premolars and canines. Later in adolescence, a final issue is third molar development. The development of these teeth can be evaluated by using periapical radiographs or a third molar panoramic radiograph (Fig. 37-14).

The adolescent should be able to tolerate size 2 intraoral films. For the child with a small oral cavity, techniques to aid in positioning are described in the radiographic section of Chapter 30.

Multiple or serial periapical radiographs are required for diagnosis of pathosis or for management of conditions that require significant follow-up, such as endodontic therapy for traumatized incisors.

Bitewing radiography during early adolescence is affected by the developing occlusion and lack of contacts. It may be that most if not all posterior surfaces can be adequately visualized until the premolars have fully erupted. The benefit of exposing bitewing films to examine two or four interproximal surfaces should be weighed against the risk. In these cases, the history of decay and a thorough clinical examination help to determine whether films are necessary.

The panoramic film has a role in adolescent dentistry as a full-mouth radiographic survey for a new patient who does not have major treatment needs. For this adolescent, who is essentially clinically disease free, the panoramic film and bitewing survey may be adequate to determine dental health. The panoramic film reveals bone pathosis and orients the examiner to the presence and position of third molars. The panoramic film also grossly displays sinuses and the temporomandibular joint (Fig. 37-15), which may be less well displayed on a multifilm intraoral survey. Table 37-2 summarizes the issues that apply to radiography of the adolescent patient.

## TREATMENT PLANNING FOR NONORTHODONTIC PROBLEMS

In the adolescent patient, attention must be paid to the long-term consequences of immediate treatment. Although the transitional dentition is considered in terms of its effect on the adult, the adolescent dentition must be considered as being that of the adult. In other words, there are no teeth to follow, only substitutes.

All phases of treatment planning should be addressed. The adolescent depicted in Figure 37-16 illustrates the complexity of problems requiring preventive, periodontal, restorative, and endodontic management.

All adolescents should receive the benefit of a preventive plan that addresses the particular needs of the adult dentition such as flossing. In addition, the preventive plan should address environmental concerns such as smoking, diet, trauma prevention, and the effect of medications on the periodontium and teeth.

Periodontal and gingival concerns are now solidly tied to restorative care. In the child, the minor inflammation around a stainless steel

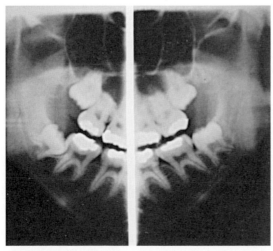

**Figure 37-14** In late adolescence, the presence and developmental status of unerupted third molars are evaluated by using periapical radiographs, a conventional panoramic radiograph, or a "third molar" panoramic radiograph as shown here.

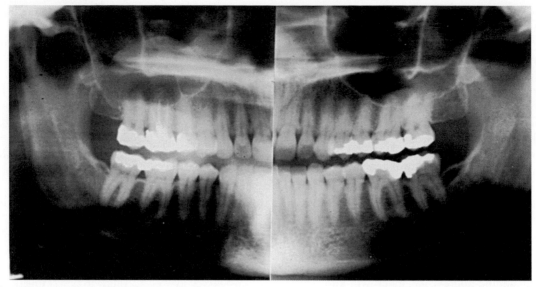

**Figure 37-15**    A large mucosal cyst in the sinus is evident in this panoramic radiograph of a 21-year-old patient. The cyst is possibly a reaction to pulpal pathosis in the permanent maxillary first and second molars.

crown on a primary tooth that is due to grossly adjusted margins is tolerated. In the adolescent, with a cast crown, the tissues must be completely healthy.

Restorative treatment planning for the teen is characterized by a number of issues[6]:

1. Pulp size is large, affecting choice of coronal coverage.
2. Anterior teeth continue to erupt, requiring consideration of various types of aesthetic restorations for traumatized or defective teeth to prevent exposure of margins.
3. Aesthetic awareness by the patient may force the dentist to undertake management of congenital or acquired discoloration or may require repeated treatment of teeth if transitional procedures are used.
4. Partially erupted posterior teeth may not serve as good abutments for protheses.
5. Decreased chewing efficiency resulting from loss of a posterior tooth may force interim replacement with a removable appliance, although this may not be the treatment of choice.
6. Planned or active orthodontic treatment may delay restoration of missing teeth.
7. Active athletic involvement may necessitate interim replacement of teeth.

The use of acid-etch composite resins and porcelain veneers has greatly improved the man-agement of adolescent restorative problems by providing aesthetically acceptable, reasonably priced, conservative interim and permanent restorations. Their consideration as treatment options in restorative treatment planning is a must.

The two remaining elements of importance in adolescent treatment planning are interrelated. They are consent and compliance. Treatment of adolescents under the age of majority requires parental consent. Payment for services also demands clarification of consent. The proposed treatment is best explained with both parent and adolescent present, although the actual delivery of care can occur with the adolescent alone in the operatory. Good one-on-one dialogue during active treatment helps to ensure compliance. Some general guidelines for communication to maximize success include the following:

1. Show the adolescent the same respect and interest as you would an adult.
2. Be sincere.
3. Treat the adolescent in privacy as an adult, separate from younger children.
4. Outline procedures and explain reasons for them.
5. Minimize or eliminate authoritarian posturing, using your knowledge rather than age as a reason for your role as a dentist.
6. Be flexible enough to adapt to a changing relationship.

## TABLE 37-2
### Radiographic Issues in the Adolescent

| ASPECT | RECOMMENDATION |
|---|---|
| **Frequency** | |
| Full mouth survey | No suggested frequency or interval |
| Bite-wing radiographs | No suggested frequency or interval |
| | Should be taken if clinical caries noted |
| | Should be taken if multiple interproximal restorations present and are being followed |
| | Should be taken if incipiencies noted on previous films and are being followed |
| | Interval for these situations should be individualized and reevaluated at each periodic examination |
| Periapical radiographs | No suggested frequency or interval |
| | Pathosis or treatment needs should dictate frequency |
| | To determine developmental status of third molars |
| Panoramic radiographs | Possible component of a full mouth survey for a disease-free new patient |
| | "Third molar" panoramic radiograph to determine developmental status of third molars |
| **Type** | |
| Full mouth survey | Number of films included to be based on tissue coverage needed |
| | *Early adolescence* (12-14 years): |
| |     Maxillary and mandibular periapicals (no. 1 size) |
| |     Canine periapicals (no. 1 or 2) |
| |     Bite-wings (two films, no. 2 size) |
| |     Four posterior quadrant periapicals (no. 2 size) to include premolars and erupted molars |
| | *Late adolescence* (16-21 years): |
| |     Complete set (21-film) survey |
| Bite-wing radiographs | Size determined by oral access, but no. 2 size used if possible |
| | One film sufficient until eruption of second molars |
| | Position varies with the location and number of posterior contacts |
| Periapical radiographs | Should be adult no. 1 size films rather than no. 2 size, used as occlusal film as in primary tooth survey |
| | An exception would be use of no. 2 film as initial trauma screen |
| Panoramic radiographs | Can be used with bite-wings for a full mouth survey and is desirable in caries-free and pathosis-free patients after a clinical examination |
| | "Third molar" panoramic radiograph can be used to determine developmental status of third molars |

## TREATMENT PLANNING AND TREATMENT FOR ORTHODONTIC PROBLEMS

Adolescent orthodontic problems create difficult treatment decisions for the general practitioner and the specialist. The nature of the malocclusion heavily influences how the problem will be managed.

### Skeletal Problems

If the malocclusion is skeletal, treatment is aimed at altering the relationship or orientation of the jaws and teeth. This can be accomplished by growth modification, camouflage, or orthognathic surgery. Because the physical maturity of the adolescent patient varies among persons of the same age, any one of three treatments may

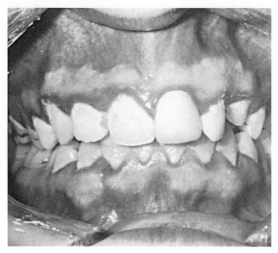

**Figure 37-16** The dentition of a 19-year-old man. The final treatment problems included caries, bone loss, defective crowns, and pulpal involvement of two anterior maxillary teeth.

be appropriate. If the developmental assessment of the patient suggests that the patient is actively growing, growth modification is a viable treatment alternative. Growth modification, previously discussed, attempts to change the actual size, shape, or orientation of the jaws to obtain an acceptable occlusion. Functional appliances and extraoral traction are used to secure these changes.

In the nongrowing, physically mature adolescent, which is most likely the case, skeletal malocclusion is appropriately treated by camouflage or orthognathic surgery. Camouflage is the orthodontic movement of teeth without changing the underlying skeletal malocclusion. Camouflage should be considered only when the soft tissue profile is acceptable and when tooth movement will not change or compromise the profile. Teeth are tipped or bodily moved on the denture base to positions considered less than ideal but acceptable for normal occlusion. For example, a mild class II mandibular deficiency with a relatively prominent bony pogonion can be managed by camouflage (Fig. 37-17). To camouflage this type of problem, the upper teeth are tipped backward and the lower teeth are tipped forward to bring the teeth together and disguise the skeletal problem. In conjunction with the tipping of teeth for camouflage, teeth in the maxillary arch can be extracted to provide more space in which to tip the upper teeth backward. Although a small amount of soft tissue change may occur and the final position of the mandibular incisors may be less than ideal, functional occlusion can be

achieved without surgery. Traditionally, camouflage of class II skeletal problems has been considered more acceptable in women and camouflage of class III problems more acceptable in men because the respective convex and straight profiles are more acceptable for these groups. Recent data indicate more acceptance among lay people.[24] The aesthetic results in males with moderately class II problems were judged to be as acceptable as those in females with class II problems, whereas the results in males with moderate class III problems remained more aesthetically acceptable than those in females with class III problems. Camouflage of class III problems usually is addressed with lingual tipping of mandibular anterior teeth to obtain an acceptable overbite and overjet while at the same time moving the upper dentition anteriorly. The mandibular tipping is often more easily accomplished when extractions are performed in the lower arch. At least for class II patients, most consider treatment by camouflage extremely acceptable even though they realize they have somewhat smaller or more retrusive chin points.[15] Skeletal malocclusion in the nongrowing patient can also be managed with orthognathic surgery.[23] The specialist works with an oral and maxillofacial surgeon to reposition one or both jaws into proper alignment surgically (Fig. 37-18). Typically, the orthodontic treatment plan calls for a presurgical period of orthodontic tooth movement to align teeth in both arches and position the teeth over the bony bases so that they will fit together following the surgery. Orthognathic surgery is performed under general anesthesia, and the maxilla, mandible, or both jaws are repositioned and held in the new position by either wire or, more commonly, surgical screws or bone plates and screws. It is possible to move the entire jaw or individual segments of the jaw in almost any direction within the constraints of the soft tissue covering. There is some restriction on the amount of change that can be achieved, and some types of change are more stable than others. Following the surgical procedure, jaw function is reduced with wire fixation or elastic traction. After healing is demonstrated, a short period of postsurgical orthodontic procedures is necessary to settle the teeth into the final occlusion.

## Dental Problems

If the orthodontic problem in the adolescent is strictly dental, conventional orthodontic treatment can be used to manage the malocclusion.

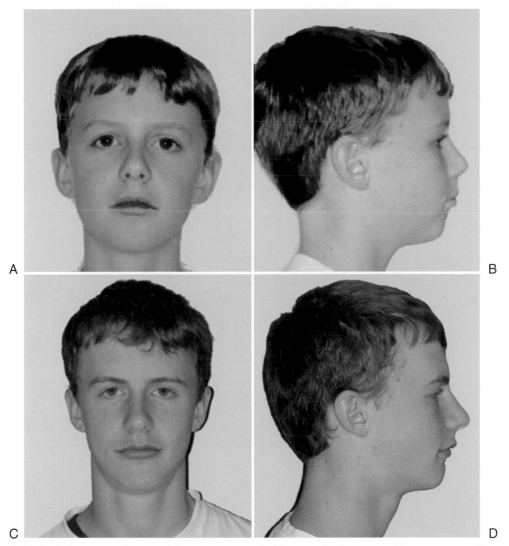

**Figure 37-17    A,** This preadolescent patient has a convex facial profile (**B**) due to maxillary protrusion. Because the facial profile is acceptable even though the skeletal relationships are not ideal, the teeth were moved to reduce the overjet and obtain a functional occlusion by retracting the maxillary teeth and proclining the mandibular teeth. **C,** At the adolescent posttreatment stage, the facial profile (**D**) remains convex but acceptable with continued maxillary protrusion.

Identification and management of dental orthodontic problems have already been discussed and basically do not change with the age of the patient. However, there is one aspect of dental orthodontic treatment that has not been discussed and should be mentioned here. Despite the preventive efforts of the dental profession, some persons continue to lose permanent teeth to decay or trauma. Other patients lose primary teeth during adolescence, which have no successors. When this occurs, a combination of orthodontic tooth movement and restorative dentistry is recommended to obtain an optimal aesthetic and functional result.

In the anterior region, orthodontic treatment is often designed to move teeth to simplify prosthetic treatment. To provide precise control of tooth movement, orthodontic brackets should be bonded to all the anterior teeth and bands should be placed on the permanent first molars. Treatment must be carefully planned so that only the teeth that require movement are affected and the other teeth remain stationary. This means that molar, canine, and midline relationships should be carefully studied and controlled during treatment. For example, if one lateral incisor is missing or if the lateral incisor is peg shaped, the space between the central incisor and the canine on that

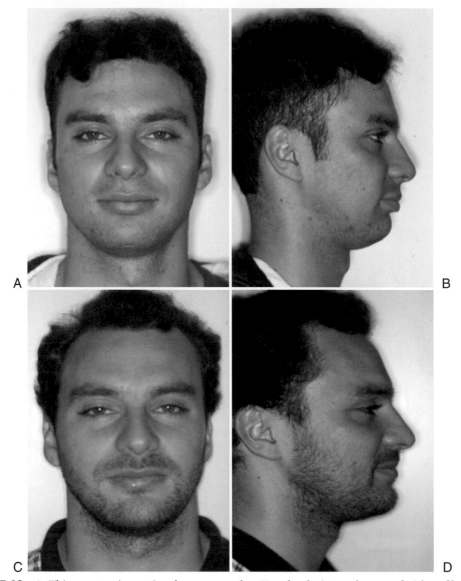

**Figure 37-18**   **A,** This nongrowing patient has a severe class II malocclusion and convex facial profile (**B**) due to mandibular retrusion. The teeth cannot be moved together to provide a stable, functional occlusion, so orthognathic surgery was performed to advance the mandible. **C,** After surgery the patient demonstrates more mandibular prominence (**D**) and facial height.

side should equal the distance between these two teeth on the other side. This ensures that the restored width of the lateral incisor matches that of the contralateral lateral incisor.

To obtain the best results, a diagnostic setup should be performed so that the final tooth position and relationships can be defined. This can be accomplished by duplicating and sectioning the teeth to be moved on plaster dental study casts. The teeth are then reset in wax to provide a treatment goal and demonstrate the goal to the patient (Fig. 37-19). Multiple setups might be

required for a single patient. Alternatively, digital study casts can be manipulated so that several treatment alternatives can be examined by the patient and dentist (Fig. 37-20).

Elastomeric chain, archwire loops, and coil springs can be used to open, close, and stabilize space (Fig. 37-21). Once the space has been opened and is nearly ideal, a closed coil spring or loops bent into the archwire are used to hold or maintain the space until the restorative or prosthetic treatment is completed. Although this type of treatment sounds simple, close attention to

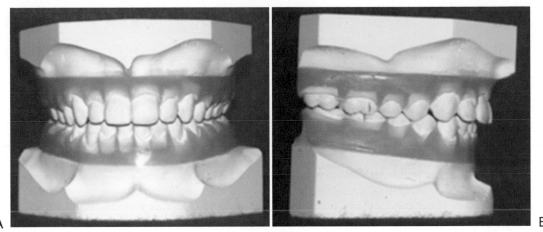

A                                                                                                                    B

**Figure 37-19**   **A,** Diagnostic setups can be used to demonstrate a treatment goal. This diagnostic setup shows a potential final occlusion where there is a maxillary anterior excess of tooth mass. **B,** Note that the molar and canine relationships are class I, but there is increased overjet because there is more upper tooth mesiodistal width from canine to canine than there is mandibular mesiodistal tooth structure.

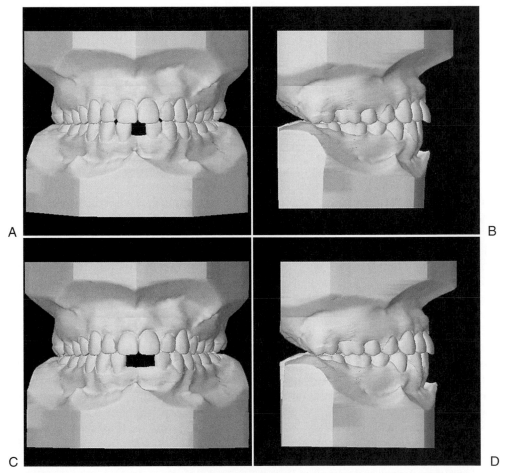

A                                                                                                                    B

C                                                                                                                    D

**Figure 37-20**   It is now possible to produce digital casts and manipulate the images to simulate setups. This series of images demonstrates options for this patient with missing lower central incisors using this technology. (**A**) An alternative is to make space for one incisor implant. (**B**) This solution positions the anterior teeth with more overbite and overjet than (**C**) a setup with space for two mandibular central incisors implants (**D**), which reduces the overbite and overjet when the posterior dental relationships are identical. (Courtesy OrthoCAD by Cadent, Inc.)

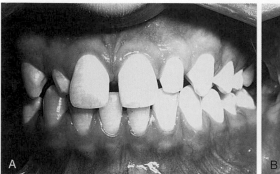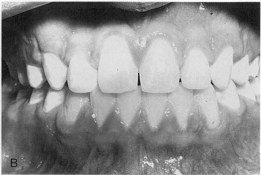

**Figure 37-21**   Orthodontic treatment is often necessary to move teeth to simplify prosthetic treatment. **A,** In this patient, the anterior space was closed and the lateral incisors were positioned to allow proper mesiodistal crown dimensions. **B,** Resin crown buildups were placed following orthodontic treatment. Retention is important to keep the space completely closed.

detail is necessary. Uncontrolled tooth movement can result in unanticipated changes in the midline, overjet, and overbite.

In the posterior region, orthodontic treatment may be necessary to upright teeth that have tipped into extraction sites after loss of permanent teeth. Typically, the permanent first molar is lost as a result of carious or periodontal involvement, and the second molar tips mesially into the extraction site while the second premolar tips distally. Both teeth next to the edentulous area may need to be uprighted to improve the periodontal and restorative potential. Orthodontically, uprighting of teeth will (1) facilitate more conservative, ideal restorations, (2) eliminate plaque-forming areas, (3) improve the alveolar ridge contour, (4) improve the crown-to-root ratio, and (5) reestablish long axis force loading of the teeth. This is best accomplished with limited single-arch, fixed-appliance treatment. Bonded brackets or bands are placed on the canine and first and second premolars. The second molar is banded. In addition, a 32-mil wire is bonded to the lingual surface of both canines to provide additional anchorage and stability during molar uprighting. There is a possibility that the arch form could change or that other teeth could move inadvertently if the lingual wire is not in place.

After the appliance has been placed, either segmental or continuous archwire mechanics can be used to upright the teeth. Selection of mechanics depends on the severity of the tipping. If the tooth is not severely tipped, a light, round, continuous archwire can be placed from the molar to the canine. Next, the occlusion on the molar

should be adjusted by reducing the length of the crown with a bur to allow the molar to erupt and upright. Finally, any periodontal defects around the tipped teeth should be thoroughly curetted to reduce inflammation and loss of attachment during treatment. Occlusal adjustments and curettage should be performed at each appointment. At subsequent appointments, the size of the archwire is progressively increased until it is of sufficient size and strength to upright and position the teeth ideally. Sometimes a coil spring placed between the premolar and molar is required to tip the molar distally and increase the edentulous space.

If the molar is too tipped for a continuous archwire to be placed, segmental mechanics are employed. The canine-premolar segment is aligned independent of the molar via a progression of archwires similar to that just described. When initial alignment of this segment is completed, an uprighting spring is bent from 19.5- to 25-mil stainless steel wire (Fig. 37-22, *A*). A helix is bent in the spring to provide more flexibility and a greater range of activation. In addition, a hook is bent into the end of the uprighting spring to allow the spring to be attached to the segmental wire just distal to the canine bracket; this allows the uprighting spring room to move distally along the segmental wire as the molar becomes upright (Fig. 37-22, *B*). The force of activation should provide approximately 75 to 100 g of force to "upright" the molar.

After the molar has been ideally positioned, tooth movement must be retained until a prosthetic replacement can be fabricated. The clini-

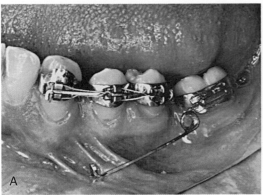
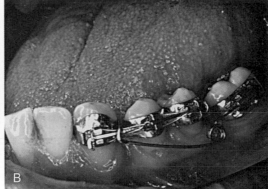

**Figure 37-22** Occasionally, a permanent first molar is missing in adolescents and young adults, and molar uprighting is necessary before prosthetic treatment can begin. The canine and premolar teeth are stabilized independently with a large segmental rectangular wire. The canines are usually stabilized further, using a bonded or banded lingual wire. After the anterior teeth are stabilized, the molar can be uprighted using a 19.5 × 25-mil helical spring placed in a bonded or banded tube on the tipped molar. **A,** The spring is passive prior to engagement of the archwire. **B,** The spring engaged on the archwire delivers the uprighting and extrusive forces to the tipped molar. Reduction of occlusal interference is necessary to allow the molar to move freely. (From Fields HW, Proffit WF: Orthodontics in general practice. In: Morris AL, Bohannan HM, Casullo DP, editors. *The Dental Specialties in General Practice.* Philadelphia, Saunders, 1983, p 327.)

cian can use either a fixed or a removable retainer. A fixed retainer is simply a 21- to 25-mil rectangular wire that rests on the occlusal surfaces of the abutment teeth. The wire should be bent down in the edentulous area to remain out of occlusion. Small rests can be placed in the occlusal surfaces of the abutment teeth with a high-speed handpiece, especially if the abutment teeth are scheduled for full-coverage restorations. The wire can be retained with either composite resin or amalgam. The major problem with wire retainers is bond and wire breakage under the stress of occlusion. If the patient does not return to have the wire repaired, relapse occurs rapidly. A removable appliance also can be used as a retainer. The edentulous area is filled with acrylic, and clasps are placed on either molars or premolars, depending on retention needs. Again, the removable appliance must be worn faithfully until the restorative treatment is completed.

Adolescent orthodontic treatment is a challenging exercise in problem solving. A good database and growth assessment are necessary to allow the proper decisions about treatment alternatives. Unless the orthodontic problem is obviously the result of dental malalignment, the patient should be referred to a specialist because of the difficulty in managing skeletal discrepancies in patients of this age.

## TEMPOROMANDIBULAR JOINT DISORDERS IN CHILDREN AND ADOLESCENTS

In 1982, the term *temporomandibular joint disorder* was adopted to encompass a range of conditions related to the masticatory system, including the temporomandibular joint, dentition, musculature, and supporting bone. Children and adolescents are susceptible to the range of conditions included under the term temporomandibular joint disorders, but the prevalence in this population is unclear. Certain afflictions of the temporomandibular joint (TMJ) are clearly identifiable, such as degeneration of the joint from juvenile rheumatoid arthritis or agenesis of the condyle in inherited conditions such as Goldenhar syndrome. These conditions usually have obvious clinical signs and can be confirmed with imaging and history. A more difficult diagnostic problem is chronic or acute orofacial pain attributable to TMD, that is, a constellation of muscle and/or joint pain and other signs with less clear-cut diagnostic criteria. However, consensus is being reached on diagnostic criteria for the more common TMDs. The diagnostic criteria of the American Academy of Orofacial Pain (AAOP) are currently the most commonly used in the clinical setting.[20]

Most authorities agree that the prevalence of TMD in children is not certain. TMD signs and symptoms are common in adults with 40% to 70% point prevalence of at least one sign of joint dysfunction such as joint noise or movement abnormality. Of adults, 33% experience at least one symptom of a TMD.[9,10,26,27] However, it is estimated that only 5% of the adult population is in need of treatment for these signs and symptoms.[9] The prevalence of TMD in children tends to be lower than in adults, with increasing frequency noted in the second and third decades.[13,17,29] The incidence of joint sounds may be as high as 17.5% over a 2-year period[30] although TMJ clicking may come and go during this time frame.[14] In spite of the difficulty in these assessments, there are several characteristics of TMD in the pediatric population that seem likely.

1. *Objective signs are common in the child population but many have no clinical significance.* Several studies identify a high prevalence of the following clinically observable findings:

- Occlusal wear or interferences[12]
- Joint sounds[8]
- Limitation of opening and mandibular deviation on opening[18]

These signs are common in children with an asymptomatic condition who have no complaints about pain. They may reflect normal variations in the child population or transient changes consistent with normal growth.

2. *Symptoms, such as pain, are not consistently associated with clinical signs.* A difficulty associated with both clinical diagnosis of TMD in individual children and determination of the prevalence of the condition in the pediatric population is the subjectivity of symptoms. Children often have difficulty in describing pain, localizing it, or understanding questions related to it.[25] At the clinical level, the younger the child, the more difficult are the localization of pain and an accurate history. Toothache, headache, ear pain, and muscle soreness are easily confused. Because children rarely seek care unilaterally, true TMD may not be addressed if parents are not concerned or can see no outward signs of illness.

3. *The relationship between signs and symptoms remains unclear.* Studies do not point to a clear etiologic factor for TMD in children or adults. The occurrence of signs or symptoms in studies of children ranges to well over 50% of subjects.[1] However, children with both symptoms

and signs who need treatment account for only about 2% of subjects. The absence of a clear relationship between signs and symptoms probably relates to the quality of diagnostic tests, a multifactorial etiologic process, as well as study limitations. Most diagnostic techniques used in research are noninvasive, nonspecific clinical examinations during function. TMJ imaging also has limitations of poor specificity and sensitivity as well as high cost. The role of psychological factors in TMD is difficult to determine in the study setting and often in practice.

The clinician should be aware of the poor correlation between TMD and a number of clinical and historical variables. Occlusal interferences, as in the adult, have little consistency in predicting TMD in children. A history of trauma has a much stronger relationship with TMD in adults than in children. Malocclusion, parafunctional habits, and orthodontic treatment have been implicated as precursors of TMD, but none of these has shown a clear and consistent relationship to TMD when scrutinized closely. The clinician is warned not to grasp these signs to support a diagnosis of TMD. None has consistently proved valuable in predicting TMD in either group or individual situations. To date, many causes have been established for TMD, but most of these have a clear and obvious relationship to their clinical manifestations. Degenerative disease, developmental abnor-

---

**BOX 37-1**

**Some Established Causes of Temporomandibular Joint Dysfunction in Children and Adolescents**

**Inherited**
Hemifacial microsomia
    Hemifacial atrophy
    Juvenile rheumatoid arthritis
    Ankylosis
    Cleft related

**Acquired**
Infectious (septic arthritis)
    Traumatic (sports injury)
    Iatrogenic (cortisone damage, surgical displacement, irradiation)
    Factitial (habits, hobbies)
    Neoplastic (tumors)
    Idiopathic

malities, and other conditions usually are obvious from historical and clinical evaluation. However, TMD in children is usually idiopathic. Box 37-1 suggests some causes of TMD in children.

4. *The efficacy of treatment for pediatric TMD remains controversial, and many techniques are unproved.* The lack of well-designed studies testing various treatment methods using randomization and clear success criteria hamper development of a reliable armamentarium. Authorities agree that irreversible removal of occlusal interferences in children is contraindicated. Preventive orthodontic therapy to eliminate risk factors has not withstood the test of time, nor has orthodontic therapy to manage existing TMD. Use of occlusal splints, which is not an invasive technique and is often an early intervention, also has produced mixed results. Early identification of a clear cause is often a mixed blessing because these causes tend often to be irreversible and have significant effects on the joint or masticatory system. Treatment often involves surgery and significant orthodontic and physical therapy. Regardless, if treatment is initiated, experts agree that all reversible therapies should be tried before irreversible techniques, such as surgery, are prescribed.

The clinician interested in TMD management should recognize that overdiagnosis and overtreatment are perhaps the most consistent aspects of dealing with this disorder in children.

### Diagnosis of Temporomandibular Joint Disorder

Every dentist who treats children should include a TMD screening examination to establish baseline function. The patient history must include a thorough medical and dental history to rule out inherited or acquired conditions (see Box 37-1). Trauma should be addressed. As with most painful disorders, especially if chronic, the pain history is critical to establishing a proper diagnosis. Information regarding, location, quality, intensity, duration, as well as initiating, exacerbating, and alleviating factors for pain should be elicited. The natural history of the pain complaint and past treatment and results of that treatment should also be obtained.

The clinical examination should include palpation of the exposed masticatory muscles as well as the trapezius, sternocleidomastoid, and posterior cervical musculature. The latter-mentioned cervical muscles may refer pain in the facial region and are frequently problematic in myofascial pain syndromes. The muscles may be palpated bilaterally and simultaneously by the clinician, who is directly in front of or behind the patient. The patient is asked whether it feels the same on both sides, if one side feels different, or if either side feels sore. The lateral pterygoid muscles are difficult to palpate intraorally and are best tested by having the patient protrude against chin resistance, which generally produces pain if the lateral pterygoid is symptomatic. The medial pterygoids are difficult to palpate. The temporomandibular joints may be palpated laterally while the patient opens and closes the mouth and moves side to side. Pain to palpation, clicking, and crepitus (grinding) are sought. Clicking is usually a sign of an anteriorly or anteriorly-medially displaced disk. Crepitus is usually a sign of joint degeneration. If limitation in mouth movement is noted, mandibular movement may be measured with a millimeter gauge placed between the right maxillary and mandibular incisors. The amount of overbite is added because that is actually the distance the mandible opens. If there is an open bite, the amount is subtracted from the maximal measurement. The child should be able to open approximately 35 to 45 mm. Generally, mild limitations in mandibular opening, especially if the opening can be increased with gentle downward mandibular pressure, is indicative of a muscular problem. A more profound mandibular opening limitation, especially if assisted opening does not produce an increase in mouth opening, is usually indicative of an intracapsular (joint) problem. The vertical position of the mandible when various joint noises occur should also be recorded. Deviation (movement away from midline that returns to midline) or deflection (persistent movement away from midline) of the mandible may also be observed.

Lateral movement of the mandible is not routinely recorded for children younger than 7 years because many of them have difficulty in following the directions, but beyond age 7 most children are able to comply. They are asked to "move your bottom jaw toward the shoulder I'm touching" or to "move your jaw side to side." The amount of lateral movement is measured in millimeters of change in the maxillary and mandibular dental midlines. The child should be able to move approximately 8 to 12 mm on each side. The amount of protrusive movement is also recorded. Severely decreased movement may indicate a permanently dislocated disk, whereas excessive movement may indicate an unstable joint due to damaged or loose ligaments or a systemic ligament laxity problem such as Ehlers-Danlos syndrome.

The age at which the full list of palpations is usually done is about 6 years, and selected palpations may be performed at an earlier age, such as palpation of the temporomandibular joints while the patient opens fully and closes the mouth. This can help to detect any irregular movement of the condyles as well as joint noises or pain. Sore or tense muscles may indicate overuse. For example, a clencher or bruxer may have sore masseter muscles. Sore lateral pterygoids may indicate a shift or slide, which requires excessive use of these muscles. A shift is the change from the first point of contact in centric relation to maximal intercuspation in all three planes of space.

### Imaging and Temporomandibular Joint Disorder

The role of imaging in TMD diagnosis has changed in recent years, but basic principles of radiographic diagnosis and test selection criteria apply. For example, joint sounds noted on routine clinical examination do not merit radiographic examination in the absence of symptoms. Examination or history should indicate that a recent change has occurred to justify any radiography done in the absence of symptoms.

A panoramic radiograph is generally regarded as the appropriate screening radiograph. When more complex imaging is needed, the magnetic resonance image is usually chosen for the good hard and soft tissue detail. Tomography is an example of a more sophisticated radiographic technique that can display excellent hard tissue detail. The selection criteria for initial TMD imaging include the following[1]:

1. Recent trauma or history of progressive pathologic joint condition
2. Significant dysfunction and alteration in range of motion
3. Significant occlusal changes (open bite, mandibular shift)

Okeson[19] has outlined a thorough examination procedure for TMD patients, and the reader is referred to this source for a more thorough coverage of this topic, which is beyond the scope of this chapter.

### Management of Temporomandibular Joint Disorder

Basic principles of TMD management also apply to the care of children. The clinician should first determine whether he or she wants to address the problem or seek further assistance from clinicians actively involved in TMD therapy. Dentists should have established referral sources that include medical and psychological professionals as well as other dentists. Nonpainful TMDs are usually not managed and monitored regularly. When pain is the presenting chief complaint, initial treatment usually consists of nonsteroidal antiinflammatory agents, soft diet, and warm, moist compresses to the face. Reversible oral treatments can then be employed with oral orthopedic appliance therapy using custom-designed full-coverage appliances. Because medication, counseling, and physical therapy may be indicated concurrently, a dentist may determine that referral to another case-managing dental specialist skilled in TMD treatment is in the patient's best interest.

Treatment of children is complicated by a host of variables not commonly encountered in adults. Compliance can be a major issue, especially with exercises or splint wear. Adolescent adjustment problems may trigger TMD, and these issues may not be readily discussed with parents or dentists. Growth, loss of teeth, and eruption of succedaneous teeth are clinical problems to be dealt with in treating the child at several stages in this period of life.

Currently, adjunctive diagnostic and treatment therapies, such as kinesiology, thermography, and jaw tracking, have no established efficacy in management of TMD in children and should be avoided.

## REFERENCES

1. American Academy of Pediatric Dentistry: Treatment of temporomandibular disorders in children: summary statements and recommendations. *JADA* 120(3):265-269, 1990.
2. Baccetti T, Franchi L, McNamara JA Jr: An improved version of the cervical vertebral maturation (CVM) method for the assessment of mandibular growth. *Angle Orthod* 72:316-23, 2002.
3. Baccetti T, Franchi L, Toth LR, McNamara JA Jr: Treatment timing for Twin-block therapy. *Am J Orthod Dentofac Orthop* 118:159-170, 2000.

4. Brady WF: The anorexia nervosa syndrome. *Oral Surg* 50:509-513, 1980.

5. Casamassimo PS: Dental and oral health problems: prevention and services. In: *Congress of the United States, Office of Technology Assessment: Adolescent Health. Vol 11. Background and the Effectiveness of Selected Prevention and Treatment Services.* OTA-H-466. Washington, DC, US Government Printing Office, 1991.

6. Castaldi CR, Brass GA: *Dentistry for the Adolescent.* Philadelphia, Saunders, 1980.

7. Chertkow S: Tooth mineralisation as an indicator of the pubertal growth spurt. *Am J Orthod Dentofac Orthop* 77:79-91, 1980.

8. Dahl B, Krogstad B, Ogaard B et al: Signs and symptoms of craniomandibular disorders in two groups of 19-year-old individuals, one treated orthodontically and the other not. *Acta Odontol Scand* 46:89-93, 1988.

9. DeKanter RJAM, Truin GJ, Burgersdijk RCW et al: Prevalence in the Dutch adult population and a meta-analysis of signs and symptoms of temporomandibular disorders. *J Dent Res* 72:1509-1518, 1993.

10. Dworkin SF, Huggins KH, LeResche L et al. Epidemiology of signs and symptoms of temporomandibular disorders: Clinical signs in cases and controls. *JADA* 120:273-81, 1990.

11. Greulich WW, Pyle SI: *Radiographic Atlas of Skeletal Development of the Hand and Wrist.* Palo Alto, CA, Stanford University Press, 1959.

12. Heikinheimo K, Salmi K, Myllarniemi S et al: A longitudinal study of occlusal interferences and signs of craniomandibular disorder at the ages of 12 and 15 years. *Eur J Orthodont* 12:190-197, 1990.

13. Keeling SD, McGorray S, Wheelser TT et al: Risk factors associated with temporomandibular joint sounds in children 6 to 12 years of age. *Am J Orthod Dentofac Orthop* 105:279-287, 1994.

14. Magnusson T, Egermarck-Ericksson I, Carlsson GE: Five year longitudinal study of signs and symptoms of mandibular dysfunction in adolescents. *J Carniomand Pract* 4:338-344, 1986.

15. Mihalik CA, Proffit WR, Phillips C: Long-term follow-up of class II adults treated with orthodontic camouflage: a comparison with orthognathic surgery outcomes. *Am J Orthod Dentofac Orthop* 123(3):266-278, 2003.

16. Moorrees CA, Fanning EA, Hunt EE Jr: Age variation of formation stages for ten permanent teeth. *J Dent Res* 42:1490-1502, 1963.

17. Motegi E, Miyasaki H, Oguka I: An orthodontic study of temporomandibular joint disorders. Part 1: Epidemiological research in Japanese 6–18 year olds. *Angle Orthod* 62:249-256, 1992.

18. Nielsen L, Melsen B, Terp S: Clinical classification of 14- to 16-year-old Danish children according to functional status of the masticatory system. *Commun Dent Oral Epidemiol* 16:47-51, 1988.

19. Okeson JP: *Management of Temporomandibular Disorders and Occlusion,* 5th ed. St Louis, Mosby, 2003.

20. Okeson JP, editor: *Orofacial Pain: Guidelines for Assessment, Diagnosis and Management.* Carol Stream, IL, Quintessence Publishing, 1996.

21. Pinkham JR, Schroeder CS: Dentist and psychologist: practical considerations for a team approach to the intensely anxious dental patient. *JADA* 90:1022-1026, 1975.

22. Poulsen S: Epidemiology and indices of gingival and periodontal disease. *Pediatr Dent* 3:82-88, 1981.

23. Proffit WR, White RP, Sarver DM: *Contemporary Treatment of Dentofacial Deformity.* St Louis, Mosby–Year Book, 2003.

24. Raj M: The perception of facial attractiveness by providers and consumers. Master's thesis, The Ohio State University, College of Dentistry, Section of Orthodontics, 2002.

25. Riolo ML, ten Have TR, Brandt D: Clinical validity of the relationship between TMJ signs and symptoms in children and youth. *J Dent Child* 55:110-113, 1988.

26. Rugh JD, Solberg WK: Oral health status in the United States. Temporomandibular disorders. *J Dent Educ* 49:398-404, 1985.

27. Schiffman E, Fricton JR: Epidemiology of TMJ and craniofacial pain. In: Fricton JR, Kroening R, Hathaway KM, editors. *TMJ and Craniofacial Pain: Diagnosis and Management.* St Louis, Ishiaku Euro American, 1988.

28. Tanner JM: *Foetus into Man.* London, Open Books, 1978.

29. Verdonck A, Takada K, Kitai N et al: The prevalence of cardinal TMJ dysfunction symptoms and its relationship to occlusal factors in Japanese female adolescents. *J Oral Rehabil* 21:687-697, 1994.

30. Wanman A, Agerberg G: Temporomandibular joint sounds in adolescents: a longitudinal study. *Oral Surg Oral Med Oral Pathol* 8:25-35, 1990.

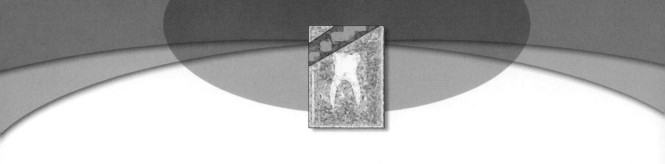

# CHAPTER 38

## Prevention of Dental Disease

*Arthur Nowak and James J. Crall*

Adolescence generally denotes the period between childhood and adulthood. However, adolescence also is known for being a period of change, rebellion, friction, and problems. It is a period when the patient progresses from junior high school to senior high school and then goes off to college, the work force, or some other aspect of adult life. It is a period of heightened involvement in peer group relationships, often at the expense of social or familial associations.

The period encompasses the completion of physical growth and development in both girls and boys. All permanent teeth have erupted except for the congenitally missing or impacted third permanent molars. The occlusion has stabilized either on its own or with orthodontic intervention. Most studies show a gradual but general increase in the incidence of dental caries during this period. Periodontal disease may become clinically evident because there are fewer routine and supervised home care sessions, less frequent professional interventions, or hormonal changes.

Dietary habits undergo dramatic changes during this period. As adolescent girls complete their maximal growth and development and begin the long process of "figure development," they begin many dietary experiments and modifications. Some of these modifications can lead to serious pathologic conditions such as anorexia nervosa and bulimia. In adolescent boys, similar modifications in dietary habits occur. During this period the boy's skeletal growth and body weight usually undergo dramatic changes, peaking at around age 16 to 18. Caloric requirements increase dramatically, and large amounts of protein and carbohydrates are consumed. In both groups, irregular meals, fast-food meals, frequent snacking, vending machine purchases, and unusual eating patterns are all common.

These changes, which have been so frequently described and routinely observed, can have profound effects on the oral environment and pose substantial challenges for the provision of professional dental care. If the individual has had the advantages of both systemic and topical fluorides, the problem of caries is usually confined to the occlusal surfaces of the posterior teeth. However, the eruption of posterior teeth into an environment of increased plaque secondary to reduced cleansing combined with frequent snacking on foods and beverages high in carbohydrates also can pose a significant risk for caries development in the immature enamel of smooth surfaces.

Therefore, periodic professional visits combined with an emphasis on continuing home care, optimal use of topical fluorides, and assistance in dietary management are both the goals and the challenges for the dentists who treat adolescents.

## DIETARY MANAGEMENT

As with younger age groups, the overall recommendations on dietary management for adolescents should concentrate on balanced intake, reduction of the frequency of snacking, and selection of foods that are not retentive to the teeth and soft tissues. Unfortunately, these recommendations conflict with the typical life-styles of adolescents. With their newly gained independence, rebellious attitude toward established social systems, and acceptance of media messages and peer group pressure, it is a difficult task for the dentist and his or her staff to communicate recommendations and instill health-promoting behaviors.

Fortunately, owing to the increasing social development that occurs in middle adolescence, there is a strong desire to look attractive; and the mouth, being the center of the face, takes on added importance. The challenge we have as dentists is to somehow make the daily care of teeth, including sound dietary habits, desirable for this group.

For the patient who has been at high risk for dental disease during the early years and has had caries in the primary or mixed dentition, dietary management is a major concern. Depending on the patient's present oral status, emotional and psychological maturity, and parental influences, counseling can be performed with the patient only or, if indicated, with the parents. At this age the adolescent may enjoy independence from the involvement of the parents. The dentist must decide whether or not to include the parents and to inform the parents about the results of the counseling.

The importance of family meals has been studied recently. In a U.S. Department of Agriculture Index Rating for the years 1994 to 1996, 94% of adolescents ages 13 to 18 showed poor-quality diets. In an attempt to understand the diet of adolescents, data from 18,177 adolescents from ages 11 to 21 who participated in the National Longitudinal Study of Adolescent Health were evaluated. The results indicated that in this age group:

- 33% perceived themselves to be overweight
- 20% ate no breakfast
- 71% reported not eating at least two vegetables a day
- 55% reported not eating at least two servings of fruit, and
- 47% reported not eating the recommended amount of dairy foods

Parents present at family evening meals exerted a substantial influence in terms of the adolescent's consumption of fruits, vegetables, and dairy products.[9]

For the patient who has active lesions in the developing permanent dentition, dietary management and modifications are definitely indicated along with a comprehensive program of oral cleaning and daily topical fluoride use. Developing a complete understanding of the importance of this approach with the patient and determining his or her willingness to cooperate is critical to achieving a successful outcome. If the patient is interested and is willing to cooperate, a dietary history is indicated. If not, it will be only a paper exercise and a waste of time for both parties involved.

Initially, a 24-hour dietary history will probably be sufficient. Based on the information provided by the history as well as from the patient about the usual daily schedules and the patient's academic, athletic, and social obligations, the dentist or staff responsible for counseling can assist in devising a preventive plan with the patient.

Having the patient acknowledge the problem and commit either orally or in writing to the recommended approach can often help improve compliance. During periodic examinations, the patient's progress or lack of progress can be evaluated. Plans may have to be modified frequently depending on the patient's changing needs. Because food preferences, social pressures, and growth changes occur frequently, this plan must allow for flexibility.

Although a 24-hour dietary history will be helpful, more insights can be obtained from a 5- or 7-day history including weekends. For improved accuracy, the patient should complete the first day's record with the dentist, paying particular attention to all liquid and solid foods consumed both at meals and between meals. Information about how much of the food was consumed and where the food was eaten will be helpful.

Once the dietary history has been received, a staff person assigned to counseling responsibilities should carefully review it with the patient. Foods high in refined carbohydrates or retentive to the oral tissues should be circled. Intake of fresh fruits and vegetables should be noted and commended. Unusual foods or dietary patterns should be identified, and the overall balance of the diet should be evaluated.

The patient should then be asked to list the problem areas and categorize them according to the ease with which they can be changed. With the problems identified and listed according to perceived ease of modification, the patient then develops a plan. It is important that it be his or her plan and not the dentist's. It is the dentist's role to guide the patient to develop a realistic plan that will build on successes. Periodic reviews can help determine the status of the dietary modifications and the need for new strategies. Reinforcements and rewards may be helpful, but in the end the patient's own perception of success will likely prove to be the most rewarding aspect for both dentist and patient. Computerized programs are also available to facilitate the analysis and guide recommendations.

An interesting web-based program, Interactive Healthy Eating Index by the U.S. Department of Agriculture Center on Nutrition Policy and Promotion (available at www.147.208.9.133), provides the opportunity to list a daily intake of all foods consumed. The diet is then analyzed for overall quality and a "score" is given. The score represents the types and amounts of foods eaten in terms of the recommended foods in the "food guide pyramid." The program also tells how much total fat, saturated fat, cholesterol, and sodium is in the diet. A number of interesting graphs are presented that assist in better understanding a diet. The program provides no information as to "dental/oral" health aspects of the diet but instead addresses the overall nutritional quality of the diet.

Dietary challenges for patients with developmental disabilities can be substantial. Depending on the severity of the disability, dietary habits may or may not be affected. For the patient with a severe neuromuscular involvement, diet and eating methods will already have been modified. Parents or caretakers must be made aware of potential problems, such as holding of food in the mouth, slow passage of food from the mouth to the digestive tract, and rumination, and their potentially devastating effects on the mouth and teeth. If management of the diet is not possible, efforts should be made to ensure more frequent and thorough cleansing as well as frequent use of topical fluorides.

## HOME CARE

Personal hygiene, like any established societal activity, is met with varying responses during adolescence. Nagging by the parent or dentist will probably lead to a negative response. When the patient understands the importance of oral hygiene and is ready to make a daily commitment, the dentist can assist him or her in developing a routine of oral hygiene that will be acceptable to the patient as well as maintaining a healthy oral environment.

During this period, dental flossing should become a part of the daily oral hygiene routine. Adolescents should have well-developed eye-hand coordination and fine-motor activity. For those who still have difficulty with the traditional method of flossing, a floss holder may be helpful.

The goal should be for the patient to perform thorough toothbrushing with fluoride toothpaste at least twice each day, ideally at the start of the day and before bed. The patient should be informed of the importance of thoroughness; therefore, a period before bed should be set aside for the routine of brushing and flossing. After meals a vigorous rinse with water should be encouraged. If orthodontic appliances are present, additional time as well as modifications of the routine will be necessary to remove not only the plaque but also the debris caught around the brackets and wires. Additional attention to the marginal gingiva is also important.

Effective daily home care is essential for the adolescent patient with a developmental disability. Again, depending on the severity of the disability, the patient, the parent, or a caregiver must take responsibility for the care. Mouth props may be necessary for some patients who are unable to keep their mouths open for oral care routines.

Chemical plaque control agents (e.g., chlorhexidine) have become popular adjuncts to daily oral hygiene. Many patients may benefit from their daily use, especially patients with special health care needs or patients with orthodontic appliances. Studies have confirmed the improvements from the use of various agents in reducing plaque, gingivitis, and gingival bleeding sites.[2,4,6] Adolescents frequently experience marginal gingivitis secondary to plaque deposits. Consideration should be given to prescribing antimicrobial mouth rinses to complement daily oral hygiene practices.[3]

For a patient with a developmental disability or an acute or chronic medical condition and who may be unable to rinse and spit, an alternative method is to apply an antimicrobial gel.

## FLUORIDE ADMINISTRATION

### Approach to the Adolescent Patient

Although most adolescents have the ability to carry out effective oral hygiene procedures, many neglect to perform these activities regularly. The key to promoting effective caries prevention during what can be a hectic and trying stage of life often depends on recognizing the predominant motivational factors operating in this age group and adopting an approach that is based on less than ideal compliance. The focus on personal appearance and hygiene in this age group can be used as a powerful motivator for developing preventive activities. Another strategy involves appealing to the adolescent's desire to be viewed as autonomous and capable of taking care of himself or herself.

Regardless of the psychological basis for the motivation, time should be taken to ensure that adolescents understand the nature of the disease processes that the preventive programs are addressing and the general mechanisms by which the prescribed measures are thought to counteract these processes. This emphasis on education is more likely to be accepted and will produce better long-term outcomes than a more authoritarian or condescending approach.

### Caries Activity During Adolescence

In spite of a well-documented decline in caries levels in children in the United States and other Western countries, adolescence still marks a period of significant caries activity for many persons. Cross-sectional data from the 1988–1991 survey of caries prevalence in schoolchildren in the United States[7] showed that the mean number of decayed, missing, and filled permanent tooth surfaces (DMFS) increased from 0.9 for 12-year-olds to 4.4 for 17-year-olds. The results of that study indicated that, on average, the DMFS index increased by 1.3 on buccolingual surfaces, 0.5 on interproximal surfaces, and 2.4 on occlusal surfaces between the ages of 12 and 17. Adolescence also marks a time of reduction in the number of individuals who are caries free. Thus, fluoride administration should continue to be an important concern during this stage of continuing caries susceptibility.

Topical fluorides (along with occlusal sealants) are the primary preventive agents of choice during adolescence because the entire permanent dentition except for the third molars normally has erupted by age 13.[5] Most studies have shown that fluorides reduce the incidence of smooth-surface caries to a greater extent than that of occlusal caries.[5] Therefore, the combination of fluoride therapy and occlusal sealants can be used to provide optimal protection for all surfaces of the teeth.

### High-Frequency/Low-Concentration Applications

As with younger children, the daily use of a fluoride dentifrice should form the foundation of a sound personal preventive oral health program, regardless of whether the person lives in a fluoridated or a nonfluoridated community. Additional protection can be provided daily by the use of a 0.05% sodium fluoride rinse for those at elevated risk for the development of caries. Frequent rinsing seems particularly advisable for those "on-the-go" teenagers who do not take the time to practice thorough plaque removal. Frequent exposures to fluoride may help to suppress the cariogenic potential of the oral flora and can help to establish an environment that may inhibit demineralization or promote remineralization.[5] As noted previously, fluoride mouth rinses also are indicated for persons who have difficulty removing plaque because of the presence of orthodontic appliances or for those with predisposing medical conditions.

## Applications of More Concentrated Fluoride Agents

Frequent applications of more concentrated fluoride gels or fluoride varnish may be indicated for teenagers who exhibit poor oral hygiene or other risk-elevating factors, or who continue to exhibit high levels of caries between recall examinations. Gels can be applied at home by brushing or by means of customized plastic trays. Custom trays are easily fabricated using vacuum-forming devices to adapt the plastic tray material over stone models of the patient's maxillary and mandibular arches. The best time to apply the gels is just before bedtime to allow the fluoride to remain in contact with the teeth for a longer time. Professional topical fluoride applications should be scheduled at least every 6 months for moderate- or high-risk individuals during adolescence as well as for those with a history of ongoing caries activity.

Adolescence is a time of heightened caries activity for many persons as a result of increased intake of cariogenic substances and inattention to oral hygiene procedures. Because fluorides have been shown to exert a greater anticaries effect in patients with higher baseline levels of caries activity and because the concurrent use of various forms of fluoride often produces greater caries reductions than when the agents are used separately, multiple exposures to a variety of fluoride sources should be encouraged during this period of elevated risk in an attempt to control the caries process.

## REFERENCES

1. American Academy of Pediatric Dentistry: Guideline on dental health of the adolescent. *Pediatr Dent* 25:36, 2003.
2. Beiswanger BB, Mallat ME, Mau MS et al: 0.12% Chlorhexidine rinse as an adjunct to scaling and root planing. *J Dent Res* 70(special issue):458, 1991.
3. Bhat M: Periodontal health of 14- to 17-year-old U.S. school children. *J Public Health Dent* 51:5-11, 1991.
4. Brightman LJ, Terezhalmy GT, Greenwald H et al: The effects of a 0.12% chlorhexidine gluconate mouthrinse on orthodontic patients aged 11 through 17 with established gingivitis. *Am J Orthofac Dentofac Orthop* 100:324-329, 1991.
5. Centers for Disease Control and Prevention: Recommendations for using fluoride to prevent and control dental caries in the United States. *MMWR Morb Mortal Wkly Rep* 50 (RR-14):26, 2001.
6. Grossman F, Reiter G, Sturzenbenger OP et al: Six-month study of the effects of a chlorhexidine mouthrinse on gingivitis in adults. *J Periodont Res Suppl* 16:33-43, 1986.
7. Kaste LM, Selwitz RH, Oldakowski JA et al: Coronal caries in the primary and permanent dentition of children and adolescents 1–17 years of age: United States, 1988–1991. *J Dent Res* 75(special issue):631-641, 1996.
8. National Institute of Dental Research: Oral Health of United States Children: The National Survey of Dental Caries in U.S. School Children: 1986–1987. NIH Publication 89-2247. Bethesda, MD, National Institutes of Health, 1989, pp 14-17.
9. Videon TM, Manning CK: Influences on adolescent eating patterns: the importance of family meals. *J Adolesc Health* 32:365-373, 2003.

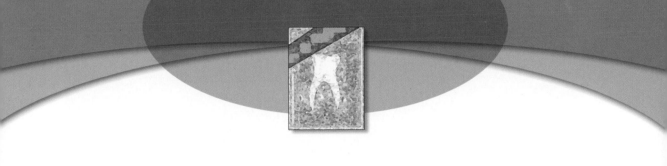

# CHAPTER 39

## Aesthetic Restorative Dentistry for the Adolescent

*Kaaren G. Vargas, Marcos A. Vargas, and John W. Reinhardt*

Having a pleasing, attractive appearance is the dream of most adolescents in our society. Great effort and expense are invested in gaining or maintaining that appearance through means such as dieting, use of cosmetics, and selection of apparel. An important component of the idealized physical appearance is a radiant smile displaying teeth that are attractive in shape and color and do not distract during speaking and smiling.

The use of dental techniques and materials to help young people obtain the most attractive appearance possible is a clinical challenge requiring knowledge, disciplined attention to detail, and skill. In return for their efforts, dentists receive the satisfaction of seeing a young person develop a healthy self-image that can have a positive effect on his or her maturation into adulthood.

Newly developed and improved composite resins along with the acid-etch technique have made it possible to restore aesthetic defects with conservative treatment. The use of visible light–cured composite resins has made the job easier. A multitude of composite resins are available and offer a choice of physical properties such as viscosity, opacity and translucency, and surface smoothness.

## FUNDAMENTALS OF MATERIALS SELECTION

Choice of materials is an important consideration for dental aesthetic factors. The clinical success of composite restorations depends on adhesive systems that provide durable bonding of composite to dentin and enamel, effectively sealing the

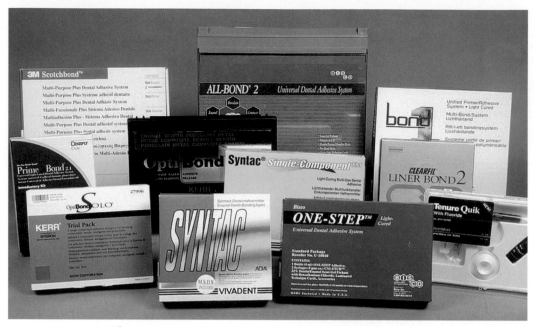

**Figure 39-1** Representative dentin-enamel adhesive products

margins of restorations and preventing post-operative sensitivity and microleakage.[13,17]

In order to achieve this, a current-generation adhesive system should be used (Fig. 39-1). Most of these systems work by demineralizing the dentin-enamel surface with an acid, which is usually 37% phosphoric. After etching, a primer resin is applied that facilitates the penetration of an adhesive resin into the demineralized dentin and enamel to form a hybridized layer of resin/tooth[13,20] as shown in Figure 39-2. In recent years, the bonding procedure has been simplified by the introduction of single-bottle primer/adhesive systems.[18] These agents combine the primer resin with the adhesive resin into a single component (bottle).[14,19]

Choice of resin composite for aesthetic restorations can be confusing because a variety of products are available with slightly different physical properties. Basically, the two types of composite resins that can be used are *microfilled* (those with filler particles averaging 0.04 μm in diameter) and *hybrid* (a blend of different particle sizes, including submicrometer [0.04 μm] and small particle [0.2 to 3 μm]). The particle size difference between microfilled and hybrid resin composites is readily apparent under magnification (Fig. 39-3). Currently, most dental manufacturers are producing "microhybrid" resin composites with an average particle size of less than 1 μm.

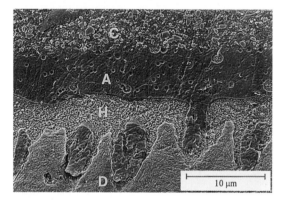

**Figure 39-2** Scanning electron microscopic view of the resin-to-dentin bond, showing composite resin *(C)*, adhesive *(A)*, hybrid layer *(H)*, and dentin *(D)*.

The mechanical and physical properties of hybrid resin composites are superior to those of microfilled resins basically because they contain a higher proportion of filler particles. Nevertheless, because of their particle size, microfilled resins can be polished to an enamel-like luster with much more ease and in less time than hybrid resins.

When considering which material to choose for a restoration, it is essential to evaluate the tooth to be restored, the location of the restoration, and the forces to which the restoration will be subjected. Hybrid resins have traditionally been chosen as a "universal restorative" since they

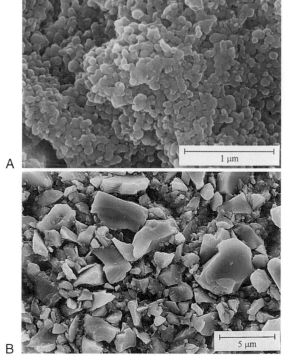

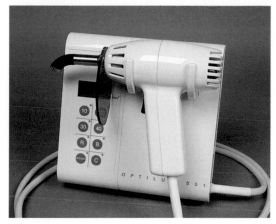

**Figure 39-4**  A typical dental composite resin light-curing unit.

**Figure 39-3**  Scanning electron microscopic views demonstrating the difference between typical micro-filled (**A**) and hybrid (**B**) composite resins.

can be used in most clinical situations. Microfilled resins, on the other hand, are primarily indicated when aesthetic restorations are required, such as class V and direct resin veneers, and when the occlusal forces permit. Aesthetically demanding but higher load restorations such as class IV can have a hybrid material used as a substrate that is subsequently veneered by a microfilled resin composite. An alternative is the use of a material containing the recently developed "nanoparticles and clusters" as fillers. These nanofillers are made of $SiO_2$, silane-coated $SiO_2$, and $ZrO_2$ with a range of 20 to 75 nm and have physical properties superior to those of microfills.

Regardless of whether a microfilled or hybrid composite resin is chosen, the use of visible light–curing products is recommended. In addition to the convenience of extended working time and rapid polymerization, these materials also have lower porosity and are less likely to become discolored than the chemically cured (spatulated two-paste) systems.

Polymerization of light-cured composite resins is accomplished by using an intense blue light with a peak wavelength of approximately 470 nm, which corresponds to the absorption peak of camphoroquinone (CQ), the most popular photo-initiator.[1,15] A typical light-curing polymerization unit uses a gun-type handpiece that contains the bulb and cooling fan (Fig. 39-4). Although manufacturers have developed other technology, such as light-emitting diodes (LEDs) to efficiently produce blue light, the emitting bandwidth of most of these LED lights is too narrow and high to produce activation of resin composites that contain CQ photoinitiators.[16] For this reason, the present recommendation is for the use of conventional halogen-tungsten-quartz (HTQ) for composite resin polymerization. The HTQ offers interchangeable light transmission tips to gain access to various areas of the mouth; however, light intensity should be periodically checked (via a radiometer) so that a minimal output of 350 mW/cm$^2$ can be maintained. Several modern light-curing units incorporate light meter devices into their bases, so curing radiometers are not needed (Fig. 39-5).

Eye protection is important when using the curing lights because direct viewing of the light is detrimental to vision.[8] Amber filters, which block the intense blue component of the light, are commercially available and can be hand held or worn as eyeglasses (Fig. 39-6). In the absence of specific protective devices, one should avoid looking directly at the light.

## FUNDAMENTALS OF CLINICAL TECHNIQUE

Shade selection is the first step to achieve an aesthetically pleasing restoration. The teeth to be matched should be cleaned with a rubber

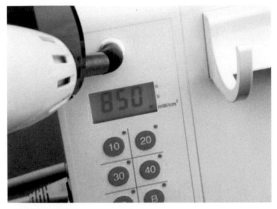

**Figure 39-5** Light-curing unit showing power output via an incorporated curing radiometer.

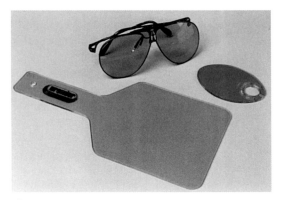

**Figure 39-6** Filtering devices designed to protect eyes when using light-curing techniques.

prophylaxis cup and flour of pumice. Tooth dehydration should be avoided because of the concurrent color change. Moistened shade tabs should be held near the tooth to be matched, using only room light or indirect sunlight. One should not use the high-intensity operatory light when selecting shades. The proper value (Munsell "whiteness") may be better determined by squinting. If shade selection takes more than a few seconds, one may need to resensitize the eyes by staring momentarily at a dark blue or gray object.

Resin composites come in a variety of shades, which are usually keyed to the Vita shade guide. Unfortunately, a perfect color match between the resin composites and the Vita guide is very uncommon, and shades among composite brands are even more variable. In recent years, the range of shades has been increased to match the shades of teeth that have been whitened or "bleached." Common names for these shades are "bleach shades," superbright shades, or extralight shades.

To overcome some of the shade matching pitfalls, many clinicians allow the patient to choose between two similar shades. Another way to verify the actual shade is to place a small portion of composite resin on the tooth surface, polymerize it, observe the appropriateness of that shade, and then remove it with a hand instrument. It should be noted that one should not etch the tooth prior to doing this or removal will be difficult. It is also generally best not to combine shades of composite resin by mixing because porosity may be introduced into the paste.

It is extremely important to maintain an uncontaminated field during the insertion of composite resins. The most reliable way to control moisture is through the use of a well-adapted rubber dam. If not using a rubber dam, one should place cotton rolls and 2 × 2 inch gauze sponges over the tongue to prevent moisture contamination. Another approach to maintaining a dry field is to use a commercially available lip and cheek retractor (Fig. 39-7). This plastic device, when used in conjunction with gauze sponges, provides excellent access and good field control.

Use of a base or liner to protect pulp tissue in deep preparations is generally believed to be important, although some practitioners are now questioning that long-held belief. Many believe that a glass ionomer liner should be used in deep areas of a cavity preparation that are thought to be within 0.5 to 1.0 mm of pulpal tissue (Fig. 39-8). The liner provides chemical adherence to tooth structure and slow release of fluoride.

After etching (15 seconds of etch and 5 to 10 seconds of rinse), an appropriate dentin-enamel bonding agent should be placed. Next, the light-cured composite resin should be inserted in layers no thicker than 2.0 mm, using at least 40 seconds of light exposure per layer. Thin layers and adequate time for light exposure help ensure the maximal polymerization. Maximal polymerization provides optimal strength and color stability of the restoration. It is important to cover the light-curing composite resin on the mixing pad so that room light does not initiate the polymerization process. In addition, it may be necessary to reduce the intensity of the operating light.

In an effort to mimic the translucency of enamel and the opacity of dentin, manufacturers have produced materials with a variety of opacities. These materials should be placed in increments in which the more opaque materials

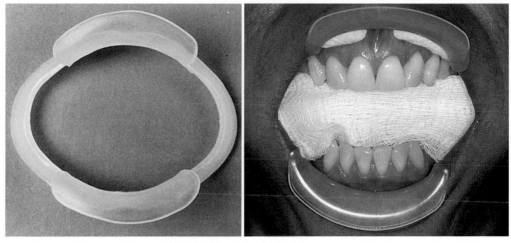

**Figure 39-7**    Isolation of teeth may be enhanced through the used of a lip-retracting device.

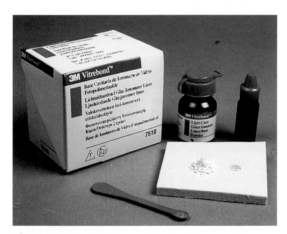

**Figure 39-8**    A light-curable glass ionomer liner.

replace dentin and the more translucent materials replace enamel to produce restorations with similar optical properties to tooth structure.

Plastic or metal instruments are useful for material placement and contouring. Fine sable or camel hair brushes allow easy contouring and blending of composite resin into the proper form. To prevent composite from adhering to the brushes and instruments, they should be lightly lubricated via gauze sponges moistened with bathing alcohol.

After the polymerization process, contouring and finishing of the restoration is accomplished using carbide finishing burs, ultrafine diamond burs, or finishing disks. Fine-pointed burs are helpful for accessing contour areas that are difficult to reach, such as embrasures. Rounded burs may be used on concave surfaces, and disks may be used on flat or convex surfaces. After

contouring and finishing, the restoration should be polished with a series of polishing disks or rubber-abrasive instruments. The final finish and polish of interproximal areas is best done with abrasive strips.

## FUNDAMENTALS OF TOOTH COLOR AND FORM

The ideal aesthetic restoration appears so natural it is difficult to discern from the surrounding tooth surface or adjacent teeth. Color and translucency must be considered together to achieve an optimal result. One may alter areas of discoloration on a tooth by applying color modifiers or opaquing agents to improve the appearance, then covering those areas with composite resin.

Composite resins with greater opacity, such as hybrid and microfilled opaque pastes, should be used in most situations. The purpose of selecting an opaque material is to prevent excessive translucency, which can allow intraoral darkness to show through a restoration and cause a dark, unappealing result.

Highly translucent materials such as nonopaque microfilled pastes should be used only for class III restorations and small class IV restorations on highly translucent teeth. In many cases, use of a hybrid composite as a foundation under a microfilled composite improves both the strength and the appearance of the restoration.

Form and anatomy of anterior aesthetic restorations can also be controlled to make the restoration appear natural. In general, embrasure spaces should be symmetric whenever possible, and contours should match those of the adjacent teeth. Adolescent anterior teeth usually show little evidence of wear and display prominent incisal embrasure spaces, rounded incisal point angles, and developmental characteristics such as mamelons on incisal edges. These characteristics are especially noticeable in young women and should be used whenever possible to enhance a feminine smile.

## RESTORATIONS FOR FRACTURED ANTERIOR TEETH

Trauma to the anterior dentition can often result in tooth fractures involving incisal edges. Injuries such as these can cause pulpal as well as aesthetic problems and should be carefully evaluated by clinical and radiographic means. Clinical findings may range from little or no dentin exposure with minimal thermal and pressure sensitivity to the acute distress of a pulp exposure. Radiographs help in diagnosing the presence or absence of root fractures. Treatment must begin with pulpal therapy as a first consideration, and if pulpectomy or pulpotomy is necessary, it should begin simultaneously with the restorative procedures.

Some clinicians consider the class IV composite resin restoration an interim restoration for adolescents until a more permanent ceramic crown can be fabricated. With modern materials and techniques, however, the strength and color stability of composite resin class IV restorations are such that they can be considered "final" restorations that will provide relatively long service. For early adolescents with severely fractured anterior teeth, these restorations can provide years of service, allowing the teeth to mature so that pulpal injury during crown preparation is less likely.

### Clinical Technique

Acid-etching techniques have lessened the need for extensive mechanical retentive features in class IV restorations. The primary retentive feature is a beveled enamel cavosurface margin of a minimum of 1.0 to 2.0 mm in length. Beveling allows maximal bond strength and minimizes leakage by exposing the ends of the enamel rods to etching. Because anterior restorations are sometimes subject to strong shearing forces that can be greater than the bond strength of the restoration to the tooth, features such as grooves, retentive points, or pins may be used to gain additional retentive strength. However, supplemental retentive features are usually unnecessary.

After administering anesthesia, the rubber dam is placed and the bevel is prepared using a medium-grit diamond bur. At this time, a base or liner may be applied to exposed dentin. Conditioning of the tooth is achieved with a 37% phosphoric acid etchant applied first to enamel and then to dentin. This is done in order to avoid etching the dentin for more than 15 seconds. After rinsing (for at least 5 seconds), the surface should be left slightly moist to prevent collapse of the exposed collagen network. The primer resin (or, in some cases, a single-component primer/adhesive) is then applied to the dentin and should be in contact with it for at least 15 seconds for most adhesive systems. Contact of the primer with enamel should not cause a problem. After 15 seconds the primer should be dried with a gentle stream of air in order to evaporate the solvent without displacing the primer. It is imperative that a shiny surface be obtained after this step; if not, most adhesive systems require additional application of primer. When using a two-component system, the adhesive resin is applied with a brush over the dried primer and light cured for 10 seconds. Care should be taken to avoid pooling or overthinning. As a final step, composite resin is applied as described previously. A wedged celluloid matrix strip can be used to prevent etching and bonding an adjacent tooth. After placing, finishing, and polishing the composite resin, one carefully checks the restoration for interferences in all excursive movements (Fig. 39-9, *A, B*). Occlusal stresses on the restoration should be minimized.

## RESTORATION OF DIASTEMAS

Many adolescents and adults consider spaces between anterior teeth (diastemas) unattractive. Historically the only restorative treatment to fill these spaces has been the construction of crowns larger than the original teeth. Even though many patients disliked their appearance with diastemas, most were unwilling to undergo the trauma and expense of crowning sound teeth simply to gain an aesthetic improvement. Improved composite resin materials and acid-etching technology now

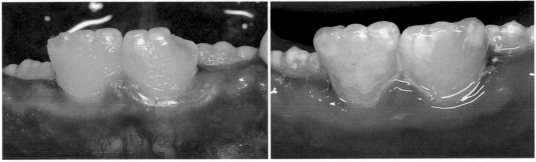

**Figure 39-9    A,** The incisal edges of teeth 24 and 25 were fractured as the result of an accident. **B,** Composite resin restorations. (Filtek Restorative Material, 3M/ESPE) of fractured teeth shown in **A.**

allow restoration of diastemas using a method that is nondestructive, reversible, and relatively inexpensive. However, patients should be forewarned that fracture and staining are possible drawbacks of composite resin diastema closures and that replacement is likely to be needed after 5 to 10 years.

When an adolescent patient wants a diastema closure, whether the spaces are the result of natural development or postorthodontic discrepancies, careful evaluation and planning are necessary prior to treatment. If the patient is nearing completion of orthodontic therapy but is still undergoing treatment, the restorative dentist may advise the orthodontist about the optimal arrangement of anterior teeth for diastema closure. The orthodontist may then complete active treatment and place the patient into a retention phase prior to closing the diastema. It is best to allow a minimum of a few months between the end of active orthodontic treatment and diastema closure therapy so that anterior teeth will be more stable and will settle into their final position. The use of diagnostic study casts is highly recommended for evaluation and treatment planning. A diagnostic wax-up of the proposed restorative treatment can aid both the patient and the clinician in envisioning the result.

Important pretreatment considerations include the size and location of the space or spaces and the size (length and width) and shape of the teeth to be restored. Normally, composite resin is added to the teeth on both sides of the space. For patients who are undergoing orthodontic treatment, one should determine if the remaining space would best be left in one place, such as the midline between teeth 8 and 9, or distributed over interproximal areas throughout the anterior segment. One must also consider the length and

width of the teeth to be restored. If the width becomes greater than the length, those teeth appear more "square," causing an unattractive result that may be as displeasing as the original diastema. Because of occlusal patterns and chewing stresses, teeth usually cannot be lengthened with composite resin without creating a high probability of resin fracture. However, light reflections can be used to create the illusion of a longer and narrower tooth when the composite resin is extended to cover most or all of the facial surface of a tooth. To create the illusion of a narrower tooth, one should form mesial and distal line angles in composite resin that are positioned slightly nearer the middle of the tooth and add definite vertical anatomic highlights (developmental depressions). In some situations periodontal crown lengthening may be considered to obtain a favorable width-to-length ratio. For some patients the best treatment is partial diastema closure, in which an existing space is made smaller by enlarging the teeth with composite resin but not making the teeth so large that they become aesthetically displeasing. In summary, aesthetic possibilities must be carefully evaluated and explained to the patient before treatment is begun.

### Clinical Technique

After cleaning, shade selection, and isolation (as described previously), treatment should begin on one tooth at a time. The space to be eliminated should be carefully measured via a periodontal probe, calipers, or Boley gauge because after one tooth is restored in an effort to eliminate half the space, it is usually difficult to determine how much of the space has actually been restored. The entire labial surface of the tooth should be etched and bonding agent applied because most of the labial surface will be covered with a thin layer of composite to allow a subtle color transition from composite to tooth. In addition, covering most of the labial surface allows the use of visual illusions that cause the tooth to look narrower or longer, as described previously.

Composite resin (preferably a resin that is viscous and opaque) should be applied, beginning at the gingival margin of the interproximal area. Using instruments and brushes, one should shape the material to allow a smooth-flowing gingival embrasure without creating an overhanging ledge. The entire proximal surface as well as the labial surface can be built up and polymerized at once or incrementally. After this buildup, one should finish the interproximal area to the proper contour and polish it. Next, the second tooth is restored similarly. A celluloid matrix and wedge are usually inserted after the gingival increment is polymerized to retain the composite resin and to prevent the restorations from bonding together. Some clinicians prefer to build the second restoration without using a matrix. In that case, the two restorations must be gently separated with a thin metal instrument using a torquing motion.

Upon completion, the matrix is removed, and contouring and polishing are completed (Fig. 39-10, A–D).

Anterior teeth that are unusually small, such as peg lateral incisors, may be restored in the same manner as teeth requiring both mesial and distal diastema closure restorations. Again, careful treatment planning is advised to determine whether the restorations should be done only on the smaller tooth or on both the small and adjacent teeth for maximal cosmetic benefit. Preoperative diagnosis is again necessary to determine whether lengthening is feasible. One should forewarn patients that the possibility of fracturing increases as length increases. In situations where fracturing is a concern, a hybrid resin should be used as a substrate and a microfilled resin placed on the surface. This technique increases the strength and aesthetic result of the restoration.

## RESTORATION OF DISCOLORED TEETH

Although there are many causes of tooth discoloration in adolescents, the most common discolorations result from trauma, enamel hypoplasia

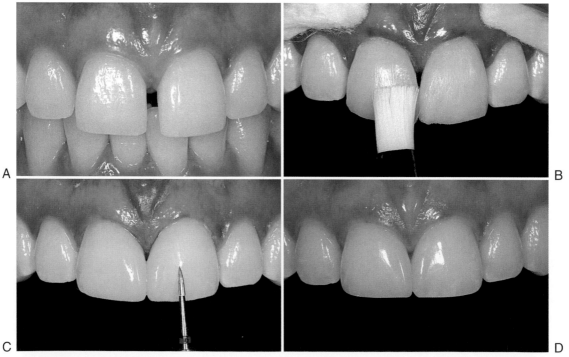

**Figure 39-10** **A,** A preoperative view of a maxillary midline diastema, which the patient found unattractive. **B,** The initial increment of composite resin being contoured with a sable brush prior to polymerization. **C,** Contouring and removing excess composite following buildup of the second tooth. **D,** A postoperative view of the completed case.

(often caused by fluorosis), and the administration of tetracycline antibiotics during childhood. These lesions vary from small white or yellowish flecking of the surface enamel, called enamel "dysmineralization,"[3] to the deep intrinsic bluish gray color often visible in tetracycline staining.

## Treatment of Hypoplastic Spots

Discrete hypoplastic white or yellow-brown spots can be improved by enamel microabrasion[3-6], or by making shallow saucer-shaped preparations in enamel to remove the intensely colored tooth structure and then restoring the enamel with composite resin. Microabrasion is the preferred technique whenever possible because it is a treatment that requires less enamel removal and does not necessitate placement of a restoration. The technique for enamel microabrasion involves application of an acidic abrasive paste by a reduced-speed dental handpiece. Microabrasion is sometimes used in combination with vital bleaching (which is described later in this chapter).

## Veneers

Composite resin or porcelain veneers provide a treatment option for patients who have moderate to severe staining of one or more teeth. Patients are most concerned about the appearance of their maxillary teeth, especially the anteriors, because they are more visible in speaking and smiling. In addition, mandibular teeth are often less likely to be successfully veneered because of limited space (insufficient overjet) and unfavorable forces at the junction of tooth and veneer during normal chewing. For veneer treatment to be successful the patient must have excellent periodontal health because the placement of veneers will result in contours and margins that require good oral hygiene to maintain gingival health. In addition, patients should be warned that biting on hard objects, such as raw carrots or pencils, may dislodge or break veneers.

Although the anticipated longevity of an aesthetic veneer restoration might be less than that of a porcelain-fused-to-metal crown, the cost is also less. In addition, veneers can be placed with minimal tooth preparation, thus preserving the natural dentition. Veneers may be made by direct buildup of composite resin in the mouth or by indirect procedures (constructed on laboratory models) using composite resin or porcelain.

### Laboratory-Constructed Veneers

The indirect veneer technique has the advantage of requiring less total chair time because the veneers are constructed in the laboratory. Excellent aesthetically pleasing contours can be achieved using porcelain or composite resin laboratory techniques. Disadvantages include the necessity of two appointments, laboratory expense, and the possibility of creating an excess bulk of restorative material.

The indirect technique usually requires the removal of some enamel (ideally 0.3 to 0.5 mm but occasionally more in severely stained teeth) from the facial surface to provide space for the veneer (Fig. 39-11). Tooth preparation is best accomplished with a medium-grit diamond bur (Fig. 39-12), with the goal of producing a Chamfer finish line throughout the surfaces to be covered. This preparation extends to the proximal surfaces just to include the contact points (Fig. 39-13). Gingivally, the preparation must extend

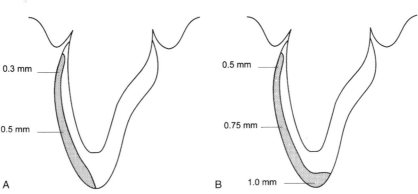

**Figure 39-11**  Cross-sectional views of a laboratory-processed veneer of ideal thickness without incisal coverage (**A**) and a veneer of greater thickness with incisal coverage (**B**).

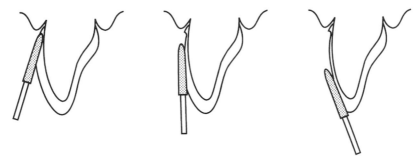

**Figure 39-12**    Cross-sectional view of the steps in diamond bur placement needed for preparing the facial surface of a maxillary anterior tooth.

far enough to cover the stained enamel sufficiently to improve the color. For better periodontal health, the finish line should be kept supragingival whenever possible. Following the preparation, an accurate impression of the teeth should be made using standard techniques and an elastomeric impression material such as polysulfide or silicone.

At the second appointment, one should isolate the teeth and clean them with pumice. After trying on (using water, glycerin, or a try-in paste to help hold the veneers in place) and adjusting the veneers, they should be cleaned with the etching gel and silanated. The preparations should be acid etched individually or in pairs and the veneers bonded in place, beginning with the central incisors. Celluloid matrices help protect adjacent teeth. Light-cured or dual-cured resins of moderate viscosity are preferred for bonding. Excess resin should be removed from margins with brushes prior to polymerization. Adequate polymerization time (40 to 60 seconds in each area) should be used because the veneers will shield some light transmission. Finishing and polishing are usually necessary only at the

margins and may be done with abrasive strips and rubber cups (Fig. 39-14, *A–C*).

### Direct Veneers

Veneers made of light-cured composite resins can be constructed directly in the mouth. Compared with the indirect type, direct veneers offer the

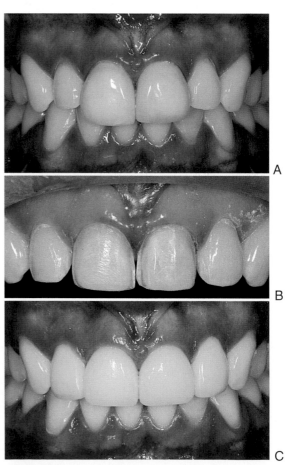

**Figure 39-14**    **A,** Preoperative view of aesthetically unpleasing maxillary anterior teeth. **B,** Teeth 8 and 9 prepared for porcelain veneers. **C,** Porcelain veneers in place on teeth 8 and 9.

**Figure 39-13**    Incisal view of veneer preparations.

advantages of improved marginal adaptation, placement in one appointment, greater operator control, and no laboratory fee. The disadvantages include the fact that direct veneers require more time, greater skill, and more patience on the part of the clinician. Also, results are more difficult to predict.

The clinical direct technique may be performed with or without any enamel removal. Darkly stained teeth usually require some enamel removal because more composite resin is needed to mask the underlying enamel. The teeth are then pumiced and individually etched, and a bonding agent is applied. Again, celluloid matrices are used between adjacent teeth. Opaquing agents may then be painted on to cover more intensely stained areas or entire surfaces. It should be noted, however, that the use of these agents can cause an unaesthetic flat appearance in the color of the final restoration. For the best appearance, opaquing agents should be used minimally and with care. When dark banding is present, an alternative approach is to remove the band with a round bur and then replace the tooth structure with an opaque hybrid composite resin. Next, the composite resin (microfilled) should be applied in a layer 1.0 to 1.5 mm in thickness and contoured via brushes. The gingival third of the restoration should usually be an opaque yellow shade, and the remaining enamel should be covered with opaque gray or universal composite, overlapping and blending the shades to create a natural-looking, gentle color transition. In many cases, a nonopaque shade can be used on the incisal one fourth to allow a natural, translucent appearance (Fig. 39-15). After all composite resin has been added to a single tooth and contouring with brushes is complete, the material should be polymerized by exposing each area to the curing light for 40 to 60 seconds. When using narrow-tipped lights, four or five overlapping exposures may be needed to cure the entire labial surface. For this reason, a wider light curing (e.g., 11 mm diameter) is recommended. Finishing and polishing are best done with burs and disks, as described previously.

## Vital Bleaching

Vital bleaching techniques involve the application of peroxide solutions to increase the value (whiteness) of teeth that are unusually dark. Two basic methods have been reported in the litera-

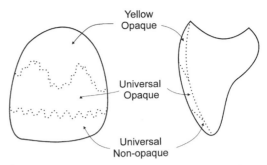

**Figure 39-15** The use of overlapping shades of composite resin to create a natural-looking directly placed veneer.

ture: power bleaching[2] and night guard (or mouthguard) vital bleaching.[9]

Power bleaching is an in-office procedure in which a concentrated hydrogen peroxide solution is applied to rubber dam-isolated teeth while heating the teeth, usually with an electric lamp.[10] This method of bleaching usually requires numerous (three or more) office visits and often causes temporary tooth sensitivity to thermal changes. Typically, patients who have had this treatment require periodic retreatment to maintain the desired color.

Night guard vital bleaching is a dentist-directed, at-home treatment. This method of vital bleaching involves a custom mouthguard and a milder peroxide solution (usually 10% carbamide peroxide) that the patient applies and wears outside the dental office, often at night during sleep, for about 2 to 3 weeks. Night guard vital bleaching appears to work as well as power bleaching and causes less thermal sensitivity. Concerns were initially raised about the potentially hazardous soft tissue effects of applying peroxide solutions in this manner, but long-term studies of the safety and efficacy of this approach are demonstrating no harmful effects.[11,12]

Peroxide bleaching methods appear to work best on teeth that are mildly discolored, predominantly yellow, and from which the discoloration originates in enamel rather than dentin.

## BONDED BRIDGES AND SPLINTS

Cast metal appliances can be bonded to enamel using composite resin cements. This procedure, in which the inner surfaces of metal are microabraded with aluminum oxide in the laboratory to create micromechanical retentive areas, is useful for attaching bridges and splints. Bridges constructed by this technique offer two advantages over conventional bridgework: greater conservation of tooth structure and lower cost. Splints can be made using the same technique for patients requiring fixed postorthodontic stabilization.

Diagnosis and treatment planning should include careful evaluation of occlusion. Ideally, the retainers would cover 80% to 90% of the lingual enamel surfaces of those teeth in order to provide maximal retention. Anterior teeth with markedly translucent incisal edges may not allow coverage to extend near those edges because metallic or resin coverage can cause an unnaturally opaque appearance. Diagnostic study models are helpful. The teeth must have adequate enamel for bonding because the presence of exposed dentin or restorations can significantly decrease retentive strength. Enamel may be reduced (0.5 mm) to provide space for the metal retainer, and occasionally opposing teeth may also be reduced slightly. For anterior bridges and splints, lingual enamel can be slightly reduced with diamond burs, ending in a supragingival Chamfer. Small proximal grooves aid resistance, retention, seating, and longevity of the restoration. Shade selection for pontics should be made prior to preparation.

An impression of the prepared arch should be made with an accurate elastomeric impression material such as polysulfide or silicone rubber. Using a sharp red pencil, the extensions of the preparations should be outlined on the working model. If preparation grooves are not used, it is helpful to request from the laboratory technician incisal rests that serve as guides for accurate seating of the appliance. These guides can be removed with carbide burs after cementation of the appliance.

The appliance should be seated to make any adjustments of shade, contour, or occlusion. It is advisable to air abrade (with aluminum oxide) the interior of the retainers. Teeth should be isolated with a rubber dam while the appliance is cleaned in an ultrasonic water bath. After pumicing and etching the abutment teeth, composite resin luting cement (autopolymerizing) is mixed and applied to the appliance. The appliance must be seated and held with firm pressure for several minutes while the resin cement hardens; otherwise, the rubber dam may push the appliance incisally, resulting in incomplete seating. It is helpful to remove excess cement with a soft brush or cotton pellet whenever access allows. Following cementation, one should carefully cut the rubber dam with a scissors and remove it. Remaining excess cement may be removed with a diamond or carbide bur (Fig. 39-16, A–D).

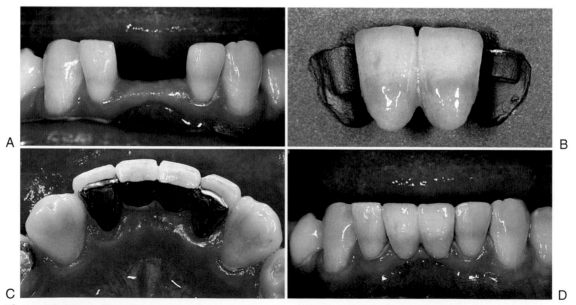

**Figure 39-16**   **A,** Preoperative view of a patient missing teeth 24 and 25. **B,** Facial view of porcelain fused to cast metal appliance that will replace teeth 24 and 25. **C,** Lingual view of bonded bridge in place. **D,** Facial view of the finished case

In the unlikely and unfortunate event of a retainer loosening from an abutment tooth, the appliance should be removed and returned to the laboratory for re-etching or abrasion roughening. It may then be reattached by the same procedure.

# REFERENCES

1. Caughman W, Rueggeberg F: Shedding new light on composite polymerization. *Oper Dent* 27:636-638, 2002.
2. Cohen S, Parkins FM: Bleaching tetracycline-stained vital teeth. *Oral Surg Oral Med Oral Pathol* 29:465-471, 1970.
3. Croll TP: Enamel dysmineralization and decalcification. In: *Enamel Microabrasion.* Carol Stream, IL, Quintessence Publishing, 1991, pp 1-102.
4. Croll TP: Enamel microabrasion for removal of superficial discoloration. *J Esthetic Dent* 1:14-20, 1989.
5. Croll TP: Enamel microabrasion for removal of superficial dysmineralization and decalcification defects. *JADA* 120:411-415, 1990.
6. Croll TP: Enamel microabrasion: the technique. *Quintessence Int* 20:385-400, 1989.
7. Dahl J, Pallesen U: Tooth bleaching: a critical review of the biological aspects. *Crit Rev Oral Biol Med* 14:292-304, 2003.
8. Ham WT: Ocular hazards of light sources: review of current knowledge. *J Occup Med* 25:101-103, 1983.
9. Haywood VB, Heymann HO: Nightguard vital bleaching. *Quintessence Int* 20:173-176, 1989.
10. Haywood VB: New bleaching considerations compared with at-home bleaching. *J Esthet Restor Dent* 15:184-187, 2003.
11. Li Y: The safety of peroxide-containing at-home tooth whiteners. *Comp Cont Ed in Dent* 24:384-389, 2003.
12. Matis BA: Tray whitening: what the evidence shows. *Comp Cont Ed in Dent* 24:354-362, 2003.
13. Nakabayashi N, Kojima K, Masuhara E: The promotion of adhesion by the infiltration of monomers into tooth substrates. *J Biomed Mater Res* 16:265-273, 1982.
14. Peutzfeldt A: Resin composites in dentistry: the monomer systems. *Eur J Oral Sci* 105:97-116, 1997.
15. Rueggeberg F, Caughman W, Curtis J: Factors affecting cure at depths within light-activated resin composites. *Am J Dent* 6:91-95, 1993.
16. Rueggeberg F: Contemporary issues in photocuring. *Compend Contin Educ Dent* (Suppl 25):S4-S15; quiz S73, Nov. 1999.
17. Tay FR, Pashley DH: Dental adhesives of the future. *J Adhes Dent* 4:91-103, 2002.
18. Tay FR, Pashley DH: Have dentin adhesives become too hydrophilic? *J Can Dent Assoc* 69:726-731, 2003.
19. Van Meerbeek B, De Munck J, Yoshida Y et al: Buonocore Memorial Lecture. Adhesion to enamel and dentin; current status and future challenges. *Oper Dent* 28:215-235, 2003.
20. Van Meerbeek B, Inokoshi S, Braem M et al: Morphological aspects of the resin-dentin interdiffusion zone with different dentin adhesive systems. *J Dent Res* 71:1530-1540, 1992.

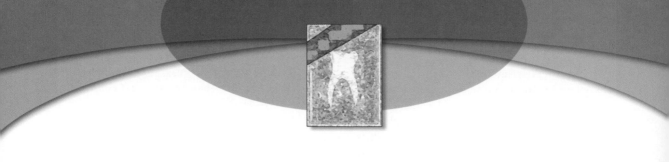

# CHAPTER 40

## Sports Dentistry and Mouth Protection

*Dennis N. Ranalli*

## DEVELOPMENTAL EVALUATION OF CHILD AND ADOLESCENT ATHLETES

### Medical Assessment

Participation in athletic activities at both the recreational and organized sports levels continues to attract growing numbers of developing children and adolescents. Many dentists who are involved in the treatment of pediatric patients are unaware of their patients' involvement in sports simply because standard medical and dental history forms do not usually include questions that elicit this type of information and parents are often unaware of the dentist's need to know. Therefore, it is advisable as part of a thorough medical history to ask parents routinely about their child's athletic activities.[24]

A complete medical examination by a physician is a necessity because several medical conditions in children and adolescents may limit or disqualify them from participating in athletics. The Americans with Disabilities Act of 1990 lists only a few conditions that absolutely disqualify an athlete. One such condition is infectious mononucleosis. Play ability must be determined on a case-by-case basis.[15]

### Growth Assessment

Another important aspect in the overall evaluation of pediatric dental patients who have identified themselves as participants in sports is the assessment of the developmental and behavioral characteristics of the individual patient. This information, together with an evaluation of the child's physical growth, can be a valuable guide to the dentist in offering sound advice to the patient and parents for selecting age-appropriate athletic activities because a prediction of athletic injuries can often be based on the child's stage of psychosocial development and physical maturity. Young children are often not ready to cope psychologically with the complex rules or physical demands associated with some team sports.[22]

Participation in sports involves many health hazards for growing children and adolescents. Parents who permit their children to engage in athletic pursuits run a calculated risk to enable the child or adolescent to achieve beneficial goals. The physical and mental health benefits that are gained, such as improving overall physical function, relieving anxiety, and improving school performance, must be evaluated by informed parents and judged to outweigh the risks of injury to the child or adolescent athlete.[15]

An Athlete's Bill of Rights suggests several factors that are necessary to improve the risk-benefit ratio in safeguarding the health of high school athletes: "Proper conditioning helps to prevent injuries by hardening the body and increasing resistance to fatigue. Careful coaching leads to skillful performance, which lowers the incidence of injuries. Good officiating promotes enjoyment of the game as well as the protection of players. Right equipment and facilities serve a unique purpose in protection of players. Adequate medical (and dental) care is a necessity in the prevention and control of athletic injuries."[9]

## Intraoral Assessment

The overall developmental evaluation of child or adolescent athletes must include a thorough oral and dental examination for accurate diagnosis and proper management of dental caries, juvenile periodontal diseases, hard and soft tissue pathology, congenital anomalies, and developmental occlusion.

Just as the long bones in young children are not yet fully formed and are more prone to fracture and dislocation during athletic activities, so too is the alveolar bone surrounding the primary teeth less dense, often resulting in traumatic dislocation injuries such as avulsion or intrusive luxation. Intrusive luxation of a primary incisor is potentially one of the most serious traumatic injuries to the underlying developing permanent

tooth bud. In addition to the possibility of ankylosis of the traumatized primary incisor, causing delayed or ectopic eruption of the permanent tooth, the underlying developing permanent tooth bud may also be displaced in the crypt. If this displacement occurs during the morphodifferentiation stage of tooth development, an abnormal curvature in the root or crown of the formed permanent tooth may result in a dilacerated tooth. If the traumatic insult occurs later during the apposition stage, when the deposition of dentin and enamel matrix takes place, a localized enamel hypoplasia of the crown of the permanent tooth may result in Turner's tooth (Fig. 40-1).

Young athletes in the early mixed dentition phase should be evaluated radiographically and clinically for the natural processes of root resorption, exfoliation of the primary teeth, and eruption of the permanent successors. Particular attention should be given to space loss associated with the premature loss of primary teeth. In the late mixed dentition phase, the presence of a class II, division I malocclusion is indicative of an accident-prone dental profile and a causal factor for sports-related dental injuries.[5] The clinical presence of an inadequate lip seal and excessive overjet place the protruding maxillary permanent incisors at greater risk for traumatic injury, especially in young athletes who participate in contact sports (Fig. 40-2). The dentist should keep in mind that the large pulp chambers close to the surface in immature permanent teeth are highly susceptible to pulpal exposures in the event of a traumatic tooth fracture.

The evaluation of developing third molars in adolescent athletes is of particular importance.

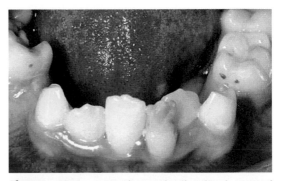

**Figure  40-1**  Turner's tooth (localized enamel hypoplasia) of the mandibular left permanent central incisor as the result of a traumatic injury during the apposition stage of tooth development.

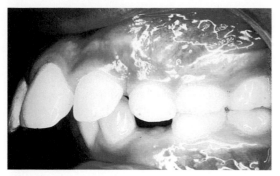

**Figure 40-2** Excessive overjet and lack of lip protection place these maxillary permanent incisors at risk for traumatic injury during athletic activities.

Not only can an athletic season suddenly be interrupted by the annoying and often painful eruption of third molars with associated acute pericoronitis, but mandibular fractures in the gonial angle region of developing third molars can also occur in adolescent athletes.[18]

The labial mucosa, specifically that in the mandibular anterior region of adolescent athletes, should be evaluated for the presence of soft tissue changes such as leukoplakia associated with the habitual use of smokeless tobacco. Snuff dipping is a common habit among athletes, and unfortunately it is occurring at an increasing rate, even among young children. Child and adolescent athletes should be warned at every opportunity about the serious intraoral and systemic dangers of this addictive habit. The use of smokeless tobacco has been associated most frequently with baseball; however, amateur wrestlers and male athletes who compete in sports that are organized according to weight classifications sometimes dip snuff to suppress appetite and control body weight.[7] Thus, an evaluation by the dentist should also include a sports-specific dietary history.

Intraoral piercing is another high-risk fad that is associated increasingly with young athletes. Postpiercing complications may result in acute medical conditions such as hemorrhage and swelling, local and systemic infections, airway obstruction, or allergic reactions. Tongue jewelry also may lead to tooth fractures, gingival recession, or alveolar bone loss and is particularly dangerous during sports activities.[19] Most athletic regulatory agencies have banned the use of tongue jewelry during participation in sports.

## Dietary Assessment

The dentist can choose from a variety of accepted dietary assessment methods to evaluate child and adolescent athletes. Whichever method the dentist selects, the special concerns related to specific sports must be kept in mind during the evaluation process.

Amateur boxers and wrestlers often practice aberrant eating behaviors and intentionally become dehydrated to meet weight classification requirements. These practices can have a negative impact not only on strength and performance but also on the cardiovascular system. On exertion in such situations, hyperthermia and even death can result. Female athletes who participate in sports such as gymnastics or ballet and engage in similar aberrant eating behaviors are subject to the same systemic manifestations. Unhealthy nutritional practices may also predispose these young athletes to the possibility of injuries such as tibial stress fractures and shin splints.[16]

Adolescent athletes who attempt to control weight through dehydration and fasting are vulnerable to hypoglycemic syncope, caused by inadequate glucose reaching the brain. Such a pathophysiologic event can be precipitated in conjunction with a stressful dental appointment. Even if observable symptoms are not present, hypoglycemia by definition is a venous blood glucose level below 50 mg/100 ml.[17]

The dentist should be alert for the following clinical manifestations of hypoglycemia: palpations, sweating, confusion, irritability, headache, seizure, and unconsciousness. To prevent such episodes, the dentist should recommend that the dieting athlete eat a light meal or snack before the dental appointment. In addition, a ready source of carbohydrate, such as orange juice, candy, or a container of cake frosting, should be available in the dental office emergency kit. Should an episode of hypoglycemic syncope occur during a dental appointment, a small amount of the cake frosting can be placed in the mucobuccal fold area for rapid systemic glucose absorption.

Especially with female adolescent athletes, the dentist should be alert for signs of the severe eating disorders of anorexia nervosa and bulimia. Enamel erosion on the lingual surfaces of the teeth, known as perimolysis, is associated with the binge-purge cycle and persistent vomiting. An accompanying clinical feature can be enlargement of the parotid glands.[8] An extreme form of this type of eating disorder may progress to a condition known as the female athlete triad. This condition includes an extended eating disorder combined with intensive training and progresses to amenorrhea and osteoporosis.[30] These severe eating disorders are often associated with psychological problems. In such instances, the dentist is obliged to recommend an appropriate referral for counseling.

At the other end of the spectrum are athletes such as football players, who desire to add bulk for increased size. This can present a dilemma for the dentist because one method of accomplishing this goal is to increase carbohydrate intake substantially. Dietary guidelines that minimize the effects on the teeth of highly cariogenic diets should be recommended. For example, it should be emphasized that the quantity of carbohydrates ingested is less critical for the dentition than the frequency of exposure or the type of carbohydrates consumed. Fruit, pretzels, and diet soda can be recommended as substitutes for sticky candy and sugar-containing soft drinks. Furthermore, these alternative foods can be consumed in greater quantities one or two times a day by those athletes desiring weight gain rather than bathing the teeth continuously with cariogenic sugars.[28]

One popular method of replacing fluids lost during athletic competition is ingesting sports drinks. The use of these electrolyte- and carbohydrate-containing drinks has not been shown conclusively to produce an advantage greater than water in maintaining electrolyte concentration or plasma volume or in improving intestinal absorption.[26] For the great majority of young athletes, cold water remains the ideal replacement beverage.

Athletes of all ages are susceptible to misinformation regarding the exaggerated benefits of "supernutrition." In particular, athletic-minded adolescents are easily convinced that miracle supplements and fad diets will give them that "competitive edge" in their selected event. Although it is true that athletes have higher than average needs for energy and water, their requirements for vitamins, protein, fats, and most minerals do not exceed those of nonathletes. Adopting a fad diet of selected foods over a long period may predispose a person to deficiencies of selected nutrients that unknowingly may be lacking in the diet. Excessive supplementation may interfere with absorption

and utilization of other essential nutrients that are equally important to the athlete. When one considers the nutritional requirements of the child and adolescent athlete, the developmental consequences of major deviations from a well-balanced diet cannot be overlooked.[28]

After a thorough developmental evaluation of the child or adolescent athlete has been concluded, appropriate advice and recommendations may be given about the prevention of specific sports-related traumatic injuries to the craniofacial and intraoral structures.

## MOUTH PROTECTION FOR CHILD AND ADOLESCENT ATHLETES

The single most important device for protecting the teeth and mouth as well as for reducing the likelihood of jaw fractures is the use of an intraoral mouth guard.[10, 11, 27] Unfortunately, only a very few organized amateur sports require mouth guards during practice sessions and in game situations. Amateur sports that mandate the use of mouth guards at the present time are boxing, football, ice hockey, lacrosse, and women's field hockey. In 1990 the National Collegiate Athletic Association (NCAA) began to require that football players use brightly colored mouth guards instead of the more conventional clear variety. This new rule was enacted so that coaches and referees could better determine whether players were actually wearing this required piece of athletic equipment. At the professional sports level, only boxing mandates the use of a mouth guard, but increasing numbers of professional athletes in other sports seem to be using mouth guards voluntarily.

Although the use of mouth guards in conjunction with helmets and facemasks has proved to be effective in reducing both the frequency and severity of traumatic craniofacial and intraoral injuries in athletes who participate in organized sports that require their use, acceptance of mouth guards in most other amateur sports has been minimal at best. For example, young athletes who participate in popular team sports such as baseball, basketball, and soccer and even in school physical education classes where mouth guards are not required continue to experience a high incidence of intraoral injuries, concussions, and even death.[20,29]

One important aspect of dental professional responsibility to our athletic child and adolescent patients is to act as an advocate with local athletic associations, school boards, and sports regulatory agencies to promote the enactment of rules requiring the use of mouth guards in these and other sports in which they are not mandatory so as to prevent future traumatic sports-related injuries and protect these young athletes.

## Types of Mouth Guards

The American Society for Testing and Materials[1] (ASTM, 100 Barr Harbor Drive, West Conshohocken, PA 19428) uses the following classification to categorize mouth guards (Fig. 40-3):

Type I: Stock
Type II: Mouth formed
Type III: Custom fabricated (over a model)

ASTM Standard Practice for Care and Use of Mouthguards[1] also lists several design considerations and special limitations. A mouth guard is best fitted by a dentist. The mouth guard should cover all remaining teeth in the maxillary arch except in athletes with mandibular prognathism. In these instances, all teeth in the mandibular arch should be covered instead. Adolescent athletes wearing fixed orthodontic appliances or those with congenital abnormalities such as cleft palate should be provided with mouth guards only under the supervision of a dentist.

In a position statement issued by the International Academy for Sports Dentistry,[12] the criteria for fabrication and the characteristics of a properly fitted mouth guard are defined. Included among these characteristics are an adequate thickness to reduce impact; a retentive fit that does not dislodge on impact; speech considerations equal to the demands of the sport; a material that meets Food and Drug Administration approval; and a wearing length equal to one season of play.

Type I stock mouth guards are popular because they are inexpensive and are readily available in most sporting goods stores. However, because they are preformed and are worn directly as manufactured, they are the least retentive, most bulky, and interfere most with breathing and speech. They must be held in place by clenching the teeth together. Because they offer the least protection, stock mouth guards are not recommended.[23] Parents should be warned against a false sense of security if their child or adolescent wears a stock mouth guard.

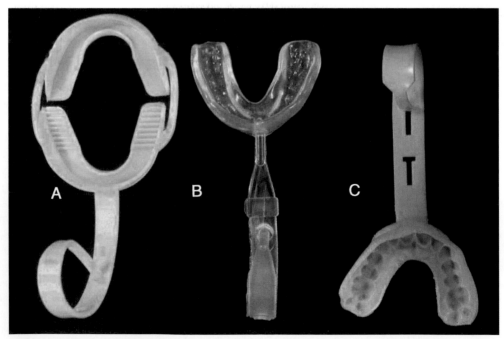

**Figure 40-3**    The three categories of athletic mouth guards include (**A**) type I, stock; (**B**) type II, mouth formed; and (**C**) type III, custom fabricated.

Type II mouth-formed mouth guards range in price, and some retention may be achieved if proper fitting is performed by a dentist. However, results are often unsatisfactory when athletes attempt to fit this type of mouth guard themselves.[23]

Two varieties of mouth-formed mouth guards are available. The thermoplastic variety is placed in boiling water until it becomes softened. After insertion into the mouth, it is molded to the oral and dental structures. To avoid burning the oral soft tissues or possible damage to the dental pulp in immature permanent teeth, care should be exercised in regard to the temperature prior to inserting the softened protector. The mouth guard should be cooler than 132°F when inserted wet and should not be inserted in a dry mouth. If a tighter fit is desired, this type of mouth guard can be resoftened and remolded. This procedure is commonly known as the boil-and-bite technique. The type II thermoplastic variety is the most commonly used athletic mouth guard, but is often bulky and distorts easily (Fig. 40-4).

The shell-lined variety of type II mouth guards offers good retention. The more rigid mouth guard shell is lined with ethyl methacrylate material. For best results, the liner should be changed before every game, although some athletes object to the taste of the freshly mixed ethyl methacrylate material.[6] Use of this type of mouth guard has declined.

Type III custom-fabricated mouth guards are far superior to types I and II in terms of adapta-

tion, retention, and protection. They are the most comfortable and interfere least with breathing and speech. Type III mouth guards are fabricated over a dental model using sheets of thermoplastic material. Because this technique requires the services of a dentist, the final product is more expensive to the consumer than the other types of mouth guards.

When information about the advantages of custom-fabricated mouth guards is presented to the parents in a consultation session, the practitioner may consider several approaches. The first and most compelling reason is the superior quality of custom-fabricated mouth guards in terms of comfort and player safety. The concept of maximal protection for maximal prevention should be emphasized. In these terms, a custom-fabricated mouth guard is in fact a cost-effective alternative. Even though the actual cost is higher than that of other types of mouth guards that are available, the relative cost is low compared with other equipment such as athletic shoes. Furthermore, the actual cost is far more conservative than the fees associated with emergency and long-term management of a traumatic athletic injury. In addition, the dental model used to fabricate the original mouth guard should be preserved so that in the event of damage or loss of the mouth guard, a new replacement can be made quickly and easily.[24]

There are two laboratory techniques in current use for the custom fabrication of athletic mouth guards: the vacuum forming technique (described in detail in the next section of this chapter) and the heat-pressure-lamination technique. The pressure-lamination technique utilizes multiple layers of material and is designed for greater adaptation (retention) as well as greater resistance to distortion over time.[25]

Regardless of the type of mouth guard finally selected, all mouth guards should be stored in a plastic container when not in use to avoid damage due to excessive heat and cold.[1] Mouth guards should be washed daily in cold or lukewarm water because the use of hot water may result in distortion. Prior to insertion, the mouth guard can be rinsed with any commercially available mouthwash to freshen the taste.[6] Mouth guards should be inspected regularly during the course of an athletic season to detect distortions, splits, or bite-through problems (Fig. 40-4). When such deficiencies are detected, fabrication of a new mouth guard should be recommended.[23]

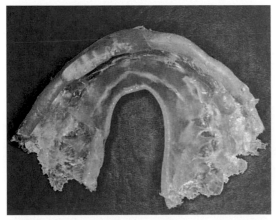

**Figure 40-4** Distortions, splits, and bite-through problems indicate the need to fabricate a new mouth guard for proper retention, comfort, and maximal protection of the athlete.

## Vacuum Forming Technique for Custom-Fabricated Mouth Guards

As with all dental procedures, universal precautions for infection control must be followed precisely. After a thorough diagnosis has been made and all necessary restorations have been completed, dental prophylaxis should be performed immediately prior to making the impression to ensure the best possible adaptation.[6]

An alginate impression of the entire maxillary arch is taken in a muscle-molded rim-lock tray. After the impression material is set fully and the tray is removed from the mouth, the impression should be washed under cold running water and then disinfected by immersing or spraying it with an EPA-registered, American Dental Association–approved disinfectant such as sodium hypochlorite. Before the model is poured, excess water and disinfecting solution should be removed with a gentle stream of air.

Following removal of these excess liquids, the dental model is poured immediately via a thick mix of dental stone. After proper setting, the impression is separated gently from the dental model. The model is trimmed, stone bubbles are removed, and voids are filled in. For athletes who wear fixed orthodontic appliances, the dental model should be relieved with plaster or heat-resistant block-out compound over the area of the appliance and prior to vacuum forming the mouth guard. The dental model also should be modified so that the finished mouth guard will not interfere with anticipated orthodontic tooth movements.[3,25]

The cold, wet dental model is centered on the vacuum former. A 5.5-inch square sheet of polyvinyl acetate–polyethylene is positioned on the vacuum machine and heated until the sheet shows a 1- to 2-inch sag (Fig. 40-5, A). The heat is switched off as the vacuum is switched on while the softened material is compressed over the dental model (Fig. 40-5, B). The vacuum should be kept on for approximately 2 minutes.

When the model is completely cool, excess material is trimmed with scissors and peeled away (Fig. 40-5, C). The palatal region is cut out in a U shape with a utility knife (Fig. 40-5, D). After soaking in water, the mouth guard is then carefully removed from the model (Fig. 40-5, E). The peripheral areas should be trimmed short of the mucobuccal fold, and care should be taken to relieve the frenum areas to avoid development of sore spots.

Final finishing of rough edges can be accomplished by using polishing stones or rubber wheels and then flaming the mouth guard lightly with an alcohol torch (Fig. 40-5, F). The completed custom-fabricated mouth guard is now ready for delivery (Fig. 40-5, G). Following placement in the mouth, the mouth guard is adjusted if necessary and then given to the athlete (Fig. 40-5, H).

## PROFESSIONAL ACTIVITIES IN SPORTS DENTISTRY

Because of the ever-increasing number of children and adolescents participating in sports, many dentists already are treating these young athletes in their practices, and many more are likely to be doing so in the future. In addition to the clinical aspects of sports dentistry, a number of other professional activities are available to dentists interested in enhancing their knowledge or expanding their involvement in this exciting field.[4]

These activities include volunteering for local mouth guard days, becoming a consultant to an athletic department, serving as a sports team dentist, or becoming a member of the International Academy for Sports Dentistry (118 Faye Street, PO Box 364, Farmersville, IL 62533, iasdsports-dentistry@cillnet.com). Some dentists may present seminars in their local communities on topics related to sports dentistry, provide information to governing agencies advocating the enactment of more stringent mouth guard regulations, or become involved in research projects studying various aspects of sports dentistry.[23,24] An excellent way to become involved is to participate in the Special Olympics/Special Smiles program.[21]

Castaldi[2] suggests that possibly the most effective role that can be played is in our dental schools, where faculty should develop a curriculum and teach the subject of sports dentistry and mouth protection for young athletes to dental students and residents in specialty training programs. Although various elements of sports dentistry, such as suturing techniques, restorations for the treatment of fractured incisors, and endodontic procedures, among others, already exist in the curriculum, few dental schools offer an interdisciplinary learning experience in sports dentistry.[14] Such opportunities are strongly

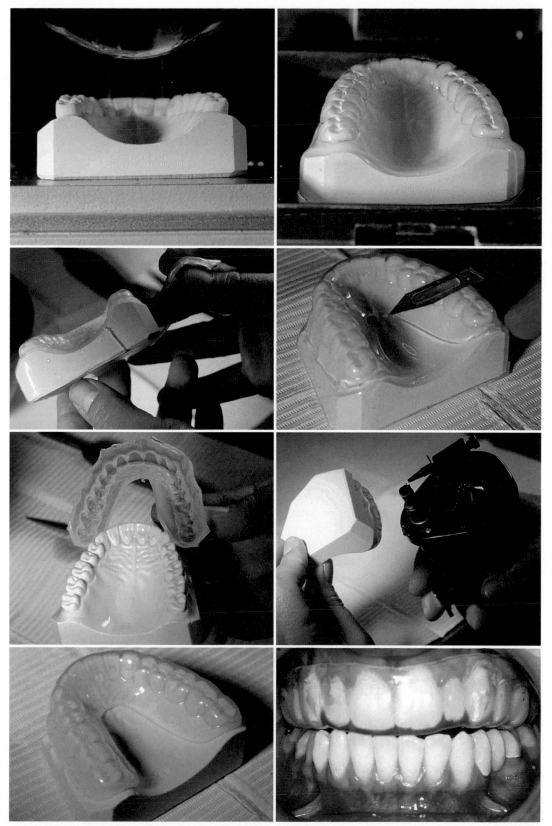

**Figure 40-5** Various laboratory procedures in the vacuum forming technique for construction of custom-fabricated athletic mouth guards. (See text for descriptive details.)

recommended in future curriculum planning and are defined by the International Academy for Sports Dentistry in a position statement on sports dentistry in the dental school curriculum.[13]

Whichever of these choices the interested dental professional makes, one fact seems certain. The field of sports dentistry will continue to expand as participation in sports in our society continues to grow. The question remains, to what extent are dentists prepared to participate in the arena of sports dentistry? We as dentists must prepare ourselves now to meet this exciting challenge.

## Why Sports Dentistry?
*William Chambers*

It's a beautiful fall afternoon. You are enjoying a great football game on television when the phone rings. It's your neighbor. His daughter, a patient of yours, was involved in a great game of her own, a soccer match. It seems she made a game-winning block to save a goal. Unfortunately, she blocked the kick at close range with her face. You now spend the next 2 hours of your nice fall afternoon in the office trying to restore a smashed smile for a beautiful young girl.

You may ask what is the point of this story. The point is that you do not have to seek out sports dentistry; sports dentistry will seek you out! With present trends, children (at younger and younger ages) and adults are becoming more and more involved in sports activities. Soccer, basketball, baseball, and softball are just a few sports that include participants with a wide range of ages and skill levels and that all too often involve frequent incidents of orofacial trauma.

Sports dentistry has two major components. The first is the management of orofacial injuries, and the second is the prevention of sports-related orofacial injuries. The management of orofacial sports injuries calls into play many different dental skills. To provide comprehensive care, a dentist must be knowledgeable and adept in the areas of oral surgery, endodontics, operative dentistry, orthodontics, hospital dentistry, and patient behavior management. The care of patients with sports-related orofacial injuries can be satisfying, especially when a positive treatment result occurs. However, what automatically comes to mind when treating these patients is the question, Why did this happen? Why do so many young athletes have to suffer such preventable injuries—injuries that can negatively affect their oral health for a lifetime? This realization brings into focus the second aspect of sports dentistry: prevention through sports safety.

My personal interest in sports dentistry evolved through a series of experiences. In college I played basketball at the University of North Carolina at Chapel Hill. Fortunately, I did not suffer any orofacial injuries, but I did witness several injuries to a number of other players. This experience sensitized me to the effect of such injuries on people I know. During dental school, while playing intramural basketball, I was intentionally elbowed in the mouth by a former tight end on the football team. Although my injury was not serious, I took this episode as a personal wake-up call to wear a mouth guard whenever I played basketball. From that day on, I have always worn a mouth guard.

Once I established a private practice in pediatric dentistry, I made many efforts to expand my practice. One effort was to inform the pediatricians I knew that I would be available, through a beeper, to cover their after-hours dental trauma cases. I soon was amazed at the number of orofacial trauma patients I treated during certain seasons of the year (i.e., basketball and baseball seasons). My initial exhilaration in treating these trauma patients eventually led to some real introspective thinking. How could I help prevent some of these injuries? My concern about the number of trauma cases I was seeing, coupled with the fact that both of my daughters were now beginning to participate in sports, certainly personalized my interest in prevention.

My initial efforts at prevention were undertaken merely in the leagues in which my children played. As a coach and league official, I urged all players to wear mouth guards. I did this though personal discussions and by sending letters to parents and coaches. Also, my own children set the example by wearing mouth guards. I also urged every patient in my practice to wear mouth guards. This was done during recall visits and in the office newsletter.

Although encouraged by the sudden large numbers of children I saw wearing mouth guards, I realized that this message had to have a broader base to truly make a difference. I then gathered all the information I could on sports dentistry and preventive programs across the country. By presenting this information and a plan of action to the North Carolina Dental Society, we have now begun

## Why Sports Dentistry?—cont'd

a statewide program to educate members of our profession and the public about the need for prevention of orofacial trauma through mouth protectors and other protective safety gear.

What has my interest in sports dentistry meant to me professionally and personally? In my community my practice is recognized for the quality of care we deliver in managing orofacial trauma. But I have received much more personal satisfaction through my efforts to improve children's dental health by helping to prevent serious dental injuries.

Dentistry has always been proud of its efforts in preventive care. We have always been advocates for any issues that represent the best interests of the public's oral health and well-being. Therefore, we have to take the lead in educating ourselves

and the public about the measures necessary to prevent and manage sports-related orofacial trauma. On the local level, this effort should take the form of encouraging coaches to recommend and players to wear mouth guards or other protective devices such as batting helmets with face shields. Effectiveness requires direct involvement of the dentist with teams, coaches, parents, and sponsors. On the national level, we can act as advocates before the governing bodies of the various sports organizations to mandate the wearing of such safety equipment.

If as a dental professional you are on a quest to be the best, the bottom line is that you must get involved; you can make a difference. Learn and do sports dentistry.

## REFERENCES

1. American Society for Testing and Materials: Standard practice for care and use of mouthguards. Designation: F697-80. Philadelphia, The Society, 1986, p 323.
2. Castaldi CR: Sports-related oral and facial injuries in the young athlete: a new challenge for the pediatric dentist. *Pediatr Dent* 8:311-316, 1986.
3. Croll TP, Castaldi CR: The custom-fitted athletic mouthguard for the orthodontic patient and for the child with a mixed dentition. *Quintessence Int* 20:571-575, 1989.
4. Elliott MA: Professional responsibility in sports dentistry. *Dent Clin North Am* 35:831-840, 1991.
5. Fos PJ, Pinkham JR, Ranalli DN: Prediction of sports-related dental traumatic injuries. *Dent Clin North Am* 44:19-33, 2000.
6. Guevara PA, Ranalli DN: Techniques for mouthguard fabrication. *Dent Clin North Am* 35:667-682, 1991.
7. Guggenheimer J: Tobacco and athletics: update and current status. *Dent Clin North Am* 44:179-187, 2000.
8. Hasler JF: Parotid enlargement: a presenting sign in anorexia nervosa. *Oral Surg Oral Med Oral Pathol* 53:567-573, 1982.
9. Hein F: Safeguarding the health of the high school athlete. In: Ryan A, editor: *Medical Care of the Athlete.* New York, McGraw-Hill, 1962, pp 16-17.
10. Heintz WD: Mouth protectors: a progress report. *JADA* 77:632-636, 1968.
11. Hickey JC, Morris AL, Carlson LD et al: The

relation of mouth protectors to cranial pressure and deformation. *JADA* 74:735-740, 1967.
12. International Academy for Sports Dentistry: Position Statement for "A Properly Fitted Mouth Guard," 1998.
13. International Academy for Sports Dentistry: Position Statement on "Sports Dentistry in the Dental School Curriculum," 1999.
14. Kumamoto DP, DiOrio LP: An interdisciplinary learning experience in sports dentistry. *J Dent Educ* 53:491-494, 1989.
15. Landry GL: Pediatric sports medicine. *J Southeast Soc Pediatr Dent* 8:12-13, 2002.
16. Loosli AR, Benson J: Nutritional intake in adolescent athletes. *Pediatr Clin North Am* 37:1143-1152, 1990.
17. Malamed SF: *Handbook of Medical Emergencies in the Dental Office,* St Louis, Mosby, 1978, pp 164-176.
18. McCarthy MF: Sports and mouth protection. *Gen Dent* 38:343-346, 1990.
19. McGeary SP, Studen-Pavlovich D, Ranalli DN: Oral piercing in athletes: Implications for general dentistry. *Gen Dent* 50:168-172, 2002.
20. Mueller FO et al: National Centers for Catastrophic Sports Injury Research, Chapel Hill, NC, Seventh Annual Report. Fall 1982–Spring 1989, pp 1-59.
21. Perlman S: Helping Special Olympics athletes sport good smiles. *Dent Clin North Am* 44:221-229, 2002.
22. Pinkham JR, Kohn DW: Epidemiology and prediction of sports related traumatic injuries. *Dent Clin North Am* 35:609-626, 1991.
23. Ranalli DN: Prevention of craniofacial injuries in football. *Dent Clin North Am* 35:627-645, 1991.

24. Ranalli DN: Strategies for the prevention of sports-related oral injuries: a practical guide for the pediatric dentist. *J Southeast Soc Pediatr Dent* 3:18-19, 1997.

25. Ranalli DN: Prevention of sports-related traumatic dental injuries. *Dent Clin North Am* 44:161-178, 2000.

26. Squire DL: Heat illness: fluid and electrolyte issues for pediatric and adolescent athletes. *Pediatr Clin North Am* 37:1085-1109, 1990.

27. Stenger JM, Lawson EA, Wright JM et al: Mouthguards: protection against shock to the head, neck, and teeth. *JADA* 69:273-281, 1964.

28. Studen-Pavlovich D, Bonci L, Etzel KR: Dental implications of nutritional factors in young athletes. *Dent Clin North Am* 44:161-178, 2000.

29. U.S. Consumer Product Safety Commission: Overview of Sports-Related Injuries in Persons 5–14 Years of Age. Washington, DC, The Commission, 1981, pp 1-47.

30. Yeager K, Agostini R, Nattiv A et al: The female athlete triad: disordered eating, amenorrhea, osteoporosis. *Med Sci Sports Exerc* 25:775-777, 1993.

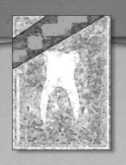

# APPENDIXES

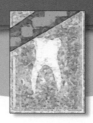

# APPENDIX A

# RECOMMENDED CHILDHOOD AND ADOLESCENT IMMUNIZATION SCHEDULE[1]–UNITED STATES, JULY-DECEMBER 2004

| Range of Recommended Ages | | Catch-up Immunization | | Preadolescent Assessment | | | | | | | | |

| Vaccine ▼ / Age ▶ | Birth | 1 mo | 2 mo | 4 mo | 6 mo | 12 mo | 15 mo | 18 mo | 24 mo | 4-6 y | 11-12 y | 13-18 y |
|---|---|---|---|---|---|---|---|---|---|---|---|---|
| Hepatitis B[2] | HepB #1 | only if mother HBsAg (-) | | | | | | | | | HepB series | |
| | | HepB #2 | | | | HepB #3 | | | | | | |
| Diphtheria, Tetanus, Pertussis[3] | | | DTaP | DTaP | DTaP | | DTaP | | | DTaP | Td | Td |
| Haemophilus influenzae Type b[4] | | | Hib | Hib | Hib[4] | Hib | | | | | | |
| Inactivated Poliovirus | | | IPV | IPV | | IPV | | | | IPV | | |
| Measles, Mumps, Rubella[5] | | | | | | MMR #1 | | | | MMR #2 | MMR #2 | |
| Varicella[6] | | | | | | Varicella | | | | | Varicella | |
| Pneumococcal[7] | | | PCV | PCV | PCV | PCV | | | | PCV | PPV | |
| Influenza[8] | | | | | | Influenza (yearly) | | | | Influenza (yearly) | | |
| ----- Vaccines below this line are for selected populations ----- | | | | | | | | | | | | |
| Hepatitis A[9] | | | | | | | | | | Hepatitis A series | | |

1. Indicates the recommended ages for routine administration of currently licensed childhood vaccines, as of April 1, 2004, for children through age 18 years. Any dose not given at the recommended age should be given at any subsequent visit when indicated and feasible. ▨ Indicates age groups that warrant special effort to administer those vaccines not given previously. Additional vaccines may be licensed and recommended during the year. Licensed combination vaccines may be used whenever any components of the combination are indicated and the vaccine's other components are not contraindicated. Providers should consult the manufacturers' package inserts for detailed recommendations. Clinically significant adverse events that follow vaccination should be reported to the Vaccine Adverse Event Reporting System (VAERS). Guidance about how to obtain and complete a VAERS form is available at http://www.vaers.org/ or by telephone, 1-800-822-7967.

2. **Hepatitis B vaccine (HepB).** All infants should receive the first dose of HepB vaccine soon after birth and before hospital discharge; the first dose may also be given by age 2 months if the infant's mother is HBsAg-negative. Only monovalent HepB vaccine can be used for the birth dose. Monovalent or combination vaccine containing HepB may be used to complete the series; 4 doses of vaccine may be administered when a birth dose is given. The second dose should be given at least 4 weeks after the first dose except for combination vaccines, which cannot be administered before age 6 weeks. The third dose should be given at least 16 weeks after the first dose and at least 8 weeks after the second dose. The last dose in the vaccination series (third or fourth dose) should not be administered before age 24 weeks. Infants born to HBsAg-positive mothers should receive HepB vaccine and 0.5 mL hepatitis B immune globulin (HBIG) within 12 hours of birth at separate sites. The second dose is recommended at age 1-2 months. The last dose in the vaccination series should not be administered before age 24 weeks. These infants should be tested for HBsAg and anti-HBs at 9-15 months of age. Infants born to mothers whose HBsAg status is unknown should receive the first dose of the HepB vaccine series within 12 hours of birth. Maternal blood should be drawn as soon as possible to determine the mother's HBsAg status; if the HBsAg test is positive, the infant should receive HBIG as soon as possible (no later than age 1 week). The second dose is recommended at age 1-2 months. The last dose in the vaccination series should not be administered before age 24 weeks.

3. **Diphtheria and tetanus toxoids and acellular pertussis vaccine (DTaP).** The fourth dose of DTaP may be administered at age 12 months provided that 6 months have elapsed since the third dose and the child is unlikely to return at age 15-18 months. The final dose in the series should be given at age >4 years. **Tetanus and diphtheria toxoids (Td)** is recommended at age 11-12 years if at least 5 years have elapsed since the last dose of tetanus and diphtheria toxoid-containing vaccine. Subsequent routine Td boosters are recommended every 10 years.

4. *Haemophilus influenzae* type b (Hib) conjugate vaccine. Three Hib conjugate vaccines are licensed for infant use. If PRP-OMP (PedvaxHIB® or ComVax® [Merck]) is administered at ages 2 and 4 months, a dose at age 6 months is not required. DTaP/Hib combination products should not be used for primary vaccination in infants at ages 2, 4, or 6 months but can be used as boosters after any Hib vaccine. The final dose in the series should be given at age >12 months.

5. **Measles, mumps, and rubella vaccine (MMR).** The second dose of MMR is recommended routinely at age 4-6 years but may be administered during any visit, provided at least 4 weeks have elapsed since the first dose and both doses are administered beginning at or after age 12 months. Those who have not received the second dose previously should complete the schedule by the visit at age 11-12 years.

6. **Varicella vaccine (VAR).** Varicella vaccine is recommended at any visit at or after age 12 months for susceptible children (i.e., those who lack a reliable history of chickenpox). Susceptible persons aged >13 years should receive 2 doses given at least 4 weeks apart.

7. **Pneumococcal vaccine.** The heptavalent **pneumococcal conjugate vaccine (PCV)** is recommended for all children aged 2-23 months. It is also recommended for certain children aged 24-59 months. The final dose in the series should be given at age >12 months. **Pneumococcal polysaccharide vaccine (PPV)** is recommended in addition to PCV for certain high-risk groups. See *MMWR* 2000;49(No. RR-9):1-35.

8. **Influenza vaccine.** Influenza vaccine is recommended annually for children aged >6 months with certain risk factors (including but not limited to asthma, cardiac disease, sickle cell disease, HIV, and diabetes), health care workers, and other persons (including household members) in close contact with persons in groups at high-risk (see *MMWR* 2004;53[No. RR-X]:X-XX) and can be administered to all others wishing to obtain immunity. In addition, healthy children aged 6-23 months and close contacts of healthy children aged 0-23 months are recommended to receive influenza vaccine, because children in this age group are at substantially increased risk of influenza-related hospitalizations. For healthy persons aged 5-49 years, the intranasally administered live, attenuated influenza vaccine (LAIV) is an acceptable alternative to the intramuscular trivalent inactivated influenza vaccine (TIV). See MMWR 2003;52(No. RR-13):1-8. Children receiving TIV should be administered a dosage appropriate for their age (0.25 mL if 6-35 months or 0.5 mL if >3 years). Children aged <8 years who are receiving influenza vaccine for the first time should receive 2 doses (separated by at least 4 weeks for TIV and at least 6 weeks for LAIV).

9. **Hepatitis A vaccine.** Hepatitis A vaccine is recommended for children and adolescents in selected states and regions and for certain high-risk groups. Consult your local public health authority and MMWR 1999;48(No.RR-12):1-37. Children and adolescents in these states, regions, and high-risk groups who have not been immunized against hepatitis A can begin the hepatitis A vaccination series during any visit. The two doses in the series should be administered at least 6 months apart.

Additional information about vaccines, including precautions and contraindications for vaccination and vaccine shortages is available at http://www.cdc.gov/nip or from the National Immunization Information Hotline, 800-232-2522 (English) or 800-232-0233 (Spanish). Approved by the **Advisory Committee on Immunization Practices** (http://www.cdc.gov/nip/acip), the **American Academy of Pediatrics** (http://www.aap.org), and the **American Academy of Family Physicians** (http://www.aafp.org).

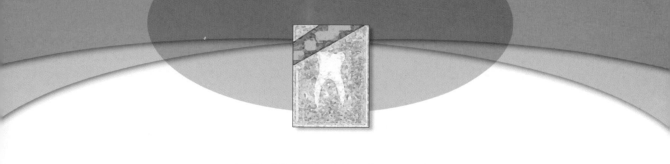

# APPENDIX B

## HEALTH INSURANCE PORTABILITY AND ACCOUNTABILITY ACT (HIPAA) OF 1996

The Health Insurance Portability and Accountability Act (HIPAA) of 1996 was signed into law by President Bill Clinton on August 21, 1996. Conclusive regulations were issued on August 17, 2000, to be instated by October 16, 2002. HIPAA requires that the transactions of all patient health care information be formatted in a standardized electronic style. In addition to protecting the privacy and security of patient information, HIPAA includes legislation on the formation of medical savings accounts, the authorization of a fraud and abuse control program, the easy transport of health insurance coverage, and the simplification of administrative terms and conditions.

HIPAA encompasses three primary areas, and its privacy requirements can be broken down into three types—privacy standards, patients' rights, and administrative requirements.

**1. Privacy Standards.** A central concern of HIPAA is the careful use and disclosure of protected health information (PHI), which generally is electronically controlled health information that is able to be distinguished individually. PHI also refers to verbal communication although the HIPAA Privacy Rule is not intended to hinder necessary verbal communication. The U.S. Department of Health and Human Services (USDHHS) does not require restructuring, such as sound-proofing, architectural changes, and so forth, but some caution is necessary when exchanging health information by conversation.

An Acknowledgment of Receipt Notice of Privacy Practices, which allows patient information to be used or divulged for treatment, payment, or health care operations (TPO), should be procured from each patient. A detailed and time-sensitive authorization can also be issued, which allows the dentist to release information in special circumstances other than TPOs. A *written consent* is also an option. Dentists can disclose PHI *without* acknowledgement, consent, or authorization in very special situations, for example, perceived child abuse, public health supervision, fraud investigation, or law enforcement with valid permission (i.e., a warrant). When divulging PHI, a dentist must try to disclose only the *minimum necessary* information, to help safeguard the patient's information as much as possible.

It is important that dental professionals adhere to HIPAA standards because health care providers (as well as health care clearinghouses and health care plans) who convey *electronically* formatted health information via an outside billing service or merchant are considered *covered entities*. Covered entities may be dealt serious civil and criminal penalties for violation of HIPAA legislation. Failure to comply with HIPAA privacy requirements may result in civil penalties of up to $100 per offense with an annual maximum of $25,000 for repeated failure to comply with the same requirement. Criminal penalties resulting from the illegal mishandling of private health information can range from $50,000 and/or 1 year in prison to $250,000 and/or 10 years in prison.

**2. Patients' Rights.** HIPAA allows patients, authorized representatives, and parents of minors, as well as minors, to become more aware of the health information privacy to which they are entitled. These rights include, but are not limited to, the right to view and copy their health information, the right to dispute alleged breaches of policies and regulations, and the right to request alternative forms of communicating with their dentist. If any health information is released for any reason other than TPO, the patient is entitled to an account of the transaction. Therefore, it is important for dentists to keep accurate records of such information and to provide them when necessary.

The HIPAA Privacy Rule determines that the parents of a minor have access to their child's health information. This privilege may be over-ruled, for example, in cases where there is sus-pected child abuse or the parent consents to a term of confidentiality between the dentist and the minor. The parents' rights to access their child's PHI also may be restricted in situations when a legal entity, such as a court, intervenes and when a law does not require a parent's consent. For a full list of patient rights provided by HIPAA, be sure to acquire a copy of the law and to understand it well.

**3. Administrative Requirements.** Complying with HIPAA legislation may seem like a chore, but it does not need to be so. It is recommended that you become appropriately familiar with the law, organize the requirements into simpler tasks, begin compliance early, and document your progress in compliance. An important first step is to evaluate the current information and practices of your office.

Dentists will need to write a *privacy policy* for their office, a document for their patients detail-ing the office's practices concerning PHI. The ADA's *HIPAA Privacy Kit* includes forms that you (the dentist) can use to customize your privacy policy. It is useful to try to understand the role of health care information for your patients and the ways in which they deal with the information while they are visiting your office. Train your staff; make sure they are familiar with the terms of HIPAA and your office's privacy policy and related forms. HIPAA requires that you designate a *privacy officer,* a person in your office who will be responsible for applying the new policies in your office, fielding complaints, and making

choices involving the minimum necessary require-ments. Another person with the role of *contact person* will process complaints.

A *Notice of Privacy Practices*—a document detailing the patient's rights and the dental office's obligations concerning PHI—also must be drawn up. Further, any role of a third party with access to PHI must be clearly documented. This third party is known as a *business associate* (BA) and is defined as any entity who, on behalf of the dentist, takes part in any activity that involves exposure of PHI. The *HIPAA Privacy Kit* provides a copy of the USDHHS "Business Associate Contract Terms," which provides a concrete format for detailing BA interactions.

The main HIPAA privacy compliance date, including all staff training, was April 14, 2003, although many covered entities who submitted a request and a compliance plan by October 15, 2002, were granted one-year extensions. Contact your local branch of the ADA for details. It is recommended that dentists prepare their offices ahead of time for all deadlines, which include preparing privacy polices and forms, business associate contracts, and employee training sessions.

For a comprehensive discussion of all of these terms and requirements, a complete list of HIPAA policies and procedures, and a full collection of HIPAA privacy forms, contact the American Dental Association for a *HIPAA Privacy Kit*. The relevant ADA Web site is www.ada.org/goto/hipaa. Other Web sites that may contain useful information about HIPAA are:

- USDHHS Office of Civil Rights www.hhs.gov/ocr/hipaa
- Work Group on Electronic Data Interchange www.wedi.org/SNIP
- Phoenix Health www.hipaadvisory.com
- USDHHS Office of the Assistant Secretary for Planning and Evaluation http://aspe.os.dhhs.gov/admnsimp/

Data from: *HIPAA Privacy Kit;* and http://www.ada.org/prof/prac/issues/topics/hipaa/index.html.

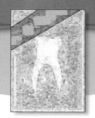

# APPENDIX C

## ANTICIPATORY GUIDANCE FOR CHILDREN'S DENTAL HEALTH

| Content Area | Dentist's Actions |
|---|---|

### Child's Developmental Age Range: 6 to 12 Months

**Milestone**
The eruption of the first primary tooth

| | |
|---|---|
| **Oral Development** | |
| First primary tooth, molar eruption | Review patterns of eruption |
| Formation of permanent teeth | Review teething facts and myths |
| | Cover oral anatomic landmarks in exam |
| | Discuss oral stimulators |
| | |
| **Fluoride** | |
| Recommendation against fluoride use until 6 months of age | Assess fluoride status |
| | Determine supplement if needed |
| Topical and systemic fluoride action | Review vehicle for delivery with parent |
| | |
| **Oral Hygiene/Health** | |
| Microflora acquisition in infants | Review oral hygiene techniques for infants with |
| Mouth-cleaning techniques | caretaker using soft brush and pea-sized amount of dentifrice or no dentifrice |
| Periodicity of dental visits | Plan for baby's next dental care visit based on risk assessment |
| | |
| **Habits** | |
| Non-nutritive sucking, pacifier use | Review pacifier use and safety and hygiene issues |
| Breastfeeding and oral health | Cover the role of mouth in infant's exploration of the environment |
| | Discuss thumb-sucking's effects on mouth |
| | Discuss breastfeeding's effects on mouth |
| | |
| **Nutrition and Diet** | |
| Nursing bottle tooth decay pattern | Encourage weaning at the appropriate time |
| Role of consistency of sugar in caries | Discuss role of sugar in dental caries initiation |
| | |
| **Injury Prevention** | |
| Oral trauma | Review what to do if infant experiences oral trauma; give parents emergency numbers |

From Nowak AJ, Casamassimo PS: *JADA* 126: 1156-1163, 1995.

*Continued*

## Anticipatory Guidance for Children's Dental Health—cont'd

| CONTENT AREA | DENTIST'S ACTIONS |
|---|---|

### Child's Developmental Age Range: 12 to 24 Months

**Milestones**
Completion of primary dentition, occlusal relationships established, arch length determined

| | |
|---|---|
| **Oral Development** | |
| Completion of primary dentition | Discuss importance of space maintenance |
| Concepts of occlusion | Discuss bruxing |
| Concept of arch length and spacing | Review molar, canine, and incisal positions with parents |
| Formation of permanent teeth | during examination |
| | |
| **Fluoride** | |
| Fluoride in food sources in and outside the home | Reassess fluoride status and determine appropriate type of supplement |
| Toxicity and safety | Discuss toxicity and how to manage accidental ingestion |
| | |
| **Oral Hygiene/Health** | |
| Type of brush | Review home oral care procedures and compliance |
| Role of dentifrice | |
| Role of child and parent in brushing | Work with parent to solve problems of oral hygiene |
| Frequency of and setting for oral hygiene | |
| Periodicity of dental visits | Plan for baby's next dental visit based on risk assessment |
| | |
| **Habits** | |
| Thumb-sucking | Review nonnutritive sucking and safe use of pacifier if not |
| Pacifier use | covered previously |
| | |
| **Nutrition and Diet** | |
| Plaque | Discuss carbohydrates and their role in plaque development |
| Role of frequency of sugar intake in dental caries | Review diet outside of home |
| | Discuss frequency of carbohydrate intake as a caries factor |
| | Discuss caries control in the framework of a healthful diet |
| | |
| **Injury Prevention** | |
| Electric cord injury | Discuss electric cord safety |
| Primary tooth trauma and its sequelae | Review normal dental and oral anatomy with parents during examination |
| Home child-proofing | Reinforce home child-proofing and use of car seats |
| | Develop plans for oral trauma management for preschool and child care |

### Child's Developmental Age Range: 2 to 6 Years

**Milestones**
Loss of first primary tooth, eruption of first permanent molar or incisor

| | |
|---|---|
| **Oral Development** | |
| Exfoliation of primary teeth | Review patterns of eruption |
| Eruption of first permanent teeth | Cover permanent molar occlusion with parents during examination |
| Molar occlusion | Point out permanent molar occlusal anatomy |
| Healthy gums | Describe healthy periodontal tissue |

## Anticipatory Guidance for Children's Dental Health—cont'd

| Content Area | Dentist's Actions |
|---|---|
| **Fluoride** | |
| Fluoride sources in water outside the home | Reassess fluoride status at periodic visit and determine both supplement and age-appropriate vehicle |
| **Oral Hygiene/Health** | |
| Child's participation in oral hygiene | Review home oral care procedures and compliance Recommend that the child begin brushing with parent supervision and assistance |
| Role of dental sealants in prevention | Discuss dental sealants Explain dental radiographs |
| | Plan child's next dental visit based on risk assessment Discuss parental separation or presence at dental visits and normal child anxiety |
| **Habits** | |
| Nonnutritive habits | If child still sucking thumb, discuss with parent how to help the child discontinue the habit |
| **Nutrition and Diet** | |
| Snacking and sugar intake at home and at school | Review diet outside the home and its caries potential |
| Use of food to reinforce behavior | Discourage use of food as a behavioral tool |
| Relationship of a healthy diet to oral health | |
| **Injury Prevention** | |
| Safety during sports activities such as bicycling and skating | Encourage use of helmets, pads, and mouthguards when appropriate |
| Permanent tooth injury | Review differences between primary and permanent teeth with parents during examination Prepare plan for home and school for oral injury and treatment options |
| Car safety | Encourage car seat use |

# Index

Page numbers followed by f indicate figures; t, tables; b, boxes.

727